NURSING CARE OF THE CHILD WITH LONG-TERM ILLNESS

EDITOR

Shirley Steele, R.N., M.A.

CONTRIBUTIONS BY

Dorothy Hoehne, R.N., M.Ed.
Donna Juenker, R.N., M.Ed.
Carol Ren Kneisl, R.N., M.S.
Mary Norma O'Hara, R.N., M.A.
Jacqueline Thompson, R.N., M. Ed.

ILLUSTRATIONS BY

Helen Ptak, R.N., M.A.

APPLETON-CENTURY-CROFTS / New York
A Publishing Division of Prentice-Hall, Inc.

Library of Congress Catalog Card Number   74-150503

PRINTED IN THE UNITED STATES OF AMERICA   0-8385-7016-X

To those who possess the courage
to look past the edge of the familiar
to the periphery of a new and challenging tomorrow.

About the Authors

MISS DOROTHY HOEHNE received her diploma in nursing from Medical Center, Brooklyn, New York. She received her Bachelor of Science and Master of Education degrees from Teachers College, Columbia. She was an instructor in pediatric nursing at the University of Oklahoma prior to coming to the State University of New York at Buffalo as an Assistant Professor of Child Health nursing.

MISS DONNA JUENKER received her diploma in nursing from Sisters of Charity Hospital, Buffalo, New York. She completed her Baccalaureate degree at D'Youville College, Buffalo, and has a Master of Education degree from Teachers College, Columbia.

Donna is an Associate Professor of Child Health Nursing and has a grant from the Department of Health, Education, and Welfare, Public Health Service entitled, "Multiphasic Self-Instruction Program on Growth and Development During Early Childhood (infancy through four years) for Baccalaureate Nursing Students" (D10 NU 00394-01).

MRS. CAROL REN KNEISL received her diploma in nursing from Millard Fillmore Hospital, Buffalo, New York. She completed her Baccalaureate degree at the University of Buffalo. She has a Master of Science degree in Psychiatric Nursing from the University of California at San Francisco.

Carol is an Associate Professor of Mental Health–Psychiatric Nursing in the graduate program at the State University of New York at Buffalo. Carol is a consultant to the Veteran's Administration Hospital in Canandaigua, New York. She is currently a co-investigator in a research project concerning attitudes of nurses toward death and dying with colleagues at the Suicide Prevention and Crisis Service, Inc., of Buffalo, New York, and is a member of the editorial board of *Perspectives in Psychiatric Care*.

MISS MARY NORMA O'HARA received her diploma in nursing from the Charles S. Wilson Memorial Hospital, Johnson City, New York. She completed a Bachelor of Science degree at the Catholic University of

America in Washington, D.C., and a Master of Arts degree from Teachers College, Columbia. She came to Buffalo from the University of Rochester where she was an Associate Professor of Maternal-Child Nursing.

MISS SHIRLEY STEELE received her diploma in nursing from the Waterbury Hospital, Waterbury, Connecticut. Her Baccalaureate and Master's degrees are from Teachers College, Columbia University. She was an Associate Professor of Child Health Nursing at the State University of New York at Buffalo at the time she wrote the book. She was a graduate student in the School of Educational Development at Ohio State University. She is a member of the editorial staff of *Nursing Forum*.

MRS. JACQUELINE THOMPSON received her R.N. and Bachelor of Science degrees from the University of Minnesota. She spent two years at Purdue University in Child Development and Family Life. She received her Master of Education degree in Early Childhood Education from the State University of New York at Buffalo.

Jackie has taught nutrition as well as normal growth and development. Her present position is Assistant Professor of Child Health Nursing and co-investigator with Donna Juenker on the training grant (D10 NU 00394-01).

Contents

Preface

Numerous advances have been made in the area of child care, which kindled a desire on the part of several nursing faculty to write this book. The book was envisioned as a supplement to current literature in the areas of normal growth and development, nutrition, and pediatric nursing. The focus of the book is the care of the child with a long-term or terminal illness, with major emphasis placed on the role of the nurse.

While the book was written with education of the undergraduate student as its principal focus, it is felt that the book will have a much wider audience.

Instructors in undergraduate programs should find the book valuable in providing learning experiences which may not be readily available in their immediate area. As it becomes increasingly difficult to provide direct learning experiences with patients, it will be especially important to have a variety of media available to help students to learn. We hope this book will be one valuable part of the additional media.

It is hoped that the book will also be helpful for graduate students in Child Health Nursing. While some of the information is very basic, to meet the needs of undergraduate students, the graduate student will find it especially helpful if she is interested in teaching or becoming a clinician in the area of long-term illness.

The staff nurse in child health should find the book a valuable reference as it pulls together much of the current literature which relates to the care of children. It may prove useful as an in-service educational tool for new staff nurses.

The authors are hopeful that the material presented will broaden the available nursing literature by expanding on selected areas in the long-term nursing care of children. We have attempted to expand on areas which are currently receiving lesser emphasis in pediatric nursing textbooks.

In most of the text, the student is referred to as "she," but only for simplicity in writing. It is meant to include all students of nursing. Also, the terms student and nurse are used interchangeably. The word student is used when the emphasis is on learning. The word nurse is used when the emphasis is on practice.

Throughout the text, we refer to parents. We have not made an attempt to cover the many family patterns which are possible, as it would be impossible in a text of this size and scope.

As medical techniques continue to develop and more and more children are spared life, we will meet many more children with long-term illnesses. Therefore, in this book, we have attempted to meet the challenges presented by these children.

The trend towards out-patient care for pediatric patients has inspired the section in the chapter on terminal illness in relation to out-patient services. These services must be improved to provide the same expert care that the child formerly received on an in-patient basis.

The chapter on terminal illness has been utilized by several students and other child health faculty. It was originally prepared as there was so little information available in this area. The typewritten material was shared with other faculty and students who used it in a variety of ways. Their many comments and positive suggestions prompted me to try to refine the material for publication.

I especially wish to thank the other faculty members who graciously contributed to this book. Their expertise in particular areas, will be well illustrated by their contributions. As editor, it has been a most rewarding experience working with them. Our professional nursing and teaching careers have spanned several years. Our writing careers have crossed paths for the first time and necessitated adjustments and concessions by all of us.

At first I hoped it would be possible to acknowledge all the clinical facilities we have used in collecting our information. This turned out to be a staggering list with the wide experiences of the contributing authors. Therefore, we wish to thank collectively all the personnel in the clinical facilities which have contributed to our knowledge of patient care. A special note of thanks is extended to the clinical facility which currently supplies the majority of our in-patient and out-patient clinical experience to our students in Child Health Nursing, The Children's Hospital of Buffalo, New York. The nursing personnel have helped us provide valuable learning experiences for students and have served as role models. Their indirect participation in this book is gratefully acknowledged.

Many parents and children have graciously agreed to have their photos used in the book. Our thanks is extended to them for their cooperation and patience.

Several of the other faculty of the School of Nursing at the State University of New York at Buffalo, have edited and criticized our chapters, while in progress. A special note of thanks is extended to Mrs. Patricia Gorzka for her reading and encouragement. Without her generous editing and suggestions, the book would not have come to fruition.

In addition, her expertise in child intensive care unit nursing has added much to the content. She also contributed time and skill to obtain several of the photos in the book. Miss Judy Bumbalo and Miss Kathleen Daniels have also edited selected chapters and I wish to thank them.

The secretarial staff, under the direction of Mrs. Reine Dowdall has done a commendable job in typing the manuscript. Despite the many requests made by us they have continued to keep their composure and meet deadlines. Their "gentle prodding" for contributions from the various faculty have aided in the completion of our task. Mrs. Dowdall has given a high priority to the typing of the manuscript and the secretaries have shown real enthusiasm for the finished product.

A special vote of thanks is extended to the Child Health Department secretary, Miss Ann Marie Kozlowski, for her many contributions to preparing the book. Ann's contributions far exceed the ordinary contributions of a secretary.

Miss Sue LaForest, friend and colleague from the Birth Defect Clinic at Children's Hospital, has been a constant sounding board for new ideas. Her clinical expertise and judgment have been most valuable. She has given freely of her time and made photos available to enrich particular chapters.

Thanks are also extended to Dr. Ruth T. McGrorey, Dean of the School of Nursing at the State University of New York at Buffalo. She originally suggested I contact Mr. Charles Bollinger about publishing the book. Dean McGrorey has shown a personal as well as a professional interest in our progress.

Collectively, recognition will have to be extended to the many students and patients who contributed to establishing the objectives of this volume. They are the true recipients of any gratitude expressed by the reader.

We have felt most fortunate to have a colleague in the Adult Health Nursing department available to do the original illustrations. Miss Helen Ptak has been unusually cooperative in meeting our many requests for illustrations.

Each of us are grateful to many other colleagues who helped us gather information or gave us encouragement. Our families and friends have been very understanding when the pressure has been high.

As editor, I would like to share with you one other item. Jackie Thompson has certainly earned the admiration of the group as she met deadlines while traveling around the country on sabbatical leave with her husband and two children. She wrote her chapters while she was driving a house bus, teaching her children, and running a household, migrant style. In addition, she introduced Allegra Carolyn to the world in July at the same time she was completing her final contributions. Her dedication to the task, despite all these factors, has been an example for us all.

The working manuscript has traveled many miles during its development. We now hope the completed manuscript will travel as many miles in helping to meet the nursing needs of children.

Shirley Steele

Introduction

The role of the nurse in the care of children is changing dramatically. Once a matter of baby sitting and diaper changing—a rather bland combination—it is now a position demanding the most critical of observations and actions. There are many reasons for the change in role. The increase in the number of children is a factor, as are the advances in medicine. The lack of qualified pediatricians is another. The more advanced preparation of nurses to assume increasingly complex roles is another. The financial support available for hospitalization also plays an important role.

The term "child health nurse" I view as all-encompassing. Therefore, it will include the nurse in the newborn nursery, the nurse on the in-patient and out-patient services relating to child care, the nurse in the child health conferences, in home-care of children, and in school health. In other words, nurses in various settings but who are concerned with the health and prevention of disease in children.

The role of the child health staff nurse is now being satisfactorily strengthened by the use of the nurse clinician. The child health nurse clinician also consults with clinicians in other specialty areas. One such nurse specialist is the nurse clinician in child psychiatry. For a more detailed account of her role, see the chapter written by Mrs. Kneisl on emotional illness in childhood. The use of specialists offers a golden opportunity to improve care to children. The nurse clinician can help to broaden the offerings of the staff nurse. It is one way of keeping the staff nurse up-to-date on the current concepts in the care of children. The nurse clinician can also demonstrate new nursing techniques. She is often called upon when children are "difficult" in the clinical area. Her demonstration of ways of delivering nursing services can serve as a model to young staff nurses.

In addition to being the "trouble shooter" she identifies areas which need concentrated nursing effort to provide improvement in nursing care. Frequently the nurse consistently and intimately involved in a particular situation feels the situation is near perfect. She is not so likely to identify weakness in the program. A nurse with additional theoretical and clinical expertise can begin identifying areas which need improvement and suggest methods to provide this improvement.

The child health staff nurse must be an actively participating member of the health team. She will not be optimally effective unless she recognizes and utilizes the special skills offered by the other team members. She must be able to be the leader of the team as well as a member of the team offering particular health services. In order to treat children effectively, the leadership role needs to shift with the needs of the child. A particular child's care may be led by the doctor at one point, by the physical therapist at another, or by the parent at another. The shifting of the leader will make care more satisfactory than always insisting that the doctor be the team leader. There is a shortage of doctors, and children with long-term conditions but who are not "sick" may not need the very specialized skills of the physician during much of their health care supervision. At a point where the doctor is necessary to lead the team, the current leader willingly relinquishes the leadership role.

In an attempt to prepare nurses for this changing role, the material in this book includes nursing tools such as the nursing history and nursing progress notes. The content included is aimed at covering the long-term conditions in greater depth than presently found in pediatric nursing textbooks.

It is important to remember that much of today's knowledge is outdated tomorrow. The creative nurse is known because she disrupts the organization. Her desire for change makes her restless. Change takes place slowly but she should not be discouraged. A satisfaction with the status quo will not be enough to guarantee excellent patient care. Today's patient is more knowledgeable and demands the best; child health nurses should be eager to provide this "best."

Children with long-term illnesses will need special understanding when attending school. The school nurse is in an excellent position to make the child's needs known. She should be instrumental in getting needed changes instituted. Structural barriers and communication barriers can be eliminated if the nurse is attuned to the needs of the child.

The child health nurse is able to contribute both professionally and as a citizen to the needs of children with long-term illness. Her knowledge can be effectively used to help get needed programs in her community.

It is with deep humility that we offer the material in this volume as a resource for the improvement of nursing care to the numerous children in our country with long-term illness.

References

Erikson, F. The need for a specialist in modern pediatric nursing, Nurs. Forum 4:24–31, 1965.

Ford, L. C., and Silver, H. K. The expanded role of the nurse in child care. Nurs. Outlook, 15:43–45, Sept. 1967.

Rudick, E. Nursing and the new pediatrics. Nurs. Clinics N. A. (Philadelphia, Saunders) 1966, p. 75–81.

NURSING CARE
OF THE CHILD
WITH LONG-TERM ILLNESS

PART I
BACKGROUND INFORMATION

1 JACQUELINE THOMPSON

Human Growth and Development: A Basis for Nursing Assessment

Can human growth and development be used as a basis for nursing assessment? The answer is obviously yes, but the implementation of this YES seems to be one of our most confusing problems. At this point in time, I believe that the problem lies in an inadequate or unusable developmental framework. We acknowledge that it is important for our nursing activities to be based upon present research from our own field and from other disciplines. Unfortunately, research reports do not come neatly packaged, so that these *pieces* of current research usually hang in limbo unless they can be based, so to speak, within a general framework. Thus, developmental framework is needed to give our nursing activities direction. With this general framework we can begin to make an assessment of the child's total development. We can establish goals centered around where we feel it is possible for him to go during our period of influence. These goals will cover, not only in the readjustment of his internal environmental equilibrium, but all aspects of his being. Thus it seems important that the nurse base her assessment of the needs of the patient within the structure of a *personally* workable concept of the growth and development of humans. It is important that this framework be dynamic so that new information or relationships can be based within it. It is also important that its structure have categories general enough that it gives security to the user. I hope that this does not necessarily mean rigidity to the reader, for this is not my intention. I believe this gross concreteness to be essential because all too often we must interact with patients without a complete analysis of his total needs. With this rather concrete and gross developmental framework we can tentatively proceed to interact and feel more secure. I believe this basic preparation will lead to better initial nursing care with fewer destructive interactions. I am also assuming that the assessment does not end there! I hope that you will come to see that a sound developmental concept with its dynamic and concrete features can be used as a tool in daily and major nursing assessment plans.

In this chapter we will discuss the development of a conceptual framework for growth and development with examples of some possibilities; it will present some broad guidelines to be considered when we are assessing the needs of the individual patients. Since most of our information about human growth and development has been documented in terms of "norms" or "averages," we must constantly question whether they do or do not correlate with any one individual's growth and development. Also included will be a short discussion of some aspects of longitudinal development, the nurse-child interaction pattern, and some of the goals and pitfalls that occur in long-term hospitalization of the child.

Toward a Conceptual Framework in Growth and Development

Previously I mentioned that the structure of the framework should be general, with categories gross enough to include a variety of related information. Before we get to this point, I wish to make an assumption which I believe must be made before a conceptual framework in growth and development can be devised by the professional nurse. That assumption is that our professional aim is to meet the total needs of the patient, insofar as it is possible, within a given set of circumstances. This assumption leads to other basic assumptions: that meaningful interaction with an individual (and for the purpose of this book, the child who will be ill over a long period of time) can take place only when all his developmental aspects or facets and their integration have been considered. This point of view is sometimes known as "holistic."

In general, human growth and development can be studied from two tacks or approaches. These approaches have been called the study of developmental crises (also "ages" and "stages") and the longitudinal approach to growth and development. The latter is an overview of the average expression of various developmental areas or aspects. Let us remember that both of these approaches consider information about large groups of individuals and this is not the same as consideration of individuals within a group (Lawrence, 1955). In nursing we are working with individuals with their own unique internal and external environments. Often these generalizations do not appear to fit our patient. There are also other problems with either of these approaches which we should keep in mind when we use them. These problems will be discussed throughout the chapter.

The developmental crises approach devises its norms by interrupting development at what the researcher believes is a critical point in human development and proceeds to enumerate the exhibited behavior. A critical point is a time when a large number of developmental areas are in disequilibrium or in change (Hurlock 1956; Ericson, 1963). I think I can safely say that we have all been exposed to this kind of approach in our basic developmental courses. Unfortunately, exposure to only this kind of approach may result in a hodgepodge of remembered facts about the physical, social, and psychological behavior of any given age. It also often leaves one with a vague notion that the children we interact with should really fit well into what we remember of his particular stage in order to be "normal" (i.e., receive his A) in development. This happens even when we know that the "norms" are not refined enough to fit any one child. On top of this we may or may not be correctly remembering the norms.

The study of developmental crises material, I believe, should be used as a vague cognitive stimulus for the professional nurse. This approach can label the child as being in a broad category (2½ years of age=negativistic stage), but it tells us relatively little about the development of an individual's specific behavioral expression of this stage. For example, will he be verbally or physically negative? We can certainly see that if child X is *verbally* negative and must have his jaw immobilized during this time it will cause a greater stress situation than child Y who is *physically* negative and has his jaw immobilized. Thus, while this gross information or broad category may be enough information for some disciplines I find it only mildly useful in our discipline, geared as it is to the needs of the individual and his uniqueness.

The second approach to the study of growth and development places its emphasis upon the longitudinal growth and development of the human. Kinds of various behavioral responses are studied in a general way to search out a basic trend or flow over the life-span. This approach is not often studied in all its aspects by the beginning practitioner and will be discussed in an abbreviated form later in this chapter. The problem with this approach is that one can get a feeling that the human is being sectioned into numerous responses, never to meet again. Although it does give us some valuable insight into where the child has been and what we may expect of his behavior in the future, it does leave the integration of behavior up to the nurse in child health.

I believe that the best answer is an exposure to both approaches with a strong emphasis upon observing the *facts* and accounting for the interaction of the various behavioral responses along with major hereditary, internal, and external or environmental influences. Thus if our professional aim in interacting with the ill child for long periods during his development is to try to meet his total needs, we must view his development from both approaches or from a "holistic" point of view. How can this holistic point of view work to our advantage when we are considering assisting the ill child with his growth and development? The expression of an individual human's growth and development is stimulated and directed by the troika: heredity, internal environment, and external environment. If this troika interacts harmoniously or works together ideally, the growth and development of the individual would be maximal. Obviously, since there is a high probability that the countless facets may interact in less than an ideal manner, we can see that the end results are rarely optimal in nature.

We can see examples of this interaction working in the newborn's activity level. The newborns in any given nursery vary in their degree of general activity and vary in their sensitivity to stimuli. After all, each child has been developing his various aspects at his own unique rate since conception—when the hereditary basis for the expression of his development was programmed. It is common knowledge that, at birth, abnormal internal and external environmental functioning may have been already maximizing, minimizing, or in some way already directing the programming set down by heredity (Carmichael, 1966; Breckenridge and Vincent, 1966; Breckenridge et al., 1958).

We see the beginning of what can be called biological functioning in the initial day and weeks of life. For example, in a very crude way we see the infant begin his cognitive (Piaget, 1932) development with the feeding process. As he is fed (a reduction of an internal need, hunger) he attaches a vague conceptual meaning to the instrument by which he is fed: the bottle or breast. How satisfied he feels by the feeding will depend upon his individual needs (i.e., the rate of growth determined by his genetic programming). He will begin his development of language in the cooing and verbal articulation of those close to him, as these activities stimulate his auditory mechanism (internal environment) to the extent that heredity has programmed the development of his nervous system. Thus we see that the troika of heredity, internal environment, and external environment enters into the expression of each piece of behavior exhibited by the infant. We view the interweaving of the developmental stimuli as they work together to stimulate the expression of the various psychological and biological aspects throughout the child's development.

The interaction of the psychological aspects with the biological aspects of an individual's development has been explored for years (Piaget, 1932, 1954, 1963; Gesell and Thompson, 1941). We know that the psychological aspects of the child's behavior intertwines with the biological aspects in positive correlation. The child cannot be physically ill without the illness' interfering in some way with his psychological functioning, and the child cannot be mentally ill without in some way the illness' interfering with his biological functioning. To some extent his whole life will be changed or modulated by his long-term illness (the theme of this book), and his subsequent hospitalization and recovery. Our role as nurses is to interfere with a series of abnormal environments, both internal and external, in such a way that the greatest degree of normality can be achieved. Subsequent chapters will detail a variety of these interventions as they pertain to particular abnormal internal and external environments.

The following is a discussion of a sample developmental conceptual framework from a holistic point of view. There are many ways of breaking down the kinds of biological and psychological behavior seen throughout life. The following seems to me to be a reasonable one for persons working with children in the intense manner necessary when the child will be hospitalized for long periods. But again let me state that each nurse must work with and develop a personal framework into which she can categorize new ideas, research, readings, etc., as she is exposed to them.

The following categories will be used:

> Body Structure and Functional Responses
> Habitual Responses
> Motor Behavior
> Development of Reality
>   a. Sensory responses
>   b. Cognitive processes
>   c. Language behavior
> Identification Behavior
> Emotional Behavior
> Social Behavior

These aspects not only influence each other as they develop but are also influenced by heredity and the internal and external environment of the individual's world. These biological and psychological aspects change through the processes of growth, maturation, and learning. These dynamic relationships interact throughout all of life, but it is during the period from birth through adolescence—that time in an individual's life when he develops his *individual reality*—that the most remarkable changes occur. It is this critical period that concerns the nurse working in the child health area. Human growth and development can be visualized as a intricate web of interrelating parts.

BODY STRUCTURE AND FUNCTIONAL RESPONSES

We can define body structure as the conglomerate of the various tissue structures: bone tissue, skin, internal organs, and so forth. Most nurses are well aware of the normally defined body and it is one of the first observations of gross growth and development made when the child is admitted to the hospital. Body function is also of immediate concern to the nursing staff since it is often some disequilibrium in this area which brings the child to the health worker. (Motor behavior can be seen as part of these behaviors or as a separate series.)

Perhaps the one most important question to be asked concerning the area of body structure and function is: "Are there any noticeable changes?" This follows because all development has a pattern and is continuous. Previous records of height and weight should be considered. Since the body grows as a unit, any abnormally slow or rapid growth of any part should be noted (Watson and Lowrey, 1968). Much of the individual information concerning this area will come from tests, doctors' reports, discussion with the patient and family, and from old records. It is most likely within this area that our first information concerning the patient's growth and development will be found. The obvious goal for this area when one is working with the child with a long-term illness is interrupting the imbalanced cycle (administration of prescribed drugs, diet, some therapy, and so forth) and bringing the body back in equilibrium. While it is true that all growth and development brings with it disequilibrium, the body normally compensates for it until it can readjust itself. For example, when the pre-adolescent growth increase occurs the child has a tendency to ingest more food and need more sleep. It is a time when the body seems to concentrate on the physical aspect of development. It is only when something goes wrong with the internal programming (e.g., giantism) or external environment (e.g., malnutrition) that the disequilibrium becomes too much for the body and it becomes overwhelmed. We should remember when we are thinking of the general overall interrelationship of the developmental areas that we more often than not will see the child in the hospital for long-term care during one of these disequilibrium phases and we can expect all areas of behavior to be modified because of this added stress. (Nelson, 1948; Williams, 1956; Anderson, 1957.)

HABITUAL RESPONSES

The second area—habitual responses—can be rather open-ended or contain only material pertaining to such things as sleeping, eating, elimination, dressing, and other daily care. These areas are biologically straightforward enough but more often than not so interwoven with emotional behavior that they can cause distress not only for the child but also for the nurse. Habit in the functional sense denotes routine sameness. Of course, immediately upon the patient's entering into a new environment, such as the hospital, old habitual responses must be modified. To say that this is stressful to the child is putting it mildly. Of course, how much distress ensues also depends upon the age, general life style of the child, and the nursing staff's tolerance of behavorial variance.

Perhaps the second most important information (sometimes it is the first) we gather about the child's behavior is the manifestation of his habitual responses. For our part we do not concern ourselves immediately in the area of norms but only in the area of what exists. Our first concern is for the child's feelings of security and comfort and this is one area where we can usually close some of the gaps between the home reality and the hospital reality. The child should know that every effort is being made to adapt the *hospital* to the habitual responses to the child. I cannot maximize the importance of having information about and being highly sensitive to habitual behavior during those first few days. The extra work will reap benefits beyond your wildest imagination.

What about later on in the hospitalization? There are, of course, suggested norms for all behavior during hospitalization. Our goals for the end of the child's hospitalization certainly will include these norms as we help the child to progress in this area of development. Sometimes these later goals can be carried out in an uncomplicated straightforward manner.

For example: The toddler learning to eat with a spoon or becoming toilet trained while hospitalized.

Please remember this word of caution! Find out the habitual response goal of the mother before you go too far. After all, the child is going back into his home following hospitalization and this will take readjustment without the undue strain of alienation from the family mores. In other words, the nurse must have an awareness of the habitual behavior of the child, his family culture, and his social group in order to set developmental goals for the hospital stay. Of course, with the parents' understanding and backing it is possible to make some minor deviations in goals. It really becomes a major concern when the child's illness interferes with the goals of the family in this area, such as special diets, unusual elimination needs, and so forth. A great deal of time can then be spent with patient and family bringing back into equilibrium or assimilating these new habits so that they do not interfere with other areas of growth and development.

MOTOR BEHAVIOR

The development of motor behavior for the well child seems to take place somewhat automatically and while hospitalization can indeed distort the pattern, there is some research to reassure us that the child can make up the differences later (Sandler and Torpie, 1968; Shirley, 1933; Chamberlin, 1966). Here again it is important to have information concerning the motor development of the child *prior* to his illness. At this time it is important to look for developmental rates. For example, if the child has been developing at a slow rate, we can expect this rate of development to continue after the child is well. Obviously our goals for this child's motor development would be much different from those for a child who had been developing at an even and rapid rate. The setting of these kinds of goals is relatively straightforward; any developmental book will give approximate normal ranges.

It is more difficult to set goals when: (1) the child has been ill all of his life and, therefore, not exhibiting his hereditary program of motor developmental patterns and (2) the child's illness will continue to interfere with his natural or hereditary programming of motor development. In both cases goals must be *very tentative;* one has almost to play it by ear. In this case it is doubly important to know in detail exactly what the child has been doing, thus permitting some understanding of the level of motor development. I stated before that there is unity in body development, but such may definitely not be true here. The illness may interfere with one aspect of motor development more than another.

If you can satisfy yourself that you have enough information concerning the child's currently exhibited motor behavior, you can then start from there with appropriate stimulation (stimulation possibilities are discussed in the chapter on play). Only by trial-and-error and listening and observing the child carefully can you time advances in stimulation toward succeedingly more complex motor behavior. After a number of weeks you may be able to set a realistic goal.

As with habitual responses, motor behavior is also set to some extent by the family's goals. Again, this must be considered in the nursing plan. These goals cannot be overlooked for the family are the ones who must give the longest-term care to the child. A realistic program of motor development stimulation should be worked out with the parents for best results (Erikson, 1963; Dennis, 1942; Gesell and Thompson, 1941; Mead and MacGregor, 1951). To some extent the child's family and social mores will have determined how much stimulation the child has had in the area of motor development. I do not think there will be as great a variance in family goals in this area as for habitual responses. There may be some, particularly when one is working with a child from one of the subcultures. Also, remember to inquire subtly about sex-difference expectations in motor development goals.

DEVELOPMENT OF REALITY

This next category is very large and could be separated, but it seems more functional to think of it in totality for an action-oriented profession such as nursing. All of the categories—sensory responses, cognitive processes, and language behavior—are based on the child's experiences with reality, as are some phases of identification, emotional, and social behavior, but to include these here would be too cumbersome.

Later on in the chapter we will discuss ways of determining the difference between hospital and outside or consensus reality. These differences will cause some consternation to both patient and nurse. Included will be a short discussion of individual and consensus reality and our commitment and responsibility to both, if we are to assist the child in his development.

Church (1961) speaks of a personal or individual reality made up of one's wishes, daydreams, inner thoughts, and of an outer or consensus reality, one which we all experience. For example: a four-year-old patient may call the nurse at night to tell a frightening tale of a large bear entering her room. Outer reality or consensus reality would tell us that the child could not have seen a large bear in her hospital room for a number of obvious reasons. It is not within our consensus reality. It is also not within the child's consensus reality which she can come to understand if we take the time to explain to her about the difference between the two. But it was definitely real to the child (as are our own "wildest thoughts"). Fortunately, we are able to differentiate between the two realities *most* of the time. I have yet to meet a person whose only reality is consensus—what a shallow, boring, limited personality he would have. It is the *individual* or *inner reality* which makes us different from each other. I make this point because we often confuse the expression of inner reality thoughts with negative things such as lying. The large bear can be brought out into the openness of our minds and talked about. The key to any discussion of the fantasies of inner reality is whether another human could have also seen it. Sometimes we are the only ones who see something and it will not fit into a reality which everyone will acknowledge. We are very understanding and sympathetic of ourselves when we have an inner thought which is so revealing and comprehensible. Of course, it may become another matter when we try to explain our wonderful concept to another individual. This is where it becomes uncomfortable and long conversations with others become necessary. Let us try to think of the large bear within this context and work with the child to grow in the knowledge of his inner or personal reality and consensus reality. I have often seen so little tolerance for the child's inner reality; perhaps it is because we have been negatively reinforced for our own inner realities. Building a rich understanding of inner and consensus reality will help the child grow and understand himself, as well as others. So much for reality or realities, since in the specific they vary from day to day, year to year, and person to person, making our culture chaotic without our elaborate system of symbols: language. It is through language that we attempt to interpret our world (inner reality) to each other and must end up being satisfied with something less than perfection interpretations (consensus reality).

This chapter will not elaborate on the longitudinal development sensory response, cognitive processes, and language behavior because any number of books exist to give you a more complete picture than could be attempted here, but I should like to point out that these processes include the interaction of the child with his external environment. To put it simply, the child uses his senses to gather material from his environment and as he gathers data he stores them. His use of the data available to him is, to a great measure, determined by his cognitive process—and this develops slowly through the years from rather concrete related interests and manipulation of concrete objects, that is, manual examination of the world around him (Piaget, 1954; Reichard et al., 1944; Baldwin, 1955; Russell, 1956; Akutaguwa and Benoir, 1959), to abstract thinking in which the child can rely on reason (mental manipulation) to understand the world around him.

Obviously, the behavior which assists the child in his discovery by organizing and labeling is language (Church, 1961). Language helps him manipulate his totally symbolic or nonconcrete thoughts into new concepts. In a real sense it is the integrating force that acts between the child and his senses and the external environment. Language is the tool which differentiates humans from other creatures. Language function can be viewed as being superimposed upon the physical structure of the human. The senses have a specific physical structure to carry out their functions, (e.g., eyes for seeing), but language must use other physical structures whose prime function is something else (e.g., lungs for breathing).

Language is not a concrete, tangible entity, but only a symbol for something in reality; or, more precisely, some concept in an individual's reality. Some kinds of words have meanings which are rather well accepted and very useful in discussion with others, but not nearly so many as one would expect.

Language is, in many respects, a reflection of our internal and external environment and the one area of development most damaged by long periods of institutionalization or hospitalization (Sandler and Torpie, 1968; Chamberlin, 1966). The solution to eradication of the problem of language retardation lies with the amount of stimulation given the child. Language development begins with the coos and smiles of the mother (or substitute) during feeding times; in the concerned babbling of the world of the toddler; or in the serious discussion during the preschool years of why there is a moon in the sky during the day. In other words, it is that part of our development which is directly stimulated by people rather than things in our environment. It is other humans who must interpret for the child what the world is all about. Language development must have human-to-human contact in a communication phase. This does not mean talking to one's co-workers or to the wall while working with children. It does mean talking *with* the child about realities surrounding him. All our communication with the child and all the experiences we plan for him should be aimed at increasing his understanding of reality and his symbolization of it. This is one of the child's prime occupations throughout infancy, childhood, and adolescence.

Because we are discussing the hospitalized child and our role as a nurse working in child health, we must remember that the hospital reality is not normal everyday reality. We must compensate for the experiences the child is missing during his hospital stay. Close attention must be given to the level of language development at the time preceding hospitalization and any signs of slowing of progress during hospitalization should be quickly noted and attempts made by the staff to compensate for them. If this comes to no avail a speech pathologist should be contacted as consultant to the staff or child, whichever role the specialist feels would be more useful to the child.

IDENTIFICATION BEHAVIOR

The exhibited behaviors of identification (emotional or social responses) are closely interrelated with each other and greatly influenced by the external environment. As with the development of language, *identification* or *self-identity* is a learned response. In a real sense we are who we are by the reaction of others to our being. This is not totally true, but the developing individual is very flexible and can change behavior which has met with negative reactions of others into behavior that will elicit a positive response. All the communication which occurs between the infant and the mother (verbal or nonverbal) builds identification behavior. The games and attention shown the child by his mother all help the child distinguish himself from his environment. This identification development continues throughout childhood and adolescence. It usually centers around those who continuously care for the child (Call, 1968; Sonis, 1968; Greenson, 1968; Epstein, 1968). There are, of course, major differences in the development of identification as there are in emotional and social responses (Greenson, 1968).

How we can in the hospital setting continue the development of identification with the parents is a most difficult task. It takes a great deal of ingenuity plus a real sense of commitment to the necessity of continuing some assemblance of the old relationship on the part of the parents and the staff. It means a number of things to me. It means reinforcing in the child's mind the existence of an absent parent even when you feel angry that the parent is not visiting as much as might be desirable. It means helping the parent to feel less guilty about the child's illness. It means helping the parents to participate, in a meaningful way, in the recovery of the child. This does not necessarily mean giving physical care but it certainly means interacting in the areas of language, motor, and reality developments. In other words, it is making sure that the child understands that all the important people in his present and past environment are harmoniously working toward the day he can be discharged. It also means stimulating the child to identify himself as an individual, apart from the things in his environment, and increasing his sense of self-integrity. (Additional content will be included in the discussion of the nurse-child interaction.) A disappointing aspect of assisting the child to develop an identification or a concept of self is that we may never see any results and therefore cannot measure our effectiveness.

EMOTIONAL BEHAVIOR

The development of emotions is closely related to family and general culture, the age of the child, the functioning of the internal environment, general maturation, and the extent to which reality is understood. (For example the four-year-old has many unwarranted fears coming from his expanding awareness of his environment and his lack of understanding of it.)

We must remember that children's emotions differ from those of the adult. They differ in the following ways:

1. Children's emotions are short-lived.
2. Children's emotions are more intense than they will be

later (i.e., to children the sun is either shining brightly or there is a downpour).

3. Children's emotions come as quickly as they go. We can elicit a drastic change in behavior by the introduction of some new toy or idea.
4. Children have more emotional outbursts than adults who frequently try to hide their emotions.
5. Children's emotional behavior can be a sign of his general feeling of well-being. If his reality does not meet his expectation he may develop nervous mannerisms, frequent hysterical outbursts, tension, restlessness, etc.
6. Children's emotions are individual (Hurlock, 1956).

It is our task to set up the hospitalized child's environment in such a way as will foster good emotional tone. Examples of environmental ingredients which foster good emotional tone are the following:

1. The child must have a feeling of confidence in himself.
2. The child must have some success in the tasks he attempts.
3. The child must recognize reality.
4. The child must have recognition of his efforts.
5. The child must have status from his peers.
6. The child must be accepted as he is, with respect.
7. The child must have empathetic understanding.
8. The child must have love and affection (Lee and Lee, 1958).

SOCIAL BEHAVIOR

Social development is often severely curtailed in the hospital situation where the child is somewhat isolated from normal peer social situations. When the child is very ill, little socialization goes on except between the adults in the situation and the individual child. Later on, as the child recovers, he will come in contact with other children in the sheltered environment of the nursing unit's playroom. When there is intermingling of children of all ages, a reasonable facsimile of normal neighborhood socialization can take place, that is, with a range of ages. This heterogeneous age group has been more beneficial to the advancement of growth and development than grouping children of the same age (Sandler and Torpie, 1968).

Obviously this socialization should be carefully planned with regard to the child's age and his physical ability. Some children will need more help with socialization than others. A general rule of thumb applies here: the larger the number of children and the younger the age of the child the more the adult must assume responsibility for interpretation of goals and intentions in the setting. Also, the larger the group of children assembled, the greater the number of activities and toys that must be available for use.

This discussion should give you ideas regarding aspects of human growth and development and how they can be encouraged at the appropriate level on an individual basis for each child during periods of hospitalization. While each area of development is unique in certain developmental constituents, there are some principles which are interrelated throughout all areas of human growth and development. Each area takes on a different context in accordance with its primary role, and when it cuts across the boundaries of differing areas of development it is called a characteristic or a principle of development. Our conceptual framework is tempered and often made more workable and rational when the observed behavior is interpreted by the use of these mediating factors.

In every development book there is a list of principles of characteristics which the author deems pertinent. There are a number of characteristics that are particularly useful for the nurse to remember as she attempts to understand her patient. Each child has his own rate of development; as we observe children growing we become aware that each individual child has his own rate of development which has its base in his hereditary programming and is directed by his environment. If the child speaks early or begins to form sentences at a very early age this has been found to positively correlate with a rapid development of more sophisticated language. It most likely will mean that other kinds of development will also tend to be accelerated, to some degree. This acceleration can be either to a greater degree than the language acceleration or to a lesser degree (Carmichael, 1966). However, all aspects will be average or accelerated, since growth and developmental aspects are also rate correlated (Hurlock, 1956).

The Individual Child

UNIQUE PATTERNS OF EMERGING ABILITIES. The child's rate of growth and development will be uniquely his own, as will the observable pattern of his emerging abilities. Some individuals will tend endlessly to practice new abilities before going on to another task. Others will appear to need no practice with the very same task but are motivated to go on to more complex behavior immediately. Of the children who go on, some may revert back to the more simple form of the particular behavior at some later date. For example, some children begin to walk independently by getting up and walking, while others take one or two walking steps with a gradual progression to walking. Others will practice activities similar to the task (e.g., walking while holding on to something for substantially long periods and then suddenly walk independently one day, as if this less complex motor exercise suffices as practice for the more complex activity). This kind of *developmental aura* is uniquely the child's own and one that we should be cognizant of when we attempt to explain his behavior. It is also relevant when we try to determine where he transects the development curve relating to the average for any specific behavioral response.

FROM SIMPLE TO COMPLEX. Behavioral changes develop from very simple, gross, or general responses to more complex, fine, or specific responses. For example, the language response to anything round first may be "ball" and later become differentiated into orange, grapefruit, or basketball (Carmichael, 1966). The infant has a general emotional response to all changes in environment and later differentiates such things as hunger, wetness, and so forth.

DIRECTIONAL PATTERN.   A great deal of information has been accumulated concerning the developmental characteristic; growth and development follows a pattern of direction. This direction has been described by many as cephalocaudal, or head-to-foot, and proximodistal, or from the center of the body toward the farthest portion of the body. Examples of this characteristic are seen readily in numerous areas of biological development. It can also be seen in areas related to the development of socialization. An example of cephalocaudal developmental direction is that the infant begins his social interaction by staring at his mother's face and only later in infancy explores her face with his hands. We can see the infant and the child's world develop proximodistally as he moves from a self-perception when he is the center of all activity into parallel play and later into small interacting groups (Hegethorn, 1968).

DIFFERENT RATES FOR DIFFERENT PARTS OF THE BODY.   Physically we see the child's head and trunk developing earlier than legs. The lower brain stem and spinal column carry on their total functions years earlier than the cerebrum (Watson and Lowrey, 1968). There is a predictable sequence of development along a longitudinal continuum which all individuals normally travel.

It can also be said that all individuals travel through all stages on the developmental continuum regardless of the particular developmental aspect and that there is a certain degree of predictability about the major stages. Shirley (1933) found a sequence example of locomotor development in the babies she observed. Erikson (1963) discusses the eight stages of man's personality development. As always, it is easier to predict development when there are groups of individuals involved. Our problem is to predict individual development.

Hopefully, the preceding will give you a start in understanding how the observation of the child's developmental expression indicates areas of nursing intervention and/or how the nursing staff can then plan patient care today with an eye on future advancement in total growth and development.

Assessing Growth and Development

With the foregoing information in mind we come to the task of growth and development assessment. There are, in today's world, numerous charts, lists, descriptions of the various categories of behavioral response, both biological and psychological, to which I refer you. I will assume at this time that the reader has indeed formulated a conceptual framework and filled it with growth and developmental information.

I should now like to discuss developmental assessment and our responsibility and commitment to it. The role or task of developmental assessment is far more complicated and critical when we are dealing with children with long-term illness. This is true for a number of reasons.

First, since the infant or child may be hospitalized for long periods of time, the nursing team has a 24-hour-a-day influence and responsibility for him. This is contrasted to other professionals who also work with children for lesser periods of time (for example, the teacher, the doctor, the social worker, to name a few). During the child's hospitalization, the child is taken out of his natural or normal environment and placed in a totally abnormal environment. A discussion of the differences between the hospital environment and the normal environment will be discussed further later on in the chapter.

Second, the new external environment is not only abnormal but the child's internal environment is also abnormal, sometimes through all or most of his stay. Obviously this brings about changes in his normal pattern of growth and development. With this in mind our first assessment problem is to find out as much as we can about this previous pattern of development. The most reliable ways of finding out this pattern is through communication with the family. All information concerning the child's previous responses to stimuli must be carefully considered. If you attempt to assess a child's development without consulting information gleaned from interviews (I emphasize the plural) with the persons involved in caring for the child previous to hospitalization, you are treading on dangerous ground not only for yourself as a professional, but more importantly, for the *child*.

The second task in assessment is detailed observation of the child's behavior and the results of tests made of areas which are not observable. It is important here not to eliminate any of the aspects since the key to adequate assessment is in an understanding of the total child. In this case the whole is often greater than the sum of its parts. Whenever a discussion of the child takes place it is important to find patterns in his growth and development and/or some clues to his unique developmental pattern which will make his behavior more understandable. When the first two steps in assessment are thoroughly covered, the nursing staff can make its preliminary statement or initial assessment of the child's needs. There should be some difference between the child's behavior as communicated by the concerned adults and the behavior seen during the first few days of hospitalization. (With some children there will be differences throughout hospitalization.) In some cases there will be marked differences in all responses (for the child whose internal environment is substantially deviating from "average" or "normal") or there may be marked difference in some responses. We may see regression to an earlier stage of average development in one or several areas. We may also see a general closure or minimalization of response behavior (e.g., silence or nonresponsiveness) as a reaction to the added stress of an abnormal external environment. We may also see the opposite or increased response behavior to stimuli (e.g., open aggression, increased attempts to manipulate the environment), or a combination of or variation upon these themes. This initial reaction should be expected and anticipated. It should be considered a normal aspect of the child attempting to come to grips with this new, very strange, and stressful reality. In fact, if the parent interviews are complete, some information about the child's normal manner of dealing with stress should be ascertained early in the hospitalization (i.e., the first day or so).

With this in mind, the nurse can take some of the deviations from "average" or "normal" behavior in her stride, without alarm or negative reactions on her part. It will help the child to adjust to the new environment if this temporary initial crisis is taken at face value and the child reassured that support will be freely and nonpunitively given. The nursing staff must have confidence in themselves and understand the child who is weathering this period in order to establish a positive kind of relationship.

The assessment of developmental behavior is something that may go on during the total stay of the child because of the dynamic nature of development. Goals may be adjusted numerous times as the web of the individual child's growth and development unfolds.

I suspect the reader may like to make some comments about the impossibility of this kind of assessment for every child. I am afraid I am rather unsympathetic of this point of view. I am particularly unsympathetic when it comes to children who will be in the nurses' care 24 hours a day over a long period of time.

Obviously, I believe that *great* care should be extended and much time spent with the child before any substantial need evaluation be made. This includes team-written and personnel-working-nonwritten evaluations of needs. I believe there should be numerous insightful but nonwritten observations or perhaps brief notations made before the formal nursing assessment, since in order to interact and work with the child some kind of temporary assessment must be made. *Please* keep them just that—temporary and flexible. When you make both kinds of notes on observed behavior, make strong attempts to include *facts* rather than judgments concerning the child's developmental expressions; they will be more helpful to you. I do not see the role of the nurse in this situation as including sophisticated developmental testing; that is the role of the psychologist. Our gathered information should result in action on our part and hopefully change on the part of the patient. But be careful about categorizing the child. This will be difficult for you since more of our life is spent placing people and things into categories. For example, let us examine notations concerning a child's eating habits: X ate his yellow carrot first; his bread second; his peaches third; one-fifth of his meat after the nurse said he could eat his peaches. After we recorded a number of days' facts concerning food ingestion, we could gain some insight into the child's dietary pattern. When a pattern such as this continues, we should become concerned about his protein intake, and perhaps calcium since no milk is mentioned and vitamins since there is no mention of green vegetables. This concern would be relayed to the nutritionist who would make the adjustment in menu content that seemed necessary. We would also be concerned that food may have been used as a usual bribe in the home. While food is sometimes used as a bribe with the "normal," "healthy" child, it is unfortunate if it is used excessively. It can be extremely harmful to the child who must adjust his food intake around some metabolic error. Of course, the bribe may not be in the food but in the personal attention a fuss in this area reinforces. Unfortunately, our society does have a tendency to connect food and love—or so it seems when we contemplate the statistics on obesity in the United States.

I hope you will see that this kind of information is more useful than what we sometimes see written: "X eats well with encouragement." The major team assessments will be constructed from looking at everyone's *facts*, not everyone's *opinions*. Hopefully there will be some observed fact in all gross categories of a team's conceptual framework for growth and development.

Here I should make some mention about possible differences between a personal conceptual framework and a team conceptual framework. Ideally, the team conceptual framework will be devised by consensus of the team. In this way, the members have time to work out any differences between personal word meanings and/or theoretical concepts. In other words, when they use a category—sensory development, for example—they will know just what will be found in the category. Are they going to include development of the five senses only or are they going to include the five senses plus kinesthetic development and vestibular development?

From the preceding discussion I hope that I have emphasized sufficiently the following points:

1. A conceptual framework for growth and development includes a gross structure which includes all aspects of human development.
2. Each professional nurse should develop her own framework with its own detailing material or find a standard one that she can live with in harmony.
3. A personal major nursing assessment plan is based upon inferences taken from the various categories of the conceptual framework and is devised from the facts collected.
4. A collection of all team members' observed facts is also one essential facet for a complete nursing assessment and plan of action.
5. Growth and development must be an understanding of both the developmental crises and longitudinal kinds of material.

6. All areas of development have traits unique to the area, but at the same time have traits or characteristics common to all.

The Interaction

In this final portion of the chapter I wish to discuss the matter of the nurse's role as one part of the total environmental influence of the child who is ill with a long-term illness. In particular, our nursing role as it pertains to the repeated and/or long-term hospitalization of the child.

When the child becomes hospitalized our influence upon his behavior becomes intensified as opposed to the nurse's role, say, in community-health, school-health, or doctor's-office. Much of the time during hospitalization the nurse is the center of the child's external environment, or she directs other persons who make up the external environment. The nurse also greatly influences the internal environment. While other members of the health team prescribe or plan (e.g., through the use of drugs or food, changes in the internal environment), their hoped-for and planned-for changes will not occur unless the drugs and food enter the child's internal environment. (More will be said concerning this role throughout the book and in the chapter on nutrition.)

From the above I am sure we can all see the vast areas of influence the nurse has as she interacts with the ill child and provides for the ingredients of his environment. I called this portion of the chapter *The Interaction* for a number of reasons. First, I believe that there must be an interacting between the professional nurse and her patient if satisfactory care is to be given by the nursing staff. Without the nurse's playing a dominant role in caring for and directing the care we cannot hope to achieve an integrated plan of action. Confusion will set in and an added stress will be placed upon the child who is *already* in stress because of his long-term illness and subsequent hospitalization. In order to have an interaction you must have the principal role players within the approximate physical environment. This means relatively low ratios of professional nurses to patients. If you are thinking this is impossible in your situation do not be surprised if the children show signs of the added stress. The little energy the child has will go into an often futile attempt to organize his environment into some assemblance of order, a task essential to his understanding of and coping with the situation (Piaget, 1954). It is not the nurse, overworked and self-seen martyr, who bears the brunt of the ensuing stressful confusion but the ill child. Thus the physical and mental nearness of the nurse is a prime positive ingredient in the hospital life of the child.

Second, an interaction brings along with it some essential ingredients for the health and well-being of both nurse and patient. It is the interaction which fosters a feeling of shared control on the part of the nurse and patient. This sharing of control will help the child to maintain his body integrity. Through interacting with a patient we pick up those important clues to his growth and development needs—changes not only general in nature but the daily small changes which also need to be made in his environments (internal and external). Needless to say, the nurse should not be satisfied to have a child leave her care no better off than he entered it. After all, he and his family should have been under the influence of a professional child care worker who should have created an atmosphere or environment for *his* unique growth and development. A positive interaction will also bring with it a feeling of worthwhileness. Infants and children seem to learn very early a sense of worth, importance, or a positive self-image. On the other hand they also learn very early the feelings of worthlessness, unimportance, or negative self-image. We cannot overestimate the emphasis the child places upon his understanding of his importance to the external environment. He makes some of his estimate of his self-worth by how much time is spent on his behalf. An ongoing interaction will give the child a feeling of integration and worthwhileness—certainly an undisputed ingredient for becoming well.

The continuing interaction with a limited number of professionals will lend security and stability to the child's environment. There is also another not so recognizable benefit from continuous interaction. Because the interaction takes concerted effort on the part of both participants, some energy from the ill child's short storehouse must be used with each new person. Obviously, the highly skilled child care worker will use many means to determine the least traumatic approach for initial interactions and strive throughout the relationship to manage her role in such a manner that little strain will be placed upon the child.

Because energy must be used by the child when he attempts to interact with each new adult, it is only rational for the staff to limit the number of new persons during any critical period or at any other time when the child is low on energy. It seems to me that staffing must necessarily be of a different routine on stations where children with long term-illnesses are cared for than on stations whose patients stay for short periods. The least that should be done is assigning the same nurses to the same patients. It not only reduces the stress of making new relationships but also gives the child a feeling of security—a feeling of knowing how this person reacts to his various behaviors (some children must find out how far they can go behaving negatively with each new interacting adult). No matter how coordinated the staff, there always exists some variance in rule importance and tolerance for minor infractions.

This brings us to another benefit of continuous interaction with a small number of persons: that of consistency. Consistency is, of course, a basic ingredient for reducing the child's anxiety about the new situation. All adults in the situation should be playing the same music, reinforcing the same rules, and building a similar internal and external environment which is based on *knowledge* of the individual child's needs. Hospital environment definitely should be considered a managed therapeutic total environment.

Throughout the preceding discussion, the nurse-child interaction has been nurturing and protecting in nature. Along with the *positive* interaction between the nurse and the child with long-term illness there should be an awareness expanding phase. The child with the long-term illness will be best assisted in his growth and development if he is helped to understand himself better as a person who is temporarily or permanently different from many other peers in the "real" or nonhospital world. The child should also be expanding in the various areas in his general growth and development.

Thus the interaction should have some demonstrable outcomes. There should be a sharing or a feeling of having a reasonable amount of control over one's own behavior and the behavior of others. Each interaction should bring with it new clues to the child's growth and development and a reinforcement on the child's part that his needs are being met by the nursing staff. He should gain feelings of worthwhileness, environmental security, and consistency.

He should also gain a better understanding of himself as a person different from many of his peers in the "real" world. This understanding of individual differences should be useful to the child in his attempt to rationalize and organize his life.

I hope I have given the impression that the planning and interaction with an individual child is a complicated, difficult task calling forth a great deal of general knowledge of growth and development plus restraint, control, and thought on the part of the professional nurse. I believe that the most difficult part of the job is the self-understanding and self-constraint which this kind of interaction demands of the adult. For these reasons I do not believe we can place nonprofessional personnel in the role of the interactor. It is too much to expect of them and the price of patient damage is too high. I also contend that this kind of interaction takes a great deal of planning. A thought *alone* with oneself after a general direction has been set forth by the nursing staff is most necessary for good nursing care. Nursing children with long-term disease who will have repeated and long hospitalization is not something one does for 8 hours a day, five days a week, and then turns off. We must think in terms of quality of care and not quantity.

PITFALLS TO CONSIDER

Interaction pitfalls are numerous, but with care many of them can be avoided or rendered harmless. In the preceding discussion of nursing assessment we talked about the child's initial reaction to the new abnormal environment. One important pitfall is that we become so accustomed to working in the abnormal environment of the hospital with children whose internal environments are abnormal that we lose track of the general, outside (consensus) reality. We then begin to lose our tolerance and understanding of this general reality. Then when the child reacts normally we are shocked and misinterpret the child's reaction, often by deeming it negatively abnormal. This is one place where our knowledge of the average or normal age behavior of the child we are interacting with comes into importance. We must keep in mind what children in the "real" world are like. I believe it is also a mentally healthy exercise to acknowledge to the child (and sometimes repeatedly to ourselves) that this environment is indeed abnormal. The child needs to know that while he is ill his needs are quite different than when he is well. Obviously, the extent to which this can be understood by the child will depend upon his age. If the child is too young for this kind of interpretation it can take place between the nurse and the parents or guardians.

In other words, the child and his parents should be introduced to hospitalization as if they were visitors from a foreign land. All the staff should be constantly reminded that even seemingly unimportant changes in reality may be very important and confusing to the child. If there is some question in your mind about the differences between hospital reality and outside reality perhaps a series of discussions among yourselves and perhaps some nonmedically oriented persons and if possible a developmentalist would sharpen your understanding of the problem.

Because of the first pitfall, that of losing track of general or consensus reality, we have a tendency to make hospital reality more different than necessary from consensus reality. I feel hospitals lose sight of the individual's rights. Individual's rights are taken away often for the convenience of hospital "routine" and expediency. Having one's basic rights taken away is a very destructive act. Of course, depending upon the age of the child, the amount of destruction will vary. The question becomes: Who is on the child's side, who is protecting the child's rights? It seems obvious that it is the same profession that is also concerned with his total developmental needs—the nursing profession. We are indeed in the best position to bring about a closure between hospital reality and consensus reality since our contact hours are so extensive.

How can we bring about closure between hospital and consensus reality? If you do go ahead with the before-mentioned discussion, I am sure you will find countless ways of making your nursing unit closer to the "real" world of the child. Another aspect which I should like to discuss has again to do with the interaction between the nurse and the patient. It is also related to that sometimes constant irritant: discipline. I call this the mine—yours—ours dialogue.

Mine—Yours—Ours

If you visit a nursing unit which has a number of patients who have been there for some time you will more often than not find children who feel and behave as if they had no rights or place to call their own and children on the other end of the continuum who seem to be "running" the unit, impinging on everyone's rights. Both of these behaviors are abnormal within the context of consensus reality. The question becomes: How can we clarify communication during our beginning interactions to place behavior less out of context with consensus reality? It is not normal for the child to feel he has no place and I do not know of any child health nurse who would not be shocked by the realization that she had communicated this idea. It is *important* for the child to have a specific place even if it is only his crib and dresser or room. In a real sense the area should be guarded as his haven, a place where he can be alone and where his possessions will not be disturbed without permission. The nurse and all personnel should understand that an invisible wall exists if a real one does not; and when you enter this area, it should be by permission—as if it were the child's home. To some this may sound a bit strange, but one of the first things one encounters in a hospital is a loss of normal courtesy and individual rights. While we cannot readjust some of the abnormalities in the hospital environment there is one important area we can readjust, that of private property. Is it all that important? I contend that it *is*, for a number of reasons. First, it carries with it a feeling of control and possession on the part of the child. It increases the feeling of being an intact unit or strengthening the child's self-image, which may be rather confused and distorted by the illness. Second, and more important for the discussion of "yours, mine, and ours," is that if we protect the child's area it is only fair that there may be areas which will be the other children's and the nurses'. The nursing staff also needs an area for their activities apart from the children—preferably a quiet place to plan and organize. It is only fair for everyone to have a protected area which is his. I believe the key to establishing a cooperative atmosphere is fairness. I do not think we need to go into what is fair and what is not fair, because it seems to change with the situation. This brings us to the *ours* portion of the nursing unit physical plant. The nursing staff will find that most of the nursing unit will be composed of *ours* space; space which may be used all the time by both nurse and patient. This space with its rules will have to be negotiated individually with each child. It is space in which there is some control by both parties. The rules of the space will be different from the *mine* space and *yours* space. In fact, the rules will obviously differ slightly depending upon the patient census, amount of disability, and general life style of the individual child. Some of you will stop here and ask how the rules can be one thing for one child and another for the next. If so, you have forgotten we are not dealing with mass care. We are developing an environment to fit growth and developmental needs of individuals. The child and his parents will understand this and be reassured. Those of us who have worked with children know how very early they can understand that people are different from one another. I have seen it in children as young as two and three. They also can understand that if the adults in the situation carefully attend the needs of the child as an individual, when he has special needs they will also be attended to—for that is only *fair*. This, of course, is based upon communication; we must let the child know what is going on and our reasons for our actions. With the very young child we often have to articulate and interpret not only our actions but also the actions of his peers and sometimes his own actions. I hope I have given you the impression that there is a lot going on at one time because there *should* be and there *will* be. The question is whether we are going to manage the nursing unit environment or whether we are going to allow confusion and chaos to manage it, for someone or something must be the leader. In other words, we not only use ourselves through the interaction as therapy and as a stimulus for the growth and development of the children in our care, but we also use the nursing unit space to stimulate and promote understanding and growth. And I dare say that the most growth-promoting areas will be those negotiable through the daily give-and-take of *ours* spaces.

Another common pitfall of the interaction are the elements of rigidity, routine, and rest. These three R's most often interfere with the mutual understanding of the nurse and patient. This is not to say there should be no structure because that does not work either. But then the rules should be few in number. A good rule of thumb is that all rules should pertain to the health and safety of the child and that a child can be held responsible for remembering as many rules as he has had birthdays. If you now go over the rules you expect your patients to follow, you may find the source of much confusion and irritation. The second R—routine—is another hangup or pitfall most nursing units indulge themselves in. I am not questioning the fact that there are certain things that must be done during the day and that sometimes they must be done at a certain time. Many kinds of routines about the "what" and the "when" of nursing care cannot be changed, but we can be creative with the "how" and "who." It is in the areas of "how" and "who" that we can use acts which are routines as tools for the growth and development of the child. The third R is rest—rest is a most important ingredient for healing the body and it needs to be encouraged. But not all children need the same amount at the same time. Some must fall asleep to rest while others rest when participating in quiet activities. An opportunity for individualization of the rest period is best accepted by the child. Again, while the routine activity is present each day, the expression of the activity is the choice of the child or the outcome is mediated by the adult if the child is unable to make a choice which leads to the goal.

Another interaction pitfall which is related to this area is how much interaction we can expect on the part of the ill child. We have said that the child's initial reaction to the abnormal environment may take many negative forms until he comes to understand and see that being in the hospital will make him feel better or fulfill some of the child's goal. In other words, the hospitalization reaps a positive reward. For the very ill child a nonverbal kind of interaction should take place.

Even if the child seems not to be responding, or may be responding very subtly, you may still be building a positive relationship. As an aside, please remember that even normal healthy children do not play the same role when making new relationships. They normally differ in their approach to adults and our approach to them must necessarily be different. (Here again the parent interviews give us many clues.) The standing rule should be that the professional nurse changes her approach to match the one which seems most comfortable to the child, not vice versa. Actually, if one tries to be flexible and uses or at least tries to use some of the current techniques of child management, the hospitalization of the child may be advantageous in many areas of growth and development.

The first question posed in this chapter was: Can human growth and development be used as a basis for nursing assessment? I hope the content of the chapter has led you to believe that when we plan and assess the areas of needed nursing intervention we do so against our background of human growth and development. An assessment of individual growth and development needs is the articulation of needed nursing intervention.

References

Akutaguwa, D. and Benoir, E. The effect of age and relative brightness on associative learning in children. Child Develop., 30:229–238, 1958.

Aldrich, C., Anderson, C., and Aldrich, M. M. Babies Are Human Beings. New York, Macmillan, 1954.

Allport, G. W. Pattern and Growth in Pesonality. New York, Holt, Rinehart and Winston, 1961.

Anderson, J. Dynamics of development: system in process. In Harris, D., ed. The Concept of Development. Minneapolis, Univ. Minn. Press, 1957.

Baldwin, A. Behavior and Development in Childhood. New York, Dryden, 1955.

Baruch, D. W. New Ways in Discipline. New York, McGraw-Hill, 1949.

Beasley, J. Slow to Talk. New York, Bureau of Publications, Teachers College, Columbia University, 1956.

Berelson, B., and Steiner, G. A. Human Behavior: An Inventory of Scientific Findings. New York, Harcourt, Brace & World, 1964.

Bowlby, J. Child Care and the Growth of Love, 2nd ed. Baltimore, Pelican Books.

Breckenridge, M., and Murphy, M. (eds.) Rand, Sweeney, and Vincent's Growth and Development of the Young Child. Philadelphia, Saunders, 1958.

———— and Vincent, E. Lee. Child Development, Physical and Psychological Growth Through Adolescence, 5th ed. Philadelphia, Saunders, 1966.

Breznitz, S., and Kugelmass, S. Intentionality in moral judgment. Child Develop., 38:469–479, 1967.

Burnshaw, S. The body makes the mind: excerpt from the seamless web. The American Scholar, 38:25–39, Winter 1968.

Call, J. D. Lap and finger play in infancy, implications for ego development. Int. J. Psycho-Analysis, 49:375–378, 1968.

Carmichael, L. Manual of Child Psychology, 2nd ed. New York, Wiley, 1966.

Chamberlin, R. W. Approaches to child rearing: their effect on child behavior

—an analysis of reported surveys. Clin. Pediat., 5:686–697, November 1966.

Christenson, C. M. Relationship between pupil achievement, pupil affect—need, teacher warmth, and teacher permissiveness. J. Educat. Psychol., LI:169–174, June 1960.

Church, J. Language and the Discovery of Reality: The Development of Psychology Cognition. MacLeod. New York, Random House, 1961.

Dollard, J., and Miller, N. M. Personality and Psychotherapy, New York, McGraw-Hill, 1950.

Denenberg, V. H. and Myers, R. D. Learning and hormone activity: I. effects of thyroid levels upon the acquisition and extinction of an operant response. J. Compar. Physiolog. Psychol., 51, 213–219, April 1958.

Dennis, W. Piaget's questions applied to a child of known environment. J. Genetic Psychol., 60:307–320, 1942.

Epstein, R. Effects of commitment to social isolation on children's imitative behavior. J. Personal. Soc. Psychol. 9, 90–95, 1968.

Erikson, E. H. Childhood and Society, 2nd ed. New York, Norton, 1963.

Gesell, A., and Thompson, H. Twins T and C from infancy to adolescence. Genetic Psychology Monograph, 24:3–121, 1941.

Greenson, R. R. Dis-identifying from mother: its special importance for the boy. Int. J. Psycho-Analysis, 49:370–374, 1968.

Harsh, C. M., and Schrickel, H. G. Personality Development and Assessment. New York, Ronald Press, 1950.

Hatrup, W. Social behavior of children. Rev. Educat. Res., 35:22–29, April 1965.

Hegethorn, B. An elementary developmental stage and its significance for the etiology of psychosis. Acta Psychiat. Scand. (Suppl.) 203, 189–194, 1968.

Hurlock, E. B. Child Development, 3rd ed. New York, McGraw-Hill, 1956.

Hymes, J. L., Jr. Behavior and Misbehavior—A Teacher's Guide to Action. Englewood Cliffs, Prentice-Hall, Inc., 1955.

Josselyn, I. Psychosocial Development of Children. New York, Family Service Association of America, 1948.

Krogman, W. M. The concept of maturity from a morphological viewpoint. Child Develop., 21:25–32, 1950.

Landreth, C. The Psychology of Early Childhood. New York, Alfred Knopf, 1958.

Lawrence, F. K. Individual Development. New York, Doubleday, 1955.

Lee, J. M., and Lee, D. M. The Child and His Development. New York, Appleton-Century-Crofts, 1958.

Lewis, M. M. How Children Learn to Speak. London, George G. Harran, 1957.

Lidz, T. The Person—His Development Throughout the Life Cycle. New York, Basic Books, 1968.

Martin, W. E., and Stendler, C. B. Child Behavior and Development. New York, Harcourt, Brace & World, 1959.

Mead, M., and MacGregor, F. Growth and Culture. New York, G. Putnam, 1951.

Missildine, W. H., ed. Feelings and their medical significance—the parent in the parent-child relationship, 9:1–4, February 1967. (Columbus, Ohio, Ross Laboratories.)

Murphy, L. Personality in Young Children. New York, Basic Books, 1956.

Neilen, P. Shirley's babies after fifteen years: a personality study. J. Genetic Psychol. 73:175–185, 1948.

Nelson, W. E. In Stuart, H., and Stevenson, S., eds. Textbook of Pediatrics, 6th ed. Philadelphia, Saunders, 1957, pp. 10–66.

Oakes, M. E. Children's Explanations of Natural Phenomena. New York, Teachers College, Columbia University, 1946.

Patter, M. C. and Levy, E. J. Spatial enumeration without counting. Child Develop. 39:265–272, 1968.

Piaget, J. Construction of Reality in the Child, New York, Basic Books, 1954.
———— Language and Thought of the Child. New York, Harcourt, Brace & World, 1932.
———— The Origins of Intelligence in Children, Cook, M., trans. New York, Norton, 1963.
Radin, N., and Kamil, C. K. The Child-rearing attitudes of disadvantaged negro mothers and some educational implications. J. Negro Educat., 34:38–146, Spring 1965.
Rebble, M. A. The Personality of the Young Child. New York, Columbia University, 1955.
Reichard, S., Schneider, M., and Rappaport, D. The development of concept formation in children. Am. J. Orthopsychiat., 14:156–162, 1944.
Russell. Children's Thinking. Boston, Ginn and Co., 1956.
Sandler, L., and Torpie, B. Improvement of residential care of infants and children from birth to age 3. Arch. Environ. Health, 17:80–90, July 1968.
Segal, J., and Luce, G. G. Now I lay me down to sleep. McCall's, pp. 88–89, October 1968.
Shirley, M. The First Two Years: A Study of Twenty-five Babies—Personality Manifestations, vol. III, Institute of Child Welfare Monograph. Univ. Minn. Press, 1933.
Sigel, I. E. The need for conceptualization in research on child development. Child Develop., 27:241–252, 1956.
Sonis, M. Implications for the child guidance clinic of current trends in mental health planning. Amer. J. Orthopsychiat., 38:(3) 515–526, April, 1968.
Speil, O. Discipline Without Punishment: An Account of a School in Action, Fitzgerald, E., trans. London, Faber and Faber, 1962.
Walters, C. E. Comparative development of negro and white infants. J. Genet. Psychol., 110:251–253, 1967.
Watson, E. H., and Lowrey, G. H. Growth and Development of Children, 5th ed. Chicago, Year Book, 1967.
Williams, R. Biochemical Individuality. New York, Wiley, 1956.
Witmer, R., and Kotinsky, R., eds. Personality in the Making, Fact Finding Report of Midcentury White House Conference on Children and Youth. New York, Harper & Row, 1953.
Zigler, E., and Butterfield, E. C. Motivational aspects of changes in I. Q. test performance of culturally deprived nursery school children. Child Develop., 39:1–14, March 1969.
Zubeck, J. P., and Salberg, P. A. Human Development. New York, McGraw-Hill, 1954.

2 DONNA JUENKER

Play as a Tool of the Nurse

Oh quench not the child's hope,
Oh do not repress one impulse of enthusiasm
                                    —FRANK LLOYD WRIGHT

A child at play is a source of delight. His evident joy in his discoveries and the intensity of his self-absorption underscore the importance of what play means to him. It is serious business—not a luxury. It is physical and it is fantasy. It can tell a child who he is or it can be a stage on which he acts out the role of the person he would like to be. Pickard (1965, p. 83) significantly concludes that "as they play, the children are the ceaseless agents of their learning, about both the outer and the inner world." Certainly then, opportunities for play should abound for all children—those who are ill as well as those who are healthy.

In this chapter, I will elaborate on the subject of play from several points of view with particular attention focused on children with long-term illnesses. After describing the meaning and value of play, I will explore the age factors that influence play behavior. An explanation of the nurse's role in establishing an environment that is conducive to play will be included along with a description of an assessment tool for identifying play needs. One section will include a delineation of the special play problems experienced by immobilized children. The chapter will conclude with the examination of the nurse-parent interaction in regard to play. Hopefully, the content will excite the reader to an enthusiastic response toward the play needs of young patients.

Meaning and Value of Play

Play is a subject open to much speculation. The existence of play has never been disputed. Systematic investigations of why and how man plays, however, are products of relatively recent times. Do people play for gain or gamble? Do they play with gusto or grin? Philosophers, psychologists, and even theologians have provided a rich collection of definitions and rationales for play. (Groos, 1901; Huizinga, 1950; Piaget, 1962; Rahner, 1967.) Any description of play must point to origins in childhood since each individual's philosophy about play and his personal style of play result from a composite of experiences that begin in infancy.

Adults may consider play in a variety of ways. Some may view it as instinctive behavior pursued for its own sake. Some see it simply as a leisure-time activity. For others, it is a means of emotional escape—a catharsis for pent-up feelings. To the child, play is much more. It is a dynamic medium through which he views himself and his surroundings. It contributes much to the development of his life-style. Play is a stable enough concept to pervade all of childhood and yet flexible enough to accommodate the child's changing needs as he grows to maturity.

How does play serve the child's needs? Groos (1901), who was one of the earliest to systematize the study of play, draws attention to instinct as the motivating factor in play. He views play as a preparation for adult activities. For example, it develops important elements of skill such as running and jumping. These initial impulses are then transferred to intellectual behaviors useful in adult living. In other words, play develops coordination and physical efficiency necessary for adult pursuits.

While not wholly supported, Schiller's (1875) surplus-energy theory of play does have some credibility. It is an obvious fact known to anyone who observes children that young people have boundless energy. They seem to have more muscular energy than they need. Consequently, the activity of play becomes a release. Spencer (1873) gave a physiological rationale for the need to release energy based on the discharge potential of living nerve cells. If a physiological need is forcing its expression, it is difficult if not impossible for the child to withhold his response. He needs outlets for these strong drives. Play experiences permit energy release in a manner acceptable to the child and to those around him. On the other hand, it is sometimes necessary to conserve energy. Play can usefully serve this end. Certain kinds of play provide a restful change of pace when either mental or physical strain causes fatigue.

There are psychological considerations in play as well. Play is satisfying for its own sake. In fact, pleasure is a dominant feature. The pleasure is derived from the play stimulus itself as well as from the pleasant feelings it arouses. It is Groos' contention that this psychological criterion is part of the essence of play.

The sociological aspect of play should also be noted. As the child grows from infancy through childhood, his social radius widens beyond the family to include peers. This opens up a richly exciting world of play. Much of it focuses on social imitation. It is extremely important to know and do what others know and do. A degree of satisfaction attends collective activity—a camaraderie resulting from united action. Play also affords good practice in communication and in the art of governing a group. It is an avenue through which social laws can be tested. Groos calls this the "cheering and humanizing effect of play."

In a more recent analysis of childhood play, Erikson (1963) describes it as an attempt to synchronize the bodily and social processes into a concept of self and as such defines it as necessary for the development of the ego. In this sense, childhood play becomes a preparation for mature behavior. Piaget (1969) stresses its value when he comments that it is a process of assimilating reality to the self. In effect, play becomes the child and the child becomes the play. To view a child without considering his play is not to see the child at all.

These benefits, while described only in general terms thus far, give testimony to the value of play. The extent to which these outcomes can be realized depends upon two basic components of play. It must be *free* and it must be *fun*. In keeping with its nature, play is a voluntary activity—one without coercions. The child must be free to direct his play within the context of his own style, that is, free to react to his own spontaneity. A child who is made to play is not really playing. He is simply performing a task assigned by an adult. His activity essentially would not differ from setting the table, emptying the wastebasket, or doing lessons for school. These tasks certainly have much to contribute to the child's learning but, as generally viewed, they do not constitute play.

The child should have a good time during play. The pleasure comes from the activity itself. In other words, the child seems more motivated by the "fun of it" than by any practical consequence the play activity may have. As a matter of fact, play often lacks a tangible outcome. It is the process of play that is enjoyed—the body movement, the fantasy, the spirit, the risk, and the excitement of mastery.

The freedom and pleasure of childhood play may seem to give it an exclusive flavor requiring no adult participation. On the contrary, the child's play will not be free and pleasurable if the adult absents himself from the play world. There are several important things that he must do. In the first place, he must encourage what is good and useful about play. In this sense, he motivates play. He should respond with interest to the child's discoveries but must not overpower with discoveries of his own. The adult provides the materials for play, controlling elements of high risk or probable danger while at the same time opening up opportunities for experimentation. Adults must allow children to explore in a variety of seetings using as many modes of expression as age and imagination permit.

I have noticed that adults vary widely in their approach to children's play. Some are obviously ill-at-ease with children. Some make it a practice to join in and play *with* the child. Others pride themselves by playing *for* the child. Some are contented to give the child "something" to play with, and then there are those who dismiss "child's play" as a matter deserving little attention. They do not feel it necessary to enter the child's world at all. There is danger in all of these approaches. The person who is ill-at-ease makes a sensitive child ill-at-ease, too. These individuals may have experienced some degree of play deprivation in their own youth and consequently lack important recollections that would permit them an entré into the child's world of play. The child, if he is old enough to perceive the problem, inadvertently is placed in a position of trying to relieve the stress of the uncomfortable adult. Those who play *with* the child all the time fail to note that this creates an unnatural play environment. Children customarily play alone or with peers. Adult-child interaction is based upon a different set of "ground-rules." Those who play *for* the child—the "here, let me show you" type—lack the capacity or the insight to permit the child the joy of making his own discoveries. Perhaps this individual is too concerned about the outcome or product of the play experience and consequently makes the child play on adult terms. In this way, he insures that the child does not "color outside the lines" or make a lopsided treasure chest. (Play suggestions, when offered, should be extensions of the child's own intent. Adults should not become impatient if the child's limited ideas do not correspond with the projected adult view based on many more years of experience.) Those who do not enter the child's world at all stand to lose the most. They miss a youthful excitement and vitality that can awaken their own enthusiasm for living and learning.

Perhaps it is unfortunate that analysis of children's play has become the work of adults. Removed, as adults are, from the personal realities of childhood, some dimensions of play are lost simply by virtue of an experience gap. Though we, as nurses, should recognize this fact, we ought not to be discouraged by it. It simply means that there is always something left to "discover" about children and how they play. Therein lies a key to success in working with children—that is, a willingness to be open to the various ways children express themselves and manifest their needs. By maximizing the play experiences of a child, nurses can literally expand the dimensions not only of the child's world but also their own.

Those of us caring for sick children are challenged to seek appropriate ways to help them enjoy the satisfactions of play in whatever circumstances they find themselves. To accomplish this, it would be helpful to explore some of the relationships between play and long-term illness.

Diagnosis and treatment of illness may require frequent and sometimes prolonged periods of hospitalization. As a result, a change in the life-style of the child and his family may be observed. The extent of the change depends upon the type of illness and the capacity of the child and parents to cope with the existing stress and make realistic plans for the future. Nevertheless, if we accept the premise that growth and development is an ongoing process marked by maturational achievements of special significance at certain ages, it quickly becomes evident that the child and family may pass through some of these developmental steps while in the hospital. Interruptions in the normal sequence of events may occur. For example, the toddler who is confined because of a dislocated hip may not be able to practice his newly acquired skill of walking; the six-year-old boy whose new school experience is interrupted by rheumatic heart disease may not have had sufficient time to work through the ambivalence normally created by dependent-independent conflicts; the teenage girl immobilized for treatment of scoliosis misses some of the important peer group activities characteristic for her age. By purposefully guiding the play experiences of these children, some of these deficits can be minimized. The toddler can experience some mobility through "action stories" and rides in a wagon. The six-year-old can continue to keep up with his schoolmates through blackboard games and word games which will maintain his interest in printing and spelling. The teenager can be encouraged to keep in touch with her friends by letter exchanges and telephone calls. She can give expression to her feelings by writing to "Dear Diary" or she can paint her feelings on canvas to hang in her room. There are many avenues through which play can accommodate developmental needs.

Long-term illness is marked by repeated periods of dependency. The child must rely on persons outside the family circle for the treatment of his illness. This often happens at a time in his developmental continuum when he is struggling to achieve or maintain his own autonomy. He may have to relate to many members of the health team because of the complexity of his illness. Yet his capacity to absorb new persons into his reality may be inadequate. The child, under these circumstances, hardly welcomes the "helpers"—especially if they perform intrusive acts that are painful or in other ways appear to invade the integrity of the body. Added to his stress is the fact that these people occupy positions of power and exercise great control over his activities. Through play, the child can "act out" fearful experiences and reduce the level of anxiety. He can recreate past events and imaginatively project future happenings which will help him to more fully understand himself and others.

Elements of freedom are curtailed during periods of illness. Freedom of mobility is often affected, favorite foods may be restricted, and the type and quantity of social interaction is limited. The frustration of these circumstances is heightened by the anticipation of repeated episodes of illness and by prospects of a long period of confinement. Play behavior is also limited to a certain extent. However, because play in confined basically only by the limits of imagination, there remains a wide range of options. With so many other limits being imposed, play can well serve as a means of providing opportunities for self-chosen activities.

There is a discouragement factor associated with the care of these sick children. The children become discouraged by the slow progress of their illness and the sameness of each day. Nurses, too, can become discouraged when the intensity of their care is not matched by a similarly dramatic improvement in their young patient's condition. Both the child and nurse can benefit in this instance from involvement in play activities. It helps the child to meet the demands of each day and gives him the satisfaction of achieving short-term goals. By watching the child in play and enjoying his accomplishments the nurse can see "small" gains and become more satisfied that some progress is being made.

In general, it could be said that many children with long-term illnesses will have to reorient themselves to a different set of lifetime goals. They will have to learn how to do two things: adapt themselves to the environment and, when feasible, effectively change the environment to suit their own special needs. This adaptive capacity does not develop intuitively. It is learned over time and through a variety of satisfying experiences. Acceptance of long-term illness and adjustment to its many physical and psychological demands will therefore require many talents on the part of the child and his family. It is in this regard that I believe that play can offer a child abundant support. I believe that one of the most significant outcomes of play is the creative behavior that such activity encourages.

Torrance (1965) suggests that creative children are stimulated by challenging problems. These children tend to probe for answers to difficult questions. Their accomplishments are self-initiated and reflect a whole-hearted commitment to a task. They do not seem to be overly intimidated by their agemates or adults who occupy positions of authority. In fact, even in relatively tense situations, they can maintain a sense of humor (Torrance, 1961). They seem better able to resist the conformity often demanded by pervading social and cultural conditions. The creative child is inclined to be independent and to aspire to long-range goals.

These qualities would well serve the needs of a child with a long-term illness. Certainly, a handicapped child would benefit by a development of a certain inner resourcefulness, a capacity for creativity that would make his satisfactions emerge from within himself. Freely selected play activities, pursued in a direction that the child elects will give him a good feeling about himself, and confidence in his ability to perform or achieve and, most importantly, he will feel capable of controlling and modifying his environment. Therefore, given the stimulus of appropriate play, the child might better achieve his potential and more fully enjoy the process of accomplishing such an achievement.

The Infant

Many long-term illnesses have their origins at birth or in early infancy. Because of the nature of medical management, the infant often requires complicated treatments and may have to undergo periods of hospitalization. Because of significant stages in development occurring early in life, hospitalization can seriously affect the behavior of the baby.

While it is true that infants lack language skills and, therefore, symbolic function, it is evident that much learning takes place during the early months of life. Piaget and Inhelder (1969) emphasize that during the first eighteen months the child constructs all of the cognitive substructures that are necessary for future perception and intellectual development.

This learning takes place at a sensorimotor level of function. These sensorimotor experiences emerge in the framework of infant play. A sensorimotor experience exists in relation to the environment—that is, it is aroused by persons and things that enter the child's reality as stimuli. In the process of reacting to stimuli, infants develop habits of play. Although initially based on reflexive behavior, these habits become very meaningful. Usually the habits are intimately related to satisfaction of basic needs such as the need for food, sleep, excretion, and care of the body. Once these habits are formed, the baby resists disruptive changes. Illness and hospitalization will certainly alter both the internal and external environment of the infant and may upset the baby's life-style. The baby who hides his face in a special blanket with a smooth binding as part of a satisfying sleeping pattern may have difficulty sleeping if he cannot repeat this behavior in the new setting.

An interruption in an expected sequence of events results in an expenditure of energy. For example, energy is used in longer periods of wakefulness in an attempt to locate anticipated events. It may take the form of fretful crying indicating general uneasiness about the unexpected situation or, in some cases, energy output becomes an angry scream testifying to the baby's awareness of the magnitude of the change in his environment. The ill child, whose illness is accompanied by physiological stress, needs to focus his body's reserve on trying to reestablish homeostasis. Therefore, anything that the nurse can introduce to her care plan that will relieve psychological stress could have a real impact on the child's recovery. The nurse has three primary sets of clues readily available to guide her selection of stimuli for a particular infant: (1) history of meaningful play activities from the parents; (2) current and anticipated developmental achievements of the baby; and (3) type of illness and consequent limitations.

Knowledge of the kind of play activities experienced by a baby and his response to those stimuli helps the nurse provide play rituals that may help to stabilize his environment. (Further comment on the use of a play profile follows in another section of this chapter.) Very likely, the kind of play that a baby engages in reflects his abilities at a given point in time. If he is able to sit up and reach for and transfer objects, he is a more independent "player" than the infant who is not yet able to support himself in an upright position. If the baby's activities are limited because of the stress of lower-extremity immobilization, for example, his ordinary play needs will be frustrated and development achievements may be delayed. By redesigning play experiences through extra provision for upper-extremity activity and upright positioning when possible, much of the loss can be compensated and energy redirected in a beneficial way.

What are some of the special play problems experienced by infants? Hospitalized infants often miss the consistent stimulation of an expressive face of another—a purposeful "locking of eyes." This very personal experience provides the infant with an explicit contact with reality. Babies can receive very good physical care that includes holding and feeding and still miss this stimulation. This may happen because the nurse shares her attention with many babies and also because she underestimates the importance of this kind of interaction. Eye-to-eye contact most often comes about through games. Games are simply styles of intraction that are usually the creation of mother and baby. Generally the game involves some manipulation of a part of the body, an accompanying verbal symbol, and an expressive face that responds to the mutual enjoyment felt by mother and baby (Fig. 1).

One classic example is the game of peek-a-boo. Maurer (1967) describes the significance of the game and connects specific learnings

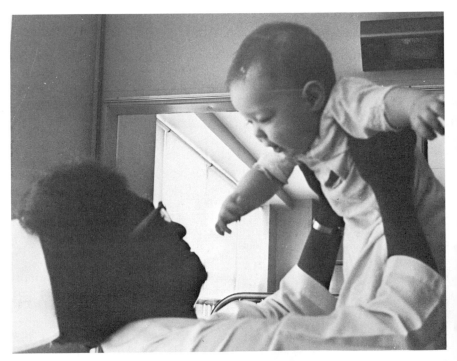

FIG. 1. This nurse and baby are having fun with a special kind of play—an infant "game."

derived from it with later ego development. In fact, she states that peek-a-boo contributes to the development of self-confidence and an early sense of identity, and even helps to allay anxiety. "The game of peek-a-boo is a replay in safe circumstances of the frightening feeling of nonbeing followed by the joyous affirmation of aliveness in the recognition accorded the child by the intimacy of eye to eyeness" (Maurer, 1967, p. 119). It is such a universal behavior that even in situations in which parents do not encourage the game, the child "invents" it himself. Other examples of early ego-supporting play include lap-and-finger play.

As previously mentioned, vocalization supports these games. Personally directed and intimate "conversations" with the baby are important, not only because the sound of the human voice can be soothing but also because it encourages the infant's own vocal response. In turn, the infant's own utterances are a rich source of amusement for him (Fig. 2).

When a baby is acutely ill, it must be remembered that his capacity to respond to new stimuli is limited. In contrast, familiar and loved items are cherished to an even greater extent than usual. The baby's "defenses" are down and he resorts to passive absorption of familiar

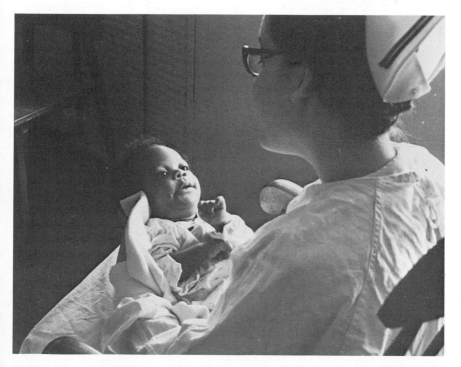

FIG. 2. This nurse and baby are enjoying an intimate "conversation." Important eye-to-eye contact is clearly evident.

sounds, feels, and smells to help him tolerate the frustrations of the situation at hand. The use of transitional objects such as favorite blankets, special toys, and familiar feeding utensils becomes very important in his adjusting to the stress of illness.

When the baby becomes more aware of his external environment, he can respond to new things with interest and enthusiasm. The color, shape, sound, feel, and movement of toys within the baby's eye and hand (and foot) space are internally satisfying. You have no doubt watched babies respond with evident delight as a bright mobile moved above their heads (Fig. 3). Of course, you cannot separate the "things" from the people who provide them—the toys offered are often loving extensions of the person and help the baby to develop trust in both people and things. Appropriate stimuli during convalescence can *increase* the baby's learning rather than merely hold fast to the status

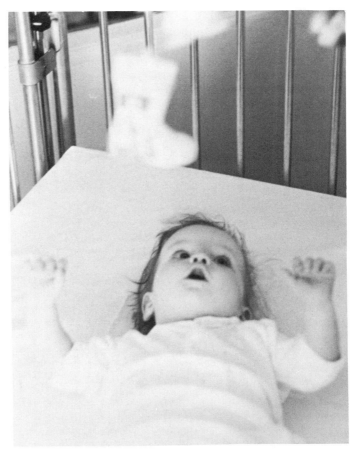

FIG. 3. This four-month-old infant is excited by the bright mobile. Her animated expression and body movements indicate responsiveness to her environment.

quo. A baby who is ill for weeks or months will need assistance in achieving new tasks. However, the baby must be relatively tension-free before he can enjoy new sensorimotor and social activities.

The timing of play is a significant factor. A baby who is very ill or who has an overpowering physiological need such as hunger must direct all his energy toward reducing this discomfort. He has little, if any, energy left for exploring his world. To play he must be capable of giving his individual attention to the matter at hand and to exercising some control over the part of the body involved in the play. When the baby is best able to play is a decision that the nurse makes in relation to the baby's overall needs. Call (1966) notes that most games in infancy are played after the feeding, when many babies have a wakeful period. At this time physiological tension is at a minimum and the baby is especially alert to the external world. Play time for the older infant, which is much broader in scope, should keep pace with expanding abilities, increasing attention span, and a widening social radius.

Bath time, whatever time of the day it might be, offers great potential for enjoyable play both for the baby and the nurse. It brings them into close personal contact. Water is a universally enjoyed play material. Splashing and kicking, unencumbered by restricting clothing, are delightful activities for the active youngster. Even for those less inclined to vigorous activity, the feel of warm water over the body creates a pleasant, relaxing sensation. The baby's own participation in the bath can be encouraged by the inclusion of bath toys such as small, brightly colored sponges. A tub bath is the best means for this kind of enjoyable play and should be much more widely used than is currently the custom. However, if the illness contraindicates a tub wash, some provision for water play can generally be provided even if it only consists of splashing the hands in the water basin.

The infant, especially the very young one, is handicapped in the sense that he is dependent on others for mobility. If he is left in the supine position, the ceiling and the sides of his crib become his world. Turning the baby to the prone position or putting him in an infant seat or playpen does much to alter a dull and narrow visual field and expand his awareness of surroundings.

While a finger has been pointed at the tendency toward understimulation, a word must be said above overstimulating experiences for the infant. One sometimes forgets about the magnitude of stimulalation in a hospital environment. There is considerable noise—both continuous and intermittent. How aware are we of the effects of the incubator motor or the sound of the mist tent? How disruptive is the noise of the page system, the voices of the doctors as they make rounds, or the clatter of dietary equipment? There are visual stimuli as well—bright lights on 24 hours a day, light reflected from metal equipment, distorted images viewed through glass partitions, and a disturbing eeriness in dim hours of twilight. Then, of course, there is the stimulus of people—people looking, people handling, people feeling, wrapping, and wiping, people intruding on the privacy of the infant's world. We must tread more carefully to preserve the infant's right to integrate his experiences at his own rate. We must be more fruitful in our attempts to reduce over abundant and disruptive stimulation.

Most of the stimuli just referred to are peripheral stimuli—all around the baby but not directed to him. The nurse also needs to be concerned about bringing meaningful objects and people within the baby's spacial limits where he can see, hear, taste, touch, and smell. Giving a rattle to a baby is helpful only if the baby can hold it comfortably, transfer it, and retrieve it if it falls from his grasp. If the baby is not maturationally able to do these things the nurse must be the active instrument in helping him enjoy and learn from the experience. A mobile or overbed toy that the baby can see and reach may be a good play tool during the nurse's absence (Fig. 4).

Although the infant delights in random body movements, his lack of control over them sometimes requires restraint in the interest of his safety and the efficacy of treatment. In cases where such restriction has to be imposed, the baby's play activity is often passive. However, this should not deemphasize its importance. The same visual, auditory, and tactile materials are used in this as in other circumstances of infant play. The difference lies in the fact that the nurse initiates the play since the baby cannot bring objects or people into his real world through his own action. Singing to the baby, stroking his body, and gentle rocking are simple activities that will help to relieve tension. A snuggle toy next to the baby may be comforting when the nurse or parent is absent.

The nurse must exercise careful judgment about the effect that a particular play stimulus has on the infant. A restrained baby who is literally "beside himself" struggling to reach a suspended toy or a nearby nursing bottle shows the effects of indiscriminate stimulation.

Periods of supervised freedom from restraint are a "must" both for physiological and psychological reasons. Arm or hand restraints are particularly frustrating to a baby experiencing intense oral drives or to one who is in the stage of exploring his body and discovering through finger play that his hands are part of him. During the latter period of infancy when locomotion skills emerge, similar frustrations are aroused by restraint of the legs. It is not unusual to see an immediate expression of relief and contentment when the baby is permitted to suck his thumb, hold the edge of a favored blanket in his mouth, or explore a toy by chewing on it. The baby need not be denied such satisfactions because of prolonged restraint. Needless to say, the nurse should use only the minimum amount of restraint necessary to achieve desired physical results.

It should be noted that with repetition of any set of stimuli, a baby will become accustomed to a certain sequence of events which he will expect to experience. Even though the "restraint" stimulus is rightly viewed as frustrating, it is somewhat consoling to know that the infant

FIG. 4. This mobile can be constructed from ordinary household materials. An infant unit should have ample supply of toys like these to provide age-appropriate stimuli.

can tolerate it if the limitation in activity does not cause actual discomfort (Dennis, 1940). Hence, if the restraint is comfortable and if other tensions such as hunger and pain are reduced, negative reactions to confinement can be significantly decreased. Parents are grateful for this encouraging information.

Parents, too, need help in playing with their baby particularly during and after an illness. They are often frightened by the baby's condition and the kind of treatment required. Sometimes this fear manifests itself in diminished contact with the baby in terms of handling or other kinds of stimulation. Their hesitancy is quite understandable and should in no way diminish feelings of motherliness or fatherliness. Nurses working with the infant can interpret the baby's need for stimulation with the parents and offer them frequent opportunities to participate actively in the baby's play. This kind of interaction and support should occur throughout the hospitalization so that the parents will have confidence to continue such stimulation at home. Babies who have visual or hearing handicaps or severe motor disturbances will need special kinds of stimulation. Therefore, parental guidance prior to their discharge has added importance.

Thus there are many avenues of play open to the infant who is ill. Of greatest importance is the intimate contact with a warm, expressive nurse whose "intimacy" touches every one of the baby's senses and sparks his awareness of surroundings and develops his capacity to trust. The "thing" world is significant, too—the mobiles, blocks, comfort items, and musical toys must always complement the "personal touch," but never replace it.

The Preschool Child

The preschool period is exhilarating and exasperating for the child and for those who care for him. Play during this volatile age has many unique and interesting facets. A dramatic transition occurs as the child moves from the parallel play of the toddler toward the cooperative play of the six-year-old. Episodic, disconnected play gives way to coherent themes. Early in the preschool period the child struggles to achieve autonomy. He acquires a new and very important dimension to his self-concept—the meaning of "I" as separate from others. In the best of circumstances, this stage has its "ups and downs." Even though a child has a long-term illness (superimposed on normally anticipated struggles), he still needs to develop independence. His pursuit of the task needs special mediations on the part of caring adults. If one opportunity for independent pursuit is cut off by illness, other avenues have to be provided. The nurse must look at the total environment and the needs and abilities of the child in order to encourage autonomy. At the same time, she must realize that illness implies dependence.

The toddler is bent on discovery. The fact that he "discovers" in a hospital or while ill may not diminish the number of his discoveries. Discovery of some limitations can really be helpful in his adjustment to a chronic illness.

Like the infant, the young preschooler continues to explore largely through sensorimotor activities. The primary differences between the infant and preschool child are the extent of mobility and the range of interpretation of new experiences. The child is no longer content with a narrow radius of interests. If he is able to be up and about at this critical stage of development, he has an obvious advantage. The child who must be confined for reasons of illness unfortunately does not always have a corresponding decrease in the intensity of his desire to roam about at will. This child challenges the nurse to find new and appropriate outlets for his boundless energy which will support feelings of independence. For example, the toddler confined to bed can enjoy vicarious locomotion activities through action stories in which he can make locomotion sounds like "swishing through the air" or running fast and "panting." Though admittedly limited in the freedom such activities provide, such expression does expand the child's inner resources to cope with his frustration.

Large muscle activity is the preschooler's forte. His muscles are growing rapidly and he is still testing his ability to control his body. Riding tricycles, pushing and pulling small wagons, and jumping off low stairs provide hours of satisfying activity (Fig. 5). Hospital corridors and playrooms as well as backyards should accommodate this equipment to a reasonable extent. If existing facilities are too cramped

FIG. 5.   These toys will interest the toddler since they encourage locomotion and hand skills.

for such an expenditure of energy, or the child's illness does not permit such activity, one should not overlook the value derived simply from walking. It is a wonderful play activity in itself. Exploratory walks are rich with excitement even if the same path is traveled each day. The child's imagination permits him to view each trip from a different perspective.

Effort should also be made to provide outdoor play. As under normal conditions, the sick child benefits through an improved appetite and sound sleep if he can spend a portion of each day in the fresh air and vitamin-rich sunshine.

Although the preschool child continues to enjoy "feeling" things, he is now more impressed with the shapes that he can form and the colors that he can blend. The hospital playroom needs simple but functional facilities for waterplay, sandbox activities, and finger painting. The hospital carpentry shop can easily construct a workable water table as illustrated in Fig. 6. A similar arrangement for sand also works well. Good for finger painting is a low table covered with oil cloth.

Attention span in the early preschool period is very short. The intensity of play may be all-absorbing but short-lasting. Consequently, a variety of materials is necessary for this age group. However, the child is better able to fix attention if he is not overstimulated by too much, too fast. A toy bag at the bedside may contain several interesting play tools but the child may only be able to handle two or three items at a time. He can then more fully experiment with all of the potentials for learning that a particular stimulus offers. I can recall a child of two-and-a-half years hospitalized for treatment of nephrosis. The nurses became concerned because the child would not play; yet, his bed was

FIG. 6. Children can enjoy water play with simple equipment. This waist-high table is a comfortable height for busy preschoolers. A plastic basin on a chair works well, too.

literally covered with toys of every description. This, it seemed, was the problem. The toys were gathered up and stored in a paper bag at his bedside. A favorite stuffed animal and several bright plastic blocks were left in his bed. The boy propped the animal in a corner of his bed within his reach and vision and then turned his attention to the blocks. He lined them up, stacked them, knocked them down, and experimented with them in a variety of ways. Intermittently, he reached out to the animal to adjust his position, pat him on the head or simply acknowledge his presence. The animal seemed to offer him enough security to permit him to explore the blocks. Too much stimulation had divided the child's attention to the point where he became so confused and fatigued that he protected himself by withdrawing.

The preschool child's increasing awareness of himself and his surroundings generally exceeds his ability to express his feelings verbally. Consequently, he often "acts out" his feelings in very physical and primitive ways. Play becomes an especially useful tool for the nurse at this time because the content of it reveals so well what the child is thinking. Enactment of family roles while the child is absent from the home environment may keep family relationships intact. Such play can also help the child to work out ambivalent feelings toward those he loves when the need to do so is most evident. He may also wish to express intense feelings of anger toward those who are caring for him. Aggressive play materials are useful in this regard because they permit the child to display his hostility in an acceptable manner without arousing guilt. It is important that the nurse or doctor carefully avoid any evidence of retaliatory behavior if they find themselves appearing in the child's fantasies. The child who "cuts up" his nurse is simply reacting to a fear about his own safety.

Regression is a common defense mechanism, especially during the early preschool period. Newly acquired skills are not firmly consolidated as yet, so that under stress the child abandons them in order to resume more satisfying, infantile modes of behavior. Regressive toys such as the nursing bottle are often favorite items in the dramatic play of the preschool child (Figs. 7A and 7B).

This age period is fraught with fears, expanding social expectations, and an inability to distinguish between reality and fantasy. The child who is ill may perceive his illness as a threat to his bodily integrity. Unable to give adequate verbal expression to his concerns, he works out his crisis by manipulating safe replicas of himself, by handling intrusive pieces of equipment, or by playing a role until it becomes manageable by use of his own resources. F. H. Erickson (1958) found that 19 of the 20 hospitalized preschool children in her study were able to dramatize or verbalize their feelings about the procedures that they had experienced. Their dramatizations involved the use of clinical equipment (such as hypodermic syringes, tongue blades, thermometers, and medicine bottles), doll figures, and a variety of small toys (such as beds, bathtubs, and guns). Erickson noted that most intrusive pro-

DOLL FIGURES

AGGRESSIVE TOYS

REGRESSIVE TOYS

FIG. 7A. Preschool children can give expression to their strong feelings in dramatic play. These "props" will encourage them to work out conflicts, allowing for both aggressive and regressive responses.

cedures (except those in the oral area) were perceived in a hostile context by the majority of the children. The play experiences obviously had much meaning for the children and she recommends that such play be encouraged as soon as possible after the hospital procedures have been performed (Fig. 8). Repetition characterizes these activities almost to the point of adult exasperation; yet the child's need to repeat an episode indicates that he has not yet worked out all of his feelings.

Miniature figures that represent both family members and hospital workers are often desired to recreate a wide range of meaningful situations. Room partitions enhance a child's imaginative doll play. The opportunity to have these props need not be restricted by the hospital situation. For the child confined to bed, a sectional piece of wood or sturdy cardboard that can be folded, as illustrated in Fig. 9, works well. It can be rearranged as the child wishes in order to serve as a hallway, a large room, three small rooms, a fenced-in backyard, or the operating room.

FIG. 7B. Brush painting and modeling with clay provide pleasant sensory experiences. The car and doctor kit are good tools as the child becomes involved in identification–imitation processes.

Dress-up clothes, especially hats, are also helpful. Hats are very serviceable for children confined to bed since they are easily handled, comfortable for the child, and highly visible—and, of course very symbolic. The nurse's "hat" takes its place with the hats of fireman and the policeman. Purses, large and small, are also good accompaniments to imaginative play. It is a very important possession for the preschool child who is wrestling with elements of ownership. Children can likewise find many exciting uses for pieces of brightly colored cloths, either as adornments for themselves or for their dolls. A boxful of such easily collected materials should be available on every hospital unit for young children. Of course, not everything that the child enacts is truly representational of what the situation "played out" really is. Furthermore, not all feelings are tied up with hospitalization and illness; some of the "plays" are the reflection of normal developmental interests. Children of this age live in a rich fantasy world and their fabrications can be expressions of pure make-believe without any link with reality. Lowenfeld (1967) reminds us that every play object is likely to have three mean-

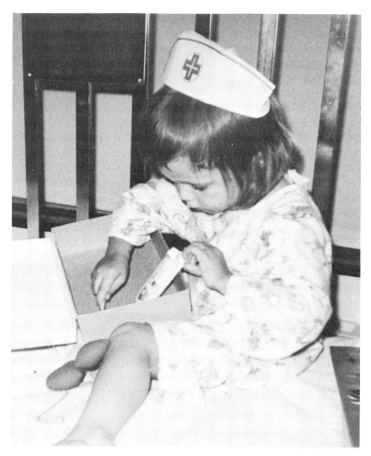

FIG. 8. This young lady is learning by *doing.* Playing out stressful situations relieves anxiety.

ings—the obvious one; the correct or incorrect knowledge possessed by the child about the object; and the significance that the object itself has for the child. Consequently, interpretation of a play episode should not be too hasty.

Play, then, for the preschool child, is a composite of many activities rich with emotional meaning. Foremost among its characteristics are the child's excursions into the world of fantasy. Through symbolic, make-believe play, the child stores sensations and perceptions that he will apply to the interpretation of future experiences. He does this in a most pragmatic way. As the preschooler delights in his "play" discoveries, he leaves physical and verbal imprints on the people and things in his environment. They, in turn, reinforce the child's desire to continue his pursuit of self-mastery.

FIG. 9. Folding room partitions can be made from any firm material and held together with plastic rings.

The School-Age Child

The hospitalized school-age child has several things going for him with regard to play. Erikson (1963) stresses that this is the age of industry—the time when the child is busy *doing* things. Physically, the school-age child has matured to the point where fine motor coordination and large muscle control permit a wide range of activities. Piaget (1969) describes this stage as that of concrete mental operations—a time when the child can become absorbed in handling immediate and tangible problems and can manipulate them by using elementary logic and reasoning.

Using these general guidelines, the nurse can call upon the traditional collection of games that have delighted children for decades. Games of chance and skill should be employed as the child desires them. Craft skills and hobbies may also occupy a good portion of the child's time. Since these things involve use of small muscles and fairly long attention spans, a hospital environment may not be too restricting (Fig. 10).

However, a word of caution ought to be introduced when one considers using such games. Energy consumption varies with the meaning that a child attaches to a particular activity. A competitive game requiring considerable skill may be quite exhausting and border on overstimulation, especially for a child who always needs to win. The circumstances under which a game is played are also important. A child who

FIG. 10. These simple materials provide the school-age child with opportunities for creative expression and for development of intellectual and manipulative skills.

is coming to grips with a changed body image or who is getting accustomed to a restriction in his activities needs an opportunity to experience a few successes. School-age children have very high expectations for themselves and can be devastated by failure, even if it is only a game of checkers that is lost. A reasonable hope for achievement must exist in any play activity. Children rightfully resent it if you "let them win;" they do not want reality altered. What I am emphasizing is the value of selecting the right activity at the right time.

Children of this age also enjoy a culture of their own. The process of growing to maturity necessarily involves participation in sustaining this culture. Adults are relatively uninformed about the characteristics of this way of life because it is nearly impossible to penetrate the peer world of the school-age child. In fact, much of the pleasure of the age comes from the fact that adults do *not* know the intimate details of this existence. Nevertheless, we do know that these children are their own best entertainers. The rhymes, riddles, puns, and songs that dance on their lips are evidence of their adherence to rituals. They have a special language all their own that spoofs reality and transmits meanings impossible to express in a conventional way. It becomes a secret code of entry into the child's world. Opie and Opie (1959) describe the "lore and language" of school children in vivid and explicit terms as they recorded it in a study conducted throughout England, Ireland, and Wales. The rhymes and riddles capture the children's views of friendship, authority, truthfulness, and humor in a unique way.

For example, Scottish children who find themselves excluded from a group jeer back at the crowd:

> Birds of a feather flock together
> And so do pigs and swine;
> Rats and mice do have their choice
> And so do I have mine.

This is an old rhyme dating back to 1844 (Opie and Opie, 1959, p. 50), yet it continues to have much meaning to the children of today.

Once the adult latches on to these phrases they cease to become important to the children. As previously mentioned, this does not seem to be an area in which adults and children can participate together. Yet I believe that an awareness of this culture has relevance to the care of the sick child.

Often the satisfaction enjoyed through peer-group activities is derived from the group's ability to test adult authority. Rhymes are often directed at persons in authority. Word tricks can be used to express legitimate aggression. Teachers are especially vulnerable to this kind of play but anyone who controls the child's environment and prescribes certain kinds of activities on a consistent basis is open to them. Nurses fall into this category, and should expect to receive a goodly amount of normal discrimination. Mimicking, making faces, and giving nicknames are all important experiences for children. The exclusiveness of play at this age should also be noted with interest. The quick act of hiding something when you enter the room, or the silly, self-conscious giggles that follow a "clique" conversation are not so much directed against the nurse as they are directed at preserving the special flavor of middle-childhood fun. Children of this age cherish privacy to an extent not often appreciated by the adult.

Hospitalization, of course, places many limits on this kind of activity. There are too many adults in the environment and there is generally too much space between children and too wide an age variation. Hopefully these factors can be modified. I believe that we sometimes overdo the necessity for close supervision of the school-age children's activities. In reality, even in play, they are seldom alone long enough to "do their own thing." This is certainly a peer-oriented time, so efforts must made to bring children into closer proximity with each other by moving beds, carts, chairs, and tables so that communication is facilitated (Fig. 11). Of course, children of similar age must be grouped together. The interests of a six-year-old boy are far removed from those of a twelve-year-old, although there will be some opportunities to share activities in common.

I have already alluded to the role of fantasy in the developmental expression of the preschool child. Fantasies are expressed quite spontaneously by young children. The older child, however, is not quite so

FIG. 11.   The closer the better for these "pals." Peer group solidarity is strong in the school years.

free. Because the child is older, he is more affected by the constraints of the "realities" of life and has a more elaborate collection of defense mechanisms. He is more inclined toward the conventional and competitive activities than toward the kind of play that might risk self-revelation.

It seems reasonable to expect that school-age children who have long-term illnesses might harbor more fears and unsettling feelings about themselves than would be experienced by healthy children. Helping the child find ways that might encourage expression of emotions without the attendant risk of losing face can become an important nursing function. Marcus (1966) successfully used the costume technique as one way of encouraging dramatic play among school-age children. He noted that these children respond better if the enactment of their fantasy is supported by props—materials related to real-life situations. Although Marcus describes the technique in relation to psychotherapy, I think that it would be a decidedly useful play stimulus for children whose age discourages their spontaneous expression. Hand puppets and marionettes are also good tools for this purpose.

Thus far I have referred primarily to manipulative and verbal activities for the school-age child. Not to be underestimated is the importance of acquiring a sense of physical well-being and adequacy through involvement to gross motor activities. The middle-childhood years do focus upon the learning of a wide variety of highly valued physical skills—running, jumping, balancing, and playing of games requiring coordination and speed. Illness at its best limits the opportunity to test and demonstrate this physical competence; at its worst, it may completely remove outlets for activity by isolation and superimposed restraint. (Reference will be made later in this chapter to specific ways that children can be helped to adapt to restrictions of illness without completely sacrificing their need for action-oriented pastimes.)

The school-age child is particularly vulnerable to what might be called the hospital culture. The activities of this age involve many significant aspects of development—developing conscience, inner control, and cooperation; learning how to think and make judgments; learning the role expectations of male and female; understanding the limitations of social class. All, in effect, move the child toward increasing independence. All of these are explored through the medium of play. Some have been described already. I should like to direct particular emphasis to the area of social class.

It is a fact that hospital clothing, room arrangements, and services tend to disguise social and economic class differences. Yet the child himself operates within the context of his past experiences. By the time he is in eighth grade, the child perceives social class in about the same way that adults do. Depending on the social class in which he was raised, certain kinds of behaviors are reinforced while others are discouraged. The hospital environment may create conflict. This is especially noticeable during long hospitalizations. Two sets of circumstances may prevail, each with its own dangers. If the child's adherence to the behavior of his social class is strong and prevails over the mores of the staff, conflicts may emerge which can be psychologically and physically disruptive. On the other hand, the child may be captivated by the hospital mores and change his behavior in order to conform and receive the system's rewards. If this pattern of response spans a considerable time period, the child may incorporate these behavioral expectations into his life-style and then the problems emerge at the time of discharge from the hospital. The child experiences a conflict between his new goals and those of his family and neighborhood. Such seeds of conflict may lay the groundwork for a troubled readjustment to his environment. I can well remember a young girl from a city slum who was hospitalized for more than a year with rheumatic heart disease. During the period of hospitalization, she became the "favorite" of many nurses. She visited their suburban homes, enjoyed many gifts for her birthday and holidays, and began a strong identification with middle-class mores to the exclusion of values held by a disrupted family. Old enough to take an active role in decision-making, she obviously resented a return to her family. She was dissatisfied with what they could materially provide for her and she became acutely aware of her own limited resources in providing the "luxuries" for herself. She obviously needed help to blend both value systems and to retain the best of each.

How can play be helpful in this regard? If the child comes from a situation characterized by economic hardship, the use of play materials that do not involve a large monetary expenditure should be encouraged. Focus should be directed on the child's resourcefulness rather than on the material itself. Activity should be based on the child's interest. It is likely that if his social class differs markedly from the nurse's, that nurse may not understand the relevance of the activities he describes. Encourage him to teach you the games and the corresponding vocabulary or jargon. This shows respect for his idea of a good and productive use of his time and also places him in the important position of making decisions about his own activities. It also will provide indirect clues about what motivates this child's behavior. This knowledge becomes valuable in helping him adjust to his illness.

I can recall receiving a thorough education from a 12-year-old patient about the dance crazes that were popular among the youngsters in a black community. Agility in performance of these dances was a mark of social acceptance within her neighborhood youth groups. The fact that some of this skill could be lost during the hospitalization was of more concern to the girl than was the fact that she was to undergo surgery for treatment of osteomyelitis. She was able to keep her interest alive and her peer position relatively secure by resorting to "pop" records and frequent visits from her friends. And, quite importantly, she derived much pleasures from teaching me about her "special thing."

As one can see, play during the school years is better organized than that during the preschool period, but it still retains imagination and inventiveness. It has an excitement of its own. The period is marked by strict adherence to rules and high expectations for one's performance. Leadership qualities emerge as the youngsters experiment with group interaction and begin to learn the meaning of altruism. Within the context of school-age play, the nurse holds a position of importance—not in the sense of becoming an active "player" but rather serving as a model of behavior. The child still looks to the adult for guidelines in choosing satisfying and acceptable modes of conduct. Play activities become a well-trod path to life in school and in the wider community.

The Adolescent

Havighurst (1952) lists no less than ten important developmental tasks that characterize physical and emotional maturing during adolescence. Acceptance of one's physique, involvement in satisfying heterosexual relationships, emancipation from parents, and some assumption of economic independence are among the important achievements of this age. Stone and Church (1962) sum up the central theme of teenagers' strivings as finding one's self. In more contemporary terms, adolescents are looking for answers to questions posed by sex, money, education, justice, conservation, peace, and war. These have been the concerns of young adults for a long time, but more and more these topics find their way into the conversations of high-school children.

Many of these learnings presuppose a certain level of physical and mental wellness and, obviously, most of them are learned in the context of a social setting. Consequently, there is no age when illness is more threatening than during adolescence. Not only is it a threat to personal integrity but it is maddeningly inconvenient to be ill during adolescence when there are so many things to do. If the illness is of long duration, involves a reorientation of life goals, or results in mutilation of a part of the body, the threat may be temporarily immobilizing.

Hospitalized adolescents have every right to be angry, distrustful, and annoyed. With their idealistic points of view, they are not accustomed to an unplanned interruption in this exciting stage of their development. Adjustment to illness and hospitalization can be eased by implementation of a thoughtfully conceived and relevant program of activity.

Peer-group activities are all-absorbing at this age. The adolescent values his ability to choose his friends and the type, scope, and duration of the activities they experience together. Hospitalization will limit this freedom—but not nearly to the extent ordinarily supposed. There are many ways to encourage spontaneous friendships. The spontaneity of the social encounter is important. The nurse's role is one that provides opportunities for young people to meet rather than one that forces social contacts.

It is best to proceed slowly in this regard. While the adolescent may feel confident and at ease with his reference group outside of the hospital, it may take some time before he can safely open himself to a new roommate or hospital group. Pushing a relationship too enthusiastically may actually retard a meaningful social experience. Teenagers are quick to be suspicious and resent situations where they feel that they are losing control. I can recall an experience involving two 15-year-old boys. One had had surgery to treat Meckel's diverticulum; the other boy was hospitalized with ulcerative colitis. They were the only teens on the unit and their rooms were at opposite ends of the corridor. The nurse who was caring for one of the boys decided to promote some social interaction so she introduced them and suggested that they meet for craft work. The boys dutifully complied but it was a strained experience for both of them. They plodded along with the task but there was little enthusiastic communication between them. After two days of this arrangement both boys found excuses to avoid the meeting. The next day both boys coincidentally found themselves sharing the game room. Left completely to their own resources, they became interested in each other's activities. One boy was a talented cartoon artist; the other was very proficient at playing pool. Each felt a certain competence in his special skill and, on this common ground, they shared their experiences. They respected each other's individuality and their friendship grew strong during the hospitalization and continued after they went home.

One way to encourage spontaneous interaction is to set up a teen "lounge" (not a playroom, please! adolescents are extremely sensitive about childish labels). Ideally, it should be equipped with a record player, radio, and simple musical instruments (guitars and bongo drums are popular and well-used). Board games of chance and skill, playing cards, a typewriter, writing paper, and magazines are also of interest to young people. A small pantry for snacks is always a good added feature. With these supportive props, teenagers can be as open to interaction as their emotional or physical state permits (Fig. 12).

The adolescent confined to bed can benefit from some communica-

FIG. 12. The adolescent is approaching adult interests. These common materials serve a wide range of abilities and help to bridge the gap between childhood play and adult recreation.

tion network that keeps him socially "in tune." This can take the form of a tape-recorded conversation passed between two patients or between himself and his classmates at school or members of his family. A weekly gossip sheet can be great fun to compile as a group activity. A sullen, withdrawn teenager can come alive as the "star reporter." The sheet can contain hospital news, "feature" articles by the adolescents themselves, announcement of coming events such as teenage luncheons or an evening "social," and birthday and graduation congratulations. A challenging crossword puzzle or a "thought for the week" might go far to relieve a little boredom and spark some animated conversation. Telephone and letter contacts both in and out of the hospital setting are other ways of preserving social awareness. Visits from other patients and school friends, while it seems almost too obvious to mention, should also be encouraged.

In planning teenage activities, it is important to remember that young people come from a media-filled world. Stereo and radio are as important to teenagers as food and water. School experiences are enriched by a variety of audiovisual techniques. Social gathering spots are accented by revolving lights and the penetrating sound of the "beat." A world-full of vicarious experiences comes to them through television. Consequently, it should not surprise us that many teenagers suffer acutely from restless boredom. The sensory deprivation of the hospitalized adolescent ought to come under closer scrutiny. Television certainly has its place in any teen activity program. In settings in which new audiovisual facilities are being proposed, consider closed circuit television. Its potential for teaching and entertainment is great. Use of movies, film-strips, and cartridge tapes are also well received if the content is *relevant* to adolescent interests.

One very important need for most adolescents (both boys and girls) is maintenance of physical strength, agility, and excellence in sports. A long illness will affect these abilities to some extent. However, in many situations, atrophy of muscles and diminished skill are needless accompaniments of illness. Weightlifting, muscle setting exercises, workouts in physical therapy, or use of an overhead trapeze or a punching bag can help to maintain a level of skill that compliments the child's image of himself. For example, I cared for a 16-year-old boy with diabetes who was hospitalized for treatment of a skin infection. He was trying out for the track team at school and was worried that his training program would suffer. After discussing the situation with the physician and the physical therapist, arrangements were made for him to go to physical therapy to "work out." I later learned that he did make the team.

It is often presumed that adolescents disregard school performance as completely irrelevant. For some of these young people this is indeed a fact. However, it is unwise to make this assumption for all. Teenagers understand well the stereotyped expectation that they "ought to" reject authority. Consequently, those who are interested in school achievement are reluctant to admit it. Therefore, it is important to provide matter-of-fact opportunities to do school work without forcing the adolescent to say that they "love" it, or otherwise draw unnecessary attention to it. On the other hand, if a teenager's interests are not scholastic, he should not be criticized. His illness probably undermines his self-confidence enough without adding another dimension—that is, failure to measure up to the nurse's "high" standards.

Every adolescent has *some* talent. Finding it might be a challenge for the nurse. When the talent is too obscure, it might be because the teenager does not feel that his interest is acceptable enough to the nurse to bring it out in the open. Whatever the talent might be—crafts, art, poetry, music, mechanics, whittling, sports, farming, or simply "hanging around with the gang"—he should be given every opportunity to continue to develop it if his illness permits. It will establish his identity in the hospital and maintain his level of proficiency when he returns to home and school.

Adolescence is a time for much soul-searching, which requires taking an inward look into the self. Consequently, solitary recreation constitutes a vital part of adolescent activity. We must respect the teenager's "right to do nothing." Time for daydreaming, thinking, and mirror-looking is necessary for all adolescents. It is even more significant if he is also struggling to accept an illness. Sometimes we overdo the tendency to keep teenagers busy. We feel compelled to keep their minds active so they won't become preoccupied with their illness. If there is no time to ponder new ideas or make sense out of the day's events, worries and fears may be so diffuse that they enter into all of the adolescent's activities—diminishing his capacity to enjoy anything.

The adolescent's room should reflect his interests. Closets and cupboards are in demand to hold the various and sundry items that teenagers cannot live without. Cork boards should be hung in prominent places so that such things as newspaper clippings, cards, art work, and cartoons can be viewed at their pleasure. Mirrors are important to accommodate the teenager's preoccupation with his body and grooming. Bright contemporary colors should predominate in room decor. (The pastels of most children's units are more appealing to adults than to children.) Bedside units with telephones and radios are also appreciated by teenagers.

While these environmental enticements do make hospitalization more pleasant, perhaps the most important part of an adolescent activity program is the role assumed by the nurse. The teenager is really anxious to respect adults but he fears deception. He is extremely sensitive to a lack of sincerity or superficial attention to his concerns. Consequently, he is cautious about opening new relationships.

There is no doubt that an experience gap exists between the nurse and the adolescent patient. Dress, language, and interests may differ but these "things" are relatively unimportant if there is a desire to help the young person think well of himself. The nurse who cares for adolescents must be someone who is convinced that teenagers are competent and can act responsibly.

Teenagers love to shock and tantalize persons in authority. The nurse should expect her share of this behavior. However, she must not retaliate by trying to "put something over on this fresh kid." Once the teenager feels manipulated, all further attempts at meaningful interaction are jeopardized. Most of all teenagers appreciate a good listener who judiciously refrains from giving "pat" advice.

In spite of the obvious experiential differences between nurse and patient, the nurse must strive for a congruent orientation with the adolescents' goals. She must not be in conflict with what he wants to achieve; nor should she feel threatened if her reasoning meets resistance. The "says-who" attitude is an understandable response from a disillusioned 16-year-old who is a newly diagnosed diabetic. The optimum benefit from the activities and facilities that I have mentioned depends upon the existence of a nurse-patient relationship that is based on mutual respect.

Environment for Play

The resourcefulness and energy that a child brings to his play comes from within, but the richness of the experience does depend in large measure on external stimuli. A suitable environment for play must be established whether the child is sick at home or in the hospital, confined to bed or visiting the ambulatory care facility. Certain environmental elements should be considered when one plans satisfying play experiences.

SPACE.   The first of the environmental elements that a child needs is *space*. Ordinarily, space is defined as boundlessness or extension in all directions. Obviously, a child's play space must have some fixed dimensions, and the sick child's world is even more confined. I prefer to think of space not so much in terms of dimensions of distance and height but rather in terms of a spacious "feeling." A relatively small area can be made to appear open and airy if walls and curtains are bright, the lighting is good, the bed has at least two open sides, and windows are low enough to "bring in the outdoors." Drab colors, poor lighting, obstructive screens, and high windows create a barrier from the real world and tone down the excitement of play. Objects that do not interest the child, such as linen and unnecessary pieces of equipment, should be elsewhere.

Spacial needs can also be considered from other points of view. Certain kinds of play activity require certain spacial characteristics. Riding a tricycle demands enough space to build up at least some sensation of speed and, of course, requires a "turn around" area. Building blocks are excellent materials for creative play. However, the preschool child often delights in saving his elaborate masterpiece until his mother or daddy sees it or until he himself is ready to destroy it. This takes not only space, but also respect for the products of the child's own ingenuity.

Bed space is also important. Games that require delicate balance may prove frustrating on an already tilted bed; board games that require an intricate layout of materials may present difficulties for a child who has a limited reaching span. Part of the excitement and pleasure of the game is to play according to the rules. Improvisation has its place but only when used at the right time. Lightweight, folding cardboard bases can be easily constructed to spread on the bed so that play materials can be balanced.

There are ways to increase the range of play opportunities for the bed-bound child. His independence is also increased since he can have more control over the play materials. Assemble the items of special interest in a reachable spot so that he can determine the focus of his play and change it at will regardless of whether adults are available to assist him. This encourages his creativity by permitting a combination of materials in new play experiments. A toy bag, a small suitcase, or a sturdy box attached to the bed can contain enough "raw material" to keep an inventive mind well stimulated for an entire day. One manufacturer of paper goods produced a large heavy-strength bag printed with bold outlines of toys and animals which the children could color as they wished. It served well as a bedside toy bag which the child could easily identify as his own (Fig. 13).

The child's "personal space" is another consideration. This is the area that he understands as his own. Both in the hospital and at home, a child needs to know what is his—that is, how far his domain extends. It becomes a source of self-satisfaction as well as an element of power and control. Furthermore, it supports his wish for freedom in that the child can change "his" things to suit his needs and interests.

If a child knows the limits of his space he can confidently speak (or fight) for what he knows is his. The hospital situation often presents elements of a community where objects are shared by everyone. Sometimes the aggressive child captures the most cherished items. By knowing what is his, the child does not have to become anxious about having to give up his possessions. Young children can become very upset when "mommy's chair" is suddenly whisked away for someone else, or when their favorite toy is passed on to another child. Realistically, many hospital toys are community property and will not go home with the child. Of course, children must be helped to accept this limitation. Understanding this reality will be less disturbing if the child knows the limits of his personal space.

TIME. The child also needs *time* to play. We must respect his interest in his own activities. Nurses sometimes find it difficult to take

FIG. 13. Toy storage is an easy matter when these containers are used. If kept within the child's reach, they provide much independence in selecting play materials. Besides, it is fun just to "put things in and take them out."

play seriously. How many times is the child interrupted in the middle of a play period to have a treatment performed, or to eat or take a bath? I do not recommend that the child's care plan revolve solely around his play needs; but I do plead that careful consideration be given to the child's own timetable of events whenever possible.

During the course of a long-term illness, the child's presence may be taken for granted. Hospital personnel may casually stop in for just a short visit—just a word or two—all with good intention. The child literally has no time to do his "work." These visitors are very important but they could be more sensitive in the timing of their visits. They should pause to observe whether the child is absorbed in play before they call attention to their presence.

The child also needs time to develop competence in his play. When suggesting an activity, one must keep a reasonable completion time in mind. If the activity such as craft or art work involves a fair amount of preparation time, be sure that enough time is allowed for some enjoyment of the activity itself before the materials have to be put away. Accomplishment is one of the outcomes of play. A child who continually gets things half done never has a chance to see himself as a successful doer.

Also important is time to terminate play. If play is afforded the respect that it deserves, we can readily understand the child's reluctance to refocus his attention on something the adult considers more essential to his care. As a matter of fact, the child may find it impossible to re-assemble his resources for a new experience—particularly if he has been fully absorbed in a re-creation of a meaningful or stressful event. However, he can adjust to limitations if he is aware of them. It is important to give a child reasonable notice about an upcoming treatment or change in routine before it occurs so that he can terminate his play partially on his own terms.

The last timely consideration is often overlooked. Every child needs time *not* to play. Judicious timing of play periods should offer opportunities to rest, daydream, plan the day's events, enjoy a pleasant view, or simply retreat to the confines of one's inner resources for refreshment and strength to face new challenges. However good play is, too much of it lessens its rich benefits. Of course, if solitary non-involvement dominates the child's play, there is just cause for concern and appropriate intervention.

FEASIBILITY.   Another factor to consider in building an environment for play is the *feasibility* of play—from the standpoint of both the player and the play material. Several questions may be posed to illustrate this point. Is the player able to perform the activity without undue fatigue? Will the time required to enjoy the activity match the time available for it? Will the materials function appropriately where they will be used? Are all essential parts of the material available for use? Let us suppose that a right-handed child has his left hand restrained while receiving a blood transfusion. In looking for a pleasant activity to occupy the time, paper and crayons are offered. It sounds reasonable since the child is right-handed. However, the activity will lead to frustration if some method is not devised to keep the paper from moving on the overbed table. The solution may be simply a large clipboard or a clamp that might fit over the edge of the table. A child is quick to lose interest and is easily frustrated when things do not work for him. A four-legged animal needs four legs *and* something to stand on. In the young child's concrete way of dealing with things, he has a difficult time seeing a reproduction-type of toy outside of its intended function. I think it unfair to make him create another function. Furthermore, it is a useless waste of energy which could be better directed in another way. Crayons that keep rolling out of reach could be stored in a box or bag that will give the child much better control of the situation. The pockets of a shoe bag suspended on the side of the crib or bed will easily keep a variety of small toys within the child's reach.

Given space, time, and feasibility, two important ingredients remain: the availability of people and things. There is no doubt that the child is the player but the nurse creates the atmosphere conducive to enjoyable play. This happens only when the nurse understands the value of play to her young patients and has the interest, ability, and time to encourage it through her own ingenuity and by consultation and collaboration with recreational and occupational therapists and volunteer play helpers. I doubt whether this nursing activity is considered fully enough when staffing patterns are evolved for children's units. If available, recreational therapists can spend only a relatively short time with a particular child or group of children for they must attend to a large number of persons. They customarily "get the child started" with an activity but cannot be expected to "follow through" with each child to determine his play needs. The nurse and therapist working together can do precisely this. The nurse can assess such factors as the meaning that a particular activity has for a child, the existence of fatigue, and the length of attention spans. The nurse can also point out the restrictions imposed by the illness and identify specific kinds of activities that may enhance a particular treatment plan. For example, a child with upper-extremity contractures from burns might well enjoy using a loom supported on a frame, suspended in front of her. She can experience the pleasure of a productive activity and also prevent the untoward development of further contractures. The therapist can assess the child's interest and skill and supply materials to match them, and the know-how to use them creatively. Both persons contribute the all-important interest in the child's enjoyment of play.

Often, the source of failure of many enthusiastically initiated play programs is a lack of materials. This can wear ingenuity to the point where it is too thin to be effective. Donated materials are, of course, encouraged but they cannot be expected to fulfill all play needs. Hospital and health agency budgets *must* reflect the essentialness of play materials to the care of young patients. Furthermore, effectiveness cannot be sacrificed in the interest of economy. Although it might serve an immediate need, the cheapest material is certainly not always the wisest purchase. It is better to consider durability and flexibility. The initial cost will be significant but, over time, the monies will have been well spent. However, many resources are available at minimal cost. Hospital carpenter shops can assemble simple yet serviceable equipment—work tables, benches, stools, stairs, bulletin boards, toy boxes, and easels—by using scrap wood left from other construction and remodeling jobs. Volunteer organizations are also very helpful in this regard. Parents, too, are ready to lend a hand. One father of a five-year-old boy constructed a special dolly to improve locomotion possibilities for his young son; he drew up a set of directions based on his design and the hospital carpenters have used it in many similar situations (Fig. 14A and B).

Obsolete hospital equipment can be adapted to serve as play materials. A good look should be taken at what disposable equipment is replacing so that useful items are not inadvertently discarded. Also, observe the "disposables" themselves. Looking at them from different

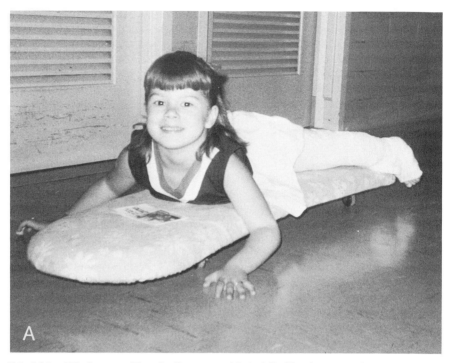

FIG. 14.A. This five-year-old really "gets around." A dolly like this permits her to participate actively in family affairs and play groups. *B.* If not available commercially, a dolly can be easily constructed as illustrated.

B

HEAVY BOARD

PROTECTIVE
RUBBER BUMPER

points of view, you might see them as containers for crayons or paints or as small toys such as hats, drums, or cooking utensils. Old bedside tables make delightful refrigerators for little mothers, with an added shelf or two and some bright paint. Unused venetian blind slats make interesting tracks for automobile racers.

PLAYROOM. One important aspect of the environment for play is the playroom itself. Every facility offering services for children should have a play area. The setting need not be elaborate but the equipment assembled must reflect the interests of the children. Otherwise, the area will not receive maximum use. Before space and equipment are selected, identify the characteristics of the children to be served. Their ages and health problems are two primary factors for consideration. Previous sections in this chapter alluded to the significance of age in determining patterns of play. The nature of the health problem is important, too. For example, if many of the children have orthopedic problems provision must be made to accommodate carts, beds, and

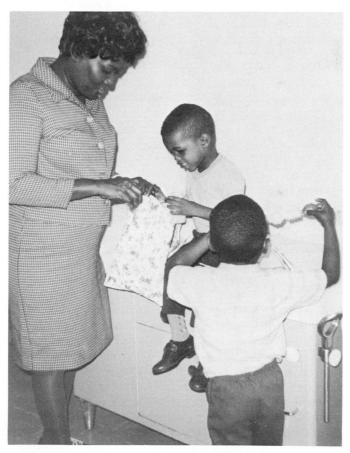

FIG. 15. This little boy is fascinated by his exploration into the toy bag that his grandmother is holding. While they wait for the doctor, learning is taking place.

traction apparatus. The height of the tables may need adjustment for children in wheelchairs. On the other hand, if the playroom is being planned in an ambulatory care facility, different considerations will be in order. A larger number of adults will be present with the children. There should be a reasonable proximity between the playroom and the waiting area so that parents can be free to participate in the child's activity whenever desirable. Because of the transient nature of the ambulatory visit, toys should not be too elaborate or require a long attention span on the part of the child.

In a clinic service, children frequently spend considerable time waiting in examining rooms. (Hopefully, with improved facilities, this time is being shortened.) The playroom concept should be broadened to extend into these areas as well. A small toy box or bag in each room can make the waiting time seem short, especially for the parent whose patience is no longer being tested by a restless child (Fig. 15). Also, the doctor will find that the toys make good conversation openers and pleasant distractions during an uncomfortable examination.

If the hospital population consists entirely of children, a logical way of organizing play facilities may already exist. Patients may be grouped according to age and type of illness. In these cases, the play area on each unit can be highly individualized. An infant unit may not

FIG. 16. This playroom is equipped for the toddler. Note the push-pull toys, rocking horse, low shelves, and plenty of space to move about. (Courtesy of Children's Hospital of Buffalo.)

require separate recreational facilities but the patient rooms should be large enough to accommodate playpens, infant swings, walkers, high-chairs, and rocking chairs for use by mothers and nurses. On the other hand, recreational and play areas are extremely important on preschool units. When facility planning can focus on one age group, play ma-terials can be scaled to the child's height and reflect his special needs (Figs. 16 and 17). Economic benefits result particularly from the pur-chase of large pieces of equipment. Homogeneous units ease the work of supervising adults since they can concentrate their efforts on the need of a particular age. Some administrative problems can be allevi-ated since staffing of play areas can accommodate the varying degrees of supervision required at various stages of development.

In most situations, however, the pediatric unit is a conglomerate of ages and illnesses. Thus the playroom will have to be very adaptable. To accommodate all, assess available space and select the largest area in the interest of flexibility. A collapsible dividing wall can make two separate play areas. One section can be enjoyed by preschool children and the other made to accommodate the older boys and girls. When necessary, the retractable wall can expand the size of the room to allow exercise of large muscles or to permit group attendance at special pro-grams (e.g., holiday parties, circus acts, or musical programs; see Fig. 18).

FIG. 17.   The three- to six-year-old enjoys these materials. House play is readily stimulated by sturdy replicas of household furnishings. The doll house is another favorite as the child explores new roles. (Courtesy of Children's Hospital of Buffalo.)

FIG. 18. A group of excited children are watching this theater troup perform. (Hamburg Children's Theatre, Hamburg, New York.)

Age of the child should be kept in mind when one is arranging the room furnishings. A possible suggestion would be to group preschool equipment on one side of the play area. The following play materials should be included: house corner (simple but sturdy wooden replicas of a stove and refrigerator, shelves, crib, small table, and chairs); a low sink or basin for water play; a stand-up sand box; a dress-up corner (with full-length mirror); a large, low table for drawing, painting, working puzzles or other manipulative tasks; a low-hung blackboard and bulletin board; and wall easels. On the other side of the room (for the older children) arrange the following kinds of equipment: game and craft tables; a tilted table for art work; cupboards containing craft and graphic materials; record player; books and magazines; puzzles; pool table with folding removable top; comfortable lounge chairs; and cork boards. A retractable movie screen is a good addition if visual programs are likely to be planned. Recessed shelves, cupboards, and drawers make storage of materials easy and keep them readily available. Bathroom facilities should be included within the play area to encourage the children to respond to the "urge," to prevent a prolonged interruption in play, and also to serve as a convenience for the supervising adult. All "middle of the room" equipment should be on wheels or casters with locks so that their positions can be easily rearranged to accommodate beds or carts or some special activity. Of course, door-ways should be wide enough to allow passage of beds as well as people. Figure 19 illustrates how such a playroom could be arranged.

An outdoor play area, either in a courtyard or on a porch, is a great asset and every attempt should be made to plan for it. The fresh air, sunshine, and freedom of movement that outdoor play provides cannot be duplicated in any other way. When a porch or yard is not available, a walk or ride around the block is a good substitute. Safety and comfort factors must receive proper consideration. Fencing might be in order if street traffic poses a threat; shading from the sun is also necessary especially around sand boxes and swings where children are likely to be absorbed in play for long periods.

One of the often-stated goals of health workers is to bring the served and the services together. By making services more personal and less threatening, persons may seek the services they need. It has been my experience that parents as well as children respond favorably to a genuine show of interest in them often expressed through the medium of shared play experiences. The hospital that has nothing to offer the child in this regard is in effect saying that it fails to respect one of childhood's greatest priorities. If play can alleviate some of the child's anxiety about his illness, and at the same time indicate to the parents that the hospital staff is concerned about the "whole child," people will encourage use of health services. For the child with a long-term illness, welcomed associations through play also mean that the inevitable return to the hospital or clinic may be less unpleasant (Fig. 20A and B).

FIG. 19.   Playroom designed for flexibility.

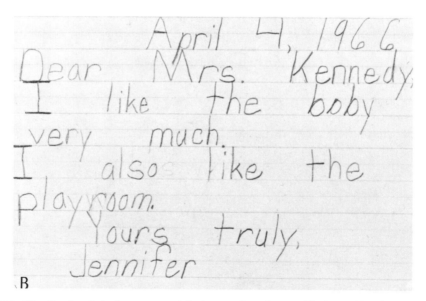

FIG. 20. The hospital playroom certainly impressed a six-year-old visitor. Her drawing (A) and her letter (B) reflect pleasant memories of her trip. (Courtesy of Children's Hospital of Buffalo, New York.)

Assessment of Play Behavior

Part of the nurse's initial and on-going assessment of her patient's status should include an assessment of play behavior—a play profile.

The purpose of such an assessment is to determine the kinds of play experience that have special meaning to the child. This allows continued benefit and satisfaction from them. By calling attention to these needs through the use of an assessment tool, play is more clearly viewed as a significant part of the child's care. The tool provides baseline information about the child so that deviations can be identified and progress recorded. The profile communicates information to all who are involved in the child's care, thereby eliminating the necessity for the child or his parents to repeat likes and dislikes and patterns of behavior to everyone who cares for the child. The profile becomes the basic framework around which to plan a balanced play program. A profile, of course, is merely an outline—it does not prescribe a course of action. Individual judgment, based on the collected data, must personalize each situation. Nevertheless, a good framework does provide a starting point.

What should the profile include? Essentially, the classic questions should be posed: Who, what, where, when, and how?

WHO? This question refers to the significant people in the child's play world. The answer to this question depends partly on the child's social radius. One can safely assume that the infant's play is solitary and oriented toward "taking in" activities with the mother as the most significant other. However, as the child grows older, assumptions are not so reliable. The child of three or four, whose social radius still has not expanded beyond the parents, will have a play style that is quite different from the child who has a neighborhood or nursery-school reference group. Presuming that the former child will comfortably enjoy an active playroom setting may be unfair to the child and introduce more stimulation than the child can handle since he has the additional stress of his illness.

The child who plays with one special friend is likely to experience some separation anxiety. If the separation is a long one, something like grief might occur. I can remember talking to eight-year-old Jimmy about his friends. He said "I hate to be away from my very best friend. We did everything together." His downcast eyes and sad expression amply conveyed the loss he felt. His feelings were intensified because the last time that he and his friend were together, the chum sustained an injury to his hand in a play accident. Now, confused by the timing of the hospitalization, Jimmy imagined himself partly responsible for the accident. He felt punished and also expressed concern about whether his friend would remember him.

WHAT? The answer to this question reveals the kinds of play activity and play material the child prefers. There are stages in development when children enjoy representational objects. Materials that invite sensory exploration and body movement—such as water, sand, clay, and paint—are preferred at other times. Table games become important when the child is able to think abstractly and develop his own strategies.

Comfort toys are important to maintain a feeling of security away from home. The loved teddy bear or blanket may be overlooked in the confused circumstances that attend illness. Queries about the existence of such things will assure that the child who needs these supports will have them. Knowing the materials that the child enjoys and handles with ease does not operate against the positive outcomes derived from new experiences. It seems logical that a familiar play activity, particularly as an initial experience in the hospital, would eliminate the need for the child to struggle with new problems right away. His energies are more properly directed toward resolution of problems related to his illness. Much time remains for developing new interests and skills.

There is interesting evidence, however, that contradicts this view. Gilmore (1966) studied a group of 18 children between the ages of five and nine who were hospitalized for tonsillectomy and matched them with 18 control subjects. He found that the children experiencing the anxiety of hospitalization preferred novel toys over simple ones and especially those novel toys—such as a doctor's kit, toy syringe, and stethoscope—that were relevant to the hospitalization. It appears from his study that anxious children wish to become familiar with the source of the anxiety. In additional studies to substantiate these results, Gilmore raises questions about the significance of the intensity of the anxiety. It seems possible from his findings that a high level of anxiety does indeed cause disruption of play. Under circumstances of extreme anxiety children selected play materials that were not relevant to the source of anxiety. Perhaps, as a consequence of this study, both relevant and nonrelevant toys ought to be available from which the child can make a choice. Careful assessment of anxiety level will provide additional clues to the child's play needs.

It is quite conceivable that the "thing" that a child cherishes most is a pet. He may feel so responsible for its care that he fears for the animal's well-being in his absence. If the animal is a dog or cat or even a larger animal it is generally not feasible to house the pet in the hospital. (I know of some exceptions to this rule—so do not overlook it as a solution to a grave separation problem.) However, when the pet is a turtle, fish, or hamster, the child may be able to continue to care for it. On the other hand, children who do not have pets at home can really enjoy an introduction to pet care. It can direct attention away from themselves and make them feel good about contributing to the well being of another. (Hospital research laboratories can be resources for interesting pets.) Whenever animals become part of the child's care, be sure that you know how to care for them in the hospital setting. Have the parents write down food, air, and water requirements or consult with a local pet shop. There is little to be gained from complicating the situation by a high rate of animal mortality!

WHERE? The places where the child customarily plays are an important consideration, too. If the illness or hospitalization is preceded by play activities that are expansive outdoor experiences, the child can be expected to have more difficulty in adjusting to the confinements of a hospital room than a child who generally plays indoors in a small apartment. How much a child is permitted to do in bed at home is another factor not often considered. The bed is frequently "off limits" for eating and playing certain kinds of games. A child who seems restrained in his play may simply be reflecting his discomfort over interpretation of his mother's command at home—"Don't use paints on the bed." Such inadvertent conflicts are important to many children but especially those who are accustomed to strict limits at home. The child has no experience by which to judge his mother's response if she should find him painting in bed.

WHEN?   The child organizes his play periods into a schedule that is satisfying for him. His routine is a reflection of many things—the arrangement of activities of daily living in his home, availability of facilities for play, and his own physical need for a balance between rest and activity. The daily morning trip to the neighborhood playground may be sorely missed—so much so that some simulation of that experience ought to be planned while he is in the hospital or convalescing at home. A trip in the wheel chair to see the day-by-day changes in a window box flower garden can be an exciting adventure for the young child. Certainly, the parents and the nurse ought to be keenly aware of the child's view of important routines.

The young child times his activities according to tangible events—things happen after breakfast, before dinner, when daddy comes home, or when it gets dark outside. He is not ordered by the clock. The hospital rest period may not coincide with his plan. His after-lunch activity may consist of a romp outdoors, so that he is not inclined to "settle in" to a new routine without some restlessness and anger.

Bedtime play rituals are also a meaningful part of the child's day. Sleep ends the day's events and the child approaches nighttime either excited by the good things that happened to him or worried and puzzled by events that had unfavorable outcomes. Loneliness overcomes some children and they often have exaggerated responses to strange noises, shadows, and even the sound of their own heartbeats. As a result there may be a reluctance to leave the state of wakefulness. Illness and the strange environment of the hospital compound and intensify feelings at the hour of sleep. Unfortunately many hospitals require that parents leave at this time. Consequently, not only does the child have to cope with bedtime problems but he often has to cope with them alone. Parents should be encouraged to stay with their young children until they are sleeping, but care must be taken to avoid deluding the child that parents will remain all night. The nurse must be careful to find out from the parents whether the child expressed special concerns so that she can be better prepared to help him cope. I have found that the nurse's attention to a child at bedtime is time well spent. She can help the child give expression to his concerns. Children seem to be psychologically more vulnerable and open at night than during the daytime. Since there are fewer external distractions the child turns inward and fantasies and worries are reawakened. The understanding nurse who tucks the child in, listens to his prayers, reads a good-night story, or sings a lullaby is in a good position to uncover fears and answer sensitive questions (Fig. 21). A teenage girl that I cared for reversed the usual circumstances and sang to me at bedtime. She had a very pleasing voice but was self-conscious about displaying her talent in front of a group. At night as I was readying her for bed, she would relax and sing. Her songs were rich with meaning. She composed many of the lyrics herself and set them to popular folk tunes. For her it was an important expressive outlet. Then, after her song she would always ask, "Do you know why I sang that?" and would launch us into a conversation about a wide variety of topics. Among other things, we discussed the meaning of love, her maturing body, and her great fascination for horses.

HOW?   Every child has his own style of play. Some children have a rich imagination. Their minds are so fertile with their own ideas that they are completely absorbed and cannot include other children until they have worked out their thoughts. Often these children move from one activity to another because one stimulus quickly sparks an idea for

FIG. 21. A bedtime story is a good close to a busy day. These girls felt a special "closeness" to their nurse for she had just prepared them for surgery scheduled the next day. They appreciated the warmth of her attention. (Incidentally, this nurse's uniform is especially appealing to her young patients—it is bright orange!)

a new project. Other children perceive more slowly and can derive satisfaction from repetitive use of simple materials. They may approach new situations with timidity and thus may not take much initiative in determining their own play activities. These youngsters may need considerable support and direct approval of their activities until they feel confident enough to fully enjoy them.

Temperament is certainly a factor in style of play. For some children emotional arousal comes easy; these youngsters are often quick to react and to show agressive behavior. They may show impatience with their inability to implement all of their ideas and express anger toward themselves and others.

Children explore their environment in many ways. A child may approach it visually first; then after the situation is surveyed carefully and he feels competent to explore more directly he might reach out to touch the people or objects. On the other hand, there are children who rush headlong into the situation only to find through trial and error that they may have acted too hastily. The first child needs encouragement and warm approval so that he can better "discover" himself and his surroundings; the other child needs help in limit setting so that he can delay his gratification in the interest of his own safety. In any event, these styles must be reckoned with so that wasteful effort will not be expended trying to fit a "round peg into a square hole."

USE OF A PLAY PROFILE

A play profile can be employed as an assessment tool at all stages of the child's illness—at the time of admission to the hospital, periodically throughout the hospital stay, at the time of discharge, and during convalescence. The profile obtained at time of admission resembles a history of information about play behavior at home as described by parents and the child. It is important to remember that this history provides only *baseline* data and therefore should not give a sense of finality to expected play behavior. The admission play profile is a guide for *initial* nursing intervention.

After the profile is determined, a plan for play is developed jointly by the parents, child, and nurse. The plan is implemented and the child's response to it is recorded. Observation of the child's behavior may validate the nurse's expectations or it may indicate that the play program needs modification.

It is a well-known fact that play behavior will change as the child's condition either improves or deteriorates. Change in play may result from the child's increasing maturation as he grows older. (This is particularly significant when children are hospitalized for a period of months.) Play behavior may also reflect everyday experiences as well as special hospital events such as surgery or transfer to another unit. Consequently, the play profile should be reassessed periodically during the hospitalization. The new profile is not derived from a history-taking process but from the nurse's own observations of the child at play. Others who have participated in the child's play add their contributions as well. The nurse then compares the new observations with the previous profile. She may find that a child who manifested aggressive behavior at the time of admission is now tending to withdraw from social contacts. The circumstances surrounding this behavior will need careful interpretation and play stimuli may need to be altered to encourage more free expression. A reassessment of an infant's play experience might reveal that a baby hospitalized for one month has gained sufficient eye-hand skill to benefit from block play. The profile in many such instances can become a tool that draws attention to the subtle clues that indicate learning readiness.

While the child is in the hospital, the profile should be available to all who care for him. Persons (including the parents) who have significant information about the child's play should be encouraged to make notations. Productive ideas can be lost through ineffective communication. Someone's good idea can generate many new ways of approaching a particular problem. However, to avoid a "hodgepodge" of information, some *one* person—such as the team leader—should oversee the plan and coordinate activities. It should be her *special* responsibility to see that play becomes a meaningful part of nursing care. Realistically, this nurse cannot note the play behavior of all of her young patients. It is not necessary that she do so. If members of her nursing team are knowledgeable about how to encourage ordinary play and what to observe about it, the team leader can direct attention to those "high-risk" children who are more likely to have potential play problems. These youngsters could be categorized into four major groups.

In the first group are those children who are mentally retarded or mentally superior. The nature and quantity of stimuli will be quite different for these children since they must keep pace with the child's maturational readiness rather than chronological age. A second group would consist of children who demonstrate psychosocial limitations in the style of their play. These children will benefit from carefully selected play materials that specifically encourage every energy release as well as interpersonal contacts that reflect awareness of the child's defense mechanisms. Children who have had or who are about to experience stressful situations comprise the third group. Play can serve as an excellent tool to prepare a child for an unpleasant event and, of course, the content of play afterwards may reveal feelings about the experience that cannot be expressed in other ways. A fourth "high-risk" group are those children with kinds of physical handicaps that could be improved through the judicious use of play. For example, the spastic hands of an infant with cerebral palsy might open more easily if the baby can support his weight in the prone position. Placing toys within reach or hanging a jingly mobile in his view will add to his enjoyment and encourage him to sustain the prone position.

Since these children have such special play needs, the nurse must rely on other members of the health team for guidance in selecting effective methods of stimulation. The occupational, physical, and recreational therapists are important consultants. In unusual circumstances in which the child's behavior reveals deep-seated conflict, a psychiatric consultant becomes necessary. A reciprocal relationship among the team members is essential if the child is to benefit from these people's individual talents. A "meshing" of goals will assure that the child will be looked at as a totality. A consistent approach must be used 24 hours a day—not just during the hours that the therapist is present.

When the child is about to leave the hospital, the play profile can become a constructive adjunct to the discharge teaching plan. The content of the profile can provide practical guidelines to parents as they anticipate convalescent play. The nurse can use the tool to illustrate how the child can be expected to behave at home. (More specific ways that the nurse can assist parents will follow in another section of this chapter.)

The discharge profile should not be discarded. It should become part of the child's record so that it can be used in a comparative manner when the child visits the clinic or is readmitted to the hospital.

Significant information from the play profile should be included when referral is made to the community health nurse so that she can provide continuity in the constructive use of play for a particular child. The community health nurse is in the enviable position of seeing the child in the home environment, where she can assess resources and suggest reasonable improvisations. She can encourage the parents, and the child if he is old enough, to compile their own profile periodically. If the whole family takes a purposeful look at play activities, their collective creativity will certainly enrich the sick child's experiences. If and when the child returns to the hospital for continued treatment, the community health nurse offers input to the admission profile—in effect, the cycle repeats itself.

The precise format of the assessment tool is not essential to its success. Many different styles can be effectively used. There is no magic arrangement of lines and boxes. The nursing staff should develop a tool to suit their own needs, the needs of the specific pediatric population that they are serving, and the needs of their particular agency. The format that is devised, however, should reflect consideration of conciseness in recording and an easy way of making changes in plans whenever necessary. If the tool is highly complicated or too time-consuming for practical use, its benefits are not appreciated. And, of course, experience dictates that when an idea fails it takes doubly long to generate enthusiasm to revive it.

For purposes of illustration, consider the following situation:

> Karen E., better known as Kari, was admitted to the pediatric unit for an open reduction of a congenitally dislocated hip that had responded poorly to conservative treatment. This girl

NAME ___Karen E. (Kari)___ AGE ___3½ YRS.___ DIAGNOSIS

CONGENITAL DISLOCATION
RIGHT HIP — CYSTITIS

PROFILE   6/1

MATERIALS – wagon, play furniture, turtle, sunglasses, rag doll *, dress-up hat

PARTNERS – parents, occasional contact with same age cousins

PLAY AREA – backyard, kitchen, bedroom (restricted in other areas of house)

STYLE – timid, watches others, not an easy joiner, long attention span, solitary play

SCHEDULE – plays midmorning, early afternoon, 2 hr. nap between 2 and 4 P.M., needs quiet time before meals

BEDTIME – prayers, rag doll in bed, sleeps in prone position (head of bed elevated)

MISC.

* CHILD HAS ITEM IN HOSPITAL

PLAN   6/1

LIMITATIONS DUE TO ILLNESS

bed rest, blood drawn each morning, fatigues easily, spica cast

Father to bring in sunglasses and hat

Wooden blocks and miniature doll play (while prone) – use doctor, nurse, child figures

Finger painting

Play with one agemate (Linda)

Water play during bath (plastic cover for cast)

Rest period in AM

Story or puzzle before meals

Bedtime prayers

Rag doll in easy reach

RESPONSE   6/2

Sunglasses in view on bedside stand. Wore hat during all dramatic play. In doll play, child doll frequently punished by doctor doll – only verbally. Very absorbed in this play.

Dabbed in paints with finger tip – wanted painting saved for mother

Parallel play with Linda – no verbal communication

Loves Magic Bunny story

Wants nurse to pray with her – "Now I lay Me Down to Sleep", goes to sleep quickly – mother not present

ADMISSION PLAY PROFILE   INITIAL PLAN FOR PLAY   RESPONSE TO PLAY

FIG. 22.   See text for explanation.

AGE __3½ yrs.__   DIAGNOSIS

PLAN 6/5	RESPONSE 6/6
LIMITATIONS DUE TO ILLNESS	Long attention to blocks
Spica cast, out of bed as tolerated, surgery planned 6/8	Shortly before leaving playroom, pushed herself to oven and opened it – said " I could cook you in here." then proudly rolled herself to her room
Playroom midmorning and early afternoon – self-propelled on dolly. Free play on floor – wooden blocks, pots and pans	
Doll figures – family and hospital doctor kit and casted doll (begin prep. for OR 6/6)	Explored every piece of doctor kit. Tried on mask. Showed to mother (prep. plan discussed with mother)
Finger painting with paper on floor	
Music with other children	Loved record player and shakers
Doctor kit in bed (add mask to kit)	
Continue story before meals	More resistive about going to sleep. Mother willing to stay until settled.
Nighttime prayers – doll in bed	

KARI'S REVISED PLAN
FOR PLAY

REPLACES
INITIAL
PLAN
FOR
PLAY

FIG. 23.   See text for explanation.

77

NAME — MARSHA B. — AGE — 11 YRS. — DIAGNOSIS RHEU...

NAME — TONY A. — AGE — 16 YRS. — DIAGNOSIS HYPERTHYROIDISM

RESPONSE

PROFILE (Marsha B.)

MATERIALS – plays piano, knits *, leaning chair *, doll collection

PARTNERS – clique of girl friends – 2 close pals, Cs and Beth, belongs to Scouts 2 younger siblings

PLAY AREA – neighborhood school, playground near home

STYLE – gregarious but enjoys solitary activities, moody when doesn't get own way, impatient

SCHEDULE – school 8 & 4, home-work after dinner, play Fri. eve, Sat. and Sun. afternoon

BEDTIME – "out like a light" 10–10:30 PM

MISC. – has a 10 day old sister

* CHILD HAS ITEM IN HOSPITAL

PROFILE (Tony A.)

MATERIALS – shoots pool, tinkers with cars, collection of model stock cars, jazz * radio * "the gang"

PARTNERS – (no special friend)

PLAY AREA – gas station, pool hall

STYLE – can't sit still, drums fingers constantly, "I'm always on the run"

SCHEDULE – no schedule "anytime I feel like it"

BEDTIME – never "socks out" before 1–2 AM

MISC. – dropped out of school last year

* CHILD HAS ITEM IN HOSPITAL

PLAN

LIMITATIONS DUE TO ILLNESS

out of bed as desired
BMR 7/2

Find pool partner. Check with play therapist about best times to play

Encourage him to help Jimmy make his car models

May like to make a card to send to guys at station

Short feature story about stock cars for newsltr. Let races for newsltr. to suggest it "editor of week"

Late night reading – sports magazine, transistor radio. Car button for transistor radio (no stimulation before BMR)

FIG. 24. See text for explanation.

of three-and-a-half had been in a double leg cast for three months prior to the admission. On the day following her arrival in the hospital, Kari developed symptoms of cystitis. The anticipated surgery was delayed until recovery from the urinary tract infection was complete. Kari was an only child who lived with her parents in an isolated rural area. Her mother stayed in a nearby motel to be with her during the hospitalization. Her favored play materials at the time of admission were a rag doll which she brought with her and a pair of green sunglasses that her grandmother had given her the week before. Unfortunately, the glasses were forgotten in the excitement of coming to the hospital. Her father brought along the low, wheeled platform that he had constructed so that Kari could scoot easily around the house. Figure 22 is the admission play profile, the initial plan for play, and Kari's response. The revised plan based on the same profile but reflecting her changing needs is illustrated in Fig. 23. (Figure 24 shows how the same basic format can be adapted to suit the needs of children of different ages.)

Problems of Immobility

Some restriction in normal activity is witnessed during the treatment of many long-term illnesses in childhood. For some children, restriction may be minimal, requiring only additional rest periods. Other boys and girls experience complete change from the customary way of living due to prolonged periods of bed rest or complete immobilization of part of the body.

Freedom of body movement has special significance during every stage of childhood. The infant responds to internal stirrings by random but satisfying body movements. It is a great achievement for the toddler to assume an upright posture (Fig. 25). The preschool child uses his body as a primary mode of expressing his feelings. The school-age child concentrates on precision and skill in manipulation and locomotion activities through which he gains acceptance in his peer group. The adolescent heartily applauds competitive sports which demand speed and agility. Thus many measures of personal achievement and self-satisfaction are derived from one's ability to move about without constraint.

Curtailment of activity introduces a high degree of frustration. Feelings of helplessness and rage are common accompaniments. The thwarting of the biological urge for activity is a highly charged situation from an emotional point of view. Several factors contribute to this emotional upheaval.

Physical constraint brings with it enforced dependency. The child's feelings may be quite ambivalent. Since he is ill, he knows that his own resources are inadequate to meet his needs, yet he will fight vigorously to retain his autonomy. The threat of regression heightens anxiety and the whole cycle perpetuates itself. The child worries about this dependency. The specific worry varies a great deal from one child to another. Some children may be concerned about not being able to play;

FIG. 25. The expression on this toddler's face reveals the excitement that freedom of mobility arouses. (Courtesy of Children's Hospital of Buffalo, New York.)

others worry about such practical matters as who will bring their food. I can recall several older children confined in body casts who expressed sophisticated concern about their safety. They queried "What will happen to me if this place burns down? How can I get out?"

The immobilized child is in a very vulnerable position. He cannot remove himself to a more protected environment. At times he may be able to do no more than turn his face toward the wall. He cannot fight to retain what he thinks is his. Indeed, he is in a precarious spot. The significant elements of power and self-control that mobility brings are notably undermined by restraint.

One primary function of movement is self-expression, and for the immobilized child this avenue of expression is limited. Physical activity is often an acceptable and satisfying way of "letting off steam." The "jumping for joy" phenomenon is well-known. Curtailed from this kind of expression, the immobilized child must rely on language to express strong emotions. Depending on the child's age, this might be a rather inefficient system of communication. For example, the preschool child finds himself in a special predicament because his language skills are not well-developed. Under ordinary circumstances the child in the preverbal stage helps himself by reverting to physical forms of acting out his frustrations—he stomps, bites, and kicks. He is simply not sophisticated enough to express strong emotions verbally. Consequently, not only does the immobilization impose a physical restriction on him but there are verbal restraints as well.

Immobility may be accompanied by social isolation. Social experiences differ in kind and duration. These children have greater difficulty seeking out friends and are restricted in the degree to which they are physically able to participate in group activities. Their social contacts are often limited to those who take the initiative to visit them. The duration of their friendships is subject to chance. Discharge from the hospital, transfer to other units, and the possibility of death may intervene to sever social ties.

These are just a few of many reasons why play is an essential aspect of care for these youngsters. There is no doubt that these children can enjoy a variety of play materials. However, I will emphasize in a special way those materials that involve freedom of movement. It is essential that the characteristic of movement be given high priority in planning any play program, but especially programs for children whose immobility clearly points to a need for an expressive outlet. In this section. I will explore the benefits to be derived from painting and music, both of which are stimuli for body movement.

ART.   Art is an excellent method of widening the range of human experiences and, at the same time, it demands exercise of a motor skill. Children's art is being studied with increasing interest—both in terms of its form and its content (Alschuler and Hattwick, 1947; Dennis, 1966; Kellog, 1967; Di Leo, 1970). Although the artistic endeavors of children can be quite revealing, accurate interpretation of symbolic content is a complex matter requiring highly specialized educational preparation. I wish to emphasize the "feeling" outcomes derived from the process of painting.

Painting and drawing require only the simplest of materials but the use of them brings rich rewards. For the very young child, the crayons, paint, plain paper, and brushes are objects to explore and nothing more. It is fun to try out new experiences. Di Leo (1970) calls this the kinesthetic stage. It is the muscular element that predominates in the scribbling done by the young child. The scribbler is not trying to give us magic insight into his conflicts but rather is interested in transferring body movements to paper. As the child does this, an observer becomes aware of expressions of joy, rhythm, vitality, and relaxation. The child derives pleasure from putting something where nothing existed before. That is why the nurse should expect the young child to paint his hands and apron as well as the paper or repeatedly to stab the brush into the paint just to make a splash. Most certainly, the young child has no intent to draw a representational object. He is helplessly confused and discouraged by the nurse whose first question is: "What is that?" The child is not being coy by refusing to answer; he doesn't know what it is either! By rewarding only drawing that conform to adult standards of excellence, the nurse is imposing a mental restriction just as confining as the immobilization itself.

Later, in the preschool period, a child's painting may reflect emotions that cannot yet be translated into words. Painting can provide

FIG. 26. A. This child is hiding behind a tilted table that provides a convenient play surface for an immobilized child. B. On the other side of the table, an artist is at work. Still clutching her mother's finger with one hand, she is gradually "moving out" to express herself in green paint.

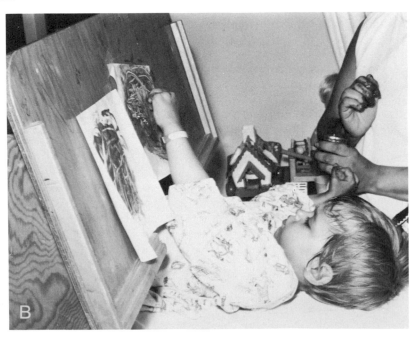

emotional release and yet the child does not fear that his adventure with the media will weaken his defenses—nor does he have to tell someone about his problems. It is not unusual for a shy, inhibited child to show much more expression during painting sessions than is evident during other activities. The child who is angry or resentful about his confinement can use artful means of expressing his discontent. Art serves as a good catharsis and permits him to advance to more mature forms of behavior. It gives the aggressive child an outlet for less-dangerous-than-other forms of explosive behavior (Fig. 26A and 26B).

Not every child will respond to the media in the same way. Take finger painting as an example. As you well know, some children literally put their whole selves into the art. Other children are anxious to wash their "dirty" hands. It is conceivable that such a difference in response may not reflect a deep-seated psychological problem on the part of the more inhibited child but rather may simply be a function of the child's social environment. Reaction to finger painting was studied in a small sample of middle- and lower-class children (Alper, 1955). The middle-class children showed a lower tolerance for getting dirty, for staying dirty, and for products they produced while they were dirty. They took a longer time to select colors of paint and to begin painting and tended to mutilate their paintings more than did the group of lower-class children. This study reminds us to be aware that not all children have the same degree of enthusiasm about commonly used play materials. Some children will need a longer "warm-up" period before they can utilize the media's full potential. If the child is hesitant to dip his fingers into paint, he can be encouraged to spread his paint with a brush at first. The greater distance between the child and the paint may permit him to become accustomed to the "messy" paint more gradually.

The school-age child has special characteristics that favor the use of graphic materials. He is capable of concentrated effort and has good mastery of the media (Fig. 27). Yet, since defenses are not fully established, paintings may reveal conflicts as the children tell their stories. Often however, the children are "self-protective" enough to describe their stories in disguised forms. Since the older child has a better understanding of the use of a variety of materials he should be encouraged to try more sophisticated graphic techniques such as collage and papier maché.

Art can be a good medium for social interaction. Children have a "feel" for each other's art and, when painting together, they can express their understanding verbally and nonverbally. Preschool children thoroughly enjoy painting with each other. They will often pause in their work to intently watch the actions of other "artists." Putting an easel on a cart between two beds stimulates verbal as well as motor activity.

Regardless of a child's age, one should remember that the child is not limited to painting what is actually visible. He can paint what he sees but he can also draw what he feels or knows. The best stimulus

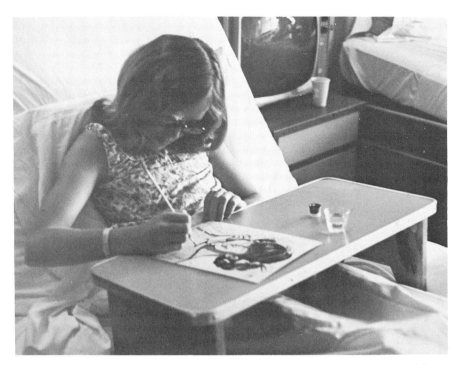

FIG. 27. The art of concentration. The fine detail of her work is satisfying to this adolescent who places a high premium on the quality of the finished product.

for this is a plain piece of paper and a crayon. Do not encourage a child to copy another image. Conformity stifles creativity.

Materials should be available whenever the child *needs* to use them—not just during specified periods of time. Restriction of time also restricts creativity. Everyone has a "best" time for work and play. A wide variety of paint colors is not necessary for the very young child but, with advancing age, selection of colors and experimentation with mixing them is part of the fun.

Inexpensive oilcloth or plastic bed covers and aprons or bibs will serve nicely as adequate protection against the "mess" that may result. Of course, some limits must be set but if they are known in advance children are usually understanding about the restriction. A large cardboard box with a few modifications makes a very sturdy easel (Fig. 28).

The nurse should make every effort to include the art medium in play since it might be the *only* way that a particular child can express his feelings—and besides, above all, painting is for *fun!*

MUSIC. Immobilized children have a special need for musical experiences; these activities, too, stimulate expansive body movements. The child can enjoy listening to music as well as making it. It has long been known that music induces relaxation in tense children and also has a beneficial effect on unhappy children. Since sick, con-

FIG, 28. This easel is so simple to construct that a pediatric unit should never be without one.

fined children are both anxious and unhappy, this should be reason enough to provide music for them. However, there are additional benefits. Music awakens the imagination. In response to exciting band music, for instance, children can mentally move to its rhythm. If the feet or legs are immobilized "marching arms" can be very expressive. A lilting melody can be accompanied by sweeping arm movements that simulate birds in flight. The child can add to his enjoyment by waving brightly colored silk scarves to the rhythm of the music. He not only enjoys the music but also the tactile pleasure of the silky scarf as it flows across his face and over his body. With the stimulus of appropriate musical accompaniment, children enjoy acting like trucks, planes, and animals and, in the process, benefit from exercise, body control, and movement. Finger plays like "Thumbolina" or "Incey, Wincey Spider" are also more exciting when done to music. For the child who cannot participate in such an active way, conversational records or those with simple lyrics can be listened to with great enjoyment.

A teenager can hardly be expected to tolerate immobilization without the aid of a stereo or radio. Keeping tempo with the beat by snapping fingers, shaking the shoulders, or wiggling the toes is a far cry from the optimum but it goes a long way toward making a bad situation somewhat manageable. Teenagers like their music loud. Unfortunately a hospital environment demands some restrictions on noise. Head sets for stereos and ear buttons for transistor radios do help this problem, but one should also consider the possibility of a music room in addition to a playroom or simply soundproofing the playroom. Even if it can accommodate only a few children it would be worthwhile. Its arrangement can be flexible enough to encompass a wide variety of uses when young musicians are not occupying it.

Music is a good stimulus for group interaction. If one patient can play an instrument, he can be the focus of a musical experience that many can enjoy. Today, a guitar is a passport anywhere. Music breaks down barriers to communication because everyone can participate in the activity in some way even if it is only to hum the melody (Fig. 29).

Musical instruments can be constructed easily. Drums and shakers can be made out of accessible materials such as tin cans and plastic bottles. Horseshoes suspended on a cord make good cymbals. Glasses filled with varying amounts of water produce interesting sounds and teach a science lesson at the same time. Having a modest collection of "real" but inexpensive instruments may provide an opportunity for a child who has not been initiated to the world of music to find a new interest. The record collection should be varied enough to satisfy the interests that a wide range of ages will demand. Young children enjoy band music and strong rhythms with full-bodied sounds. Repetitious lyrics and melodies encourage them to join in singing. (Incidentally, adult choices are not necessarily those of the children.) The teenager is the "pop," "rock," and "folk" fan and so the library also should include a collection of these albums. Of course, most adolescents have their own collection which they can be encouraged to share with their hospital agemates.

FIG. 29. These boys take their music seriously. Folk tunes can be good expressive outlets for youthful ideals and concerns.

Give the child freedom to respond to the music in a way that seems natural for him. Occasionally some direction may be necessary but generally most children will select a mode of expression that is peculiarly their own. They may even assume regressed but comfortable body postures and infantile activities like rocking and sucking. What is important is that the child respond in his own style.

In addition to providing the stimulus, the nurse can assist the child in another way—by her own active participation with the child. The child will be comfortable and more likely to throw himself into the activity if the nurse's spontaneity is evident. If she assumes the role of spectator, she places a restraint on the child's activity. Her involvement is a key to the successful use of music.

While the points that I have mentioned have special relevance for immobilized children, all sick children should have opportunities to enjoy experiences with art and music. A further comment about the value of these media relates to their usefulness for nonEnglish-speaking children. These children often feel frustrated when they cannot make their needs understood. In a sense, art and music are universal languages through which they can express themselves in a manner similar to their peers. Both the nurses and the children may feel comfortable communicating via these media when the spoken word arouses confusion and anxiety.

The Nurse, The Parents, and Play

It has been repeatedly emphasized throughout this chapter that children enjoy play. It is a time when they are truly themselves. That parents and other family members participate in the enjoyment of play should be a foregone conclusion. However, it is likewise well-known that parental anxiety is increased when children are ill.

Many parental prerogatives are weakened or totally removed by the presence of an illness. Much of the "caring" component of the parental role is accomplished by specially educated professional persons. Because so much depends on doing the "right thing," parents become increasingly sensitive about the possible consequences of their actions.

For instance, they are uncertain about the limits of play. When asked about play during a clinic visit, I have heard them say "I wasn't sure that he could do that without becoming sick again," or "I didn't want to take any chances." This lack of confidence may be reflected in two courses of action: parents can be too visible to their child so that the child's personality development is squelched, or they can withdraw necessary support so that the child will learn to "stand on his own two feet." Both of these reactions can be different ways of manifesting anger, disappointment, guilt, fear, and helplessness.

If the illness is severe and has many observable signs, the parents' attention may be wholly directed towards the child's limitations. His assets, while certainly present, may be overlooked in the parents' grief and disillusionment. As a result, play deprivation may occur. The nurse can be instrumental in helping the parents evolve a positive viewpoint about play and, in so doing, revive interest in its beneficial outcomes (Fig. 30).

In speaking about the nurse in this section, I wish to make pointed reference to the fact that nurses in all settings—hospital, out-patient service, and community—can provide the support that I will describe. Each has a particular contribution to make by virtue of her position. (Hopefully, the future will see more nurses moving freely among all of these settings to better coordinate the child's care.) In the hospital, the nurse has the opportunity to observe play behavior over an extended period of time. The community nurse is in the position of seeing the

FIG. 30. Daddy is obviously enjoying this "little farmer's" play. A noninterfering, appreciative adult reinforces the child's "good feeling" about the arrangement of the animals.

child in his home setting where parental guidelines for play will have greatest practical significance. The clinic nurse, bridging the hospital and home, can evidence on-going interest in the child and note changes in play behavior occurring over time. Communication among these nurses is essential so that continuity in planning a meaningful play program can be achieved.

EVALUATION OF PLAY RESPONSES

What are some of the things that parents will find helpful? Realizing that play should be fun, many ask how they can know with some assurance that the child is really enjoying his play. There are some reliable clues. Watch for facial expression and body posture. Expression reveals absorption in the activity and the child who is enjoying his play is generally relaxed and moves his body freely. Listen for verbalization during play. Children will use all avenues of expression to convey excitement and pleasure. Parents who are good listeners encourage play simply by giving a sympathetic, interested ear to the descriptions of the "great things" their children do or imagine themselves doing. Look for indications of pride in accomplishments and be alert to assure that there are more successes in play than failures. Note how much adult assistance is required. If parental presence is needed a great deal of the time, look to see whether the complexity of the activity exceeds the child's capabilities or whether it simply reflects the child's need for the personal presence of a supportive adult. If the latter explanation seems accurate, perhaps the play should be interrupted so that the parent can stay with the child for a while. This will reduce the energy expended to call someone every few minutes. A short period of undivided concentration on the child's primary concerns can provide the child just enough support and encouragement to enable him to proceed on his own to independent play. Time and effort is saved in the long-run for both child and parent. Also, note whether play is restless or aimless. This may indicate that the child is not ready to play, has too much to play with, or, possibly, too little stimulation.

Parents can expect this age-old rainy-day question from their children: "What can I do now?" The question certainly poses a challenge to parents, especially since play options will be somewhat hampered by the child's illness. Helping the parent to select play experiences that are balanced in scope is important. A bit of preplanning does not really limit the spontaneity of play. Look ahead for a month or so to see if there are any special events. Perhaps a holiday, a birthday, a visit of a relative, or a family excursion is forthcoming. The child who is ill must have his activity properly paced so that he is not stretched beyond the limits of his endurance. If one month contains a birthday and a holiday, perhaps the family excursion could be planned for a less busy time. Preplanning helps in another way, too. It provides a wellspring of ideas for play activities. If a holiday is coming, some activity to prepare for it might appeal to the child; if daddy's birthday is on the horizon, the child can make plans for the celebration or even make his "present." The parents should know that periods of quiet play should alternate with physically active play so that release of tension can be accommodated. The aspect of finding an aggressive outlet for the child often presents a major problem for parents. They do not always realize that anger, hostility, and fear are normal responses to the frustrations of illness. Materials such as clay, paint, pounding boards, and punching bags are good for draining off excess energies.

SELECTION OF PLAY MATERIALS

Criteria for selection of play materials can be useful information for the parents. Qualities of safety, durability, washability, color, and appropriate size and weight should be emphasized. Consideration of family resources must take high priority in this matter. Reasonable suggestions are fine but unrealistic expectations are likely to meet with understandable resistance, since they make the parents feel inadequate to satisfy the child's needs. If guilt is already a problem, this merely magnifies it. Stress the idea of constructing toys from available household materials. Many parents feel that a toy is not a good one unless it comes from a toy store. Actually, simple household materials can bring many hours of delight to the child. Pots and pans, plastic bottles, spools, pieces of linoleum and rugs, sewing remnants, and discarded clothing provide endless opportunities for imaginative play. Making play materials also gives the parents something constructive to *do* for their child when other avenues of "caring" may be thwarted because of illness.

FAMILY PARTICIPATION IN PLAY

Parents of a child with a long-term illness often need to be reminded that the child will be returning to a *family*. Therefore, he should have a visible role to play in family life and should share in family responsibilities. Participation in family-centered activities may require a rearrangement of space and furnishings to permit accessibility to the conduct of family affairs both indoors and out. A child who is confined to an upstairs bedroom misses a good deal of the interaction.

A child whose activity is grossly and permanently limited will place many strenuous demands on all members of the family. The child will consume an extraordinary amount of time and space and will tax the emotional reserves of the family. If serious social and economic constraints are also present, the stress is proportionately greater. However, although some of the problems will exist in the best of circumstances, satisfying outcomes can result.

Sibling acceptance of a child's handicap will affect how the ill child views himself. Unless the brothers and sisters are given assistance in coping, siblings may be uncomfortable in the presence of a sick child either because of the way he looks or acts or because they are afraid of the illness itself. It is not always easy to find common interests for them to share. Yet a mutually satisfying experience is absolutely necessary for the child's integration into the family unit. The shared activity does not have to be elaborate but all members must have significant input. For example, each of the children could select a dinner menu each week or, on occasion, the whole family could participate in preparing a meal. The bedbound child might make the placemats, shell peas, or peel the potatoes. The well child's responsibility might be the arrangement and serving of the dinner for the sick brother or sister. It can be an exciting and festive occasion with lots of opportunity for creativity for all involved. Another idea might be to have a continuing "art exhibit." All the children can use graphic materials in their own way and then display them in some visible area. Paintings can be exchanged so that brothers and sisters can "exhibit" each other's work. This encourages appreciation of their individuality.

A child whose mental ability is grossly below that of his siblings or whose physical movements are bizarre presents an added challenge. One such child, who had cerebral palsy with multiple handicaps, was learning elements of balance and equilibrium. It was suggested that he roll around the yard in the center of a large cylinder. His brother and sister really enjoyed their participation in this activity of tumbling him round and round. The handicapped child obviously enjoyed the fun and the siblings felt satisfied that they were a part of his laughter. Family members themselves may come up with many more ideas if they are encouraged to do so. Persistence in the face of discouragement pays in this significant area of family play.

The reality of the illness sometimes remains obscure to family members. Consequently the child's real limitations may not be fully realized. For example, I met a 13-year-old with rheumatic heart disease when the girl visited the clinic for a reevaluation of her condition. In response to queries about her play, she quickly replied that she didn't have time for play. She was too busy cooking and cleaning. As it happened, she lived with an elderly infirm grandmother and four younger brothers. Since she was the eldest child and had assumed this responsibility before her illness, she returned to the customary role, since, to all appearances, she seemed well.

The nurse can also be instrumental in encouraging play experiences outside of the family. Peer relationships are important to children, so when close friendships have formed during a hospital stay, it might be beneficial to sustain them. Make sure that the parents are aware of the new chum and know how he can be contacted. Also, parents are not always aware that organized groups such as Scouts and 4H clubs can adapt activities for chronically ill children. The child's participation in such groups, even though limited, is ego-supporting and socially beneficial.

Incidentally, school activities, though not strictly in the province of play, must not be overlooked nor should the family overlook the services of the school nurse. Parents can be encouraged to use the assessment tool previously described. Using the listed categories as guidelines, the parents can periodically observe their child at play and when the nurse makes her visit they can describe the positive outcomes and point more clearly to the problems that still seem to exist. The use of the profile is an aid to memory and reinforces the important role that play should be assuming in the child's way of life.

Overall, it is important to realize that not all parents have an intuitive feel about children's play. They will appreciate some concrete suggestions. To be most helpful, the nurse must convey to the parents that she has confidence in their ability to meet the child's needs. She must respect their own personal resources and the sincerity of their efforts. The nurse must also be convinced about her own ability to offer worthwhile guidelines but she must be flexible enough not to cling tenaciously to *her* plan. Perhaps the most valuable contribution that she can make is to help the parents feel a genuine respect for the creative urge that exists in every child and for the freedom of expression that the creative urge demands. This represents the child's most important "play right."

Summary

Children learn about themselves and the world in which they live through intense involvement in play. They discharge physical energy while enjoying pleasantly satisfying sensory experiences; they expand and intensify social relationships; they explore the environment while actively manipulating materials in creative ways. Play is a freely chosen activity that, above all, is fun.

Each child has a style of play that is uniquely his own. Factors such as age, past experience, degree of physical limitation, and suitability of environment influences the way in which a child plays.

When a child faces a stressful experience, such as illness or hospitalization, he can work out many of his concerns and frustrations through the medium of play. He can recreate situations that aroused anxiety under circumstances in which he has control. Play can be used in preparing a child for a new experience. And, of course, play can simply be fun-filled activities that occupy the many hours of confinement that illness implies.

The nurse who hopes to meet the physical and psychological needs of her young patients must understand the child's view of play. Play behavior becomes an important part of the nursing assessment of the young patient.

In order to satisfy the child's play needs, the nurse must know what materials the child likes to use, who his play companions are, where and when he prefers to play, and the kinds of interactions that typify his play. By learning about the child's style of play, the nurse will be able to provide a rich play environment that will be a pleasurable experience for the child and will also serve to relieve the stress of illness and hospitalization. The nurse's role extends beyond the child to include the parents since play is an ongoing activity that is useful and necessary during every stage of illness—including convalescence.

Play is a major resource for resolution of the psychological conflicts that accompany illness. Provision of appropriate opportunities for play encourage intellectual and creative abilities that will help the child to cope with his illness in a constructive way.

If the nurse is impressed with the importance of play and sees that her convictions are expressed in operational terms, she can be instrumental in adding a dimension of enjoyment and learning to the lives of children under her care.

References

Alper, T., Blane, H., and Abrams, B. Reactions to finger painting as a function of social class. J. Soc. Abnorm, Psychol., 51:439–448, 1955.

Alschuler, R. H., and Hattwick, L. W. Painting and Personality: A Study of Young Children. Chicago, University of Chicago Press, 1947.

Barton, P. H. Play as a Tool of Nursing. Nursing Outlook, 10:162–164, 1962.

Blake, F. The Child, His Parents and the Nurse, Philadelphia, Lippincott, 1954.

———— Immobilized youth—a Rationale for supportive nursing intervention. Am. J. Nursing, 69:2364–2369, 1969.

Caillois, R. Man, Play and Games, Barash, M., trans. New York, Free Press of Glencoe, 1961.

Call, J. D. Games babies play. Psychology Today, 3:34–37+, 1970.

———— and Marschak, M. Styles and Games in Infancy. J. Am. Acad. Child Psychiat., 5:193–210, 1966.

De Nevi, D. Fantasy and creativity. Child and Family, 6:23–27, 1967.

Dennis, W. Group Values Through Children's Drawings. New York, Wiley, 1966.

———— Infant reactions to restraint. (Abridged from Trans. N. Y. Acad. Sci., 2:202–217, 1940.) In Dennis W., ed. Readings in Child Psychology, 2nd ed. Englewood Cliffs, N. J., Prentice Hall, 1963.

Di Leo, J. H. Young Children and Their Drawings. New York, Brunner/Mazel Publishers, 1970.

Erikson, E. H. Childhood and Society, 2nd ed. New York, Norton, 1963.

Erickson, F. H. Play Interviews for Four-Year-Old Hospitalized Children. Monographs of the Society for Research in Child Development, Inc. 23:No. 3, 1958.

Frailberg, S. The Magic Years. New York, Scribner's, 1959.

Fink, P. J., Goldman, M. J., and Levich, M. F. Art therapy—a new discipline. Pennsylvania Med., 70:61–66, 1967.

Friedenberg, E. Z. The Vanishing Adolescent. New York, Dell, 1959.

Gallagher, J. R. Medical Care of the Adolescent, 2nd ed. New York, Appleton-Century-Crofts, 1966.

Gilmore, J. B. Role of anxiety and cognitive factors in children's play behavior. Child Devel., 37:397–416, 1966.

Goldberg, S., and Lewis, M. Play behavior in the year-old infant: early sex differences. Child Devel., 40:21–31, 1969.

Groos, K. The Play of Man. New York, D. Appleton and Company, 1901.

Hartley, R., Frank, L. K., and Goldenson, R. M. New Play Experiences for Children. New York, Columbia University Press, 1952.

Hartley, R. E., Frank, L. K., and Goldenson, R. M. Understanding Children's Play. New York, Columbia University Press, 1952.

———— and Goldenson, R. M. The Complete Book of Children's Play. New York, Crowell, 1963.

Havighurst, R. J. Developmental Tasks and Education. New York, McKay, 1952.

Huizinga, J. Homoludens: A Study of the Play-Element in Culture. New York, Roy Publishers, 1950.

Jersild, A. T. The Psychology of Adolescence, 2nd ed. New York, Macmillan, 1963.

Jolly, H. Play is work: the role of play for sick and healthy children. Lancet 2:487–488, 1969.

Josselyn, I. M. The Adolescent and His World. New York, Family Services Assoc. of America, 1952.

Kellog, R. The Psychology of Children's Art. New York, Random House, 1967.

Kramer, E. Art Therapy in a Children's Community. Springfield, Ill., Charles C Thomas, 1958.

Lewis, H., ed. Child Art: The Beginnings of Self-Affirmation, Berkeley, Calif., Diablo Press, 1966.

Lowenfeld, M. Play in Childhood. New York, Wiley, Inc., 1967.

Marcus, I. M. Costume play therapy—the exploration of a method for stimulating imaginative play in older children. J. Am. Acad. Child Psychiat., 5:441–452, 1966.

Matterson, E. M. Play and Playthings for the Pre-school Child. Baltimore, Penguin Books, 1967.

Maurer, A. The Game of Peek-a-Boo. Dis. Nervous System, 28:118–121, 1967.

Morgenstern, F. S. Facilities for children's play in hospitals. Develop. Med. Child Neurol., 10:111–114, 1968.

———— Psychological Handicaps in the Play of Handicapped Children. Develop. Med. Child Neurol., 10:115–20, 1968.

Noble, E. Play and the Sick Child. London, Faber and Faber, 1967.

Opie, I., and Opie, P. The Lore and Language of School Children. London, Oxford University Press, 1959.

Piaget, J. Play, Dreams and Imitation in Childhood, Cattegno, C., and Hodgson, F. M., trans. New York, Norton, 1962.

———— and Inhelder, B. The Psychology of the Child, New York, Basic Books, 1969.

Pickard, P. M. The Activity of Children. London, Longmans, Green, 1965.

Pickett, L. K. The hospital environment for the pediatric surgical patient. Pediat. Clin. N. A., 16:531–542, 1969.

Rahner, H. Man at Play. New York, Herder and Herder, 1967.

Sapora, A. V., and Mitchell, E. D. The Theory of Play and Recreation, 3rd ed. New York, Ronald Press, 1961.

Schiller, F. Essays, Aesthetical and Philosophical. London, George Bell, 1875.

Slovenko, R., and Knight, J. A., eds. Motivations in Play, Games and Sports. Springfield, Ill., Charles C Thomas, 1967.

Spencer, H. Principles of Psychology. New York, D. Appleton and Company, 1873.

Stone, L. J., and Church, J. Childhood and Adolescence, 2nd ed. New York, Random House, 1968.

Takata, N. The Play History. Am. J. Occup. Therapy, 23:314–318, 1969.

Torrance, E. P. Constructive Behavior: Stress, Personality and Mental Health. Belmont, Calif., Wadsworth, 1965.

——— Problems of Highly Creative Children. Gifted Child Quart., 5:31–34, 1961.

Winnicott, D. W. Playing: Its Theoretical Status in the Clinical Situation. Int. J. Psyscho-Analysis, 49:591–599, 1968.

3 SHIRLEY STEELE

General Ideas in Relation to Long-Term Illness in Childhood

The child with a long-term illness can be a real challenge to nurses, as well as other medical personnel and to his family. The child develops some unique qualities which are formulated as a result of living with an illness.

In planning nursing care, the student should keep in mind that these factors will influence the overall plan of care. Too frequently nurses have a tendency to respond only to immediate pressures rather than planning care to incorporate expected behaviors. Some of these expected behaviors are included in this chapter for your consideration and utilization in planning and executing patient care.

PROFILE OF THE CHILD. The child with a long-term illness is more likely to want to know the nurse's name. He very often prefers to call the nurses by their first names. However, he will abide by the customs of the institutions.

He also expects everyone to know his name and he delights in showing the other children how popular he is.

He is well aware of his rights on the hospital unit. He is often very authoritative when demanding or asking for things. He frequently finds a very prominent place, such as the nurses' station, to spend a great deal of his day. Another favorite spot is by the elevator, where he can watch everyone get off and on. If there is an acutely ill child on the unit, he frequently guards that door to learn all he can about what is going on.

HOSPITAL VOCABULARY. The child who is hospitalized a great deal develops a hospital vocabulary although he does not always know exactly what he is verbalizing. The terms may sound very convincing, but if you explore further with him he frequently does not really know what he is talking about. The child uses his hospital vocabulary to impress people. He especially likes to use it when new students of every discipline arrive. He uses terms like NPO, OR, and OT as though every child knows them. These terms are less impressive, however, than his very scientific-sounding description of his medical condition and its treatment.

Despite his apparent satisfaction gained from using hospital jargon when it meets his needs, he will pretend he does not understand you when you use it. An example is when you tell the school-age child he is NPO for blood work. The blood work is late and he gets hungry. He decides to eat a piece of candy from his bedside stand. When you ask him about it, he says you did not tell him he could not eat. You point out the NPO sign on his bed and he explains he does not understand what it means.

BREAKING THE RULES.   The child will also know the rules of the institution and frequently learns how to break them. He delights in "outsmarting" the authority figures, such as the nursing supervisors. He learns their schedules and plans his wayward activities around them. He soon learns that he can be mischievous without much chance of being caught. In his planning he usually uses children with less knowledge about hospital routines. He seems to feel that children who are less well-known are less likely to get reprimanded. His need to be independent and explore are usually met during these escapades.

An illustration follows. Ed was a teenager who was hospitalized for physical therapy and fitting of braces. During the early part of this hospitalization he was in a wheelchair. He was allowed up most of the day, with the exception of an enforced afternoon rest period and an early retiring time—much too early to meet the needs of the adolescent. Ed knew the time the evening supervisor made rounds. He knew the rounds were started at his end of the hall. He also knew it was rare to see the regular staff nurses for a few minutes following the supervisor's rounds. He mapped out a plan for the two school-age children in the next room to get out of bed immediately after the rounds and go across the hall and push the elevator button. (The elevator was frequently still there as the supervisor got off.) Ed quickly got himself into the wheelchair and scooted out to the open elevator. All three children went to the main lobby and wheeled around innocently exploring the area. Approximately 10 minutes later they entered the elevator and returned. Not much was accomplished by adult standards but for these children it was fun and exciting to "outsmart" the nurses. It was also fun to tell "understanding" adults about the excursion.

HOSPITAL ROUTINES.   The child also may become very involved with hospital routines and he may get quite upset when the routines are not carried out on schedule. He is used to having his wishes granted immediately because of the large number of helping adults surrounding him; when these wishes are not granted he may become very disturbed.

The child is quite aware of the treatments he should receive and he likes to direct the nurse with these procedures. As a means of manipulating his environment, he may refuse to have them done by certain individuals. Any deviation from the usual way of performing his treatment may result in great anxiety to the child. If he has had a tracheostomy for a long time he may prefer to suction and clean it himself. If the nurse attempts to do this it may result in any number of unfortunate circumstances. The child may also wish to have his parent perform his treatments to simulate his home routines as much as possible. The child with a long-term illness frequently is much more dependent on his parents than is the normal child.

TATTLING. The child also has a tendency to "tattle" on professionals. When you are doing his dressing he tells you: "Miss Jones did not use the forceps when handling the 4 x 4 dressings." He watches you eagerly to see if you react to this piece of information. If he gets a response he is likely to continue to tell you "items" whenever he has the opportunity.

He also spends a great deal of time "tattling" on other children. This should be discouraged so that the child does not begin to act as the unit "security officer." A certain amount of "tattling" is normal for children but it is easier to handle when the child is not hospitalized with so many people as the recipients of "information."

SEEKING INFORMATION. The child with a long-term illness also feels free to question how much you know about his particular problem. He has had a great deal of experience with people with varying degrees of competency and has learned to fear those who are least expert in the field. This is especially true in relation to blood work, injections, and other painful procedures. He likes and demands the most skillful person. This may present problems to the nursing student who is just learning child health nursing techniques and may show a degree of hesitancy.

PLACEMENT IN THE HOSPITAL. The child with a long-term illness may also develop a desire to be on a specific unit or in a specific room. He may be far less comfortable when put in an area which is not his choice. As he gets older it may be increasingly difficult to make him happy in his hospital placement. He may resent being in with toddlers or hearing them cry. As an adolescent, he frequently does not fit in with adult patients as he is often less mature than would be normal for his age. An adolescent unit would be ideal for meeting his needs. Conversely, sometimes a change in hospital placement results in an improvement in the child's behavior.

I am reminded of a child, Lenny, who had hemophilia. He was frequently hospitalized on a general pediatric unit. He was a "behavior problem" during much of his hospitalization. He knew all the personnel on the unit and the contribution each one made to his care, directly or indirectly. His hospitalizations were often "planned" to coincide with certain predictable changes in the staff. He would try to be admitted on or near the first of July when the medical house staff changed. He took great delight in "scaring" the new physicians. He knew the rotation schedule of the student nurses through the unit. He often had "an accident" so as to see a favorite student nurse before she rotated to a new unit. This type of abnormal and manipulative behavior was a definite pattern of this child's life style. (Unfortunately, there were many complicating factors, which I will not discuss here, that precluded psychiatric help for this child.)

The child continued this pattern during his school-age and early adolescent years. Despite several serious illnesses, he reached adolescence. He had an injury and needed hospitalization when the pediatric unit was filled to capacity. The decision was made to admit him to an adult unit. As he was cared for as a service patient, he was admitted to an adult area which frequently had the "sickest" patients. It was a busy time on this unit, and there was little opportunity to select the "best placement" for the adolescent. He was admitted to a four-bed room. As was his usual pattern he screamed loudly, as he was moved from the wheelchair to the bed. He started screaming about his incurable disease and how much better everyone else was in the hospital. At first, the other men frowned and felt sympathy as well as dismay at their new roommate. However, these patients were also quite ill and their impatience quickly overtook their immediate emotions. First one and then another complained quietly to the nursing personnel about their noisy roommate. The nurses tried, in vain, to control him. Then the doctors tried to quiet him, first by "friendly persuasion" and then by medication. All this failed. They called the nurses from the pediatric area to come to their aide. Lenny seemed to be happy to see them but he was acting much as he did on the pediatric area, so their presence did not improve the situation. It may have even worsened it! Lenny continued his plan to disrupt the unit and get attention. The other patients were becoming increasingly impatient. They began to yell back when Lenny yelled. They shouted "shut-up" or "quiet-down" and their booming voices startled Lenny. He was more used to a nurse suggesting he be quiet so as not to disturb the babies or other sick children. The shouts of the men were very similar to the commands he received from his alcoholic father. Lenny began to "settle in" and the men took increasing interest in him. His change to an adult area actually improved his mental status. His admissions to the hospital decreased and it would seem that Lenny had actually "grown-up" as a result of his change in the long-term care he received.

In the foregoing illustration the child seemed to have benefited from his change in medical environment. This is not always the case, however, and the child may have to undergo several different placements before he is able to adjust.

CHANGING HOSPITALS.   The child who has received medical supervision from a children's hospital may find it disturbing to be ineligible, by virtue of age, to continue with his familiar health care. On the other hand, some children with long-term illnesses are eager to change their care so they do not have to tell their friends they are going to a "children's hospital." The reputation of the facility in the community also has a bearing on how the child perceives it. This is especially significant to the adolescent. If the hospital has a positive program for adolescents, the child may be more content to continue going to it. If the adolescent is treated as a second-rate citizen, he may be eager to change.

AS A FAMILY MEMBER. A child who is hospitalized for long periods may have a very superficial idea of what it actually is to be a member of a family. He has frequent or long periods away from the family, which loosens his ties. The family may consider the child as a burden, financially or socially. They may use the periods of separation caused by hospitalization to recuperate from the strain caused by the long-term illness. This separation is often interpreted by the nursing personnel as lack of interest or even neglect. The staff, who has become very attached to the child, may become resentful of the family. This can result in a very poor nurse-parent relationship. The child gets in the middle of this and begins to try to get the staff to side more and more with him and create a bigger gap between the staff and his parents. The child then decides to ignore the parents when they do visit. The child's attitude makes the family further deny their importance to the child and their visits are made even less frequently.

PRIVACY. The child needs an area that he can identify as his own. The child with long-term illness does not feel so comfortable if he is moved frequently to "make room" for new admissions. There should be an area where he can have his private belongings and not worry that they will be moved when he is not present. He should be encouraged to clean his own area, and if the nurse needs to assist she should only do so with the child present.

POSSESSIONS. The child's possessions can be very important to him and their true significance is rarely appreciated by the nurse.

If any of the child's possessions are taken home by the family, it should be with the child's full knowledge. This will save a great deal of searching for missing objects.

SIMPLE CHORES. The child will also benefit by having simple chores which help him feel a part of the hospital. He may be expected to put the tablecloth on the table, or distribute the mail, or help compile new charts. If he has a chore it is important to insist that it is done. Also, the chores should be changed periodically so he does not become bored. He may request certain tasks to do but he easily tires of them. Competition with other children with long-term illness may be healthy. Children are used to competition and it can be beneficial if the child is not consistently the loser. He needs to have some positive experiences in order to be willing to become involved in competition.

HANDLING MONEY. The child will also need help in learning to handle money. He has fewer chances than the "normal" child to spend money. If he is hospitalized for long periods, he should have an allowance like his peers. This is especially important for the late school-age child and the adolescent. They can use their money to buy newspapers, magazines, or small purchases in the gift shop. If they are interested they may buy supplies and make small articles to sell or give as gifts. The child will not always buy wisely, but this is also part of the learning experience. The child should not be allowed to "solicit" money from visitors. This will establish a pattern which is difficult to break. The child needs to know how to make his money "safe" and precautions should be taken to insure the money is not stolen.

SCHOOL.   School is an especially essential experience for the child with long-term illness. If there is no school provided in the setting, the nurse is responsible for setting aside a time for the child to do schoolwork. If it is not possible to get books from the child's teacher, books with very explicit directions are readily available in stores. The child should be encouraged to do an assignment a day. In addition there may be school activities such as drawing which will increase his interest. To study, the child needs an area comparatively free from distractions. It is usually more interesting if more than one child is studying together. This more closely assimilates an ordinary class situation.

CHURCH OR CHAPEL.   Depending on the institution, chapel or church services may or may not be easily accessible. Most institutions have an area provided for quiet meditation. However, many do not actually have church services conducted. If the child is used to attending Sunday school classes he will usually miss them. Inexpensive, illustrated books of children's prayer and hymns can provide a substitute. An area supplied with children's hymnals and an altar can also be made available for the children to hold their own church services. If the nurse feels comfortable participating with the children she should feel free to do so. The children enjoy learning simple hymns and prayers. These can also be said at bedtime either as a group or individually. In addition, representatives of major faiths are usually available to most institutions. Many church-affiliated hospitals have very active participation in the children's area. The parents will usually be helpful in contacting the religious advisor of their choice.

The adolescent may be able to leave the hospital and attend a local house of worship. This, of course, requires a doctor's approval.

ADMISSIONS OF OTHER CHILDREN.   Admissions of other children to the unit may pose a threat to the child. He may view them as infringing on his territory or his adopted family. The new child may require extensive care, and this cuts down on the time given the child with less acute problems. The new admission may also receive a great deal of parental attention as well as gifts, and this makes the child with a long-term illness further resent him. The child who has been there a long time may greet the new parents and he often will request gifts and favors from them. He learns that parents easily feel sorry for children who are hospitalized for long periods or children who do not have visitors. Frequently the child is able to manipulate the parents so much that they have difficulty visiting with their own child. The parents may feel obligated to bring gifts of toys and food to the child. This often complicates the nurse's role as she tries to discipline the child or maintain a therapeutic diet. The parent who becomes involved with long-term children on the unit may need to be consulted and informed about the needs of the child with the long-term illness. This consulting need not be considered as a violation of the child's privacy. It is rather a necessary part of the medical and nursing supervision needed to guarantee the best possible care to the child who is hospitalized for long periods.

I can best illustrate with an example. John was 12 years old when he was diagnosed as having a malignant tumor. The medical plan was to have John receive radiation therapy. He lived in a shack in a rural area. The shack did not have running water or toilet facilities. It was not adequately heated and John shared a floor with several adults.

Because of poor transportation and the above conditions, John was hospitalized many months. The family did not visit him, and he was very lonely. He became friends with children of all ages. He helped the younger children accept bed-rest by spending time playing with them or getting them needed supplies. The children eagerly introduced their new friend to their parents. John was most appreciative of the attention he received. The parents began asking him about his family and they were amazed at the conditions John described. They often checked with the nursing staff to see if all John described was true. Then their next move was to buy things for John. This generosity confused John. He did not know how to respond. It was felt that the parents' gifts could be better spaced. When a parent asked about John the nurse took the opportunity to explain that he was not used to receiving gifts, and he actually did not use many that he received. The nurse suggested that if a parent wished to donate toys that they be used in the play area and John would benefit, mutually, with the other children. In this way, John did not have to wonder why he was being singled out to receive numerous unsolicited gifts from people he had just met.

If the parents were still interested in giving directly to John, a suggestion such as contributions to his holiday celebration or to his wardrobe may have helped to cut down on the daily contributions he received—thereby providing him with special surprises when the other children also received them. This would make the gifts seem more natural. Another practical suggestion would have been to have the parents send cards to John rather than gifts. Then he would receive mail, like the other children.

DISCHARGE OF OTHER CHILDREN. Discharges can also be a stress situation for the child. He sees children admitted after him returned to home, and he wishes he could be discharged. He also makes friends from within the hospital and his group relationships are broken each time a child is discharged. While he may long to go home, he may fear losing the security he feels in the hospital. The hospital may protect him against many of the inflictions he receives on the outside. This is especially so in relation to physically handicapped children who are stared at or made fun of in the outside world. They like the security of medical personnel who are not so likely to be "shocked" by their appearance.

ACTIVITIES OF DAILY LIVING.   The child who is hospitalized for long periods may lack many of the outside experiences of daily living. The child who is physically handicapped may be more deprived in this area, as even when he is sent home he may not receive enough stimulation and exposure to everyday happenings. Every attempt should be made to take these children out for walks or to give them weekend passes so they do not become completely deprived of normal experiences. Utilization of volunteers would be especially helpful in this area, as they offer another valuable aspect: they are not related to the medical or nursing profession.

VOLUNTEERS.   The volunteers utilized in the care of children with long-term illness should span the population. The grandmother or grandfather is as important as the young high-school student. The college student serves another function. The role of the sexes cannot be underestimated. The boy with a long-term illness needs male figures who do not constantly hurt or examine him. He needs the attention of healthy males with male roles to model after. He needs to see ordinary street wear of the male. He benefits by the male slang. Diversity is extremely important for both the girl and boy with long-term illness. They are exposed to more than the average amount of medical personnel, and it will take many nonmedical persons to balance this exposure.

STREET CLOTHES.   The child with a long-term illness may benefit from wearing his everyday street clothes as opposed to hospital garb or pajamas and robe. The more natural attire may make it easier for him to retain his contacts with the outside. It also helps the nursing staff and visitors relate to him in a more ordinary fashion. Somehow, the child seems "less sick" if he is up and dressed (see Fig. 1).

Wearing his own clothes will also give him a reason to look after his belongings, which more closely resembles his responsibilities at home. Throwing hospital clothes down the laundry chute each day does not encourage responsibility in the child. The child can be responsible for washing out his socks or small items. This may serve as his chore that we discussed earlier in the chapter.

HOBBIES.   The child can also be encouraged to continue with hobbies he had at home. Tropical or gold fish can easily be accommodated in his hospital unit. Children frequently respond quickly to new pets that are easily maintained in the hospital, such as turtles or hamsters. These smaller animals can sometimes take the place of the bigger, more familiar pets the children have at home.

Another means of supplying pets to children with long-term illness is to have a program similar to a lending library. The animal is brought in for a few hours from a veterinarian to visit in the playroom or hospital lobby. The animal is specifically chosen for his love for children. A responsible adult is present for the entire time the children are visiting

FIG. 1. Teens together help to pass the long hours of hospitalization. Note the child who is ambulatory dresses in her own comfortable attire.

the animal. Children who are used to having pets will gain a great deal from this exposure. The period can also be used to introduce children to animals they did not previously know or have close contact with.

TRIPS.   The child with a long-term illness can also be taken to the local zoo to see animals. A museum visit may also be beneficial. This trip might stimulate an interest in a hobby of collecting pictures of animals such as butterflies. The trips to these areas can be less expensive of professional time if volunteers are effectively solicited for the project. Frequently volunteers are more knowledgeable about these areas than the professionals. Any activities planned outside the hospital will, of course, require permission of the physician and the child's parent or guardian.

LIMIT-SETTING.   The child should be exposed to reasonable and realistic limits while hospitalized. This should also be carried on even after discharge. Limits are very important to the child so that he knows his boundaries and feels free to function within them. He should not have free reign as this does not adequately prepare him to live in our society. (See the Chapter on normal growth and development for further guidelines.)

WATER PLAY.   The child's care should be planned to be as homelike as possible. The use of water play with children with certain disease conditions has been described by Erickson in her *Play Interviews*

With Hospitalized Children. I believe that water has real significance to all children and should be utilized effectively for their care. The normal child is rarely used to being bathed from a basin. He is more used to the bathtub or shower. If his condition warrants it, the home routine should be continued. This bath period can be a water-play period for the preschool child who delights in water play. For the older child it is a close association with home.

RECREATION AND PLAY. Play activities are covered in Chapter 2. They are an important component of the nursing plan for the child. The nurse will utilize other available team members such as the play therapist, volunteers, and occupational therapists to provide this component. Recreation is an essential element and other interested citizens can provide movies, slides, or film strips for evening entertainment. The more adequately equipped facilities will have swings, slides, and monkey bars provided for the children. Hospital excursions can also be planned. A planned scavenger hunt collecting inexpensive hospital items such as tongue blades, cotton balls, and soap can be great fun. With a little preplanning these items can be satisfactorily hidden in the area chosen for conducting the hunt.

SETTLING-IN. I believe we sometimes underestimate the differences between home and hospital. The child admitted from a white suburban community may receive a "cultural shock" when first admitted to an integrated hospital setting. He may quickly be exposed to children of many cultural and ethnic backgrounds. This experience can be very valuable to the child. However, he needs help in adjusting to the situation. A child who has heard bigoted remarks about another race may begin to incorporate this into his own thinking. He may find it extremely difficult to find himself sharing a room with a child of a different race. Fortunately, children seem to accept others for what they really are and adjustment periods usually turn into keen friendships. The exposure the child has to other cultural and ethnic groups can prove to be one of the most positive factors derived from his long periods of hospitalization. The sharing of experiences during periods of stress, with children from all backgrounds, may make him better able to face the outside competitive world.

The child from an all-black community may be extremely uncomfortable living with and being ministered to by numerous whites. As more integration is achieved these situations will hopefully lessen.

MATURATION. An important factor to keep in mind is that this child will grow socially, mentally, emotionally, spiritually, and physically during his hospitalization and illness if we provide an adequate environment. This implies that we must adjust our plan of care to meet his changing needs. It also means that we must not always remember all the unpleasant things the child did when he was younger. Each time he is seen, a new evaluation of his progress should be made. It is also falsely assumed that if a child has a large comprehensive chart that everyone knows all about him. It has been my experience that large charts are often avoided as it takes too much time to read them. So, despite a good resource, people may know very little about his past medical or nursing history and even little about his present reasons for hospitalization. An outsider who does not know the child may be a valuable asset to a team conference on the child. Some very significant things can easily be overlooked when the child stays around a long time. An outsider, who has no vested interest in the child, may see other approaches or suggest further evaluation or treatment.

GOAL-SETTING. The short-term and long-term goals of nursing care should be spelled out specifically. We are too prone to rely on day-to-day care rather than spelling out our plans and trying to meet them. These goals can be made independently by the nurse, or in conjunction with the patient and his family, or in conjunction with other members of the professional team.

An example of this goal-setting follows. A child with a long-term illness is admitted to the unit. His parents live 60 miles away and have four younger children. Your goal is to maintain as close a child-parent relationship as possible. An approach is to have the parent plan to telephone at a certain time on a definite day of the week. Another approach is to provide the child with postcards and stamps to write to the parent. Still another approach is to have pictures of the entire family taped to the inside foot of the bed so he can easily see them. You have thus specified the long-term goal of maintaining the child as part of the family unit. You have also identified short-term goals which can easily be met. If this is done on admission, you are more likely to take care of this because it is fresh in your mind. If it is put off, a significant gap in the child-parent relationship may already take place and neither the child nor the parent may have any interest in starting the program.

NURSES' NOTES AND PROGRESS REPORTS. In addition to daily nurses' notes, we must begin to keep progress reports which identify how we are contributing positively to the child's overall care. Otherwise we may fall victim to providing only custodial care for the child with a long-term illness. The progress notes in relation to the foregoing goals of nursing care would relate items such as the child's response to the parents' telephone call or the child's enthusiasm or lack of it for sending postcards. They could note also whether the child reacted positively or negatively to suggestions offered by the parent. They should also include information about whether the parent wanted to talk to the nurse about the child's progress or whether this information had to be given to the parent without a specific request. The progress notes should also include new ideas for maintaining a child-parent relationship. An example would be scheduling a visit from the parent and any request the parent has for this visit, such as an interview with the physician or a financial counselor. The progress notes should include nursing intervention taken in relation to these requests.

PARENTS OF CHILDREN WITH LONG-TERM ILLNESS. The parents of the child who is hospitalized frequently are not well-informed about hospital policies. It is often falsely assumed that repeated exposure to a situation makes one extremely knowledgeable. This is not true and it is especially important to help the parents receive the information they need or desire. One very important area of concern to parents is the use or misuse of "specialists." Frequently, a specialist in a particular field of pediatrics is utilized. The parent may not be aware that a new physician is being utilized. They may not realize the need for the physician and, in their ignorance, they may be opposed to having him on consultation. The specialist may be known to the parents only by a bill they receive for services rendered. This type of incident rarely occurs with acute illnesses but is quite common with children with long-term illnesses. It is imperative that parents receive the same consideration and information when their child is in continual need of medical supervision.

The Family of the Child with Long-Term Illness

To understand the implications of long-term illness to the family, one must draw upon the work of sociologists and social psychologists. They help to put into perspective the family as it exists in our present-day society. We can then more easily understand some of the reasons that families react the way they do to illness. It is not my intention to try to break down into minute categories the various types of family structures in our country. The discussion may seem to fit the middle-class white segment better than any other, only because the other segments of our population are less well-known to the writer and are therefore covered in much less detail. The student should consult the work of sociologists and anthropologists who are dedicating their talents to understanding these other groups.

First, I should like to discuss the family as a unit. The unit may be comprised of many small systems depending on the numbers and types of participants. Within this unit there are a number of interrelationships which exist. Anything which affects one member of the family, directly or indirectly, affects all the other members. The degree to which people are affected varies from member to member. We must assume that the family is not an entity unto itself. It is also affected by and altered by the environment in which it exists.

These factors are especially important to professionals working with children with long-term illness. They are probably even more significant when the long-term illness is acquired rather than congenital. In an acquired illness the role of the child in the family has already been established and has to be adjusted to the new illness. The interrelationships the child has in the family may be drastically changed due to his illness, whereas the child who is *born* with a long-term illness derives his role in the family with the condition being considered. This does not mean, however, that his condition makes the role of the other family members in relation to his illness any easier.

To understand this more thoroughly we will now look at roles within a family structure. Spiegel (1957) has stated that interrelationships of roles are crucial, as no role exists in isolation; it is always patterned to fit the complementary or reciprocal role of a role partner. He states that as long as the role each family member occupies is complementary with and conforms to the role expectations other members have for him, the family lives in dynamic equilibrium.

This explains why it is important to understand what the family feels about the child with a long-term illness. If they assume that he is going to live a long productive life and this is not the case, the family equilibrium may be shattered when the child does not succeed. If the family has cast the child in the role of a helpless individual and the child assumes an active role, this may shatter the family equilibrium. If another sibling reacts negatively to the role of the child with the long-term illness, this can interrupt the family equilibrium.

Why worry about family equilibrium? Spiegel (1957) states that the equilibrium which is brought about by complementary roles is a rewarding state of affairs. He further contends that the disequilibrium serves to motivate family members to attempt some form of resolution of existing role discrepancies.

The rewarding nature of equilibrium stems from the fact that when roles are clearly defined and mutually agreed upon, the individual is spared the necessity of almost constant decision-making about the acts he performs.

This can be illustrated by the child with a cardiac condition. A mother casts the child in the role of a "cardiac cripple." The child feels well enough to go to school and participate in nonstrenuous sports. The child assumes a role not consistent with the one another vital family member has for him. The mother writes a note to the school forbidding her son to participate in any sports. The school acts as the environmental factor. The principal requests a note from the physician. The mother tries to influence the physician to take her side. The physician intervenes in favor of the son. The son participates in sports. The mother then is faced with a role which is not conducive to the one which she has established for her son. Disequilibrium results and role expectations must be modified if equilibrium is to be reestablished.

The role a parent ascribes for a particular child may also influence the way the other family members accept that child. A child with a cardiac condition is often "coddled" by his siblings because they take their clues from their parents. Consequently, the other siblings may wait on the child with the cardiac problem and lessen his chances of establishing independence. The child with the cardiac condition may then "expect" that his needs will be consistently met in this way. When he gets to school, he finds it difficult not to have his siblings able to continue their indulging role.

Spiegel (1957) states that there are four principal ways in which an individual acquires his social role. In each case the individual can accept the role assigned to him or he can refuse it, such as in the case presented above. Some roles are *ascribed*, that is, universally accepted —such as age and sex roles. Other roles, such as occupation, have to be *achieved* and others *adopted*. The fourth role he calls *assumption*, when the role has playful qualities. Such assumed roles are taken in make-believe and it is important that all members concerned realize the playful character of the assumed role. The adoptive roles are informal in character. They are adopted by one member and usually relate to another member. This can be illustrated by a 10-year-old sibling adopting the mother-role to the child with a long-term illness, rather than the sibling-role usually adopted by two children in the same family.

There are two other terms used by Spiegel (1957) which are useful in this discussion. One is the term *allocative discrepancy* and the other *goal discrepancy.* Allocative discrepancy is used when the individual refuses the role allocated to him or when others fail to complement his role. Goal discrepancy exists when the goal of one family member is to obtain some form of gratification from another, but the other fails to meet the demand because his goal is related to withholding or because he is unable to gratify the demand, for some reason. Goal discrepancy is especially significant, as long-term illness can cause a member not to be able to gratify the demands of other family members. A number of examples can be cited. The child born without limbs cannot achieve his father's desire for him to be a football player. The child with advanced cystic fibrosis cannot take dancing lessons. The daughter with asthma will not be able to exist comfortably in the frilly bedroom signifying to the mother the height of femininity.

The severity of the discrepancies between what is expected and what is attained can greatly influence the family equilibrium. The severity of the discrepancy may vary from family member to family member. What may be a severe disappointment to the mother may be only a minor disappointment to a brother or sister. However, the degree to which it interrupts the relationships within the family is of major importance.

CURRENT ROLES OF FAMILY MEMBERS

In the foregoing discussion we have talked about roles in the family. It is useful to examine some of the present roles that influence the care given the child with a long-term illness. Again, the roles described are most appropriate to the white middle-class population.

Mother role. The role of the mother has always been concerned with the health of the children. Recently the roll has changed from being not only one of concern with physical health but also the psychological well-being of the child. This expanded role has put new and more demanding responsibility on the mother. She is forced to read about new developments in child care and to keep up with advances in medical practices. Formerly, it was sufficient for her to get to a doctor when the child was ill. She is now faced with understanding preventive medical practices and responsibility for the emotional components of development.

The more educationally advantaged the mother, the greater are the demands for her to be informed. I am reminded of a nurse in a master's degree program who had to conduct a parent discussion group as part of her requirements. She found herself reading copious amounts of material to keep up with the parents' questions. She did not find herself in the role of disseminator of material, but rather as a person who could compare one authority to another or discuss controversial ideas and clarify ideas.

In comparison are those mothers who have little or no education and derive their roles by modeling after a mother or grandmother, or by word of mouth from some other educationally disadvantaged mother.

When looking at the mother role in relation to illness, Bell (1966) states that the middle-class mother usually assumes the role of mediator between the impersonal rational role decision of the medical expert and the application of those decisions within the highly emotional contexts of her relationships to her husband and children. This mediating role of the mother further extends the impersonal relationship between the medical personnel and the patients.

This is dynamically illustrated by the adolescent patient with a long-term illness. The medical person usually feels an obligation to talk to the parent before talking to the patient. The parent then makes some decisions which are not always the best for the patient. The medical person then proceeds, incorporating the parent's decision. The relationship between the medical personnel and the patient may suffer as a result. The decision that directly affects the adolescent has been mediated by an outside source, and the adolescent frequently has to live with this decision. It is fortunate that the adolescent has the capacity to rebel, as this rebellion may provide an opportunity for him to be consulted about his own care.

An example of an adolescent whose own thoughts were not originally included in plans for medical intervention follows.

An adolescent boy was paralyzed from the waist down in an automobile accident. Prior to this time, he was an outgoing, well-developed male with superior intelligence and ability. Immediately after the accident, a Foley catheter was inserted for incontinence. The Foley was kept in place until John developed repeated infections. A change of medical supervision was sought and a new regimen of care instituted. After a trial of medical management, the doctor felt an ileoconduit was indicated. The parents were approached and the operation was explained. The father declined surgical intervention because he felt that urinary drainage via the Foley catheter was more "manly" than a urinary diversion. The medical personnel tried on several occasions to have the family understand the implications of this decision. The parents would not reverse their decision and repeated infections caused kidney damage. Each time tests were performed and the results were more severe. The family was asked again to consider the surgery. John's severe kidney damage was shortening his life expectancy and he was not consulted about the operation, a decision that influenced his future life. John's mother visited daily and spent a good portion of the time telling him how wonderfully he was doing under the present conditions. Any information given in relation to the surgery was biased. John had a real crisis period, with scant urinary output, high temperature, and chills. He became extremely frightened and for the first time started questioning on his own. After much preparation and a long lapse in time, John finally received the surgical intervention he needed.

John did not verbalize his father's fears of losing his masculinity due to the reconstructive surgery. He had been used to making serious decisions for himself prior to his accident. He had successfully emancipated himself from his parents and was well on his way to adulthood. His accident occurred at a time when he had a very positive relationship with his parents. After a period of time, John realized he had been deceived by his parents and he began to distrust their judgment. He was very disappointed to learn they had not been telling him the truth. His physical deterioration was a result of their decision to change the role they had previously established with their son. This change in role was actually encouraged by the medical personnel who chose to deal with the parents at the exclusion of the patient who was capable of being included.

It is important when a child's trust in his parents has been crushed to help him to reestablish trust and to give him the support he needs during the time he is trying to reestablish this trust.

This very dramatic illustration can be contrasted with the role of the lower-class mother. This mother is frequently the head of the family and shoulders many responsibilities. She is so strained by other responsibilities that she has little or no time for illness. According to Rainwater, as cited in Bell (1966), her attitude toward illness even when it becomes chronic is apt to be a tolerant one. People in lower socioeconomic families learn to live with illness rather than using their small stock of interpersonal and psychic resources to do something about the problem.

These attitudes about illness are influenced by the degree to which the family members regard the crisis as a threat to the present or future life of the family. The parent responding to an ill child is responding to both the illness and our society's dependency role of the child. In other societies, in which the child is less dependent, the parents' need to protect the child may be less.

The mother with a child with long-term nutritional anemia may bring the child to the hospital only when the child is dangerously close to death. The child is treated and responds. The mother is counseled on the dietary requirements of the child and seems to understand. However, the child is readmitted a few months later, in the same condition. The mother again is responding only when she considers herself incapable of handling the situation. She is not worrying about the sequale of the frequent brushes with death. Her aim is to keep the child alive but the overall well-being of the child may be an unknown concept to her. Even if it is known, she may have so many overwhelming crises to handle that she is not physically able to respond to them all and handles each one as she interprets its importance.

In my short visit to Paraguay, South America, as a consultant in Child-Health Nursing, this was very vividly illustrated. The children that were brought to the city for medical supervision were frequently close to being moribund. I was advised that the parents lived long distances away, that transportation was limited, that families were large, and financial resources limited, so parents did not quickly seek medical aid when one child became ill. They would frequently wait until another child also needed care, or until their "folk medicine" seemed to fail completely. These families did not have a great deal of faith in modern medical techniques and, therefore, did not eagerly seek them. They also were used to having children die and more readily accepted this fate than do people in middle-class white America.

Also, when they did bring in their child for medical care they were less apt to disassociate themselves from the child's care and continued to be actively involved. This reflects not only the difference in delivery of health services but also the family's involvement with their family members.

Implications of Long-Term Illness to Parental Roles.   Bell (1966) has stated that some families have the tendency to resist the facts that a problem really exists. However, he has found that the parents of children with long-term illness tend to be less sociable and more withdrawn than the parents without such children. He found the mothers less likely to work outside the home than "normal" mothers. He also found that the community of "normal" families was not supportive of the revised norms of child care that must be established by families with severely handicapped children. Furthermore, the norms and values regulating participation in the community of normal families are hostile to the demands made upon the parents of severely handicapped children.

An illustration of this point is found in this picture given by a parent of a child with severe cerebral palsy.

> I was young and a newly married college graduate when I moved into the community my husband grew up in. I quickly settled into his friends and family and felt right at home. Our only child was born less than two years later. It was a difficult birth and Janie was 'brain-damaged.' The fight she put up for survival deserved everyone's praise and exultations. My period following delivery was filled with complications and necessitated an extended hospitalization. Everyone was very kind and extended themselves to include visiting me and my infant daughter as well as extending meals to include my husband.

Since that early time many adjustments have been made in our lives to accommodate our severely handicapped daughter. Our opportunities to be with friends and family have decreased as baby-sitters are difficult to find or keep. When friends visit our home, we must alter our lives to make them comfortable. Few friends accept our dinner invitations, as they do not like to eat with our daughter whose awkward movements make eating seem primitive. Our friends are not sympathetic to her needs, when their own needs seem more important. Even our families do not understand why we eat at the same table with our own daughter, when she makes such a mess. Why don't we feed her? Why don't we put her in a nice home with other children with the same problem?

These questions and other similar questions serve to illustrate that other families do not have patience with the revised life-style of the family with a handicapped child.

The hostility is not always overt but may be of a much subtler nature—such as when the friends merely refuse or find excuses not to accept another dinner invitation to the involved family's home. The hostility can further be manifested by the invited guests' telling other friends about their experience "to spare you from the same ordeal." This form of hostility tends to further isolate the family with the handicapped child and decreases their motivation to try to keep ties with their former close associates.

In discussing implications to family roles, it is necessary to keep in mind that people raise their children according to their own standards. These standards include those regarding what is health and what is illness. What is "normal" may be very different for one family than another. A minor handicap due to a long-term illness may not have any implications to roles in one family, but in another it is a major crisis.

The comparison of two families with children with phenylketonuria will illustrate the last statement. One mother learned her child had this condition. She did not see any reason to be alarmed. The girl was 12 years old and functioning at a moderately retarded level. The mother did not change her role. She always let the child get her own meals and eat what appealed to her. Meals were never a source of enjoyment and the family did not come together for them. The child was told of her medical condition and for a short period she tried to comply with the medical management. Her role reverted back to the one she was comfortably occupying prior to the medical discovery, and the phenylketonuric diet was discarded.

The second mother learned the medical diagnosis and immediately set out to control the diet of her daughter. She became an amateur dietician, nurse, detective, and all around "commander-in-chief." She experimented with new ideas for preparing the limited diet and willingly shared them with other parents and medical personnel. Her role as mother was being camouflaged by her desire to be a crusader for her daughter's cause. Needless to say, the role of the child changed dramatically. She found her mother less capable of giving the love and support needed to her daily growth because she was too busy with her newly found chores. The change in the mother-child relationship influenced the entire family. The mother began quizzing her husband on his observations of increased intellectual functioning of the child. The other sibling resented the restricted dietary intake enforced upon her sister. The size of the family was also stabilized as a result of this long-term illness. It would be possible to go on and on about the implications of this illness to this family and its place in the community, but I believe what has been said adequately illustrates the point.

Implications for Sibling Roles. A fair amount of material has been written in relation to the changes in parents' roles in relation to illness. The effects on the other siblings has been less well-defined. In the chapter on terminal illness I have included some thoughts in relation to the other children, but I would like to include a few more in this section.

As the emphasis in child-rearing has focused on the individual rights of the members of a family, children have tended to become more egocentric. Their individual demands are frequently granted until a crisis arises. In time of crisis, the individual's rights are relegated to a lower level of priority and the crisis situation emerges with top priority. Let us take, for example, a family with two children. Henry and Mary have been treated with equal concern by their parents. Their needs were individual but easily met with a degree of give and take by the family. Henry has an accident and is severely injured. His developmental level regresses to that of a toddler. The family begins to expend all their energies on behalf of Henry. Mary's "normal" requests and demands are now considered unreasonable. The parents have no time to spend on the ordinary activities of daily living. They are burdened by going to the hospital, seeing that the best doctors are brought in, obtaining and maintaining private duty nurses, getting people to donate blood, checking on medical insurance coverage, etc. Mary is very much in the background of the medical crisis. She is painfully on the other end, where living conditions have deteriorated. Her meals are forgotten or thrown together, her clothing is neglected, no one is available to answer her questions or to ask her about her day. The phone rings frequently but the calls are always about Henry. In her childlike way she tries to adjust her sibling-role to meet the crisis, but she becomes more and more painfully aware of her own desires and needs.

This traumatic beginning influences the way Mary will be able to handle her new role in relation to Henry with his long-term illness. Her role of equal competitor may change to one of hostility. Her position may be further in jeopardy when Henry returns home in a more dependent role. She may be asked to assume some of the responsibility for his care, casting her in a mother role or nursing role. She may adopt the role of mother willingly, and compete with her mother for this position with Henry. She may assume a role of a cheerful happy young lady while in reality she very much resents her new responsibilities. Her exterior facade gives her parents confidence that she is delighted with her new responsibility. This creates a comfortable feeling in the parents and they do not look past it into Mary's true feelings.

This example illustrates why I believe that medical care must be family-centered rather than patient-centered. The needs of Mary may well get to crisis proportions before anyone is aware that they even exist.

The changing role of siblings can be detrimental to the children's normal life pattern. With some degree of predictability, Mary might experience loss of normal activities of her age group. She might resent the premature role of mother and choose never to accept it again. She might become hostile toward her parents and not be able to establish a warm and loving relationship again.

A professional person, working with the family, might identify some of the clues to Mary's unhappiness and help her to handle her feelings.

In families that attend clinics for long-term medical supervision, it is becoming evident that siblings have an increase in emotional problems. These emotional problems have been manifested in obesity, nail-biting, school failure, etc. The severity of the symptoms is not necessarily correlated with the degree of disturbance.

If it is unrealistic to have all the siblings included in the medical supervision of the child with long-term illness, we might at least plan group sessions in which they can get together and ventilate their feelings about their roles and responsibilities. These sessions could be planned in the evening, so they do not interfere with school. Another possibility is for the school nurse to assume the leadership for these sessions. They can be successfully integrated into the health education program.

Hospitalization of the Child

Hospitalization of a child with a long-term illness becomes an expected event. Periodically his life-style is interrupted and hospitalization is instituted. The nurse is one of the first professional workers to meet the child. Her admitting evaluation can aid the team greatly.

EVALUATION OF CHILD'S ASSETS: NURSING HISTORY

The use of the nursing history in hospital and out-patient settings is starting to be instituted. I have included a form (Table 1) which has been developed by using formats suggested by other nurses and by adopting this form to get the information needed in a particular setting.

The excuse that a form does not fit a particular institution or

TABLE 1. SUGGESTED FORM FOR NURSING HISTORY

UNIVERSITY HOSPITAL
U.S.A.
NURSING HISTORY (IN-PATIENT PEDIATRICS)

Name:_____

Date:_____

Number of hospital or home care admissions

Duration of hospital admissions

Age(s) during hospital stay(s)

    I. Appearance

   II. Patient's understanding of illness—preparation for hospitalization

  III. Events leading up to present hospital admission

  IV. Place in family constellation—identification of family members

   V. Significant information relative to:
  a) feeding
  b) toileting
  c) sleep
  d) play
  e) language development
  f) independent and dependent activities of daily living

  VI. What is important to this child to make him feel secure in this situation?

 VII. What are the policies of this agency which will interfere with or promote the well-being of this child?

VIII. What is the medical plan of care that will influence the nursing plan of care?

  IX. What are the short-term goals for this child?

   X. What are the long-term goals for this child?

  XI. What methods can be identified and tried to meet these goals?

 XII. What are the significant principles of growth and development which will be incorporated into my plan of care?

XIII. What community or team resources will be utilized or approached to meet my nursing objectives?

XIV. What nursing intervention needs to be done with the family at this time?

agency's needs and, therefore, is not being used, is an outdated idea. The form is just a suggestion and should be tailored to meet your current needs. It is merely a guide for collecting data. If it is a deterrant to getting data then it should be discarded in favor of another method.

Any child admitted to the hospital feels much more secure if he realizes that you know and understand him. One way to get to know the child and his parents is to do a *nursing intake history*. This history will help to identify significant factors to develop a realistic nursing care plan. The history will be taken on admission for most long-term patients. However, if the child is admitted in an acute crisis, the information may be more easily obtained a day or two after admission. Table 1 is a guide for obtaining pertinent nursing information. If the information is stored easily, some of it can be saved from admission to admission and just be up-dated.

Pertinent information obtained from this interview should be immediately placed in the child's chart for utilization by the entire health team. Some of the aspects are gathered specifically for the Kardex. Other information, such as use of community resources, is utilized for instituting proper referrals.

Of the information gathered, some—such as feeding, toileting, and so forth—will need to be further evaluated by direct observation. An example would be: Mrs. Jones says that two-and-a-half year old Johnny feeds himself. When you make out his Kardex you include this fact. Johnny experiences regression due to hospitalization and refuses to eat. The Kardex should be revised to read: encourage self-feeding, needs assistance.

The question in relation to policies which interfere with meeting certain objectives may lend itself to changes in policy. For instance, you find that Johnny is very attached to his six-year-old brother. The hospital does not allow children under 14 years of age to visit. If you gather enough information indicating that the child's progress is hindered by being separated from his siblings, a change in policy may be considered.

Physicians have always identified, on admission, a plan of care and things to be tried in relation to this plan. Nurses should also identify their care plan and ways they intend to facilitate this care. The physician then keeps progress notes in relation to things he has tried and their results. Then he adds more ideas and ways to meet the revised plan of care. Nurses seldom keep progress notes and rarely do we spell out why we changed our plan or what our future plans will be. Let us take as an example Mary, who is admitted with myelomeningocele with paralysis of her lower extremities. She is admitted with a decubitus ulcer on her ankle. Presently we begin a plan of care and chart on the nurses' notes in relation to size, location, discharge, and treatment given. A few days later we chart a different treatment given. Our only clue to what the treatment may be is the doctor's order sheet. However, nowhere is the independent nursing function charted. We may have tried to leave the area uncovered for three days without apparent improvement. We may have tried treatment by a heat lamp. We may have used a bedcradle or footboard to eliminate pressure from bedclothes. We may have positioned the child at night to keep her from rolling over and getting the decubitus on the sheet. We may have bathed the area in warm water three times a day. All of these independent measures should be charted with their results or lack of results and when a new approach is started the rationale clearly stated so everyone reading the chart can easily see that the independent nursing needs as well as the medical needs of the child are being met.

Needless to say, gathering of information is only one step in the process of improving care. Ways must be devised to disseminate this information to make it readily available and to eliminate some of the duplication that exists. We do not want to follow the medical profession's policy of several levels of medical personnel all gathering the same information. The use of computers to conveniently store and retrieve information will greatly improve our present methods of sharing information. It is imperative to establish how to identify pertinent nursing information, so we can identify what we can contribute to the computer input.

TABLE 2. THE EXPANDING ROLE OF THE NURSE IN HISTORY-TAKING

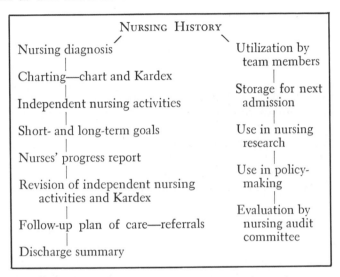

When one studies Table 2 it becomes evident that the role of the nurse is greatly expanded and encompasses a longer span of time than it did formerly. The nursing history just sets the stage for more dynamic types of nursing intervention. The information gathered helps the nurse to identify areas of care which are uniquely nursing or are shared by nursing. The nurse makes a nursing diagnosis and then formulates the plan of care to meet the patient's needs. Patients with long-term illnesses may have so many medical diagnoses that we hesitate to add a nursing one to the list. However, this nursing diagnosis is somewhat different. The diagnosis is partially derived from factors relating to growth and development and normal developmental tasks (see Chapter 1). It is made by considering constraints made by the hospitalization process. It is made by considering the medical diagnosis and the scientific limitations imposed by this diagnosis. It is made by considering the child as an integral part of a family unit. It is made by the social forces which are present. It is made by the types of services available for aiding this child. It is made by the time element we have available to minister to the child.

An example might be that you make a nursing diagnosis of extreme environmental deprivation causing failure to thrive. You would like to have the same nurse care for this child each day on each shift. You would also like to provide the child with consistent visitation of the parents. You would like the parents to participate in the care of the child, especially in regards to feeding and handling. After the diagnosis is made and plans tentatively formulated you learn from the parents that they live far away and they will not be able to visit consistently. You also find the staffing of the unit is inadequate for the next few days and per diem nurses will be utilized to supplement the regular nursing staff.

It is now necessary for you to revise your thinking in relation to this child and to see what other resources you can draw on to supplement the care. You then decide that a volunteer may be used with this child, that she could provide the cuddling necessary for the child, that she would have more time to rock the child, and that she might even be in a position to feed the child. You will also want to be sure that the per diem nurses have the benefit of a very complete Kardex or verbal report to utilize when caring for the child so that they know the parents will not be there, so that they do not wait feedings if the volunteer is not there, and also that they will provide some of the stimulation the child will need during their tour of duty.

In addition you decide that toys should be used to assist you in your plan of care and you put up a mobile, or you use some musical wind-up toys that can be wound up periodically and used as auditory stimulation for the child. You also provide the child with a toy to cuddle. Another valuable resource to be utilized in the care of a child who needs additional attention because his parents are not available is the student of nursing. Frequently she has more time available to spend with the child and is eager to give the additional attention needed. She is also well-equipped with some of the new theories about child-rearing and will appreciate an opportunity to try out some of them.

In line with Table 2, the next step—in addition to getting information in the Kardex in relation to this child—is to be sure that the charting states exactly how the child responded to the additional handling, to the toys, to sound, to feeding, etc. It is especially important that the chart shows when the child begins to eat better, what types of things contributed to his eating better, and if there were particular conditions under which he ate better. It is not unusual to have the child, even with additional handling, eat poorly at the beginning of his hospitalization. A child who at home has his bottle propped may not like the change of being held to be fed and may take quite some time before he begins to respond, and to like having somebody hold him and perhaps rock him while he is eating. The fact that the child seems to like having his bottle propped better than being hand fed does not mean that the nurse should use the propping procedure. It merely means that the child becomes programmed to propping and because he knows no other way, he has learned to adjust to this. However, we know because the child fails to thrive that he is not getting the full value out of feeding. The nurses' notes should clearly indicate when the child begins to improve or at what points the child might regress. We should be able to pinpoint very clear on the notes some of the factors that contributed to progression or regression. We should also begin to accumulate a number of things that the child likes or dislikes in the way of food in his diet.

In designing goals for this child, it has already been indicated that we have established some short-term goals. The long-term goals may be in sending referrals to the local community health nurse to visit the home and to help the mother with feeding the child, or in listening to the mother to see what types of things have contributed to the poor—or what seems to be poor—mother-child relationship.

The referral to the community health nurse should be made early so that she can provide the hospital team with information that may be very valuable while the child is hospitalized. She may have known the family for a long period of time prior to this hospitalization. The mother may need a great deal of reassurance while the child is hospitalized, and perhaps the mother might even have some guilt feelings about this child, especially if anyone has told her that it is the result of her behavior that the child has poor feeding habits and failure to thrive. This is not an unusual occurrence when a child with failure to thrive is admitted to the hospital.

The nurse's progress report should clearly state that she has contacted the community health nurse in the area and should also indicate any information that she has collected by this resource so that other members of the health team can also utilize this information. The independent nursing activities and the Kardex must be revised frequently in order to give the best possible care to the child. Having outdated information is no better than an empty Kardex.

We should also put in the Kardex some of our follow-up plans for the child. They may include such things as return to clinic so that we know that the child does have some after-care, or it may include the name of the physician to whom the child will be referred on the outside and, of course, the name of the community health nurse who can be contacted easily in the child's community. It is very important also to include in our charting a discharge summary of this child, indicating the progress the child has made during hospitalization and also some of the key nursing interventions that were made in order to meet the nursing needs of this child. This discharge summary should be sent to the community health nurse in the area and to the follow-up medical care, wherever it will be given for this child.

CONCLUDING STATEMENT

The foregoing information is only of value to the student of nursing if it is utilized as a guide in delivering nursing services. Each child must be considered on an individual basis and treated within his own particular set of circumstances. The general ideas are given as guidelines for what the student might expect in learning the specific skills needed to deliver the best nursing services to the child with long-term illness.

Case Study Presentation and Study Questions

PRESENTING DIAGNOSIS: BLINDNESS

Bobby was 12 years old when I first met him. He was blind from birth. Bobby was a premature baby tipping the scales at a brief 2 lb. He was the fifth child in four years for this young Irish couple. He was born in a city hospital with a medium-sized obstetrical department. (Size judged on admissions prior to "the pill.")

The family doctor delivered Bobby. The delivery was quick, uncomplicated, and performed without episiotomy or anesthesia. There is no Apgar score, but by the mother's recollection the child was "lifeless." A great deal of attention was already focused on the hazards of oxygen therapy to the eyesight of prematures. According to the records, the physician ordered higher concentrations anyway, as he expected the child to die soon.

The physician felt a great deal of guilt regarding Bobby's blindness and gave Bobby free medical supervision and care. The parents were very upset when the physician died (when Bobby was two-and-a-half years old) and it was at this point that they began to feel the real burden of having a child who was blind.

The parents were contacted by someone from a preschool facility for blind children. They enrolled Bobby at three years of age in this school. Bobby was not ready for this socialization process and did not adjust to school. He was termed "retarded" by the professional personnel and the family was counseled to keep him home until he showed more signs of school readiness.

The history is vague regarding Bobby as he came to be the middle child in a family of 10 children. Mrs. G. did not write down developmental achievements and therefore was not able to keep one child's record straight from another. Bobby received less and less of his parent's individual attention as they attempted to stretch their attention to reach 10 active children. Mr. G. took a second job to help with the expenses of raising his large family. This made his personal contributions to his family decidedly fewer.

Bobby received individualized attention from an elderly aunt who was a retired elementary school teacher. It was her creativity that was responsible for Bobby's early educational endeavors. Miss W. taught Bobby the alphabet by designing boards with small-shell-macaroni letters. Bobby traced the letters with his fingers and after much persistence and dedication he could print his alphabet. Miss W. had no formal training with the blind, but she read everything she could get in regard to teaching. She played the piano and decided to teach Bobby how to play. After many hours of practice, he achieved several beginning piano pieces. At this time, Miss W. bought a piano for Bobby to have at home. Prior to this, he played only on Miss W.'s piano. Her home was within walking distance but approximately three quarters of a mile away, making it seem inaccessible to the less ambitious members of the family.

It seemed like an excellent idea to have Bobby demonstrate his ability at the piano. None of the other siblings could play and this seemed like Bobby's opportunity to excel. However, it turned out to be a sad situation. Bobby was asked to demonstrate his talent for anyone that came to the home. His minimal talent was blown up out of proportion to his actual achievement. Bobby began to resent this and eventually he lost interest in playing the piano for anyone other than his aunt.

A routine type of check was made of all blind children and Bobby was "rediscovered" by the school authorities. He had passed the most appropriate ages for achieving particular developmental tasks and he lacked many simple skills needed for entering school. The school officials suggested Bobby be thoroughly evaluated by an interdisciplinary team concerned with handicapped children.

When the evaluation was completed, it uncovered some interesting factors and raised several questions. After a conference with the parents, Bobby was enrolled in a special school and a tutor was hired by the school to work specifically to teach Braille to Bobby. Her individualized teaching was greatly responsible for the many educational advances made by Bobby. In addition, he needed to have his large muscles more thoroughly developed. This was partially achieved by swimming and gym classes. It was at swimming that Bobby's skills regarding dressing and undressing were perfected. Bobby was also taken on walks outside and was taught to cross the street by pushing the traffic control button and listening for the cars to stop. Bobby's walks were also used to introduce him to grass, flowers, curbs, people, and weather. Teaching Bobby was a challenge and a pleasure and occasionally frustrating. It is difficult for a sighted person to describe things without including sight. It is too easy to take words for granted and assume they are self-explanatory. For instance, one day we were walking and a voting booth had been put on the sidewalk where we ordinarily passed freely. The booth was green, wooden, and rather plain. Before reaching the booth I explained to Bobby that the booth was there and to be careful as he approached it. Bobby got to it and started feeling it. He asked, "What did you say it was?" I replied, "A green house." "Oh, no," said Bobby, "a greenhouse is glass."

The same type of things can happen in the hospital setting. What seems to be a perfectly logical and simple explanation can be misinterpreted or rejected by the blind child because it is not consistent with his past experiences.

The needs and accomplishments of Bobby could fill many pages but he is introduced here only to raise questions for nurses involved in the care of blind children. I pose the following questions for consideration:

1. How much can a family be expected to do on its own in seeking care for a handicapped child?

2. What can a community health nurse do to enhance the learning of a blind child excluded from formal schooling?
3. What clues would suggest the child is ready to be taught self-feeding?
4. How can nurses teach blind children to feed themselves?
5. How can a nurse provide needed stimulation for a hospitalized blind child?
6. How does a child "compensate" for being blind, or does he compensate?
7. What tasks could the other children in this family be delegated to help teach Bobby?
8. What types of information about Bobby's life style could be obtained by interviewing one or two of the other children in the family?
9. If you were the one who uncovered Bobby's semi-isolation, what agencies would you contact for help and guidance?
10. What other types of activities could be suggested for developing Bobby's large and small muscles?

PRESENTING DIAGNOSIS: GRANULOMATOUS COLITIS

Harry is a 13-year-old white male and John is a 16-year-old white male. I introduce them as their long-term illness is the same: granulomatous colitis. Harry is presently hospitalized and receiving hyperalimentation therapy.[1] John is hospitalized on the same unit and is receiving medication therapy that presently consists of Imuran, ozulfadine, prednisone, multivitamins, and Librium. Harry has been through the medical route and has had a combination of medical and surgical therapy but his disease has progressed to the serious condition which necessitated this admission.

Let us look at Harry's 13 years in more detail. Harry is the youngest of two children. His brother is 19 and has a spina bifida. His father has diabetes and his mother has anemia and a coagulation disorder. Harry's early years were without history of illness. His development is noted as normal, but little is known of the parent-child or sibling relationships. At age seven his life-style was changed by serious illness which was diagnosed as colitis.

Hospitalizations occurred at age seven, age ten, age twelve, and age thirteen. Treatment during these confinements included medical regimens, surgery resulting in an ileal colectomy and closure of a ileal rectal fistula, and tracheostomy for respiratory distress resulting from laryngotracheobronchitis.

His present hospitalization followed a period of months of medical management which did not control rashes, fever, loss of weight, or the diarrhea. For nearly a year, schooling was impossible and a tutor came to Harry's home.

Harry is in a private room and one of his parents is allowed to room-in. The mother stays the majority of the time and assumes the majority of Harry's physical care. Mrs. J. is considered "overprotective" by most of the nursing staff. She has been accused of "interfering" with the occupational thera-

[1] Parenteral administration of glucose, amino acids, vitamins, and electrolytes through a catheter into the child's right atrium (other hospitals report using the superior vena cava). Heparin is added to the IV solution to decrease the possibility of thrombosis formation.

pist's plan of care for Harry. When Mrs. J. leaves the room, several professionals have described an "improvement in Harry's attitude." He seems to open up and is willing to vent his feelings regarding his illness and hospitalization.

An example of Harry's interaction with a student nurse while his mother is present follows.

Nurse: "Do you have any friends visit?"
Harry: "No."
Nurse: "Are any of those cards from friends?"
Harry: "Yes, from James age ten, Mary age thirteen, Joe age fourteen."
Nurse: "Would you like paper to write to them?"
Harry: "No, nothing to say."

Even open-ended questions resulted in short answers, and attempts to encourage interest in games were in vain.

Mrs. J. left the room and the following conversation took place.

Harry: "I'm tired of this routine (hyperalimentation). I know it's essential but I miss not eating."
Nurse: "I can appreciate that."
Harry: "I'm tired of being in the hospital. The worst part about being in the hospital is going home. All the kids laugh at me because I'm sick. They tease me because I can't keep up."

It is obvious from Harry's conversation that he needs more opportunities to be with a professional person without his mother being present.

There are several other factors which are significant in making Harry's hospitalization tolerable. He is retarded in growth due to the large amounts of steroids he has received over the years. The hospital school teacher knows his age and grade placement but relates to him as a younger child. Harry resents this and finds the school work too easy. He needs to be challenged more on his intellectual level.

Harry's hyperalimentation therapy requires diligent and continual monitoring. The hourly check of the intravenous bottle does not guarantee Harry quality nursing care. The child frequently takes second place to the bottle. People frequently enter the room with their eye contact being made with the bottle high over Harry's head. Harry's morale is an important consideration in his therapy. During one hospitalization it was necessary to discharge him because of his "profound depression."

John's history includes several hospitalizations for medical management. He is currently having several bloody stools a day and requires transfusions for replacement. John is fully informed of his disease and knows about Harry's hyperalimentation routine. John does not feel he needs this therapy. He knows that Harry has had surgery without success and he doubts that surgery is the answer for control of his own disease.

John's parents doubt that he has colitis despite his long history and feel it is really "dysentery." John dropped out of school as a freshman in high school. He states he was an honor student and bored. He lives in an apartment with his brother. The brother is teaching him a trade.

John has visited Harry at Mrs. J.'s request. John feels Harry "lets his disease get to him." He feels Harry gives in too easily to cramps. John says, "I take my pills and stay up and go to work. That's why I do better than him."

Both boys show an adolescent understanding of their disease process. Both have a large hospital vocabulary. Both show effects of a long-term illness on peer relationships; neither seems to have many close friends. While John's parents continue to deny his disease, Harry's family is intimately involved in learning all they can about the disease and passing the information on to their local medical personnel. Both boys live a fair distance away and come to this hospital—"Where the experts are," according to John.

The effects of the long-term illness on Harry are quite obvious. His ability to express himself is greatly impaired when his mother is present. He spends much time picking lightly at his arms and face. His eye contact with people is infrequent. He smiles very little and perhaps with good reason.

John seems much more self-sufficient despite his long-term illness. He knows he feels better when he takes sitz baths during periods of acute diarrhea. He swabs xylocaine viscus on his mouth ulcers when needed, and discontinues it when the ulcers are improved. He chooses his own diet which is liberal but discourages large amounts of roughage. He has definite likes and dislikes in food and feels free to order meals. He refuses to let the hospital routine interfere with his ordinary personal hygiene habits. He is used to bathing in the evening and continues this practice in the hospital. He feels free to question his medical management. One example is in relation to giving blood for laboratory examination. He felt he needed a blood transfusion because the laboratory technician took so much blood. In an attempt to show him he was wrong, an empty intravenous bottle was filled with water from the blood tube. This demonstrated that even eight test tubes of blood would not necessitate a replacement transfusion.

John also showed some rebellious traits. He refused to save stool specimens needed for collection. He was allowed out of bed and used the toilet instead of the accessible bedpan. He did seem, however, willing to keep track of the number of stools he had a day. John also had difficulty relating to or empathizing with his 13-year-old roommate. This boy was newly diagnosed as having multiple sclerosis. He had sudden and profound loss of muscle tone on the left side and needed a great deal of assistance. John considered him "a baby" and told anyone that would listen. John and his family monopolized three-quarters of the two-bed room leaving only one-quarter for the other boy and his family. In addition to space, John had the advantage of the window and close proximity to the bathroom.

John and Harry illustrate how two teenage boys are reacting to an acute stage of their long-term illness. Their acceptance of some of the therapy is an example of a positive response of honest interpretations by medical personnel. Their difficulties in adjusting to school may be a result of how others view their illness or it may be the result of their own personalities. The emotional predisposition to their particular disease cannot be underestimated. How they interact with their peers and family may be a major link in their disease process. No less important during hospitalizations is how the nurse interacts with them.

Nursing intervention should focus on how best to meet their emotional needs during hospitalizations. I pose the following questions for consideration.

1. Is rooming-in a desirable practice for teenage boys?
2. What can be done to compensate an adolescent on NPO for approximately 30 days?
3. Are selected diets a way to make the child feel he has some "control" of the situation? (Selected diet is one the child chooses.)
4. How much "support" does an adolescent with a milder form of a disease need when he is exposed to an adolescent with a more serious form of the same disease?
5. In what ways can the nurse be instrumental in channelling the child's educational pursuits? Or should the nurse get involved?
6. What types of recreational activities can be utilized during a child's bed-rest to help him mature?
7. Is the room placement of either of these boys adequate? What would you consider a realistic placement on the unit?
8. Are there any other team members who seem essential for the quality care of these boys?
9. What role can a student nurse assume in her short experience in the clinical area? Should she assume any role, and why or why not?
10. Are the medical routines being used consistent with providing emotional support, or by their nature should we expect the child to be depressed? Why?

Nursing intervention is also concerned with the nursing tasks necessary for providing safe care. I pose the following questions for consideration in relation to these nursing tasks.

1. Who can safely assume responsibility for collecting, observing, and recording stools?
2. Is it possible to have the adolescent assume responsibility for recording his own intake and output? What factors would influence this decision?
3. Who is responsible for monitoring and recording the fluid administration? When the fluid is administered into the atrium, does this make the situation "too charged" for the usual consideration given an intravenous?
4. When the child is allowed out of bed only to be weighed, are there any special precautions necessary?
5. Who should be responsible for doing the urine specific gravity tests? Can the family be utilized for this task?
6. What special considerations are necessary when taking blood pressure readings? What significance do you think the taking of blood pressures has to these adolescents?
7. When the medication routine is changed, how much explanation should you give the child? Should adolescents with long-term illness be candidates for self-medication routines in the hospital or at home?

Children's Misconceptions and Interpretations

The jargon of the hospital easily becomes known to the child with long-term illness. However, the child is like every other child during his original orientation to the hospital. Children's misconceptions are easily made when a nurse fails to explain things in understandable language. Some illustrations follow.

Nurse: On admission, the child is seen by the *intern.*
Child's interpretation: I'll be seen in turn but for what? I hope it doesn't hurt. Whose turn is first? We take turns in school but the teacher tells us for what. I hope the bell rings before my turn comes up.
Nurse: John is to have *blood work* and a *CBC* and *x-ray pictures.*
Child's interpretation: What is this blood work? I know a needle. I hope the doctor doesn't come. I need my blood. I hope I don't die. See Bea See, sounds like they think I'm a girl. Wonder what they want me to see. Hope it is nice. Pictures I like but these x-ray pictures, I don't know. Wonder why they want my picture? Do they keep a family album of all the kids that come here?
Nurse: We need a *urine specimen* from John.
Child's interpretation: What is this your in? In what? Specimen, wonder what this means? Better ask mom.
Nurse: John should put on his *Johnny shirt.*
Child's interpretation: This isn't my shirt. Why did she call it Johnny's shirt? What a funny shirt all opened down the back. Why do I have to wear a shirt? Where are the pants? Look how short!
Nurse: Here is your *call light.*
Child's interpretation: Why call a light? Where is the bulb? Does the light talk? Must try to call the light but what do I do with it?
Nurse: This is your *bedside stand.*
Child's interpretation: Why do I have to stand by the bedside? That looks like a cabinet to me. Wonder what's in there? Why does she call it mine? I never saw that before. I don't even like it.
Nurse: Visiting hours are from 11 A.M. to 8 P.M., for parents only.
Child's interpretation: Where are my parents going? Isn't daddy going to work? They didn't tell me they were going away. Imagine putting me in here and then leaving town. I think I'll put up a fuss. Maybe it isn't so bad—Alice will have that terrible old baby-sitter.

The next day John is introduced to several other confusing situations. He looks around the room and sees the following signs on the children's beds.

NPO
Child's interpretation: Must be some kind of sign language. Good, a secret language, these kids are really cool.

HOLD
Child's interpretation: Hold what? I'll just watch and see why they hold that kid. Maybe it's part of this secret game.
Late Breakfast
Child's interpretation: Oh no! Just when I'm starved they decide to serve breakfast late. Mom always has my breakfast ready when I come downstairs. Wonder how late it will be?
Force Fluids
Child's interpretation: Wow! Wonder what they do for force. Hope it doesn't hurt. Feel sorry for that poor kid. Fluids, that sounds familiar but really don't know why they'd force lighter fluid. Mom says it's dangerous.
Save Urine
Child's interpretation: That urine is really going to the bathroom. I learned that yesterday. But, why save the urine? Wonder what they do with it. Supposing someone flushes the toilet when you're not looking? Do you get punished? Or maybe you use that urinal thing. Hope it doesn't overflow, that would be awful!
Daily Urine
Child's interpretation: Guess they like those urine specimens. I better get ready if you have to do it daily. Hope that nurse doesn't look, it's hard to go with her standing here.
Note Bleeding
Child's interpretation: Gosh that poor kid's in rough shape. I wonder when he bleeds? I don't like to see blood. Wonder why they want us to watch. I'll just cover over my head with the sheet.
OR
Child's interpretation: That's a funny sign. Or what? This place has to be nuts. Nothing makes sense.

The nurse enters the room and talks to John.

Nurse: John, I will take you to the *treatment room* for a *finger prick.*
Child's interpretation: Treatment room, what's that like? I like my room. I'm scared to go there. And a finger prick—I don't want to get stuck. That's all they do here everytime a guy turns around they give him a shot. Wish mom were here to go to this awful place with me. Wonder how I get there, on an elevator, by wheelchair?
Nurse: The *doctor's orders* state that you must have blood work done by the *house officer.*
Child's interpretation: Orders. I guess they give out a lot of those around here. The doctor seemed like a nice guy in his office. Why did he have to give orders to hurt me? I'll get even with him. I won't talk to him. Big bully! House officer sound like the cops are around. Anyone can see this isn't a house, it's a hospital. A big mean old hospital and I hate it. I want to go home; wish mom would come. I'm real mad at her; she left me here, left me and went on vacation. Forgot to ask her about that, wonder when she'll be back. Anyway, she wasn't going

until 11 A.M. Maybe she'll come here just in time to save me from this blood-sucking monster. But, what good will it do? She'll never know where this treatment room is. Bet it's down in the basement, down in a dark dungeon! Wish I was home, I miss Alice. Alice is my very best friend. Maybe she'll run away and come find me.

As the nurse and John walk down the hall the nurse begins to identify things for John.

Nurse: That is the *linen chute.*
Child's interpretation: Linen shoot, linen shoot. Shoot is something you do with a gun. Why would they want to shoot linen? Maybe they shoot people, too. Or maybe it's a shoot like a slide. Yes, that's it—a slide. Wonder if the kids can slide down it? But, linen that makes it a special slide. I haven't seen a tablecloth anywhere, wonder where the linen is. Perhaps there's a dining room with these linen tablecloths. Maybe that's where they serve the late breakfast. I hope she shows it to me soon.
Nurse: That is *the dumbwaiter* that goes to *Central Supply.*
Child's interpretation: I knew that waiter was dumb before she told me. Late breakfast when a guy is starving! Central supply must be the place where they keep the food, wonder why they don't call it a kitchen or pantry like mom does. That door seems awfully high for that dumb waiter to pass through. Maybe he has a stool or they wheel away the stairs like on an airplane. Or maybe he's like Superman, magic. Gee, I hope I get to meet him. Maybe he's not such a dumb guy after all.
Nurse: There are two people you will see a lot while you're here, John. The *cleaning lady* and the *security guard.*
Child's interpretation: Cleaning lady—she doesn't look like Minny. Wonder what she cleans, maybe it's the other kids. Not me though, Mom will clean me. Minny irons the clothes but anyone can see they don't iron these terrible Johnny shirts. Glad I have my bathrobe to cover it up. I don't want anyone to see me running around in this thing. It must have shrunk in the wash. Maybe if she irons it, it will be longer. I'll ask her next time I see her. And that security guard. What a spooky place, your very own policeman walking around looking in the rooms. I see him smiling at the kids but I won't smile back when he gets to me.
Nurse: That boy is in the *oxygen tent.*
Child's interpretation: Fine tent that is, you can see right through it. How does the poor guy sleep? I don't like the tent—it's so small the bed doesn't fit all the way in. Wonder what that pipe is doing shooting fog into the tent? Maybe they're trying to kill the kid. He doesn't look so good. Hope his mom comes to save him. That tent makes an awful lot of noise, wonder how the other kids sleep? Maybe they get soundproof tents at night.
Nurse: This is the treatment room John. That is an *intercom* to use in an *emergency.*

Child's interpretation: Emergency, boy I knew things were getting rough. Maybe I better use it now to call mom. I'd rather go home, this emergency stuff is not for me. This whole room is filled with terrible things. Just look at that—hard table, wonder what they're for. Surely, not breakfast. Who could eat in here anyway. I feel sick to my stomach just looking at all those tubes and needles and machines. Even that scale is big enough to weigh a giant! There's a refrigerator, I guess it must be the dining room after all or maybe that central supply place —wonder where the dumb waiter is? Here he comes now with the white jacket. He doesn't look too dumb.

Nurse: Hello, Dr. Jones, this is John.

Child's interpretation: Foiled again, it's not that house officer guy or the dumb waiter. It's not my doctor, either. They must have me mixed up with some other kid. I'll just set them straight and beat it out of here.

The doctor prepares to take the blood and John complains he feels faint.

Nurse: I'll have *oj* ready for you as soon as it's over.

Child's interpretation: Imagine, a real live football player waiting to see me after he sucks out the blood. Maybe this place isn't so bad after all.

Nurse: Doctor, would you like to talk to John about going to the *OR, recovery room,* and possibly the *intensive care* unit?

Child's interpretation: Intensive care, wonder why you get that. No one cares here. They just stare at you and take urine and put up signs on beds. OR—that must be one of those words they don't want me to know. Just like all the other big people, they spell when they don't want you to know what they're talking about. But, what's this recovery bit? How can I recover when I haven't even seen a ball being thrown. Imagine a whole room for ball games. Maybe they'll take me there after breakfast. Gee, but I'm hungry. I should have read that sign on the bottom of my bed. Maybe it said, no food, ever. If I could only get some of that intensive care or just someone who cared even a little when a guy is hungry.

The foregoing examples are given to emphasize to the student that teaching the child about the hospital is more than relating facts. The child will interpret information by utilizing experiences in his life experience. It is difficult for him to understand new concepts without help. Time must be spent to help the child interpret facts in a new way. The child enjoys learning new things and will be more comfortable when he gets the meanings intended, rather than his garbled interpretation. There are numerous examples which can be cited. The student must be certain to communicate with the child on his own level, and then spend time being sure the child really understands what is being said.

References

Bell, R. R. The Impact of Illness on Family Roles: A Sociological Framework for Patient Care. New York, Wiley, 1966, pp. 177–189.

Bright, F. The pediatric nurse and parental anxiety. Nurs. Forum, 4:30–47, 1965.

Bowlby, J. Grief and mourning in infancy and early childhood. Psychoanal. Stud. Child, 15:9–52, 1960.

Diller, L. Psychology of disabled children. In Rudick, E., ed., Pediatric Nursing. Dubuque, Iowa, Wm. C. Brown Co., 1966, pp. 11–17.

Farber, B. Family: Organization and Interaction. San Francisco, Chandler, 1964.

Green, M., and Durocher, M. A. Improving parent care of handicapped children. Children, 12:185–188, Sept.–Oct. 1965.

Illingworth, R. S. The increasing challenge of handicapped children. In Rudick, E., ed., Pediatric Nursing. Dubuque, Iowa, Wm. C. Brown Co., 1966, pp. 6–10.

Parad, H. J., and Caplan, G. A Framework for studying families in crisis. In Parad, H. J., ed., Crisis Intervention. New York, Family Service Assoc. of America, 1965, pp. 53–72.

Rapoport, L. Working with families in crisis: an exploration in preventive intervention. In Parad, H. J., ed. Crisis Intervention. New York, Family Service Assoc. of America, 1965, pp. 129–139.

Ross, A. O. The Exceptional Child in the Family. New York, Grune & Stratton, 1964.

Rubin, M. Caring for children with illness requiring long-term hospitalization. In Current Concepts in Clinical Nursing. Saint Louis, The C. V. Mosby Co., 1967.

Shore, M. F., Geiser, R. L., and Wolman, H. M. Constructive uses of a hospital experience. Children, 12:3–8, Jan.–Feb., 1965.

Smith, Margo. Ego support for the child patient. In Rudick, E., ed., Pediatric Nursing. Dubuque, Iowa, Wm. C. Brown Co., 1966, p. 60–70.

Smith, D. A clinical nursing tool. Am. J. Nurs., 68:2384–2388, Nov. 1968.

Spiegel, J. P. The resolution of role conflict within the family. Psychiatry, 20:1–16, 1957.

4 DONNA JUENKER

Child's Perception of His Illness

The life-span of a child consists of a multitude of experiences that he assimilates into his reality. His "reality" depends to a larger extent on how he *perceives* those experiences. Perception is the process of organizing and attaching meaning to the raw changes that occur in the brain following stimulation of the end organs of sensory receptors (Nash, 1970). This attachment of meaning to stimuli is a complex process for the child. When one compares the relative insensitivity of the newborn infant with the sophisticated modes of perception that characterize the adolescent, one is immediately aware of the magnitude of change in perceptual development.

The baby first perceives *emotional* significances (Stone and Church, 1957). The *meaning* that an object has is perceived well in advance of the characteristics of the object itself. Later on, an awareness of "action" relationships is added to "feeling" associations. Objects are perceived in relation to what they *do* to the child. As the objects in the child's world assume more stability and permanence, visual perception dominates. With increasing sophistication in visual abilities, the child learns to perceive objective properties.

The child is aided in his perceptual development by the fact that specific language labels are applied to objects. Once he learns that "dogs" have properties that are different from "cats" or that "yellow" and "orange" are different shades of color, he is more likely to note the distinction the next time he sees these stimuli.

When confronted by an unfamiliar stimulus, such as a picture of an unusual object, the young child tends to react to the entire stimulus as a whole rather than to its parts. The older child, on the other hand, can see distinct aspects of the same new stimulus. His initial perception will include a more complete description of the details in the picture.

Perception is affected by the intensity of the stimulus—that is, the degree to which it absorbs the child's attention. A very strong stimulus blocks out distracting influences. Such intense involvement or absorption in an experience can open one's sensory receptivity to a point at which maximum learning can take place. However, if the stimulus is very stressful, the perceptual field can become extremely narrow so that attention is directed solely to the alleviation of the stress.

The child's perception is also affected by the scope of the stimulus —that is, the number of parts in the whole. If his senses are simultaneously penetrated by many stimuli such as sights, sounds, and internal stirrings, he is likely to select out from the total those parts that have special meaning or are in some way connected to a familiar past experience. While this selectivity is an understandable way of coping with a new situation, the child's perception of the experience may not conform with consensus reality. He may have missed many significant aspects that were quite evident to onlookers.

In spite of perceptual constancy in areas such as shape, color, and depth, perception is a very individual matter since it is constantly being altered by past experience. Throughout the evolution of perceptual development, experience broadens the child's repertory of cues so that he can be increasingly adept at recognizing similarities and differences among the objects in the environment. As the child grows older, a stimuli perceived earlier can have increasingly complex meanings because of the child's ability to see new properties in a particular object or to see new alternatives in a particular problem situation. By repeated experiences involving seeing, hearing, tasting, smelling, and touching, the child improves his powers of discrimination and gradually his perceptions become more objective. This process is an important part of cognitive development.

Many children face the experience of being ill. Illness brings with it an endless combination of disquieting symptoms, variation in intensity of objective stress, and marked changes in the social and physical aspects of the external environment. Each of these components constitutes a unique experiential phenomenon which the child assimilates into his reality as best he can. Each new experience is somehow linked to previous ones. Early experiences serve as preparation for those that follow. A child who is confronted by a situation such as illness that is unlike any previous experience is left without a ready response. He has to call on what may be a limited number of mental configurations or images and immature psychological defenses to accommodate the new experience.

The long-term aspect of an illness influences the child's perception of his confinement in at least three distinct ways. The factor of time has special significance. Although each stage of illness is different from the preceding one, the chronic nature of an illness does permit the child and parents to perceive and assimilate the illness and its effects more gradually. There is more time to prepare for new experiences and to inquire about areas of concern. There is more time for productive teaching within a moderately paced schedule. Misconceptions can be identified and more easily corrected.

Another important factor is the increased exposure to illness that children with long-term health problems experience. Each time they are hospitalized or visit the doctor's office or clinic, they see a variety of illness among other children. Conversational focus centers on illness. Depending on the nature of the illness and the attitudes of parents and health workers, disease can become a dominant feature in the lives of these children. Overemphasis on health and illness has the potential for arousing fantasies and fears about the child's physical integrity. It naturally heightens self-concern and may dramatically influence how the child perceives his illness.

A third factor is that long-term illness, by its very nature, sustains contact between the nurse and the patient and family. Because she sees the child over an extended period of time, and because she knows what the child experiences, the nurse can help the child interpret illness in a manner that is realistically appropriate to his level of understanding. This opportunity to provide on-going support must not be overlooked. upright posture further extends feelings of "you-ness" and "me-ness." what the child thinks about his illness.

This chapter seeks to identify and describe the factors that influence the child's perception of illness. Emphasis will be placed on those factors that are most essential in planning nursing care. For example, it is well known that illness alters body image to some degree. To understand the impact of change in body image, it is important that the nurse knows how the body-image concept evolves in childhood and how important such a concept is to a child.

Another section of the chapter examines the child's view of the structure and function of the body. It is obvious that the child's reality is different from the way an adult understands body function. When a health professional with sophisticated knowledge about the body attempts to communicate with a child about his illness, many false assumptions can be made. Misconceptions on the part of both frequently result. If the nurse understands what the child thinks about the healthy body, her communication can be guided by the level of knowledge which the child possesses. She is in a better position to help the child interpret the bodily changes that accompany illness. If she is aware of common misconceptions that children have, she is not likely to presume that they have a realistic grasp of their problems.

Every child attaches a wide range of meanings to his illness. The variety of factors that determine his interpretation will also be discussed. The influence of age and past experience will be emphasized.

Still another section of the chapter will explore the impact of hospitalization. Viewed as one aspect of illness, the hospitalization experience will be examined primarily in relation to the marked alteration in the child's environment that it produces.

Since one of the primary factors affecting the child's perception of illness is attitudes and actions of parents, the chapter will conclude with an analysis of parental influence.

This collection of information will hopefully increase the nurse's awareness of the perceptual process as it relates to a child's view of illness. An important by-product of this awareness is an increased empathy for her young patients and their families. With empathy serving as a motivational factor, she can draw upon this body of knowledge to serve as a base for meaningful interaction about a very significant experience for any child—illness.

Concept of Body Image

Gorman (1969) defines body image as the concept of one's own body, based on present and past perceptions. Body image is a dynamic concept—constantly undergoing changes in keeping with one's perceptions. The ability to give one's body the characteristics of unity and distinctness from others requires an integration of external stimuli and internal sensations. The concept of body image evolves over a lifetime, with its beginnings traceable to infancy.

The young infant, of course, cannot grasp the concept of his separateness. He perceives himself and the world to be identical. One of his important tasks, then, is to learn about his distinctiveness. Because of the body's concentration on oral activities, it seems likely that the infant begins to note the differences between things coming into the mouth from the outside and the internal feelings that ingestion of food brings with it. The constancy of the mouth and tongue as opposed to the changing nature of the solids and liquids entering the oral cavity serves to identify the mouth as a body boundary. Increasing observation and use of arms and legs and fingers and toes along with the assumption of an upright posture further extends feelings of "you-ness" and "me-ness." The "out-of-sight, out-of-mind" cognitive stage gradually gives way to the realization that the extended arm or leg can be maneuvered into the range of vision, that its function remains constant and that it is "me." Thus maturational changes affect body image. Posture, for instance, involves steadiness and stance as well as adaptive movements of locomotion and prehension.

There are several other factors that contribute to the infant's "body feeling." One mechanism is pain (Schilder, 1935; Bender, 1963). Pain felt in a particular body area helps the infant in the orientation of his body parts. Although the young child may not be able to verbalize the location of pain, pain is *felt* as a localized phenomenon and consequently it is associated with the organization of the body image. When there is pain on the surface of the body, that body part becomes over-emphasized. The individual's attention is drawn to it. Through repetition of painful experiences, the baby not only learns about his own body boundaries but he also comes to realize that only he can feel "his" pain.

Another mechanism that contributes to the body-image concept is touch (Anthony, 1968). Touching one's own body arouses a different sensation from that experienced when touching the body of another. Being touched by another is yet a different experience. The infant who chews on his own fingers evokes a feeling state that is quite different from that achieved by chewing on his mother's fingers.

Anthony (1968) also describes a third mechanism in the process of self-differentiation—the mirror image. By looking into a mirror, the infant sees himself in the way that others see him. As social awareness increases the child recognizes the reflection as his own image.

Psychosexual stages in development have considerable bearing on concepts of body image in the young child. For instance, the child develops erotic interests in particular parts of his body—especially the oral, anal, umbilical, and genital zones. The satisfaction derived from exploring these areas draws attention to body configuration and helps to consolidate concepts of unique body boundaries.

With increasing age, language becomes an important contributor to body image. Body parts are named and classified. The frequency with which certain body parts become a part of the approved vocabulary makes the child attach a certain level of significance to them. If a part of the body and its accompanying terminology are purposefully avoided or are spoken about in hushed or emotional tones, the child may learn to repress this knowledge or consider it taboo.

Learning control of body functions occupies much of the toddler's energies. This preoccupation and "fussing" with the body may resemble a hypochondrical reaction. The power over elimination symbolizes power over all body processes and is another mark of differentiation between the self and others.

One of the preschooler's most significant discoveries about his body is finding sex differences. This discovery gives rise to the Freudian concept of the castration complex. The little boy's "pride" in his penis coincides with his extreme fear of losing the organ (as he thinks happened to girls). Girls, on the other hand, feel cheated and deprived and may wish to grow a penis. Recognition of and response to these concerns may have a bearing on how these children perceive the male-female aspects of their body image.

The ordinary social experiences of the young child, including body contact with others, also helps to determine where the body leaves off and another body begins to function.

Children continue to expand their awareness of body dimensions as they progress from the early stages of development when initial discoveries about the body are of great magnitude. They still perceive the body in terms of what it can *do* for them. However, as they move into the school years (and perhaps even before), these concrete body concepts are modified by more subtle interpretations of the meaning of body type. For example, Staffieri (1967) studied 90 boys between the ages of six and ten to determine the extent to which they associated body build with social-personal behaviors. Responses differed depending upon whether the children were viewing silhouettes of mesomorphic (muscular), endomorphic (fat), or ectomorphic (thin) body types. All of the adjectives that the children assigned to the mesomorph figure were favorable. For example, among other traits, they were rated as strong, healthy, good looking, brave, smart, and as having lots of friends. Characteristics assigned to the endomorph and ectomorph figures were generally either socially or personally unfavorable. The fat child was often viewed as naughty, mean, ugly, dirty, and stupid. On the other hand, the thin silhouette evoked descriptions that included words like quiet, afraid, sad, and weak. Although the boys in the study had a reasonably accurate perception of their own body type, they showed a clear preference for looking like the mesomorph image. This preference began to be evident between six and seven years of age.

Accuracy of the perception of one's body appears to increase with age. Nash (1969) studied a group of seventh- and ninth-grade boys to determine the extent to which they could recognize photographs of parts of their own bodies and those of their acquaintances. Self-recognition accuracy exceeded chance levels for most of the body regions investigated. The facial regions (forehead, eyes, mouth) were better recognized than other parts of the body. In this sample, because of the age (puberty), recognition of some of the features seemed to be related to developmental factors such as acne and changes in body proportions.

The group studied was racially heterogeneous. The greatest accuracy of self-recognition was found to be among the minority group children. Majority race children also tended to be more accurate in recognizing minority group children than they were in recognizing their same race acquaintances. The accuracy of recognition seemed to be related to stereotyped concepts associated with the anatomical features of minority races. While the results of the study are certainly not conclusive, they lead one to speculate that a child's personal interest or concern about his body is sustained during the school years and possibly heightened at times when normal physical changes in the body become evident, especially at the time of puberty. The study introduced a point that needs further exploration. It seems possible that a child's membership in a stigmatized group may also heighten body concern. One might wonder whether alteration in body image is more disturbing to these children whose bodies are apparently well scrutinized by themselves and others.

It seems reasonable to conclude from the foregoing statements that one's concept of body image evolves from multiple factors—biological configuration, physiological function, developmental maturation, and social reinforcement. The intensity of the child's interest in his body varies but it seems obvious from the literature that body perceptions are quite keen fairly early in life. This should lead us to examine more closely what a young child thinks about his body when it undergoes unanticipated changes during illness.

Perceptions About the Inside of the Body

While children appear to have some sophistication about the external dimensions of the body, the internal organs and tissues of the body are shrouded in considerable mystery. The fact that there is substantial ignorance about the inside of the body is really not too surprising when one realizes that most bodily sensation is concentrated on the body surface. When the body systems are functioning normally, children are not acutely aware of organic activity. The lungs, heart, and intestines are not in the mainstream of consciousness as they carry out their daily activities.

Nevertheless, in spite of a vague awareness of body organs and little theoretical background, children do construct frameworks of body functioning—sometimes very elaborate ones, indeed.

Schilder and Weschler (1935), among the earliest to describe children's concepts about their bodies, asked children what was inside of the body. Most of them (especially between the ages of five and ten) replied that the inside of the body contained food. This answer seems logical since children are well aware that food enters the body. Some used more concrete terms and pictured themselves filled with bread, milk, or meat. One boy of eight-and-a-half expressed a combination of ideas when asked what was in his belly. In response to the query, he replied: "Food, my stomach, sweets, and ice." The children expressed interesting ideas about the self. When one child was asked to describe what was under his skin he answered "me." For some it seemed to be an envelope of the self. In other words, if the skin were peeled off, the whole self would be revealed.

This five-year-old boy's discussion with his teacher reveals his thoughts about his skin. (Words in parenthesis are comments of the teacher.)

> (Inspecting his abdomen as he dresses after nap.) You know a thing? There is something funny about my skin. It fits all smooth mostly, but when I do this, there are extra skin in crumples. What is that for? (It's loose so you can move and stretch, etc.) No it is not loose or it would show. It would hang down. It would be too big. (Like a rubber band.) Would it break if you pulled it too much? (Can stretch a lot.) I had this same skin when I was a baby. It fits very nice. It is me. (Stone and Church, 1957, p. 160.)

Concepts about body processes were studied by Nagy (1953). She focused on brain function, breathing and digestion. The children in the sample ranged in age from about four to twelve years. Nearly all of the children associated the brain with intellectual activities. It was not until the age of eight that other functions began to appear in the children's descriptions. Predominance of mental function over emotional and physical factors is not surprising because children are often reminded to use their brain when mental effort is required. Nerves—with functions such as feeling, working, and moving—were mentioned by some of the older children but such sophisticated answers occurred rarely throughout the study sample.

Children did not refer consistently to the *process* of breathing (i.e., taking in and expelling of air) until around nine years of age. The nose, mouth, and throat were frequently mentioned in relation to breathing. This seemed to indicate that children believed that air circulated in the head region, primarily between the nose and mouth. A high percentage of children believed that breathing was necessary for life but generally did not know why.

The digestive tract was thought by most to consist of the mouth and stomach. The stomach was the place for "keeping our food" or for "eating;" the purpose of eating was very vague—"to live," "to grow," and "to keep healthy."

Gellert (1962) also conducted an extensive study aimed at examining children's perception of the content and functioning of the human body. The children ranged in age from four years nine months to sixteen years eleven months. All of the children were hospitalized, so it is likely that their ideas about their bodies were affected by their illnesses. Gellert's study differs from some of the early ones in the sense that she not only compiled quantitative age-by-age data but also made a qualitative analysis of the children's responses. As in the Schilder and Weschler study, she found that younger children listed food, blood, and excretia as being inside of the body. As age increased, digestive, urinary, nervous, and respiratory systems were mentioned with greater frequency. The numbers of body parts that children could name dramatically increased at about age nine. For example, children between five and seven years could name an average of three parts; those between nine and eleven would list an average of nine parts.

When children were asked about the most important part of the body, the heart was given this distinction by most of the children in all age categories. Organs associated with nervous, sensory, and intellectual activity were next in order. The importance of an organ was generally rated on the basis of its capacity to "run and/or control vital functions." It was interesting to note that some of the very young children associated importance with the amount of care and attention given to a particular body part. One youngster claimed that his toes were the most important part of the body "because you have to scrub between [them] which is real hard" (Gellert, 1962, p. 320).

The children were asked to describe the parts of the body that they consider dispensable. Doing without a part of the body was inconceivable for some; 20 percent of the children quizzed firmly believed that they needed all their parts and could dispense with none. (All of these children were under the age of eleven.)

Of the dispensable parts recorded by the children in Gellert's study, it was surprising to note that arms and legs were mentioned with greatest frequency in spite of their importance in the daily life of the children.

There is some evidence in the study to support the influence of the mass media on concepts that children have about the body. For instance, Gellert discovered that several children were aware of the existence of organ transplants. The impact of illness was also evident since many children attached special significance to the diseased parts of their bodies.

The methods used to gather the data in the aforementioned studies included interviews, graphic representations, written essays, and paper-and-pencil tests. A variety of methods had to be used in order to accommodate the cognitive abilities of the children. The investigators are careful to point out that the findings reveal only what the children are willing to talk about or write down. Very likely the information given does not reflect all that they know. As mentioned before, certain parts of the body may be considered as "forbidden" areas and the child may not express his knowledge because he thinks it is unacceptable to do so.

Children's human figure drawings reveal a great deal about how children view their bodies. The head predominates in the child's first recognizable drawings and arms and legs appear as projections from the head (Di Leo, 1970). The head, arms, and legs are significant in the child's life since they are primary foci for sensory input. They serve locomotion needs and permit exploration and experimentation with people and objects in the environment. Generally speaking, the trunk is ignored. Eyes are the dominant facial features, appearing as large circles in the head. The frequency of their presence in early drawings suggests the importance to the child of expressive eyes. Other facial features will be added before the body is consistently included in the drawing. It is not until about age five that the trunk is added.

As the child grows older, he perceives more of the fine details of the body and has the manipulative ability to depict his perceptions. Yet, his figure drawings do not truly reflect actual body dimensions. Rather, they seem to coincide with body image—not as we see the child, only as he conceives himself (Gorman, 1969).

Child's Interpretation of His Illness

Illness has meaning for every child. His interpretation depends upon a wide range of factors: age, the nature of the illness and its treatment, family relationships, and past experiences. Illness is stressful at all ages—even when illness is mild, family relationships are satisfying, and past experiences are basically untraumatic. However, each child experiences his own set of concerns to a degree of intensity that is uniquely his.

PERCEPTIONS ABOUT CAUSE OF ILLNESS. A primary concern of the ill child is resolution of responsibility for the illness. It is commonly assumed by children that illness is a punishment. Sometimes the child can recall a specific deed that he perpetrated that is of sufficient magnitude to cause illness. Recollection of mother's warning "If you don't wear your rubbers, you'll get sick" suddenly becomes very meaningful. That blame and illness or injury go hand in hand in the child's mind was readily noted when a young boy of eight reacted to a picture of a child with a bandaged head by saying, "It was his fault. He probably didn't watch the cars when he crossed the street."

The idea of punishment is not just related to bad deeds. Illness can also serve as a retribution for bad thoughts. During the preschool years, for instance, children are known to wish their parents dead because of competition for affection. There is much ambivalence about this notion so that they also experience guilt. When illness or injury strikes, they can associate this discomfort with "evil" thoughts. Feelings of anger often accompany the guilt but sometimes the opportunity to "suffer" relieves some of the child's anxiety.

The school-age child associates the cause of illness with "germs" (Nagy, 1953). Many children believe that germs are animals, identified especially with insects such as flies and spiders. They are commonly thought to enter the body through the mouth and once inside the body children say that they invariably cause illness. Germs are believed to have properties such as walking around inside the body, eating and breeding. Although the child connects disease with an external causative factor, he may continue to hold himself responsible for the entry of the germ into the body. Sometimes, children will extend the blame to parents and peers.

CONSEQUENCES OF ILLNESS. The sick child can be visibly concerned about the tangible consequences of his illness apart from the physical aspects of his disease. For instance, the child may worry about a loss of position in the family. This might be an especially critical issue if his status is already a bit shaky because of the arrival of a new sibling or if an older brother or sister has just returned from college. In the case of the new sibling, however, the illness may provide the child with the added attention that he craves.

School absenteeism accompanied by interruption in the social and competitive aspects of peer activities are also major worries for the sick child. If the duration of the illness is prolonged, the child may be fearful about his ability to resume normal activities. Not "measuring up" to his own expectations and the expectations of others is an age-old concern of all children in the middle years of childhood. However, if residual effects of illness complicate the situation, the problem can be enormous.

The restrictions of movement and diet that often accompany illness can exert hardship on the child. During the acute states of an illness, a child may be content to reduce his activity and the intake of food. However, once he begins to feel better, these restrictions are increasingly difficult to bear. Of course, the reaction to these limitations is affected by the meaning that they have for a particular child and family. An active, sports-minded, outdoor enthusiast will experience more stress than a child whose interests are more sedentary. In a family in which enjoyment of food plays a dominant role in its life-style, restriction of foods presents a problem not only for the sick child, but also for the mother who must enforce the restrictions. Many mothers judge the effectiveness of their mothering role by how well they feed their children.

All illness brings with it a certain degree of dependency. In moderation this is good because it permits the individual to focus attention on himself and conserve energy that he might otherwise expend in trying to sustain independent function. If the degree of dependency is great, it becomes threatening. Dependent-independent conflicts are frequent occurrences in childhood. The autonomy for which the toddler strives hinges on the achievement of a variety of important developmental tasks such as walking, bowel control, self-feeding, and talking. When illness disrupts the normal progression of these developmental landmarks and robs the child of new-found independence, the effects are clearly visible and the child takes backward steps in all of these areas. This regression wounds the ego, and it requires sensitive handling to reestablish self-satisfying independence.

The dependency problems experienced by the older child are not quite so obvious. Dependency on others, after a period when the child has mastered complete control over his body, arouses feelings of shame and embarrassment. Strong feelings of modesty conflict with the invasion of privacy that attends bodily illness. The adolescent resents dependency in a special way. In some ways the intensity of his feelings and his self-interest parallel that of the toddler—but there is a difference. The adolescent, in his search for identity, is concerned with how he appears in the eyes of others as compared to his view of himself. Dependence, in this instance, can be devastating because it puts the adolescent out of touch with his peers and places the reins of control in the hands of authoritarian adults from which he is trying to loosen ties.

The older child who is sick can be very conscious of the hardships that his illness exerts on the members of the family. He may struggle with the realization that his own needs are in conflict with family needs. In his sincere attempt to reduce his demands on family resources, he may inadvertently appear to reject his family's attention. Youngsters also worry about the financial burden that the treatment may impose. The father who has to work a double job to make ends meet is a reminder to the child that he has strained family resources. The concern is especially acute during the school years when contributions to and responsibility for family affairs is an important aspect of social development. A child who thinks that he is not doing "his share" thinks less of himself.

Family vacations and other activities may be postponed in deference to the needs of the sick child whether he is treated at home or in the hospital. The child's needs may require someone in attendance at all times. Parents can well understand the need (although they realistically experience disappointment when anticipated plans are changed) but siblings have greater difficulty in handling the conflict of interests. The sick child is often quite aware of the turmoil he thinks that he has caused and this may intensify already present guilt feelings.

PHYSICAL ASPECTS OF ILLNESS. I have just pointed out that the behavior of a sick child has many psychosocial determinants. It is also important to discuss the relationship between behavior and physical aspects of the illness itself. This concept is not quite so clear, although the existence of some type of relationship seems likely.

Infants and toddlers do not perceive the significance of altered body function in its real sense; rather, they view it as an interruption in the usual sequence of the meaningful events to which they have become accustomed. To them, illness amounts to a collection of deprivations and overstimulations. No doubt these children experience internal stirrings that beg for satisfaction along the tension-relaxation continuum. Frustration of oral drives and restriction of movement are major sources of tension.

The toddler, of course, perceives more of his body than does the infant, but as yet he has not incorporated the concept of self and therefore does not see himself clearly as a separately functioning unit. While it is true that toddlers can identify visible parts of the body, especially facial characteristics, they do not have the cognitive faculty of associating illness with threat to body function.

The preschool period brings with it increased awareness of body structure and function. Control of excretory function draws attention to the body and its products. The child attaches great significance to physical sex differences and, generally, is taken up with the notion of physical identity. Fear of injury to the self, including castration anxiety, is common. Any part of the body is essential to its wholeness. Thus a break in the skin or a removal of a body part such as the tonsils fragments the child's concept of his unity.

Stone and Church (1957, p. 161) record the following comments made by a five-year-old boy, which well illustrate feelings about being complete:

> Once there was Stuart with a tooth and in it there was a hole. So it was fixed. The man had many little streams there, very nice. There was a pain, a bright pain. It was bright when he pushed with a noise and a bar. But there was no blood. No blood. . . . Can I get a hole in my hand like the hole in my tooth? Will it have to be filled with a loud noise? . . . The queen was in the garden hanging up her clothes, there came along a big thing to snap off her nose. . . . Her nose was not. It bled and bled and she died. Humpty Dumpty did die, too. He fell off and couldn't put together again. . . . When I have my tonsils out— what will happen when I have my tonsils out? Will it bleed?

Will I be dead? Being blood is being dead. Why do I have my
tonsils out?
    *I do not like myself not to be myself, and that is what will
happen if even my littlest tonsils is taken away from me.*
    . . . Sad it was to have a nose taken off. So it will be sad to
have a tonsil out. Blood, blood, blood. When the nose—the
tonsil is out.

Older children have more realistic conceptions of their bodies.
However, because they can connect illness with impaired body function
and then relate impaired function with a threat to their well-being,
bodily changes can arouse marked anxiety. This is especially true if
misconceptions go undetected. Death fantasies are quite common during later childhood. The consequences of illness such as physical limitation or dietary restriction are more impressive to children in this age
group. This may contribute to the increased incidence of withdrawal
and depression.

At all ages, certain parts of the body have symbolic significance.
Diseases of the heart, brain, and eyes seem to cause a high degree of
anxiety (Blom, 1958; Langford, 1961). This coincides with the importance attached to these organs by children themselves. Anna Freud
(1952) postulates that genital operations arouse castration fears at
virtually all levels of development. Of course, *any* part of the body can
be charged with libidinal significance if, for some reason, it is made the
focus of an unusual amount of attention.

The visibility of the illness may also be a factor in determining
the child's reaction. Bergmann (1965) describes differences between
children with orthopedic illnesses and those who had cardiac conditions.
The orthopedic patients, as a group, seemed to adjust to their illnesses
in a more positive manner than did the cardiac children. Part of this
reaction seemed to be due to the fact that the malady was so tangible.
The child and his roommates could see the evidence of the disorder and
the apparatus that was used to treat it. The illness, in effect, could be
touched and manipulated. In fact, it could *not* be hidden even if there
was a desire to do so. Explanations about the illness could be given
matter-of-factly with a predictable timetable of progress. The undeni-
able reality of the illness seemed to discourage excessive use of fantasy.
The realization that other children were in the same circumstances also
seemed supportive.

Bergmann proposes an interesting basis for acceptance of the illness. She suggests that children might view their period of immobilization as a time of "suspense" in a way similar to atonement in fairy tales
in which "a happy ending is reached only after great hardship has been
endured, such hardship not only being accepted but sought after and
endowed with pleasurable anticipation" (Bergmann, 1965, p. 61).

She goes on to point out, however, that although these children
appeared to adjust well to the period of immobilization, they behaved
in quite a different way when ambulation was begun. The slow progress

of ambulation undermined their magical expectations. Once the element of freedom was reintroduced, they were unwilling to be patient with any further restriction no matter how slight it was.

Cardiac patients, on the other hand, were generally depressed and discouraged and tended to be hypochondrial. In the absence of clear-cut evidence of illness, these children had to find something on which to focus their attention. Often, they became preoccupied with their heartbeat and identified even normal variations in it with a deterioration of their condition.

Part of the children's problem in dealing with this type of illness seemed to be related to their inability to comprehend the nature of heart action. The progress of their recovery was not predictable and they constantly compared themselves with others and viewed relapses as premonitions of their own fate. Their mental construct of the importance of the heart often had ominous overtones.

It seems likely to me that the staff's own attitude toward a particular illness could have an important bearing on the attitude of the child. The staff could probably be more open about orthopedic illnesses than they were about cardiac conditions. When the outcome of an illness is obscure or when treatment is unpleasant or introduces a threat to life, the medical and nursing personnel can experience much ambivalence in interacting with the child. It is always easier to tell a child that he is getting better than to explain why he is not.

The extent to which ill children look alike or different from other youngsters may also affect how they view their own illness. In Gellert's study, it was noted that children verbalized that arms and legs were dispensable parts of the body. However, when other children were confronted by a child with an amputation, they had difficulty identifying with the disability (Bergmann, 1965). The impact of the reality of the situation overshadowed the intellectual awareness that, indeed, one can live without an arm or leg.

The existence of scars is a significant factor to consider when one is trying to assess the child's reaction to illness. The adult's perception frequently centers on the scar's appearance. The older child, especially the adolescent, is concerned about appearance, too. However, the scar may cause great upset because of the alteration of function that may result or because of such a seemingly inconsequential matter as the strange numbness that may occur around the scarred area.

I remember caring for an 11-year-old girl who was badly burned on the upper trunk and legs. She was a black child and the extensive skin grafts left very unsightly changes in the pigmentation of her skin. Her primary concern, however, was not the scar itself but rather that the scars would restrict development of what little breast tissue remained after the burn. She was likewise very anxious about the fact that she would not have any breast nipples.

SIGNIFICANCE OF PAIN. The kinds of symptoms associated with an illness may also affect the type and intensity of the child's reaction.

One of the physical consequences of illness and treatment is pain. It is generally assumed that very young infants lack a sophisticated mechanism to perceive and respond to painful stimuli. Evidence to support this assumption from a physiological point of view is scanty. Although it is generally agreed that the fetus and the newborn (at least for a few hours) have a high degree of tolerance for pain (Pratt, 1954), it has also been noted that there is a developmental decrease in electrotactual thresholds of infants as early as one day of age (Kaye and Lipsitt, 1964). Therefore, it seems that sensitivity to pain increases quite rapidly. It does not take long before the infant withdraws the part of his body that has encountered a noxious stimuli.

The physiological basis for pain involves the functioning of a complex interwoven network of fine, beaded, subcutaneous nerve terminals, chemical substances that activate nerve impulses, and an intact central nervous system (Crowley, 1962). However common this physiological make-up might be to all individuals, children do react in various ways to what might be considered the same intensity of objective stress. Many reasons for these variations have been proposed.

People attach considerable psychological meaning to the experience of pain. These meanings are derived largely from experiences in early childhood. I have already pointed out the significance of pain in determining body boundaries and, consequently, its contribution to body image.

Engel (1962) states that early in childhood, pain and punishment become linked. This is understandable if one remembers that a considerable amount of childhood pain results from such stimuli as spankings when one is bad. Guilt is associated with the pain of punishment. If the experience of reconciliation after punishment constitutes the only love and support that a child receives, it is probable that some children may actually enjoy the pain of punishment because they anticipate love and forgiveness. If an insecure child notices that his complaints of pain call forth expressions of concern and sympathy from usually undemonstrative parents, the child may *use* pain as a means of getting love from them (Hardy et al., 1952).

Children can also associate pain with aggression and power. Threatening or inflicting pain can give the child control over persons or objects in the environment.

Child-rearing practices (often determined by the past experiences of the parents) can condition response to pain. In Western culture, sex roles determine the limits of acceptable responses to pain. Boys generally are discouraged from crying in the interest of avoiding "sissylike" behavior; girls, on the other hand, are expected to be more emotional, so that a show of tears is seldom punished. Apart from this cultural determinant, the parent's own attitude toward pain affects how the child will behave. If the parent attaches great significance to the slightest bodily hurt, the child will likely respond with a heightened sensitivity to pain. Lack of protection from pain will be just as detrimental and will also result in a low pain threshold. Total avoidance of painful experiences is certainly improbable and actually unwise. However, when a child experiences pain he obviously needs support from significant persons. Given such support, it is probable that repeated exposure to moderately noxious stimuli helps the child to cope with the stress of pain.

Any one or any combination of these factors may be operating when a child's illness has the element of pain associated with it. They must be considered in evaluating the significance of the pain. The child who screams from pain following a finger prick deserves attention as does the child with severe incisional pain following surgery. In both cases, the child's pain is real to him and it must be dealt with in terms of his experience.

Recognition of the existence of pain has always been a nursing dilemma. The very young child has difficulty expressing feelings of pain and localizing it partly because of maturational factors and partly because of fear. The nurse must rely on nonverbal cues to spot evidence of pain. Tense body position, inability to be comforted by ordinary means, rolling of the head, rubbing or pulling on a part of the body, and restlessness and overreaction to the environment are indications of the child's discomfort. The older child can be more explicit in his description of pain but he is also more sophisticated in covering up real pain when he feels that it might be to his advantage to do so. A child anticipating discharge from the hospital, for instance, might withhold a complaint of pain since it may become an obstacle to leaving.

In the same sense, the older child can also willfully exaggerate pain to serve his own needs. The presence or absence of strained facial expression, unusual quietness, and disinclination to move a part of the body are subtle indications which even the older child finds difficult to hide especially if "no one is looking." Pain causes tension of skeletal muscle and if it occurs for prolonged periods of time it produces fatigue, lethargy, and additional aches and pains elsewhere in the body. Consequently prompt relief based on early recognition is important.

When illness is accompanied by diarrhea or vomiting, children may experience a psychological as well as a physical insult. Especially to the preschool child, it represents loss of control over a function of the body that had previously been managed at his discretion. Signs such as pronounced edema and severe postural defects are of special concern to adolescents whose self-identity hinges on the body's appearance. Dizziness, nausea, and dyspnea are frightening sensations for which the child is unprepared. He feels strangely different but has no way to judge the degree of threat posed to his well-being. Treatments such as intubation, enemas, rectal temperatures, spinal taps, and forcible administration of medicine can be viewed by the children as purposely intrusive acts.

PERCEPTION OF TYPES OF TREATMENT.   If the treatment involves motor restraint, the nurse can expect heightened aggression in some children; in others, there may be increased docility. Restraint of one part of the body may inhibit nonaffected parts (A. Freud, 1952). A deficient or malfunctioning part of the body, wherever it might be, will capture the child's attention. For the period of illness, that part stands isolated and will distort the body image to some extent.

Illness, especially if it requires surgical treatment, arouses the child's fantasies. As previously mentioned it might bring to the foreground ideas about being attacked or castrated. These notions appear most frequently in the conversations of young children. Anna Freud (1952) suggests that an operation might be experienced as mutilation in punishment for penis envy or masturbation. Other fantasies may center around episodes of abandonment and uncontrollable animated properties associated with diseased parts of the body. The elaborate construction of a body model can be illustrated by the case of a five-year-old boy described by Anthony (1968). He was referred for treatment of severe constipation, headaches, sinus trouble, and a dry cough. The little child explained these symptoms in the context of this coherent framework: "The 'plops' that didn't come out were turned back and wandered instead into his chest (to give bronchitis), into his face (to produce sinus trouble), and into his head (to produce headaches)" (Anthony, 1968, p. 111).

The child's age and past experiences will play a part in his fantasies. As children grow older and enter middle childhood, they are concerned with how the world really is. They are preoccupied with how things work and the concrete outcomes that result from their endeavors. Fantasy, while still present, is modified by added experience. There is an increased awareness of the difference between fact and fantasy so that, when fantasy occurs, the child tends to repress it. To the casual onlooker, it is sometimes difficult to sort out the fantasy in the child's expression because he has so well incorporated it into a quasi-realistic framework. A child's preoccupation with a function of his body or his constant testing of the limits of bed rest may be deeply rooted in fantasy. For instance, he may imagine, as did a child in Gellert's study that "if you didn't have ribs, somebody could hit you and you'd collapse like a feather." A child with this impression may be overwhelmed with fear if he was about to experience chest surgery. Fantasy, of course, is a well-recognized coping strategy. It can be a very acceptable way of tolerating a stressful experience (Murphy, 1962). It is a rather common way of adjusting to losses of body parts and injuries such as severe burns. However, when it becomes a dominant mechanism of defense, fantasy leads to isolation (Lidz, 1968).

Langford (1961) describes a type of anxiety experienced by sick children that he calls "organismic." It is an unconscious phenomenon in which the child perceives a threat to the life or integrity of the organism. Evidence to support this idea comes from Langford's observations of children who developed neurotic symptoms prior to the onset of physical illness. Acute overwhelming anxiety that is out of proportion to the stress is sometimes reported by parents before signs and symptoms appear. Anna Freud (1952) explains this as resulting from the heightened demand of the ill body for libidinal cathexis.

COPING MECHANISMS. Each child responds to these stressful feelings with a unique pattern of behavior. In essence he learns a series of coping strategies to fit a variety of environmental demands. Murphy (1962, p. 274) defines coping strategies as "the child's individual patternings and timings of his resources for dealing with specific problems or needs or challenges."

Although the strategies are first learned in early childhood, they are likely to be sustained, though perhaps under better control, through adulthood. The same coping mechanism can be used in a variety of stressful situations. It is helpful to know how a child reacts to stress because when he is ill he may use the same defenses. Many of the techniques used by young children have been extensively described by Murphy (1962). Some of the common mechanisms can be summarized as follows:

The child can sort out those aspects of a stressful situation that he can reasonably handle. Some children are hesitant in facing a new situation and proceed one step at a time; others are eager to explore many aspects of an unfamiliar situation simultaneously. The little child who fights to "put on his own Bandaid" may not only be concerned about keeping himself intact but may also be saying that his involvement in a familiar activity relieves some of his stress. Older children may show exorbitant concern about a minor defect such as an old scar or birth mark rather than focus on the uncomfortable symptoms of their illness.

Children can avoid a stressful situation by denying reality. By resorting to fantasy, they can make their illness temporarily less real. This gives them time to absorb the effects of the stress more gradually. Sometimes children will insist that they are completely well. Langford (1961) reports the case of one boy who had gangrene of the foot. He insisted that his mother not be told of the impending amputation until after his foot had grown back on. Forced gaiety is another manifestation of denial used as a temporary defense mechanism.

Another method of reacting to unwelcome pressures is simply to escape from them. "You never told me, so how was I to know?" Excuses give the child some tentative control over a situation when he feels that he is losing ground. The teenager who turns off potentially stressful conversation by burying himself in a book or television is using this mechanism. Other children, when faced with the stress of an unpleasant procedure literally run away from it. Children have fled the hospital on more than one occasion in obvious rebellion against what they considered a hostile environment. Stalling and other delay tactics are also common devices used for escape.

The tension in some anxiety-producing situations can be contained by exercise of insight or through conscious evaluation of the nature of the threat. If the stress is not overwhelming and the child is assured of appropriate support, he can tolerate an uncomfortable experience. A young child may lay quietly in bed as directed by the doctor but may be sullen and noncommunicative about it; on the other hand, another child faced with the same restriction might creatively look for new ways to pass his time. An older child may tolerate—but certainly not enjoy—his injections. Some are convinced only that "shots" constitute an inevitable evil but others do see their connection to a greater good, eventual recovery, and consequently endure the pain with good-natured resignation.

Stress can be managed through compulsive repetitions or continued practice of elements in the situation. The child expends extra effort in mastering the particular task. Moderate practice generally consolidates a skill. However, if a child feels compelled to repeat an activity over and over again, his attention may be so fully absorbed with the task that he loses his ability to cope with even minor additional stresses.

Ritualistic behavior, such as repetition of body movements (foot-tapping, scratching, etc.) can facilitate release of tension.

Children may balance a threat with security measures that include reassurance. In effect, they protect themselves with available gratifications. "Can I go to the playroom after I take my medicine?" is a query that children often make. An affirmative reply cushions the discomfort and helps the child to cope with an unpleasant situation. Children visiting a clinic in which I work are given a candy sucker to take home with them. On repeat visits, many youngsters head straight for the sucker box. A tight hold on the sucker stick while they wait to be examined seems to give them a tighter hold on themselves.

Children frequently regress under tension. Resorting to earlier patterns of behavior reduces the level of anxiety to a more manageable proportion. A lower level of operation is less demanding intellectually, socially, and emotionally. By allowing others to assume responsibility for care, the child feels more secure. Regression in the face of illness is a common manifestation, especially in young children, and can be almost invariably predicted in situations involving hospitalization. The young child's classic regression in areas such as toileting, eating, and sleeping is well known. However, the older child, too, can manifest behavior such as whimpering, baby-talk, and demands for show of affection.

Some children are able to change or transform elements in a situation in order to deal with it constructively. This is often evident in the child's play experience. In coping with the stress of being a patient and consequently the recipient of the intrusive actions of doctors and nurses, the young child will reverse roles so that he can have the experience of being the doctor or nurse himself. This manipulation helps him to better tolerate the patient role.

The older child may react to anxiety by a show of depression. Often this is related to the fact that the child blames himself for the illness. He tends to feel hostile toward himself and unconsciously wishes to be punished. Nothing is worthwhile and the well-meaning attempts to help are met with further withdrawal. The juvenile period itself contains its share of "normal" anxieties and depression; illness simply exaggerates the situation.

Hypochondriacal reactions are sometimes evident in older children. This overconcern with bodily functions directs feelings to the self. Many times the parents of these children are themselves hypochondriacal and symptoms of illness are frequently discussed in the home. Often it results from a convalescence that is unnecessarily prolonged or from an overemphasis either by parents or physician of a particular type of symptom. Children who are labeled "potential cardiacs" because of a murmur are examples of a particularly susceptible group. Anxiety and unconscious fears and fantasies may also lead to hypochondriacal behavior.

Sublimation is a more sophisticated way of coping with stress. With appropriate support, the ill child can be helped to employ this mechanism. It is a device whereby a socially unacceptable activity is redirected into a more approved channel. The child with rheumatic heart disease who desires to be the running back on the football team will have to make a goal-substitution in order to cope with his illness.

The Impact of Hospitalization

The reactions to illness described thus far may occur in response to any illness and may happen whether the child is treated at home or in the hospital. If the illness does require hospitalization, stress is likely to be intensified in all the dimensions already discussed. Added to these factors is another set of unique variables which hospitalization, by its very nature, imposes.

IMPACT OF SEPARATION. Hospitalization implies separation—separation from loved persons and familiar environment. For the young child (especially under three years of age) separation from the mother is the most frequently mentioned source of psychological upset. The effects of this kind of stress are well documented (Robertson, 1958; Bowlby, 1960; Spitz, 1965; Fagin, 1966; Branstetter, 1969). Since the child is too young to interpret the reason for hospitalization properly, he can see it only in terms of the loss of his mother or at least of mothering care. He feels abandoned and lonely. Loss of the mother's care interferes with the fulfillment of basic needs for affection, food, elimination, and sleep. The young child thinks that his parents are all-powerful and expects their protection when he is threatened with harm. Their absence at what is for him a critical time, arouses hostile feelings which the child cannot deal with comfortably. The child's conception of comfort and protection as synonymous with love seems contradicted in his mind and this confusion is psychologically disrupting.

Bowlby (1960) and Robertson (1958) describe the behavioral results of such stress. Three phases of disturbed behavior are noted during periods of separation—protest, despair, and detachment (denial).

> The initial phase, that of Protest, may last from a few hours to a week or more. During it the young child appears acutely distressed at having lost his mother and seeks to recapture her by the full exercise of his limited resources. He will often cry loudly, shake his cot, throw himself about, and look eagerly towards any sight or sound which might prove to be his missing mother. All his behaviour suggests strong expectation that she will return. Meantime, he is apt to reject all alternative figures who offer to do things for him, though some children will cling desperately to a nurse.
>
> During the phase of Despair, which succeeds protest, his preoccupation with his missing mother is still evident, though his behavior suggests increasing hopelessness. The active physical movements diminish or come to an end, and he may cry monotonously or intermittently. He is withdrawn and inactive, makes no demands on the environment, and appears to be in a state of deep mourning. This is a quiet stage, and sometimes, clearly erroneously, is presumed to indicate a diminution of distress.
>
> Because the child shows more interest in his surroundings, the phase of Detachment which sooner or later succeeds protest and despair is often welcomed as a sign of recovery. He no longer rejects the nurses, accepts their care and the food and toys they bring, and may even smile and be sociable. This seems satisfactory. When his mother visits, however, it can be seen that all is not well, for there is a striking absence of the behaviour characteristic of the strong attachment normal at this age. So far from greeting his mother he may seem hardly to know her; so far from clinging to her he may remain remote and apathetic; instead of tears there is a listless turning away. He seems to have lost all interest in her . . . (Bowlby, 1960).

Disruptive behavior often extends into the posthospitalization period. It is important that parents be apprised of this fact so that they can better respond to the child's needs.

Fagin (1966) found that young children who were separated from their mothers during hospitalization continued to show regressive behavior one month after discharge from the hospital. The children demonstrated behavior such as emotional dependence, food finickiness, resistance to going to bed, and regression in urine training.

Older children may show an emotional coldness at first and then follow this by intense and demanding dependence on the mother. Jealousy and outbursts of anger are also common posthospitalization behaviors.

Prugh et al. (1953) also noted that infantile behavior persisted for several months in many children under the age of five. Nightmares, bed-wetting, and undue fear of needles were found in older children, but these behaviors disappeared more quickly than in younger age groups.

While there is considerable agreement that sustained behavioral changes can result from hospitalization, it is likewise generally agreed that the emotional and physical environment of the hospital can be constructively modified to minimize such ill effects. Permitting maternal attendance during hospitalization reduces the number and intensity of adverse reactions for the young child (Fagin, 1966). When the mother cannot be present in the hospital, substitute mothering will reduce trauma since it is possible that some of the emotional distress experienced by the young child results from need deprivation rather than from separation anxiety per se (Branstetter, 1969).

Relaxed admission procedures, liberal visiting hours, early ambulation (to minimize effects of immobilization and sensory deprivation), play programs, and purposeful preparation for traumatic procedures are additional ways in which the environment can be modified to reduce the child's anxiety level (Prugh et al., 1953).

For the older child, more sophisticated techniques can be used since anxiety can be dealt with in a different way. Group discussions seem to be a profitable method of managing anxiety. Psychotherapy sessions in which children are encouraged to explore their concerns and fantasies seem to have more long-range benefit than mere information-giving tutorial meetings (Rie et al., 1968). Although the latter group "learned," communication in this type of setting tends to be unilateral and demands a singular response from the children. When anxieties are confronted directly and actively explored by the children themselves, there may be no actual reduction in anxiety; however, through this open method of interaction, older youngsters can reduce their need to cope with anxiety in a defensive manner. In effect, this method tends to encourage a child to search for a solution to his problems in an independent way.

PREPARATION FOR HOSPITALIZATION. There is scarcely anyone writing on the subject of effects of hospitalization who does not emphasize the importance of preparation for the new experience. The concept of preparation needs elaboration. Often it seems to imply a specific beginning point and a definite conclusion. Preparation for illness and hospitalization is an on-going process and is a part of every new experience. Often it is presumed that because a child has been in the hospital before or has had a doctor's examination on many occasions, he does not need much preparation. Two factors make this an unfair assumption. In the first place, each time a child returns to the hospital he is literally a different person. He is at a wholly new stage of development with correspondingly different fears and expectations that must be dealt with at his present level of comprehension. Secondly, the past experiences with illness may have been upsetting ones which he imagines will be repeated. It is therefore essential before any preparation is attempted, that the nurse find out how the *child* views the circumstances of his illness. Once this information is obtained, the nurse has a sound basis on which to begin.

Age is an important factor in determining the method and style of preparation. The preschool child thinks primarily about himself— how he feels, what will happen to him. He is in the animistic or magical stage of thinking in which reality and fantasy are indistinguishable to him. He also thinks in very concrete terms. However, his capacity to understand far exceeds his verbal limitations. Therefore, when preparing him for hospitalization or treatment, one should keep a few simple rules in mind. The preschool child requires only about two days' advance notice of an upcoming hospitalization or operation. A longer period of preparation awakens fantasies and arouses unnecessary fears. Yet he does need some time to absorb the idea of a new venture and to ask questions. Keep the actual preparation simple. Direct attention to what will happen to *him* and how he will *feel* when things happen. Playing out anticipated events gives the child something tangible to cling to as he faces new and strange situations. Do not hesitate to explain things even though the child has not verbalized his curiosity and concern. Because the preschool child considers adults to be all-knowing, he expects that those caring for him understand what he is thinking.

The thinking of the school-age child begins to be based on logic. He is able to classify and label objects. He has more realistic concepts about his body and its functions. Consequently, he requires and seeks a more detailed explanation of the illness and its treatment. He can benefit from more time to prepare so that he can make some decisions about controlling his environment. He can decide, for example, what to bring to the hospital, and how to tell his friends about the hospitalization. Bringing his own clothes and other familiar items helps to preserve his own identity. Proper timing will also permit him to voice his inevitable concerns which are often quite realistic. Questions about possible death and residual disability are not infrequent. While these youngsters appreciate a fairly comprehensive preparation in keeping with their increasing knowledge about the body, care must be taken not to *over*emphasize self-control. The discomforts and anxieties that illness will arouse may cause a temporary breakdown in the child's emotional control, which is very understandable. Children must not be made to feel that they are "failures" because of this.

The adolescent is capable of abstract thought and conceptualization and can assume initiative in solving his problems. He should have considerable "say" in making decisions that affect his own welfare. If the hospitalization is elective, he should be involved in the decision about timing. Social and academic affairs might reasonably have priorities over hospitalization in certain situations such as graduation, a swimming meet, or a Senior Prom. Again, avoid falling into the trap of omitting important information because the teenager gives the impression of knowing all about everything. Do not be discouraged when the adolescent greets your efforts by a blasé, disinterested "ho-hum"! It is not a valid indication of the real impact that the teaching had.

Repetition may be necessary at all age levels, depending upon the reason for hospitalization and the extent of personal threat involved. When preparation has to be hurried, it is generally advisable to give less detailed information and supplement the gaps by being present during the experience so that on-going explanation and physical and emotional support can be given.

The use of props or teaching tools is recommended for all age groups. Puppets, coloring books, storybooks, and doctor and nurse kits are appropriate for preschool children. Older children appreciate simple diagrams of the body or diseased organ. Instructional films, videotapes on closed-circuit television, or self-instruction materials are all effective media. Self-instruction tools are especially beneficial because the child can learn at his own pace. There are few child-oriented materials available for this purpose. More attention could well be directed to their development.

HOSPITAL ENVIRONMENT.   Hospitalization introduces the child to a wholly new environment. Hall (1959) has expounded on the idea that when persons move from one country to another, they experience a condition known as "culture shock." He defines this phenomenon as "a removal or distortion of the many familiar cues one encounters at home and the substitution for them of other cues which are strange" (Hall, 1959, p. 156). Gellert (1958) comments that in the child's eyes the hospital is like a foreign country. It is a place with its own customs, language, and schedules to which the child must adapt. Certainly, the familiar cues that help a child feel secure are either absent or distorted —sometimes beyond recognition. Established routines for daily care that provide continuity from day to day are altered to suit hospital protocol. Equipment is often noisy and overpowering. This is especially true if the child is hospitalized in an institution primarily geared to the care of adult patients. Consequently, the child can view hospitalization as a type of "culture shock."

The child tries to attach meanings to unfamiliar vocabulary and often misinterprets what is said. "Diagnosis" can be mentally construed to be "dying noses"; children can give a literal interpretation to the doctor's statement that he will "sit on" the case until morning; "resolution" of pneumonia easily turns into "revolution"; "blood work," for a child unfamiliar with the jargon and still in the stage of animistic thinking, can mean that his blood is "working" inside of him.

There is a considerable amount of sensory distortion in the hospital environment. Normal cycles of day and night are not always clearly discernable, particularly in special-care units in which windows are high-set and often at a premium and bright lighting is maintained around the clock.

Auditory stimuli may consist of the continuous sound of the respirator, isolette, or mist tent, or the unintelligible garble of distant voices. A very disquieting sound is that of the cries of another child.

Visual stimuli take on an unnatural perspective, too. Sometimes, because of confinement to bed or to a particular room, range of vision is limited. If the child is immobilized the restrictions are even more severe. What the child does see leaves much to be desired—the same four walls, the same arrangement of furniture. As the child peers into the hospital corridors, sometimes through several glass partitions, the people he sees are often distorted and literally unrecognizable.

Interpersonal spatial distance is also distorted in the hospital. It is well known that the spatial distance between interacting persons is a cue to the type of social relationship existing between them (Hall, 1959). As the degree of acquaintance increases the distance between members of a dyad decreases. This connection between physical close-ness and closeness of interpersonal relationship is understood by children as young as the age of eight (Blood and Livant, 1957). Such ideas are quite clearly utilized by age 11 or 12 (Guardo, 1969). Since children do use these cues of physical proximity to interpret relation-ships, I wonder what difficulty is posed for the child when perfect strangers assume positions of considerable intimacy. Often, the child has no time to develop an acquaintance with the many people who take care of his body. A real friendship with them is a rarity. Since children do value personal space, it would seem likely that close physical contact with the school-age child ought to be used with discretion. Of course, it must be remembered that these children were not studied under conditions of stress.

The same set of circumstances does not seem to operate for the young child. Rosenthal (1967) introduced preschool children to an anxiety-provoking situation and studied their dependency behavior in relation to their mothers and to strangers. Under nonstressful cir-cumstances, dependent behavior was observed with mothers more fre-quently than with strangers. However, anxiety increased dependency behavior toward *both* mother and stranger. This appears to conflict with the common notion that when under high anxiety, a child will withdraw from strangers. Therefore, the diminished ability of young children to cope with stress such as that of hospitalization demands behavior from the nurse that is physically comforting and responsive to the child's dependency needs.

One of the most unsettling aspects of hospitalization is the in-consistency of care. The number of interpersonal contacts in the course of a single day is phenomenal. Many persons who enter the child's world come for a very specific purpose and once it is accomplished they are gone. This kind of disturbance, though it raises the fear of repetition, is relatively self-limited in its effect. However, inconsistency among the nurses who have prolonged contact with the child is less well tolerated. After a certain number of unsettling, confusing ex-periences, the child realizes that he really cannot prepare himself for the next day's plan of care because each nurse approaches him dif-ferently. In an environment in which interruptions and surprises are frequent occurrences at best, the child is robbed of one element of consistency that he could come to depend upon: his nurse. In the interests of scheduling limitations, one nurse cannot work around the clock nor take care of a child with a long-term illness without interruption. However, the child can feel more secure if he knows one nurse in a special way. He can adjust to the inevitable changes on her days off because he knows where she is and that she will return. Gradually, the space barrier between them can be broken down so that meaningful matters will come up for discussion.

Hospitalization is often necessary because surgery is planned as a part of the treatment. An operation brings with it many anxieties. One obviously relieved child told me that "I had my operation today. That means I won't have to have it tomorrow." The anticipated loss of or entry into a part of the body is very threatening especially for the preschool child. If the surgery will result in disfigurement, anxiety is heightened and self-image is significantly altered. The operating suite itself is the object of many fantasies for children of all ages. Because it is largely unknown to them and even to those who must prepare the children, it takes on ominous and mysterious characteristics, and when they are actually confronted with the environment, it is admittedly austere and impersonal—with masked faces and gloved hands. Children fear anesthesia not only because of the traditional mask and "smelly gas" (which incidentally are seldom used for induction) but also because they fear losing self-control and consciousness. The postoperative presence of such things as oxygen, drainage tubes, and intravenous tubing is quick to arouse anxiety. The taking of medicines, both oral and parenteral, are compounded by fears of being attacked or of having the body penetrated. The preschool child frequently is convinced that "his insides will run out through the hole" made by the needle. The insistence on Bandaids following intramuscular injections is often based on this conviction.

All of the environmental variables mentioned thus far have been stressful. While the subject has not been extensively studied, there is some indication that, for some children, psychological *benefit* may result from hospitalization (Jessner, 1952; Solnit, 1960; Shore, 1965; Rie, 1968). Shore cites several areas in which benefit has been noted; encouragement of normal growth patterns; support in parent-child relationships; provision of refuge in emotional storms; provision of identification models for parents and child; and assistance to the child in developing self-mastery. Langford (1961) comments that children who come from unstable family circumstances may find that the hospital provides them with more consistent care and acceptance than they receive at home. He recalled one child's appreciative exclamation, "Gee, sheets and a pillow!"

Hospitalized children, particularly those who have a long-term illness, have occasion to see more illness than do healthy children. They see children in all stages of illness and, undoubtedly, during repeated hospitalizations, have witnessed some catastrophies. The sight of many people and strange equipment coupled with an atmosphere of tense urgency arouses all sorts of fearful fantasies concerning the child's own safety. A sudden upsetting event may leave the child no time to support himself through anticipation of it.

Care ought to be taken in planning room assignments so that children are not introduced to more stress than they can tolerate. A child with an amputation should not be indiscriminantly placed with a preschool child whose normal fantasies concern mutilation. It will only confirm his worst fears. An older child can be expected to have difficulty adjusting to such a disabled child but he can be better supported because of his appreciation of reality. The situation obviously needs to be discussed so that misconceptions do not brew under the surface. Placement of a child severely scarred with burns requires the same considerations.

Careful judgment has to be exercised when children with the same illness are placed together. Sometimes it can be mutually beneficial, but inevitable comparisons will be made. If the condition of one child is precarious, comparisons between the two children could undermine the progress of each. The sick child can become jealous of the other's progress and the other can fear that a setback is bound to happen to him.

Young children suppose that other children harbor the same fears that they do (Lazar, 1969). If they are highly anxious and therefore believe others to experience the same kind of fears, the child may see no avenue of help for himself in the stressful situation. The child can become fearful through close contact with anxious people. Older children gain in their ability accurately to predict other children's fears so they do not project on to every other child the intensity of the fears that they are experiencing. Likewise, when other children are obviously frightened, they may be better able to separate out those feelings as distinct from their own. The child who hears another patient cry plaintively for his mother may be as frightened as the crying child. This factor of fear transmission and fear interpretation must also be considered when one is assigning patients to rooms.

Because of the emotional aspects involved in meeting the needs of sick children, on-going staff education is essential. Staff members may often experience high levels of anxiety as they attempt to support parents and children through very traumatic experiences. All staff members have certain biases about children stemming from their own attitudes toward child rearing. Consequently, some behavior in children and in parents can arouse strongly charged reactions in the nurses who care for them. Recognition that this situation is natural and not something to be ashamed of is part of realistic nursing intervention. When such attitudes go beyond the nurse's control and directly interfere with effective function, outside assistance should be requested without shame. Group conferences where feelings can be "aired" openly and without fear of reprisal do improve the level of care. Inappropriate attitudes and inappropriate skill in working with children accentuates the child's adverse reaction to the stress of illness.

Parental Influence on the Child's Perception of Illness

"Like father, like son"; "he's a chip off the old block"; as the tree is bent." These phrases are common clichés pointing to parental influence on the child's behavior. Through the experience of early mother-infant and father-infant relationships, the child learns to recognize cues that express parental approval and disapproval and adjusts his behavior accordingly.

CHILD'S INCORPORATION OF PARENTAL EMOTIONS. The theory of symbiosis helps to explain how the child incorporates the emotional reactions of his mother. The symbiotic relationship existing during pregnancy enhances feelings of motherliness. The hormonal changes occurring with pregnancy arouse libidinous feelings of well-being that are intimately related to motherliness. During this time, the mother's fantasies not only incorporate her desires for a child but also include wishes and ambitions that she hopes to fulfill through the child (Benedek, 1949). Thus, the child is viewed in terms of the mother's predetermined goals before he is born.

After birth, the need for symbiosis continues in the mother. The woman's desire to care for the baby and to experience the close bodily contact that symbiosis implies, really represents the *original* symbiotic relationship for both the infant and the mother. The motherliness that develops when needs are gratified expands the mother's personality and, in a cyclic manner, enhances her capacity to meet the infant's demands. The resulting closeness affords the baby the opportunity to experience a transfer of the physiological effects of a warm, relaxed body, and the psychosocial effects of her smiling face and soothing voice.

As experiences accumulate, the baby becomes able to distinguish between tension and relaxation; between anxiety and contentment; between fear and confidence. His cues may take the form of voice change, muscle tightness, facial expression, or spatial distance. Whatever form they take, the child's early and sustained scrutiny of his mother makes him uniquely sensitive to her moods.

As he develops, the child's interpersonal relationships envelop the father and the siblings. When the process of imitation and identification becomes dominant, sensitivity to the behavior of others increases correspondingly. The child begins to see himself as a "contributor" to their reactions and experiences "good" feelings or "bad" feelings depending on his perception of the outcome of the interaction.

When a child becomes ill, he has a great need for parental support. His search for their assurance heightens his sensitivity to parental behavior. If the parents appear very anxious or seem to lack control over the situation, the child's fears about his well-being will be accentuated. For example, if a baby is ill and cannot accept or even appears to reject (by crying, vomiting, diarrhea, etc.) the mother's ministrations, the symbiotic relationship referred to earlier is weakened. The baby lacks confidence in the mother's ability to meet his needs and the mother also loses confidence in her ability to assume her idealized mothering role.

A similar phenomenon occurs when the child is older. The pre-school child believes that his parents are all-powerful and that they will protect him from harm. When they appear to condone painful experiences, the child may express anger and resentment toward his parents. Parents often react by becoming overindulgent. The child, consequently, is unsure of their expectations from him. He may become quite unsettled when previously unacceptable behavior is suddenly rewarded or at least overlooked.

What is happening in this "feedback" mechanism is that changes in both parent and child behavior affect responses in each other and complicate ability to interpret the behavior with objectivity. If the behavior of one could be guided toward some degree of consistency, the behavior of the other might be more comfortably stabilized.

Parents have the capability of mature thought and hence can respond to rational interaction. Therefore, nursing intervention directed toward reducing parental anxiety would be a very productive means of allaying the fears of sick children. If the child had not learned to be so "in tune" with parental feelings, parents could have more latitude in the expression of their worries. As it is, parents are called upon to exert great self-control under difficult conditions. To carry out this responsibility, they will appreciate opportunities for expression which the nurse can provide.

CHANGES IN PARENTAL BEHAVIOR DURING PERIODS OF ILLNESS. Before the nurse can respond to the parent's need for help, it is important to know what factors are likely to contribute to a change in parental behavior.

Parents are not always fully aware of the so-called normal behavioral changes that are concurrent with childhood illness and hospitalization. Consequently, it is easy to understand why parents may misinterpret their child's behavior.

For example, many mothers view the child's demanding behavior as "being spoiled." Consequently, they may react by vigorous attempts to correct this, which the child in turn can interpret as rejection. Parents sometimes have a difficult time seeing things from the child's point of view. From their adult perspective, many of the events that provoke aggressive or "naughty" behavior are not of sufficient consequence to cause such violent outbursts. They expect the child to demonstrate more control over his feelings than is possible for his age or condition.

The rejecting child is another source of parental concern. Children can withdraw from their parents just when the parents wish to be most consoling. This may happen for a variety of reasons. Sometimes the child is simply disappointed or angry with his parents because they do not "rescue" him from the strange, unpleasant environment. Other children may fear losing self-control if they give free expression to their feelings. So, they withdraw into themselves. This frightens parents and accentuates feelings of guilt and helplessness.

The child's "misbehavior" threatens the parent in another way. Parents are well aware of their dependency on the members of the health team and they do not want to risk losing their good favor. If the child misbehaves, parents may feel that the disruptive behavior will alienate the staff who will then retaliate by withdrawing attention. This is, perhaps, one reason why parents tend to worry more when their children are troublesome and aggressive than when they are quiet and fearful.

Children in the hospital sometimes manifest behavior characteristics that are completely different from their "at-home" personalities. Parents are genuinely at a loss to explain the change and if it is a "change for the worst" they are embarrassed and concerned that the staff will consider them unsuitable parents. We all know the frustration of trying to defend a situation when the evident circumstances do not reflect "the way it *really* is."

Occasionally, parents must bear some of the responsibility for their child's maladaptive behavior. Parents may inadvertently contribute to the stress of hospitalization because of unfortunate associations they have created in the child's mind. Often parents assign punitive meanings to going to bed, confinement to a room, or food restrictions. Thus, when the child faces these circumstances during the course of his illness, it is not unreasonable for him to attribute his confinement to punishment for "bad" acts or thoughts. And, of course, any child can find something in his real or fantasied past that deserves retribution. This may confirm the child's fear that even his most "secret" thoughts will somehow be punished. Another common threat voiced frequently by parents is "to stop crying or I'll have the nurse give you another shot." This does little to cement friendly nurse-patient relationships but however much the nurse cringes at this unfair description of her role, she must understand that the parent is generally motivated more by a strong desire to stop the child's crying than by any conscious attempt to undermine a therapeutic relationship.

HOSPITAL RULES AND REGULATIONS. Other contributors to parental anxiety are hospital rules and regulations. They can readily upset parents by seeming to interfere with their style of child care. Food restrictions and limited visiting hours are perhaps the most obvious recipients of criticism but they might serve as available scapegoats for more subtle concerns. There is a code of conduct or hospital protocol to which parents feel obliged to adapt. Unfortunately, the "code" of expected behavior is not always explicit. *Whom* to ask for *what* thing can become a real challenge. How to get needed information without becoming a bother is often an important parent concern. Another question parents ask themselves is, "How far do I go in ministering to my child's needs before I assume the nurses' prerogatives?" How frequently are parents unsure about whether to stay with their child during treatments? Placing the burden of such decision-making solely on the parents predisposes to the development of a lack of self-confidence. Failure to find reassurance from others further heightens the anxiety that can be so readily transmitted to the super-sensitive child.

Inflexibility in management of some units occasionally presents grave hardships for parents which are not always evident to the staff. I can remember one father whose desire to be with his sick child some distance away from his work, caused him to lose his job because work and "visiting hours" conflicted. A call from the physician explaining his absence reinstated him but this would have gone undiscovered had not the nurse been interested enough in the total family to make the significant inquiry about employment.

SOCIOECONOMIC AND CULTURAL FACTORS.   Socioeconomic and cultural factors may intensify parental anxiety. A significant experience gap may occur between parent and nurses. It is important to bear in mind that persons in the low-income strata generally have different ideas about health and illness than do those in the middle-income group. The fact that parents may bring a child for treatment when it seems to be too late may not be due to neglect but rather may be a function of their definition of illness. Among the poor, symptoms of physical discomfort do not always constitute sickness. Actual incapacitation is viewed as a more realistic criteria (Koos, 1954; Rosenblatt, 1964). Also, poor mothers tend to be less concerned with detecting children's illnesses or taking precautions to prevent them (Mechanic, 1964). Mere toleration of such unseemly behavior is quickly transmitted to parents and they can react either with hostility or self-beratement—both of which elevate the level of tension.

Persons who live in poverty have goals and values that differ from those who live in a more affluent environment. The effects of economic deprivation are expressed in four life themes: fatalism, orientation to the present, authoritarianism, and concreteness (Irelan, 1967). It becomes difficult for persons with this orientation to make plans for the future since they are more concerned about immediate happenings and sensations. If they consider their destiny to be controlled by fate, it is unlikely that they will look seriously at the consequences of their actions. Authoritarianism is based on belief in the validity of strength; decisions are made on the basis of authority rather than reason. This attitude can pervade health and child rearing practices.

Child-rearing practices have many cultural variations which the nurse must consider. It becomes especially important in providing anticipatory guidance to parents, which is such an important part of the nursing role.

I can recall a situation in which the clinic nurse was having a conference with a Puerto Rican mother about her daughter's nutrition. The seven-year-old child was convalescing at home following a bout of rheumatic fever. The mother reported that her appetite was poor. Among other things, the nurse encouraged social interaction at mealtime, and more variety in choice of foods, implying that the predominance of rice, beans, and starchy vegetables typical of Puerto Rican diets was nutritionally inadequate. The mother seemed uninterested in the well-intentioned information. Had the nurse first explored cultural preferences, her advice could have been more meaningful.

The benefits of making mealtime a social exchange are not necessarily appreciated in Puerto Rican families. As a rule, meals are not eaten by all the family together. Usually the father is served alone out of respect for his position in the family. While the mother may prepare some "American dishes" for her children since their taste has been tempered by the new environment, the youngsters are likely to eat separately according to their custom (Padilla, 1958). There is little conversation at the meal. Disruptions of any kind may be met with severe punishment. Some parents consider eating, "like praying, a time for seriousness, quiet and devotion" (Landy, 1959, p. 104).

Instead of trying to change the cultural dietary pattern, some slight modifications can improve nutritional quality without changing the existing framework of preferences. For example, white polished rice is highly valued by the Puerto Rican. Consequently, attempts to persuade the purchase of unpolished rice are not likely to be successful. Rather, the nurse can encourage fortified rice enriched with vitamins. The red kidney bean is a valuable source of protein but the nurse can suggest the addition of other beans such as soy and chick beans which are far more nutritious. *Cafe con leché* is the universal drink for all ages from childhood up. Rather than discourage young children from the drinking of any coffee, encourage *minimal* coffee and more milk in view of the child's need for protein. These examples illustrate the concrete value of cultural awareness.

Oriental parents are sometimes accused of aloofness and lack of feeling that seem out of keeping with the stress of the situation. Unless it is realized that restraint and self-discipline are prized traits and have no relationship to depth of feeling, the nurse cannot be truly supportive (Opler, 1955).

It is important that the reader give proper interpretation to this kind of information. The examples just described should not in any sense encourage the stereotyping of particular socioeconomic and ethnic groups. There is great danger in ignoring the diversity of individual life-styles within groups. Certainly not all poor people are fatalists and many Puerto Rican families are so "Americanized" that any resemblance to island culture is remote. Nor does every Oriental parent have a sober, constricted temperament. Unless one's ordinary biases are balanced by a genuine openness to individual differences, meaningful communication is blocked.

If the nurse is aware of the existence of such anxiety-provoking factors as inevitable changes in child's behavior, environmental insecurity, and experiential gap between parent and health worker, she can then plan how to intervene constructively.

PARENTAL PREPARATION AND SUPPORT. Preparation for any new experience enriches the learning that can come from it. The occasions of illness and hospitalization are no exceptions. Parents play an important part in the child's preparation. Nursing intervention ought then to assist parents with this task. Perhaps the most meaningful part of the intervention takes place long before the actual illness. I am referring to the anticipatory guidance that is part of well-child supervision. While preparation at the time of crisis is important, studies have indicated that the number and severity of adverse reactions to hospitalization depend to a great extent on the quality of the parent-child relationship prior to the illness. For instance, children who are poorly adjusted emotionally before surgery have more severe postoperative reactions even though they have been thoroughly prepared (Jessner, 1952). Emotional trauma prior to illness seems to predispose the child to a stronger reaction. Therefore, through anticipatory guidance designed to assist parents in developing sound, mutually satisfying relationships with their children, the nurse is actually "preparing" the child to weather the crisis of illness with less upset.

When actual hospitalization is anticipated, specific preparatory intervention is important. The parents, physician, office nurse, and clinic nurse should participate in the process. Before the parents can be helpful, they must have a reasonably accurate idea of what will happen. The physician should explain in detail the reason for the hospitalization and what the treatment regimen will entail. The nurse can reinforce the doctor's statements and add her own unique knowledge about illness and hospitalization to the parents' repertory of background information. She can explain the hospital environment. Booklets that describe hospital policy and procedure should be given in advance of the time of admission so parents can become familiar with them. Very often such brochures are handed to parents when they arrive at the hospital. This can be wasted effort because the parent's natural focus at this time is on the child—not on hospital policy. The nurse can also be helpful in suggesting teaching methods that parents might use. Books designed for children with colorful pictures about the admission procedure or the trip to the operating room are good tools, but only if they depict the situation realistically and appropriately to the particular hospital environment to which the child will be exposed. Suggestions about role-playing episodes and timing of preparation are also appreciated by parents. Office and clinic nurses ought to have a collection of props available for parents. Caps, masks, tongue blades, and bandages can be given out when appropriate; "nurse-doctor" hand-and-finger puppets can be loaned out for use in the home. Arranging for an actual visit to the hospital and/or group teaching of parents commonly involved in a particular situation such as open heart surgery are well within the range of nursing intervention.

A telephone call to the family shortly before admission to the hospital would give the nurse an opportunity to allay some of the last-minute apprehensions and to answer questions which inevitably arise as plans are made for a stay in the hospital. The nurse may not be able to do this for all patients, but she can set priorities. Families about to experience treatment that has a high degree of risk or families that are already known to be highly reactive to stress would be selected for such contacts. All families, however, should be encouraged to make telephone contacts with the nurse whenever they feel the need to do so.

Once the child is in the hospital, on-going support is essential. Roy (1967) describes three very practical ways in which the nurse can intervene. The nurse's actions are aimed at supporting the mother's adequacy in relating to her hospitalized child. I believe that these actions could be employed in interacting with any significant person in the sick child's environment. The supportive interaction techniques are *congruent orientation, involvement,* and *role reference.* Congruent orientation means that the nurse aligns the focus of her attention with that of the mother. For example, if the mother is concerned about her own fatigue, the nurse would focus her comments on this area, too. Involvement refers to specific communication with the mother about the child's condition. The nurse, in this case, might tell the mother that the child slept well or that he ate a good breakfast. Role reference is used when the nurse defines for the mother what she can do for the child. Teaching the mother how to apply a dressing is an example of this. When mothers are supported in these direct ways early in the course of hospitalization, they demonstrate a greater degree of adequacy in meeting their child's needs. By introducing to the mother these cues for care, the nurse indicates her understanding and acceptance of parent needs. By taking the initiative in these traditional areas of parent concern, she removes the burden of inquiry from the parents.

Skipper and Leonard (1968) also describe the value of purposeful social interaction between the mother and the nurse in reducing the anxiety level of the hospitalized child. They measured the effectiveness of the interaction in terms of somatic measures of children's stress such as temperature, blood pressure, pulse, postoperative vomiting, and oral intake of fluids. Communication of information and emotional support to mothers especially when begun at the crucial time of admission significantly reduced the child's manifestations of stress. This study reinforces the need to give more than just "lip service" to the social process between parent and nurse as a means of reducing adverse effects of stress in the child.

The way in which these cues are offered is important. Avoid cutting off communication by the thoughtless use of professional jargon.

Parents are sometimes hesitant to admit their ignorance of medical terminology and consequently valuable information can be clouded with distortion and half-truth. Also, do not judge parents solely on the basis of first impressions. As has been pointed out, parents are not themselves when their children are ill. Their usual calm objectivity often melts into emotional subjectivity when they are faced with a personal crisis.

Parents can also benefit from informal group discussions designed to help them explore their concerns about their sick child or hospital policies or any of a number of issues which may arise in the course of hospitalization (Glaser, 1960). Such conferences, if properly guided, offer direct benefit to parents not only because of the information they receive from the hospital staff but also from the support that they receive by sharing experiences with each other. It can be a valuable teaching tool for continuing education of the staff since it reveals how parents view the hospital environment. Suggestions by the parents as consumers of health services can also stimulate constructive administrative changes in unit management. In order to achieve these benefits, however, it seems important that an open, nonpunitive atmosphere be maintained by selecting a group leader who is not directly involved in the management of the unit or the care of the children.

Summary

The way in which a child interprets illness depends upon his concept of body image, his view of body function, and also on such variables as age, nature of the illness and its treatment, family relationships, and past experience. Consequently, a child's view of his illness is a very individual matter.

The child may view his illness in the light of psychosocial consequences. Absence from school, loss of position in the family, threat of dependency, and financial strain on the family are examples of common concerns.

Physical aspects of illness determine, in part, how the illness is perceived. The symbolic significance attached to the diseased part of the body, the visibility of the illness, and the symptoms associated with it all contribute to the child's mental construct of his illness.

Through experience every child develops his own strategies of coping with stress. These mechanisms range from complete escape or denial to temporary regression to a positive "restructuring" of the stressful situation into manageable dimensions.

Hospitalization during the illness crisis introduces a new set of variables. It causes separation from loved ones. This induces behavioral reactions that include tearful protest, hopeless withdrawal, remote disinterest, and regression in normal age-appropriate activities.

The hospital setting introduces the child to a new environment with which he is often ill prepared to deal. The familiar cues that help a child to feel secure are missing. Sensory distortion is a common occurrence, as is inconsistency in care.

Much of the stress of hospitalization, especially for the young child, can be minimized by maintaining a close mother-child relationship during the confinement. Provision of appropriate support is important in order to assure adequacy of the mother's role. Also, the nurse can ease the child's stress by carefully planned and implemented preparation for new experiences.

Parental feelings and actions also influence the child's perception of his illness. A child is extremely sensitive to the changes in his parents' behavior that inevitably accompany his illness. Parental anxiety can stem from unexplained changes in the child's behavior, hospital rules and regulations, socioeconomic and cultural gaps between parent and health worker, and lack of confidence in ability to assume the parental role. Involvement of parents in the care of the child along with provision of cues to help them participate effectively is an important way of relieving some of their anxiety. Encouragement of self-expression through group discussion is another productive way of improving the hospital environment and thus indirectly lessening the stress of hospitalization for the child.

The nurse who understands the many possible ways that illness can be perceived is in a position to deal with the stress in a manner that is appropriate for the family and also satisfying to herself.

References

Anthony, E. J. The child's discovery of his body. Physical Therapy, 48:1103–1114, 1968.

Bakwin, H., and Bakwin, R. Clinical Management of Behavior Disorders in Children, 3rd ed. Philadelphia, Saunders, 1966.

Bartoleschi, B., and Novelletto, A. The influence of severe bodily illness in early childhood on mental development. Intern. J. Psychoanal., 49:294–297, 1968.

Bender, L., and Faretra, G. Body image problems of children. In Lief, H., et al. eds. The Psychological Basis of Medical Practice. New York, Harper and Row, Hoeber Medical Division, 1963.

Benedek, T. The psychosomatic implications of the primary unit: mother-child. Am. J. Orthopsych., 19:642–654, 1949.

Bergmann, T. Children in the Hospital. New York, International Universities Press, 1965.

Berman, D. Pediatric nurses as mothers see them. Am. J. Nurs., 66:2429–2431, 1966.

Blau, A. et al. The collaboration of nursing and child psychiatry in a general hospital. Am. J. Ortho-Psych., 29:77–93, 1959.

Blom, G. E. The reactions of hospitalized chillren to illness. Pediatrics, 22:590–599, 1958.

Blood, R. O., and Livant, W. P. The use of space within the cabin group. J. Social Issues, 13:47–53, 1957.

Bowlby, J. Maternal Care and Mental Health. Geneva, World Health Organization, 1952.

———— Separation anxiety. Intern. J. Psychoanal., 41:89–113, 1960.

Branstetter, E. The young child's response to hospitalization: separation anxiety or lack of mothering care? Am. J. Publc Health, 59:92–97, 1969.

Breckenridge, M., and Murphy, M. Growth and Development of the Young Child, 7th ed. Philadelphia, Saunders, 1963.

Coffin, M. Nursing Observations of the Young Patient. Dubuque, Iowa, Wm. C. Brown, 1970.

Crowley, D. Pain and Its Alleviation. Regents of the University of California, 1962.

Davidson, A., and Fay, J. Phantasy in Childhood. New York, Philosophical Library, 1953.

Di Leo, J. Young Children and Their Drawings. New York, Brunner/Mazel, 1970.

Engel, G. Psychological Development in Health and Disease. Philadelphia, Saunders, 1962.

Fagin, C. The Effects of Maternal Attendance During Hospitalization on the Post Hospital Behavior of Young Children: A Comparative Survey. Philadelphia, F. A. Davis, 1966.

Freud, A. The role of bodily illness in the mental life of children. In Eissler, R. S. et al., eds. The Psychoanalytic Study of the Child. New York, International Universities Press, 1952.

Friedman, D. B. The parent in the parent-child relationship. California Medicine, 86:25–28, 1957.

Garrard, S., and Richmond, J. Psychological aspects of the management of chronic diseases and handicapping conditions in childhood. In Lief, H., et al., eds. The Psychological Basis of Medical Practice. New York, Harper and Row, Hoeber Medical Division, 1963.

Gellert, E. Children's conceptions of the content and functions of the human body. Genetic Psychology Monographs, 65:293–405, 1962.

———— Reducing the emotional stresses of hospitalization for children. Am. J. Occup. Ther., 12:125–129, 1958.

Glaser, K. Group discussions with mothers of hospitalized children. Pediatrics, 26:132–140, 1960.

Gorman, W. Body Image and the Image of the Brain. St. Louis, Warren H. Green, 1969.

Guardo, C. Personal space in children. Child Development, 40:143–151, 1969.

Gutelius, M. Child-rearing attitudes of teen-age Negro girls. Am. J. Public Health, 60:93–104, 1970.

Hall, E. The Silent Language. Greenwich, Conn., Fawcett Publications, 1959.

Hardy, J. D. et al. Pain Sensations and Reactions. Baltimore, Williams & Wilkins, 1952.

Hirt, M., and Kurtz, R. A reexamination of the relationship between body boundary and site of disease. J. Abnorm. Psychol., 74:67–70, 1969.

Howe, J. Children's ideas about injury. In ANA Regional Clinical Conferences. New York, Appleton-Century-Crofts, 1968.

Irelan, L. (ed.) Low-Income Life Styles. Washington, D. C., U. S. Dept. of Health, Education and Welfare (No. 14), 1968.

Jessner, L., Blom, G., and Waldfogel, S. Emotional implications of tonsillectomy and adenoidectomy on children. In Eissler, R. S. et al.; eds. The Psychoanalytic Study of the Child. New York, International Universities Press, 1952.

Kangery, R. Children's answers. Am. J. Nurs., 60:1748–1751, 1960.

Kaye, H., and Lipsitt, L. P. Relation of electrotactual threshold to basal skin conductance. Child Development, 35:1307–1312, 1964.

Kessler, J. W. Impact of disability on the child. Physical Therapy, 46:153–159, 1966.

Kliman, G. Psychological Emergencies of Childhood. New York, Grune & Stratton, 1968.

Koos, E. The Health of Regionville. New York, Columbia University Press, 1954.

Landy, D. Tropical Childhood, Chapel Hill, N. C., University of North Carolina Press, 1959.

Langer, J. Theories of Development. New York, Holt, Rinehart and Winston, 1969.

Langford, W. The child in the pediatric hospital: adaption to illness and hospitalization. Am. J. Ortho-Psych., 31:667–684, 1961.

Lazar, E. Children's perceptions of other children's fears. J. Genet. Psychol., 114:3–11, 1969.

Lidz, T. The Person. New York, Basic Books, Inc. 1968.

MacGregor, F. Social Science in Nursing. New York, Russell Sage Foundation, 1960.

McCandless, B. R. Children: Behavior and Development, 2nd ed. New York, Holt, Rinehart and Winston, 1967.

McNeil, E. Human Socialization. Belmont, Calif., Brooks/Cole Publishing Co., 1969.

Mechanic, D. The influence of mothers on their children's health attitudes and behavior. Pediatrics, 33:444–453, 1969.

Mellish, R. W. P. Preparation of a child for hospitalization and surgery. Pediatric Clinics of North America, 16:543–553, 1969.

Murphy, L. B. The Widening World of Childhood. New York, Basic Books, 1962.

Nagy, M. The representation of "germs" by children. J. Genet. Psychol., 83:227–240, 1953.

————. Children's conceptions of some bodily functions. J. Genet. Psychol., 83:199–216, 1953.

Nash, H. Recognition of body surface regions. Genetic Psychology Monographs, 79:297–340, 1969.

Nash, J. Developmental Psychology, Englewood Cliffs, N. J., Prentice-Hall, Inc., 1970.

Olshansky, S. Chronic sorrow: a response to having a mentally defective child. Social Casework, 43:190–193, 1962.

Opler, M. Cultural values and attitudes on child care. Children, 2:45–50, 1955.

Orsten, P., and Mattsson, A. Hospitalization symptoms in children. Acta Paediatrica, 44:79–92, 1955.

Padilla, E. Up from Puerto Rico. New York, Columbia University Press, 1958.

Piaget, J., and Inhelder, B. The Psychology of the Child. New York, Basic Books, 1969.

Pickett, L. The hospital environment for the pediatric surgical patient. Pediatric Clinics of North America, 16:531–542, 1969.

Pratt, K. C. The neonate. In Carmichael, L., ed. Manual of Child Psychology, 2nd ed. New York, Wiley, 1954.

Provence, S., and Lipton, R. Infants in Institutions. New York, International Universities Press, 1962.

Prugh, D., et al. A study of the emotional reactions of children and families to hospitalization and illness. Am. J. Ortho-Psych., 23:70–106, 1953.

Rie, H., et al. Immediate and long-term effects of interventions early in prolonged hospitalization. Pediatrics, 41:755–764, 1968.

Robertson, J. Young Children in Hospitals. New York, Basic Books. 1958.

Rodrigue, E. Severe bodily illness in childhood. Intern. J. Psychoanal., 49:290–293, 1968.

Rosenblatt, D., and Suchman, E. Blue collar attitudes and information toward health and illness. In Shostak, A., and Gomberg, W., eds. Blue Collar World. Englewood Cliffs, N. J., Prentice-Hall, 1964, pp. 324–333.

Rosenthal, M. The generalization of dependency behaviour from mother to stranger. J. Child Psych., 8:117–133, 1967.

Roy, Sister M. Role cues and mothers of hospitalized children. Nursing Research, 16:178–182, 1967.

Scahill, M. Preparing children for procedures and operations. Nursing Outlook, 17:36–38, 1969.

Schilder, P. The image and appearance of the human body, Psyche Monographs: No. 4, London, Kegan Paul, 1935.

———, and Wechsler, D. What do children know about the interior of the body? International Journal of Psycho-analysis, 16:355–360, 1935.

Shontz, F. C. Perceptual and Cognitive Aspects of Body Experience. New York, Academic Press, 1969.

Shore, M. F., Geiser, R. L., and Wolman, H. W. Constructive uses of a hospital experience. Children, 12:3, 1965.

Shrand, H. Behavior changes in sick children nursed at home. Pediatrics, 36:604–607, 1965.

Skipper, J., and Leonard, R. Children, stress, and hospitalization: a field experiment. Journal of Health and Social Behavior, 9:275–287, 1968.

Simmel, M. Developmental aspects of the body scheme. Child Development, 37:83–95, 1966.

Smith, M. Ego support for the child patient. Am. J. Nurs., 63:90–95, 1963.

Solnit, A. J. Hospitalization. An aid to physical and psychological health in childhood. Am. J. Diseases of Children, 99:155–163, 1960.

Spitz, R. The First Year of Life. New York, International Universities Press, 1965.

Staffieri, J. R. A study of social stereotype of body image in children. J. Personality and Social Psychology, 7:101–104, 1967.

Stone, L. J., and Church, J. Childhood and Adolescence. New York, Random House, 1957.

Torrance, E. P. Constructive Behavior: Stress, Personality, and Mental Health. Belmont, Calif., Wadsworth Publishing Co., 1965.

Vernon, D., et al. The Psychological Responses of Children to Hospitalization and Illness. Springfield, Ill., Charles C. Thomas, 1965.

Walters, C. E. Interaction of the body and its segments. Am. J. Phys. Med., 46:280–289, 1967.

Wolff, S. Children Under Stress. London, The Penguin Press, 1969.

Wu, R. Explaining treatments to young children. J. Nurs., 65:71–73, 1965.

5 JACQUELINE THOMPSON

Current Nutritional Considerations: Manipulation of the Internal Environment and the Role of the Nurse

The primary focus of this chapter will be an attempt to take a look at current nutritional information, particularly as it effects children through their growing years (through adolescence). Also considered will be the role of the nurse in relation to the nutritional aspects of care as seen in a variety of nursing settings.

The following general topics will be discussed throughout this chapter. First, a short discussion of the nurse's commitment to the manipulation of the patient's internal environment. Second, the normal nutritional needs of well children from infancy through 18 years of age—with a short discussion of the various nutrients, their function, and interrelatedness. Third, an exploration of various kinds of stress experienced by ill children and its effect upon their normal nutritional needs. Fourth, a look at several current nutritional problems and its influence upon the growth and development of the child. Finally, nutrition, nursing, and how we can find this aspect of nursing more reinforcing to ourselves and our patients.

Manipulation of the Internal Environment

When one first considers the title of this chapter, one might fall into the trap of believing that manipulating and stimulating the internal environment of an individual is less complicated than manipulating and stimulating the external environment of an individual. To my mind, the gross numbers of variables which must interact, all in their

173

own unique way, to achieve "normal" internal functioning are neither less varied nor more stable than the variables which interact within the child to achieve "normal" external functioning.

The human body with its multitude of functioning cells may be best visualized as a free-form mass. Its constructs and very existence are bombarded with *internal* and *external* stimuli. These stimuli may be so destructive or negative that they change or threaten the very existence of any or all of the constructual parts. Or the stimuli may be so constructive or positive that they strengthen and enhance any or all of the constructual parts. We can consider this *barrier* of functioning cells as *life*. Our task is then to define the nurse's role as it interacts with and mediates the stimuli on either side of this "barrier."

The professional nurse seems to have little difficulty understanding her role as an interactor with respect to the *external* stimuli. The nurse is able to interact and mediate even external stimuli which are only mildly negative. Thus she is able to manipulate relatively small changes in the external environment. Unfortunately, some nurses feel great reluctance when interacting with and mediating stimuli which are *internal*. These stimuli must largely be manipulated by changing various ingested materials, usually food nutrients. The internal environment is generally adjusted either by drugs that bring the internal environment back within the normal viable range or by manipulation of ingested nutrients. I realize that the administration of a yellow pill can be less trying than getting a child to eat his lunch. In fact, one of the most unrewarding times of the day for many nurses is when they are attempting to manipulate the internal environment through food intake. In a real sense this is one of the nurse's dilemmas. It is not that the nurse does not understand the importance and purpose of food in their patient's recovery but many will not or cannot define their own role in this area in positive terms. More often than not, the whole role centers around who is going to "pass the trays." This is hardly the most paramount issue.

Why is there such an obvious rejection of this manipulation of the internal environment? It is certainly just as important as any found in the area of external environment. What is there about the feeding situation that makes many of us reject any positive thoughts about our involvement?

Let us reflect for a moment on the subject of food in our world— particularly, the concrete experience of being fed. Both "love" and "food" will have some impact upon our attempts to "set a scene" for the ingestion of food during that dreaded lunch time. Fortunately or unfortunately, since an interaction is a reciprocal relationship, the impact of our own previous experiences related to feeding must not be overlooked. I sometimes wonder how aware we are of the impact of our own early feeding experiences on our current day's action! To reiterate my point, how significantly do our *feelings* about food interfere or enhance our ability to "set the scene" for the manipulation of the internal environment through the ingestion of nutrients?

Another area of concern along with our own feelings about food and the kinds of foods that we considered good to eat is the difficulty of separating the role of the nurse from the role of the dietician. Many believe that our role should be very limited when a dietician is a member of the team. Justification for our limited role is based on the assumption that the dietician has greater expertise in the area of nutrition. This assumption is certainly granted; she may also have greater or as great technical knowledge in the area of feeding and the two roles augment and interact daily. However, despite this expertise, most often success or failure to change the internal environment lies in creating a positive atmosphere at meal time which is entirely dependent upon the nurse's overall relationship with the child.

As adults we know that the same menu served by candlelight with people we enjoy is more palatable than an identical meal eaten hurriedly with less congenial people. We must recognize this is also true for the child. If the child is not feeling well, if he does not like the person he is with, and if the environment is new, strange, or hostile, the likelihood of his eating is lessened.

Normal Nutritional Needs of Well Children

The field of nutrition has undergone rapid advancement within the last decade. As Philip L. White (1969) in his address to the 54th Annual Meeting of the National Dairy Council at Cleveland, pointed out, we now have enough knowledge concerning human physiology that we can determine the food intake each individual in our society needs for optimum health. White believes that nearly every aspect of human development can now be to some extent controlled by nutritional manipulation during the first months of life and thereafter.

This startling statement certainly encompasses the world but the logistic possibilities of delivering this kind of service to each indivdual is minute. While it seems, academically, to be a very interesting point of view, it actually is not very useful at this time. However, it does point out the knowledge explosion in the area of normal nutrition and the rapidity with which it is changing. Nutritional books are sometimes outdated by the time they are published. White therefore recommends that the subject of normal nutrition be taught through the readings of current published articles. If this suggestion is not practiced, the chosen text should be heavily supplemented by current published articles.

The rapid unfolding of new information in the area of nutrition is exemplified by new recommended daily allowances that are released every few years. The food and nutrition board of the National Academy of Science, National Research Council, publishes a recommended daily allowance which is designed for the maintenance of good nutrition of practically all healthy people in the United States. The last revision was in 1968 (see Table 1 for pertinent excerpts from these recommendations). When one reviews the recommended daily allowances it is im-

TABLE 1
Food and Nutrition Board, National Academy of Sciences—National Research Council
Recommended Daily Dietary Allowances[1]

Age (Years From Up to)	Weight Kg	Weight (Lbs)	Height Cm	Height (In.)	Kcal	Protein Gm	Fat Soluble Vitamins: Vitamin A Activ- ity I.U.	Vita- min D I.U.	Vita- min E Activ- ity I.U.	Water Soluble Vitamins: Ascor- bic Acid Mg	Fola- cin[2] Mg	Nia- cin[3] (Mg Equiv.)	Ribo- flavin Mg	Thia- mine Mg	Vita- min B6 Mg	Vita- min B12 μg	Minerals: Cal- cium Gm	Phos- phorus Gm	Iodine μg	Iron Mg	Mag- nesium Mg
Infants																					
0–1/6	4	9	55	22	kg x 120	kg x 2.2[4]	1500	400	5	35	0.05	5	0.4	0.2	0.2	1.0	0.4	0.2	25	6	40
1/6–1/2	7	15	63	25	kg x 110	kg x 2.0[4]	1500	400	5	35	0.05	7	0.5	0.4	0.3	1.5	0.5	0.4	40	10	60
1/2–1	9	20	72	28	kg x 100	kg x 1.8[4]	1500	400	5	35	0.1	8	0.6	0.5	0.4	2.0	0.6	0.5	45	15	70
Children																					
1–2	12	26	81	32	1100	25	2000	400	10	40	0.1	8	0.6	0.5	0.5	2.0	0.7	0.7	55	15	100
2–3	14	31	91	36	1250	25	2000	400	10	40	0.2	8	0.7	0.6	0.6	2.5	0.8	0.8	60	15	150
3–4	16	35	100	39	1400	30	2500	400	10	40	0.2	9	0.8	0.7	0.7	3	0.8	0.8	70	10	200
4–6	19	42	110	43	1600	30	2500	400	10	40	0.2	11	0.9	0.8	0.9	4	0.8	0.9	80	10	200
6–8	23	51	121	48	2000	35	3500	400	15	40	0.2	13	1.1	1.0	1.0	4	0.9	0.9	100	10	250
8–10	28	62	131	52	2200	40	3500	400	15	40	0.3	15	1.2	1.1	1.2	5	1.0	1.0	110	10	250
Males																					
10–12	35	77	140	55	2500	45	4500	400	20	40	0.4	17	1.3	1.3	1.4	5	1.2	1.2	125	10	300
12–14	43	95	151	59	2700	50	5000	400	20	45	0.4	18	1.4	1.4	1.6	5	1.4	1.4	135	18	350
14–18	59	130	170	67	3000	60	5000	400	25	55	0.4	20	1.5	1.5	1.8	5	1.4	1.4	150	18	400
Females																					
10–12	35	77	142	56	2250	50	4500	400	20	40	0.4	15	1.3	1.1	1.4	5	1.2	1.2	110	18	300
12–14	44	97	154	61	2300	50	5000	400	20	45	0.4	15	1.4	1.2	1.6	5	1.3	1.3	115	18	350
14–16	52	114	157	62	2400	55	5000	400	25	50	0.4	16	1.4	1.2	1.8	5	1.3	1.3	120	18	350
16–18	54	119	160	63	2300	55	5000	400	25	50	0.4	15	1.5	1.2	2.0	5	1.3	1.3	115	18	350
18–22	58	128	163	64	2000	55	5000	400	25	55	0.4	13	1.5	1.0	2.0	5	0.8	0.8	100	18	350
22–35	58	128	163	64	2000	55	5000	—	25	55	0.4	13	1.5	1.0	2.0	5	0.8	0.8	100	18	300
35–55	58	128	160	63	1850	55	5000	—	25	55	0.4	13	1.5	1.0	2.0	6	0.8	0.8	90	18	300
55–75+	58	128	157	62	1700	55	5000	—	25	60	0.4	13	1.5	1.0	2.0	6	0.8	0.8	80	10	300
Pregnancy					+200	65	6000	400	30	60	0.8	15	1.8	+0.1	2.5	8	+0.4	+0.4	125	18	450
Lactation					+1000	75	8000	400	30	60	0.5	20	2.0	+0.5	2.5	6	+0.5	+0.5	150	18	450

Courtesy of the *Dairy Council Digest* (November-December, 1968). Revised 1968; designed for the maintenance of good nutrition of practically all healthy people in the U.S.A.

[1] The allowance levels are intended to cover individual variations among most normal persons as they live in the United States under usual environmental stresses. The recommended allowances can be attained with a variety of common foods, providing other nutrients for which human requirements have been less well defined. See text for more detailed discussion of allowances and of nutrients not tabulated.

[2] The folacin allowances refer to dietary sources as determined by *Lactobacillus casei* assay. Pure forms of folacin may be effective in doses less than one-quarter of the RDA.

[3] Niacin equivalents include dietary sources of the vitamin itself plus 1 mg equivalent for each 60 mg of dietary tryptophan.

[4] Assumes protein equivalent to human milk. For proteins not 100 percent utilized, factors should be increased proportionately.

perative to keep the goals of the Council in mind. These recommendations were devised for planning food supplies and as a guide for the interpretation of food consumption records of large groups of people. Therefore, you may see individual diets which you believe are inadequate when viewed in context with the recommended allowances. This does not necessarily mean that for a particular individual it is an inadequate diet since the recommended allowances are standards established to meet the needs of most of the people. Because individuals have their own internal and external environmental needs, we find that for some people the food recommendations are too small and for others they are too large. The recommendations include enough nutritional value so that daily allowances are aimed at what the Board considers optimal health for persons needing the maximum. All biochemical functions can be maintained with desirable *storage levels*. It is not merely providing enough nutrition to avoid deficiencies.

With the above in mind, let us consider some of the nutrients that we find included in the recommendation for infancy through 18 years of age. Let us also consider a brief review of the various functions and in some cases the important interrelatedness of one nutrient to another.

CALORIES AND ENERGY EXPENDITURE

Let us first discuss the recent information in relation to the area of caloric and energy expenditure in the child. As you look at the recommended daily allowances you will note that the period of infancy has now been broken up into three age levels. The recommended allowances for the various ages are based largely on the general composition of breast milk and on the general intake of thriving infants because there is a real lack of information of normal infant needs. Unfortunately, from age 1 through 18 the recommendations are based on rather scant available experimental information when compared to adult nutritional requirements.

When we consider energy metabolism, we should recall that the daily need for energy fluctuates within the individual from one day to the next as the body attempts to maintain its equilibrium with the external environment. Watson (1967) talks about the clinical signs of an *increased pulse rate* as reflected in an increased heat reduction and muscle action resulting in increased energy need. *Climate* also makes a difference in the day-to-day fluctuations of energy need. Hot weather will decrease the body heat production while cold weather increases it. *Food intake* itself will influence energy expenditure by raising and lowering the basal metabolism rate. An insufficient diet will tend to lower the basal metabolism rate while a regular diet will raise it approximately 6 percent, and overfeeding may raise it as much as 40 percent. *Growth*, of course, tends to increase heat production. The individual child's ability or inability to adequately maintain normal body temperature will affect metabolism and thus energy expenditure. Temperature decreases during infancy will increase metabolism rate. This process is called *thermogenesis*. Thermogenesis in infants is similar to shivering in adults. Examples of factors which interfere with thermogenesis are respiratory distress syndrome, extreme prematurity, the ingestion of some drugs, and so forth (Watson, 1967).

There are a number of rules of thumb which can be used when calculating caloric needs. Caloric needs can be predicted best on the basis of body height. Caloric intake closely correlates with the various stages of growth. Peak energy intakes coincide with the highest growth rates. Unfortunately, current studies tend to lump children together by age groups and do not take into account growth patterns—thus discounting, for example, the changes that occur during the preadolescent growth spurt. The studies particularly miss the high energy needs of the adolescent girls at menarche. Another significant factor is that of energy expenditure resulting from physical activity. Energy expenditure through physical activity in the child from four to six years of age is 35 percent of his total energy intake, while energy expenditure of the child from 10 to 12 years of age is 32 percent of his total energy intake in physical activity (Heald et al., 1963). Sex-based caloric need variances must also be considered. For example, in late childhood the boy exceeds the girl by a very small caloric margin—up to 13 years of age when the boy begins to increase his caloric intake and the girls begin to decrease their caloric intake.

While age specified by year grouping is not a very reliable indicator of caloric requirements, we do see some similarities in the various phases of growth and development. The caloric requirements of the infant are high when compared with his body weight. By body weight, infants are more active metabolically than adults but less active than the toddlers one through three years of age. The infant uses energy for his activities and stores large amounts of calories for growth and loss of heat. Heat loss is great because of his large skin surface in comparison to his body weight. His growth process is marked by increased cell number and sizes, cell mass and to some extent cell function (*Dairy Council Digest*, March–April, 1969). One group of experimenters found that the caloric intake of the four- to six-month-old infant was more closely related to the degree of activity than to the size of the infant. Energy is also lost through the specific dynamic action of foods (approximately 5 to 7 calories per kilogram) and loss through excretion of body wastes (8 to 10 percent in breast-fed infants). We can extrapolate from this information that individual infants vary greatly from one another in their actual daily use of calories because of their *varying energy expenditures*.

Individual calorie needs and daily allowances will not be appropriate for every individual, but the recommendations can be used as a general guideline just as those connected with the basic four food groups. As the child grows from toddler age through adolescence, his energy needs are determined by his genetically programmed body size and growth pattern, as well as by his sex and his activity level. The child's basal metabolic rate reflects his high cellular activity and high body surface. The basal metabolic rate decreases slowly year by year with a temporary increase during adolescence with resultant decrease to the adult maintenance level. The basal metabolic rate is higher for boys than girls because of the higher muscle mass. Males increase their rate of muscle cell growth over females, actually having a greater number of muscle cells at maturity.

Calories during the growing years are needed to compensate for expended body energy. Because of their critical role, deficiencies as small as 10 calories per kilogram body weight can result in failure to grow and decrease nitrogen retention. Excessive calorie intake will be discussed later in this chapter, as will lack of calories in undernutrition. Unfortunately, our ability correctly to estimate specific caloric requirements is not very reliable and becomes impossible when energy disturbances come into play; a well-known example is obesity (Heald et al., 1963; Proudfit and Robinson, 1967).

PROTEIN

As you will recall from your earlier study of normal nutrition, protein functions as an essential ingredient for proper growth and development. It forms the basic building-block material needed for tissue growth. Protein is also used by the body in connection with various enzyme systems. An example of this function is seen in the infant's use of trytophan or phenylalanine in the production of antibody responses.

It must be remembered that the recommended daily allowances for infants are calculated on normal breast milk. While cow's milk has more protein by weight than human milk, it is not so well utilized because human infants do not have the proper enzymes for efficient digestion. Obviously, cow's milk was made for calves and not for human infants. However, some increase in utilization of cow's milk does result from the milk being pasteurized and homogenized. For example, one-half the protein in breast milk is lactalbumin, which is quickly digested by the infant. Only one-fifth of the cow's milk is lactalbumin. In the child, approximately 12 to 14 percent of the total caloric need is supplied by proteins. Some investigators believe that the current protein intake of children and adolescents provides more than the recommended daily allowances and that there may be some question that an overabundance of protein is being provided in the child's diet.

The need for protein tends to parallel such maturational events as growth spurts and sexual maturation during adolescence. Recommendations regarding protein must take into account sex differences, as they did for calorie intake. Boys tend to reach a peak of protein intake at about 15 years of age and gradually fall off until 18—when the adult maintenance level is reached. Girls' protein intake raises gradually to 12 years of age and then begins to decline. Here again, information concerning protein and nitrogen metabolism in the normal adolescent is scarce. However, researchers have found that nitrogen retention is related to menarche in adolescent girls and that there is a greater retention of protein during the period of accelerated growth preceding menarche. Following this growth spurt in girls, nitrogen retention diminishes. Unfortunately, we have no acceptable data for boys during the period of the preadolescent growth spurt (Heald et al., 1963).

VITAMINS

Vitamins function in a myriad of biochemical systems. The vitamin interrelates in a weblike fashion with the functioning body tissues and with all other nutrients. For example, vitamins function within the brain itself. They facilitate the transportation of amino acids across brain cell membranes. They serve as a co-enzyme in the enzyme system which is involved in the formation of catecholaminines. They participate in the formation of single carbon fragments that are incorporated into the chemical structure of nucleic acids, affecting their synthesis and limiting protein biosynthesis (Coursin, 1967).

VITAMIN A. One important aspect of Vitamin A and the next vitamin to be discussed (Vitamin D) is that large amounts will produce toxicity and in small infants this is a most acute and dangerous side-effect. Deficiencies in Vitamin A result in faulty bone and tooth development, night blindness, and keratinization of the epithelium and mucuous membranes, as well as skin and xerophthalmia.

VITAMIN D. Vitamin D is most often synthetically fortified in modern-day foods. Vitamin D functions in the regulation of calcium absorption. Deficiencies of Vitamin D have been quite common in children in the past. The most widely known result is, of course, rickets. Classical ricket symptoms are rarely seen today in industrialized countries, although subclinical states may be more common than supposed. These subclinical states may be revealed by serum calcium, phosphorus, and alkaline phosphatase tests. Of course, patients suffering from renal insufficiency must be immediately suspect. Individual needs of Vitamin D vary markedly because of differences in absorption and utilization, exposure to ultraviolet radiation, skin pigment, etc. (*Current Aspects of Infant Nutrition*, 1962). Vitamin D deficiency can also cause convulsions in children.

VITAMIN E. Vitamin E was included for the first time in the recommended daily allowances of vitamins in 1968. Its inclusion in the recommendations occurs primarily because of an increase in dietary polyunsaturated fats. As the intake of polyunsaturated fats increases, so does the need for Vitamin E. Also, part of the problem is that Vitamin E is not stored in the body to any extent and must be taken in each day. There are some questions as to whether the body can synthesize Vitamin E in the intestine, but more research will have to be done in this area. The main source of Vitamin E are the plant tissues, rice germ, wheat germ, green leafy vegetables, and so forth. It functions in the body by reducing oxidation of Vitamin A, carotenes, and polyunsaturated fatty acids. It also functions in hematopoiesis. Research has established that in experimental animals Vitamin E also functions in the normal reproduction cycle and in the development of cholesterol. It also assists in the utilization of sex hormones.

There is a diversity of opinion concerning the amount of deficiency of Vitamin E in the population at the present time. Some studies indicate that there is no deficiency so long as there is not a large amount of polyunsaturated fats in the diet. Other studies have found that there are indications of Vitamin E inadequacy in infant diets, particularly in premature infants. This, again, depends on the amount of polyunsaturates in the diet. For example, some workers found a Vitamin E deficiency syndrome which is characterized by edema, hemolytic anemia, and thrombocytosis. This deficiency was found in premature infants given commercial formulas high in polyunsaturated fatty acids. As Vitamin E now is included in the recommended daily allowances, it is likely that more studies of its activity will be published shortly.

VITAMIN K.   Vitamin K, another fat-soluble vitamin, is not mentioned in the current recommended daily allowances. Vitamin K is found in a diversified array of food. There is also some question as to whether Vitamin K is not synthesized in the gastrointestinal system. The Committee on Nutrition of the American Medical Association did show some concern about Vitamin K levels in the newborn infant. They believed that infants diagnosed as having hemorrhagic disease of the newborn definitely exhibited a deficiency of Vitamin K. They also found Vitamin K deficiencies in older children due to such diseases as obstructive jaundice, and biliary and pancreatic insufficiencies. Vitamin K is required, of course, for the synthesis of prothrombin or for blood clotting.

VITAMIN C.   Vitamin C is found in its greatest concentrations in the most active tissues. It forms and maintains intercellular substance. Vitamin C is used in the metabolism of some amino acids and it facilitates absorption of iron in the conversion of folic acid to folinic acid. Deficiencies of Vitamin C result in cutaneous hemorrhages, improper bone development, weakened cartilages, muscle degeneration, anemia, stunted growth, susceptibility to infection and, of course, the well-known disease of scurvy. By and large Vitamin C is found in most fruit and vegetables.

Folacin is used in the synthesis of protein and as such is necessary in the regeneration of blood cells. Folacin also regulates the metabolism of a number of amino acids. Folacin interrelates with ascorbic acid since ascorbic acid is used by the body to transfer folic acid (which is the dietary form of folacin) into the biologically active folinic acid. Deficiency of folacin is not likely to be found in normal man, but it may occur secondary to disease. Examples of diseases in which folacin deficiencies are found are macrocytic anemia, diarrhea and malabsorption, and so forth. It can also be present in infancy and pregnancy. Sources of folacin are widespread in the food stuffs.

NIACIN, RIBOFLAVIN, AND THIAMIN. Niacin functions as the active constituent of enzyme systems primarily used to transform hydrogen. Its deficiency disease is the well-known pellagra, which causes changes in the gastrointestinal, skin, and neurological systems. Niacin is found in all of the basic four food groups. Riboflavin, another water-soluble vitamin is primarily used as the constituent of enzyme systems. It assists in the transfer of hydrogen from one metabolite to another. Symptoms of deficiency of riboflavin include cracks at the corner of the lips, inflammation of the lips and tongue, burning and itching of the eyes, photophobia, and blurred vision. Riboflavin is primarily found in green leafy vegetables and in rich foods such as liver, kidney, and milk. Thiamine functions primarily as part of the enzyme system, carboxylase. Deficiencies of thiamine result in lack of appetite, nervous instability, depression, fatigue, gastrointestinal atony, constipation, and the well-known deficiency disease beriberi, which ellicits symptoms of polyneuritis, cardiac failure, and edema. The committee on nutrition of the American Academy of Pediatrics discussed several experiments with children in connection with the vitamin, thiamine. One author described symptoms of thiamine deficiency in breast-fed infants. He found that the infants failed to gain weight, were constipated, and vomited frequently. By and large the committee did agree that thiamine deficiency in infants was less frequent than thiamine deficiency in preschool and school-age children.

VITAMIN B_6 AND B_{12}. Vitamin B_6 functions in the carboxylation from amino acids, transamination from one substance to another, and transulfuration from tryptophan to niacin. It also participates in the conversion of linoleic acid to arachidonic acid. Deficiencies in Vitamin B_6 are usually not seen in adults. Investigators have observed in Vitamin B_6 deficiencies in experiments in which infants received a formula deficient in the vitamin. Disorders observed during the experiment were impaired growth, hypochromatic anemia, and convulsions.

Vitamin B_{12} is involved in purine metabolism and the synthesis of linoleic acids and nucleoproteins. Vitamin B_{12} is essential for the maturation of red blood cells in the bone marrow, synthesis of methionine, and the metabolism of nervous tissue. Vitamin B_{12}'s level of absorption into the body is dependent upon the intrinsic factor, a mucoprotein enzyme secreted by the stomach. For years it was believed that Vitamin B_{12} was needed for growth in infants and children. Recently there have been a great number of studies concerning the effects of Vitamin B_{12} on the growth of infants and children. Primarily, those persons studying the premature infant found that there was not beneficial growth on the part of the infants fed Vitamin B_{12} supplements. Experimenters studying normal infants generally found the same results. The same lack of positive results was found in experiments dealing with older children (ranging from age 7 to 14). A conclusion was drawn from these studies by the Committee of Nutrition of the American Academy of Pediatrics, which stated that these workers thought it was clear to them that Vitamin B_{12} did not encourage appetite so as to cause growth increase in children. Pernicious anemia, macrocytic anemia, and degenerative changes of the nervous system result from Vitamin B_{12} deficiency (Hill et al.,1958; Proudfit and Robinson, 1967; McWilliams, 1967; Witkop, 1967; *Dairy Council Digest,* March-April 1969; Blumberg et al., 1961, 1963).

MINERALS

General minerals function in the following ways: (1) Minerals in ionic form are components of all body fluid; (2) minerals are components of essential compounds within the body; (3) minerals regulate the metabolism of many enzymes; (4) minerals maintain the acid-base balance; (5) minerals influence osmolarity; (6) minerals facilitate membrane transfer of essential compounds; and (7) minerals functioning as ash are found in bones and serve as structural support and as hemostatic mechanisms.

The major prerequisites for mineral functions is that they be in the right place at the right time and at the right concentration. An example of the interrelatedness of the inorganic compounds with other nutrients is their relationship with proteins and calories. We see in protein calorie malnutrition such conditions as reduced length of bones, decomposition of matrix and total ash, and increased reabsorption of other nutrients effecting bone growth. The interrelatedness of Vitamins A, C, and D and the minerals magnesium manganese, copper, zinc, and phosphorus is seen in mineralization and modeling of bones. It appears as though the bonds between the nutrients are more important than the absolute amount of each of the nutrients in the body. It is believed that an inbalance in minerals will not occur unless one of the elements is missing or is deficient in the diet.

New to the field of mineral research are studies of the relationship of the internal environment and its influence upon the inorganic elements. There is some evidence to indicate that the interrelationships of the various minerals, as well as their absorption and excretion and their internal functionings, will affect the dietary needs of other nutrients. For example, the enzymes needed for the breakdown of glucose are influenced by the body's calcium and sodium level. Deficiencies of most minerals or their absence is rarely seen in normal man. However, when the body is under stress of infection or disease clinical evidence of mineral deficiencies may emerge (*Dairy Council Digest,* September-October, 1968).

CALCIUM. Calcium functions in the building of bones and teeth, in muscle contraction, normal heart rhythm, nerve irritability, activation of some enzymes, and blood coagulation. The absorption of calcium into the body is regulated by body need and aided by Vitamin D, ascorbic acid, and lactose. Oxalic acid, phytic acid, and certain highly saturated fatty acids interfere with the absorption of calcium. When we discuss the metabolism of calcium, consideration must be given to a wide variety of differing opinions on the subject. First, it has been found that high intakes of calcium correlate with increased bone density —which one might assume. It has also been found that during periods of inactive growth the amount of calcium needed to maintain the balance reflects the previous calcium intake. For example, if a child has a high calcium intake during infancy, this same child will need more calcium to maintain his balance during the next period of low growth than the child who has gone through the growth period in a deficient state. Second, calcium is absorbed more efficiently at lower rather than higher levels of intake. For example, the retention of calcium at a low dietary level is 90 percent while the retention of calcium at a high dietary level would be something around 27 percent. With this taken into consideration, it has been found that chemical and histologic examinations of the bone fail to reveal any difference between high and low intakes of calcium. An increase of absorption does not necessarily mean increased retention. It appears that the problem with current studies is that they may be reflecting only the availability of calcium within the subjects. In any case, results of calcium studies may certainly be seen to be in conflict with one other.

The need for calcium throughout the child's life varies depending upon growth. The infant's need for calcium has been studied by Beal (1968). His study found that the maximum need for calcium during infancy was four times as high as the minimum need. He also found that during the first six months of life the need for calcium is at its highest. The median need for calcium was about six to seven months for girls and seven to nine months for boys. It has also been found that calcium is generally low in adolescent girls to a lesser extent than in adolescent boys. Of course, this may be merely reflecting a greater intake in calcium in adolescent boys than in adolescent girls. Experimenters have found a relationship between estrogenic secretions and calcium. They administered gastronic substances to normal girls. This depressed both the calcium and the nitrogen retention. They found an abrupt depression of calcium retention following menarche after which some girls recovered to values higher than before menarche, whereas others did not.

Another problem in estimating the individual's need for calcium lies in the area of maturation timing. For example, we see rapid gains in skeletal mass in early maturing individuals. This is in contrast to continuing long-term growth in late-maturing individuals. Obviously, the calcium needs of these divergent groups of individuals would be in error if the values were calculated by age alone. When we are dealing with the problem of calculating calcium intake for individual children we run into large numbers of problem children. These are usually boys with high calcium requirements because of tremendously increased bone growth, and late-maturing girls who are concerned with their figures, i.e., their fat stores, so that their calcium intake is often inadequate. Unfortunately, discovery of low calcium stores is difficult. Inadequate intakes of calcium in combination with calories adequate for growth may have no discernible effect on the outer bone growths but it definitely will effect the tubular of the bones, and the size of the skeletal mass. Good sources of calcium are found in the dairy products and vegetable group (Proudfit and Robinson, 1967; *Dairy Council Digest*, September-October, 1968; Pfeiffer, 1968; Garn and Wagner, 1967; Heald et al., 1963; McWilliams, 1967; Beal, 1968; *Dairy Council Digest*, March-April, 1969).

PHOSPHORUS.   Phosphorus functions in the building of bones and teeth and is used as buffer salts. Phosphorus is a compound needed by every cell. It is seen in biological material such as DNA, RNA, and so forth. Phosphorus is also important in the pH regulation of the body. Phosphorus absorption is aided by Vitamin D, thus interrelating with Vitamin A. Deficiencies of phosphorus are not likely to occur, particularly if an adequate amount of protein and calcium is ingested. However, in individuals subjected to prolonged therapy with certain antacids we may find a deficiency in phosphorus. Such a deficiency can be manifested by poor mineralization of bones, poor bone growth, or rickets.

IODINE.   Iodine, a constituent of theroxin, regulates the rate of energy exchange. There is, of course, iodinization of table salt in this country. This practice is particularly recommended in areas in which food is low in natural iodine. A symptom of iodine deficiency is, of course, a simple goiter or an enlargement of the thyroid gland. A deficiency occurring prenatally results in a condition called cretinism, but this is very rare in the United States.

IRON.   Iron is a mineral found in hemoglobin and myoglobin. Iron is also present in serum transferrin and certain enzymes. It can be found in all of the body's cells. Information regarding iron tends to suggest that the substance is deficient in most of our population. For example, investigators recommend double iron for infants of low birth weight or of low iron endowment. A number of studies have found that iron in infants and in preschool children is lower than the recommended intake. Andelman and Sered (1966) believe that iron deficiency anemia is a common and prevalent disorder throughout our environment, and that it contributes to infant mortality despite our advanced knowledge in the area. They also held that hospitalized infants had a higher rate of anemia. The rate ranged from anywhere between 25 and 44 percent of hospitalized infants categorized as low socioeconomic, of whom 76 percent were anemic even when their diets were recommended by a pediatrician and they were receiving pediatric supervision. The true incidence of iron deficiency is unknown, but the Committee on Nutrition of the American Medical Association maintains that the incidence of iron deficiency is relatively high in pregnant women and infants under one year of age. One study of children under six years of age in rural Tennessee found 10 percent to be anemic. Children under one year old were even more anemic.

Since iron is not easily excreted by the body, iron level regulation comes from absorption capacity. As the child grows older the ability of his body to absorb iron increases. This increase usually happens from about 7 to 10 years of age. In the older child, iron losses come from menstruation in the female and from fecal loss. Unfortunately, there are very few studies of iron requirement during adolescence although we do know that the need for iron increases at this time. Boys' needs are increased because of the rapid growth of body mass. This is accompanied by increased blood volume, muscle mass, and respiratory enzymes. There is a real question as to whether girls above 10 years of age are able to ingest, through dietary means, an adequate amount of iron. Recent studies have disclosed that iron stores are reduced or absent in about two-thirds of menstruating women. A number of investigators recommend eating fortified foods as a desirable means of combating iron deficiency.

The average full-term infant has enough iron at birth for about the first six months of age. If the infant then has an optimal food intake, he will derive enough iron from his dietary sources alone. The term infant with a deficient body iron at birth may require iron as early as three months and the premature infant as early as two months. The premature infant requires more iron than the term infant because of two factors: (1) lower total iron and (2) a proportional and greater growth rate postnatally. The absorption of iron by infants has been studied by a number of investigators. Some found that such absorption by infants under three months of age was faster than at any other age during life (*Dairy Council Digest,* March-April, 1969; Committee on Iron Deficiency, February 5, 1968; Heald et al., 1963; *Dairy Council Digest,* November-December, 1968; Schulman, 1961; Andelman and Sered, 1966; *Dairy Council Digest,* September-October, 1968; Proudfit and Robinson, 1967).

MAGNESIUM. Magnesium influences almost all of the bodily processes. Deficiencies are largely unknown in man, with the exception of secondary deficiencies caused by alcoholism, cirrhosis, severe renal disease, absorption syndromes, loss of body fluids, and some surgical procedures. Because magnesium is interrelated with numerous other minerals, its deficiency has a profound effect on the body. Magnesium is largely found in whole grain cereal and in dark green vegetables.

SODIUM. Sodium functions in the regulation of osmolarity. It is used as buffer salts and as an enzyme activator by the body. It assists in the maintenance of water balance and regulates muscle and nerve irritability and is a constituent of hydrochloric acid. It is found mostly in the extracellular fluid, but a small amount is also found inside of cells. Deficiencies of sodium rarely occur. If they do, the symptoms are nausea, diarrhea, and muscle cramps. There are some investigators who believe that there is an increased need of sodium by the body during pregnancy. Sodium is primarily found in the meat group, milk, eggs, and also table salt.

CHLORIDE, POTASSIUM, SULFUR, ZINC. Chloride is found mostly in the extracellular fluid, along with sodium. Deficiencies are rarely found except in patients who have experienced prolonged vomiting. Chloride is found in the same food group as sodium, and is also found in table salt.

Potassium is found in the intracellular fluid with only small amounts in the extracellular spaces. It functions in the regulation of pH, osmolarity, cell membrane transfer, and carbohydrate and protein metabolism. Deficiency in potassium is rather unlikely, but conditions of secondary deficiencies may be found in patients with kidney diseases and diabetic acidosis.

Sulfur is present in sulfur-containing amino acids, in oxidation reduction reactions, and in the synthesis of a number of essential metabolizers. It also functions with thiamine, biotin, and other inorganic sulfurs. Sulfur is a constituent of hair and nails. It is found in eggs, cheese, milk, and meat.

Zinc functions as a constituent of carbonic anhydrase, for the transfer of carbon dioxide, and is a constituent of the digestive enzyme for the hydrolysis of protein. Zinc may also be important in the metabolism of nucleic acid. Zinc deficiency has been demonstrated in the population of some underdeveloped countries, particularly in persons whose diets are also deficient in proteins and iron.

COPPER. Copper functions in the absorption of iron and in the metabolism of ascorbic acid; it also acts in normal hemoglobin synthesis, in the oxidation of fatty acids, and in the oxidation of tyrosine to melanin pigments. Some experimenters believe that copper may also be an integral part of the DNA or RNA molecules. The deficiency of copper will lead to retarded hemoglobin production, but it rarely occurs within our society. Copper is found in liver, shell fish, the meat group, and whole grain cereals.

MANGANESE, FLUORINE, COBALT, MOLYBDENUM. Manganese functions in the body in the formation of urea and in thoroxin formation. Manganese is related to lipotropic active enzymes in the Krebs cycle. Deficiencies in manganese are not known in man. Manganese is found in whole grain cereals, in meat groups, and in green leafy vegetables.

Fluorine is used to increase the resistance of teeth to decay. It appears to affect teeth due to its combination with bone crystal in the forming of more stable compounds.

Cobalt, a constituent of Vitamin B_{12} is essential in the normal function of all cells, particularly cells of bone marrow, of the nervous system, and of the gastrointestinal system. Primary deficiency disease is rare, except in persons in whom no animal products are consumed. Secondary deficiencies may be found in conditions such as lack of the gastric intrinsic factor, gastrectomy, and malabsorption syndromes. The source of cobalt is found in Vitamin B_{12}.

Molybdenum is a constituent of essential enzymes. There is little information about this micromineral (*Dairy Council Digest*, September-October 1968; Proudfit and Robinson, 1967).

Recommended Daily Allowances

When I considered writing this chapter on nutrition, I first thought that I would not even mention recommended daily allowances. I felt this way because I have found too many nurses who have had poor educational experiences concerning nutrition, and who promptly suppressed the information after it was "learned." But after reconsidering the total chapter I wanted to make an attempt to put the daily recommended allowances in their proper place—that of a *base* or *starting point* from which we can consider the individual's needs. It can serve as part of our concrete conceptualization of human nutritional needs along with the basic four food groups. Both of these suggested aids can be used as a core content to weigh the current literature on nutrition.

I was recently asked to recommend a book on nutrition for distribution to several cooperating agencies. Rather than recommend a book, I recommended a notebook which would contain current copies of pertinent articles. Nutrition is indeed a *dynamic* discipline, but unfortunately many professionals still remember all the outdated information they "sweated blood" to memorize many years ago. My hope is that this chapter will give the reader a taste of the current information so that she can begin to translate her new information into new nursing practices.

STUDIES AND THEIR RESULTS

Now that we have at some length examined the recommended daily allowances for the average child, let us consider *reality* for a moment. Since the mid-1960s numerous experimenters have been working, trying to evaluate the nutritional status of the American child. Large numbers of children have been studied ranging in age from two years through adolescence. Several methods of study have been used —ranging from interviews; food records; height, weight, skinfold thickness; attitude scales; and chemical analysis to circulating levels of thiamine, hemoglobin, ascorbic acid, and so forth.

One study of children two to six years of age found the children's intake of iron sufficiently below the recommended daily requirement and in sporadic instances low amounts of the other nutrients, particularly ascorbic acid. These results are even more startling if one considers that 71 percent of the children were receiving vitamin supplements and had parents of a high educational level.

Another study of 150 children of six to twelve years of age from Burlington, Vermont, recorded height, weight, skinfold thickness, plus other clinical and biochemical measures in order to determine nutritional status. Besides these measurements, social adjustment, parental attitude, and dietary intake were determined. The investigations found that there were low-average intakes of calcium, Vitamin A, and ascorbic acid. Other pertinent factors were that children of average weight rated higher on various tests of social adjustment and nutrient intakes than children who were either overweight or underweight. A study conducted in two suburbs in a Minnesota community examined 136 children. The children studied were nine through eleven years of age. Methods used in this study were dietary data collected from the children, and socioeconomic and attitudinal data collected by children, teacher, and parent questionnaires. The results showed that, on the average, the children were fairly well fed, but large segments had very low or very high intakes of Vitamin A and ascorbic acid.

A multiracial study in New York City studied 642 10- to 13-year-old children. These workers investigated the levels of thiamine, biotin, riboflavin, pantothenate, nicotinic, carotin, ascorbic acid, total cholesterol, triglycerides, and Vitamins B_6, B_{12}, A, and E. This study found that 12 percent of the children received protein below the amount accepted as adequate. It also found an association between diets low in protein and lower-than-average blood values of thiamine, biotin, and ascorbate. Another multiracial study was conducted in Onondaga County, New York, with 400 12- to 15-year-old children. The methods used in this study were biochemical analysis of blood and urine samples, interview data on race, age, father's occupation, and breakfast, as well as food supplements. The results of this study were as follows: the data on height and weight, skinfold thickness, and certain biochemical criteria indicated poorer nutrition in Negroes than in white children; also, girls were less well nourished than boys and were more likely to be overweight.

In a study done in 1965 in Burlington, Vermont, 401 school children of varying socioeconomic levels and from ages 12 to 15 were subjected to biochemical measures of nutritional status; hemoglobin, hematocrit, and thiamine, riboflavin, and ascorbic acid levels. It was found that overall nutritional status of these children was good. Although hemoglobin and thiamine were found to be rather low or deficient in the highest number of children, with girls rating poorer than boys. Most of the children came from moderate to more affluent residential areas; 22 percent of the boys and 29 percent of the girls came from low-income areas.

In the late 1960s there were two studies of high-school students— one in Berkeley and one in a town in Iowa. The Berkeley researchers studied seven-day food diaries. Children were classified by degree of body fat, and it was noted that: (1) the calcium and iron intakes were low, especially for girls; (2) highest intakes of calories and nutrients were found in average-weight boys and in lean girls; and (3) Negroes and lower-socioeconomic-level whites tended to have lower intakes of nutrients than others. The Iowa study of 2045 high-school students conducted physical examinations of all the students, made biochemical analyses, and collected clinical and dietary data from 252 of the students. They found the average teenager was healthy and well-fed, but a substantial minority omitted breakfast and ate diets which were not well-balanced. They also found that some individual diets were poor—not because of socioeconomic status, but rather because of diet fads and food preferences.

From these studies we can get some indication that even children from average families—children who are considered healthy and well—may indeed have nutritional deficiencies or may have a nutritional index that is borderline. From this we must assume that today we can no longer automatically state that if a child lives in America he must automatically have an adequate nutritional status. If we believe this assumption to be true, how will it change the nursing role when caring for children? How can we begin to evaluate, in terms of our nursing role, the adequate nutritional status of our patient?

First let us consider what we would look for in a cursory visual evaluation of the child in our care. Proudfit and Robinson (1967) elaborated on several of the observations we can make when we are grossly evaluating nutritional status. One thing that stands out in most peoples' minds, when they consider the usual behavior of well-nourished children, is energy and vitality. Most children exhibit a high activity level throughout the day. They exhibit their ability to recover quickly from fatigue and fall asleep quickly at night after a long, rush day. Well-nourished children are usually happy, interested in activities, and generally have a sense of well-being. Their posture is appropriate for their age, and teeth are usually straight and free of cavities. Their gums are firm and pink, without any signs of bleeding; they are slightly moist and have a healthy glow. The eyes, one of the major areas to observe, should be clear and bright—with no circles of fatigue around them. The well-nourished child's hair should be lustrous and shiny, with a healthy scalp. The well-nourished child will have a good appetite and eliminate regularly. His attention span will be appropriate for his age and he will tend to get along easily with others. The child's weight should be normal for his height, age, and body build. For ill children, weight-height information can be obtained from the chart. Signs of crying and irritability and restlessness are significant signs of a disturbed or ill child. With the above in mind one should consciously make attempts to evaluate the children whom he sees in the hospital. (Proudfit and Robinson, 1968; *Dairy Council Digest*, November-December, 1967).

NUTRITIONAL ASPECTS OF THE CHILD UNDER STRESS

We have discussed the recommended daily allowances and the general nutritional status of normal healthy American children. Now we must look at the changes in nutrition which occur when the child comes under "stress." What is stress? The *Dairy Council Digest* (May-June, 1966), defines stress as ". . . the wear and tear on the human machinery that accompanies any vital activity and, in a sense, parallels the intensity of life." This body wear-and-tear includes such things as increased physical activity or decreased physical activity, immobilization of the body for any length of time, obesity or underweight, extreme hot and cold environments, infections and malnutrition, trauma or stress of psychological origin, surgery, various gastrointestinal disorders, and drugs.

Some stress is not necessarily harmful to the individual, particularly if the individual is physically and mentally prepared to adapt to the stress. We all know that the body has a number of adapting mechanisms; the major one is the endocrine system. The nervous and endocrine systems help to keep the body structure functioning in equilibrium during times of stress. For example, the body's reaction to moderate to severe trauma is a net loss of protein. There is an increased secretion of glucocorticoid hormone which increases catabolism of tissue but is useful to increase the body's defenses in times of stress. On the other hand there may be disturbances within the endocrine system itself which will affect the nutritional process and may consequently alter the needs of the tissue for the various nutrients. "An increase or decrease in the release of hormones is reflected in cellular metabolism and affects the cellular requirement for certain vitamins and other essential nutrients" (*Dairy Council Digest*, May-June, 1966, p. 13). For example, in hypothyroidism there is an increase in metabolic rate which increases the caloric needs of the body as well as the requirements for almost all of the water soluble vitamins.

PHYSICAL EVENTS AND CHANGES IN NUTRITIONAL NEEDS

Increased physical activity affects the body's requirements for energy-yielding nutrients. The amount of change in the need of energy-yielding nutrients is proportionate to the intensity of the physical activity. Along with this, an increase in thiamine, riboflavin, and niacin are recommended with increased calorie expenditure. Vitamins are particularly susceptible to changes in physical activity and the ability to perform work is impaired by vitamin deficiency. Of particular note in the studies was the decreased work capacity suffered with severe Vitamin C deficiency.

IMMOBILIZATION.   Immobilization is one stress which we find prevalent in the hospitalization of children. Immobilization produces alterations in the metabolic balance leading to a net loss of certain nutrients. Protein breakdown and excretion of nitrogen are drastically increased above normal during immobilization. Take for example a person immobilized for seven weeks; he has an average daily loss of 2.3 g of nitrogen and requires another seven weeks to recover from this stress. Nitrogen losses in persons immobilized with fractures are found to be even greater than this. One study found that 8.13 g/day of nitrogen was lost on an average with fracture patients.

Calcium is another nutrient which is lost in large amounts during immobilization. It seems as though the body needs a certain degree of stress on a skeletal system to maintain its calcium balance. For example, a patient immobilized for seven weeks might have a total loss of 13.1 g of calcium. Following bed-rest he would continue to lose calcium or to be in negative calcium balance for the next three weeks—even though he was actively losing approximately 4.4 g of calcium per day. Unlike protein the calcium loss may take years (one to four years) to restore balance. Apparently bone that does not receive stress from the weight of the body or the pull of the muscle loses calcium. There are other negative balances in the area of electrolytes which also occur during immobilization. The whole area of nutrient loss during immobilization suggests the real need to look into passive exercises or isometric body position which increase gravitation pull on the skeletal structure of immobilized patients. How much good reinstituting the passive range of motion exercises during a bed-bath of the immobilized patient is something that might make an interesting and useful study for the nurse.

OBESITY. Obesity must be considered as one of the body stresses. The problem lies in the oxygenation of so much adipose tissue. There is a high prevalence of impaired glucose tolerance or hyperglycemia in obesity. Now we find that diseases of bones and joints are complicated by excessive weight. (Obesity will be discussed at length in a later section.)

HOT AND COLD ENVIRONMENTS. We rarely think of an increase or decrease in environmental heat as a stress, but it certainly does change the need for certain nutrients. This must be considered one of the normal stresses of life. We can all recall that large amounts of sodium are lost during a heat wave, particularly if in addition to the heat the person is also doing physical work. But I believe that many of us fail to recognize that nitrogen is also lost in large amounts in high temperatures (anything above 70 to 80°F). Studies of moderate physical activity have found that the large amounts of iron are lost in tropical kinds of climate as well as calcium, copper, manganese, phosphorus, and potassium. It has been stated that nitrogen loss in sweat may be one of the several contributing factors to the high prevalence of protein malnutrition or kwashiorkor in tropical areas.

INFECTION AND MALNUTRITION. The combination of infection and malnutrition often leads to more severe diseases than when either one is found alone. Some groups of Americans suffer more from this combination than others. Such persons are food faddists, elderly persons, or those on desired reducing diet, teenagers with erratic food habits, and individuals with depressed appetites or who are debilitated from chronic diseases. It must be remembered that all infection, no matter how minor, brings changes in the nutritional requirements in the individual body. The malnutrition connected with infections is brought about by three major faults: (1) faulty intake; (2) faulty digestion, absorption, or excretion; and (3) faulty metabolism.

Sebrell and Goldsmith (1967) found that malnutrition in the United States was usually secondary malnutrition—that is, secondary to physical, mental, or psychological stress of the variety we have been discussing. The recommended daily allowances we discussed earlier were not devised for the ill, although they may form a buffer against increased needs during severe trauma. Health workers of the future must consider the metabolic status of every patient and correct the nutritional and metabolic imbalances produced as a result of some other disease. Unfortunately not much information has been produced concerning the prevention and treatment of this kind of nutritional deficiency. One disease which we have seen frequently is acute diarrhea. Acute diarrhea and other disorders which grossly interfere with gastrointestinal functioning are often fatal, particularly in malnourished preschool children. Experimenters have also found that kwashiorkor usually follows from four to six weeks of acute diarrhea or acute infections in those undernourished individuals living in underdeveloped countries. Diarrhea occurring concurrently with the weaning of children in underdeveloped countries is an outstanding example of the synergistic interaction of malnutrition and infection.

One nutrient that is involved in the areas of infection and malnutrition is protein (nitrogen retention). There is usually a decrease of 10–15 percent nitrogen retention in severe cases of diarrhea. If the child is fed nothing but gruels and starchy solutions, this also results in protein malnutrition. This high carbohydrate kind of diet can also perpetuate the diarrhea even after the infection has passed. It is far better to feed a child with diarrhea adequately since the absorption of nitrogen and fat increases quantitatively with intake even though it is less efficient because of the diarrhea. Vitamin A during an infection is greatly reduced in the blood. Childhood diseases frequently precipitate keratinization of the epithelium, particularly in underdeveloped countries. The same phenomenon may also occur in our own depressed areas, although the subject has not been studied.

Borderline thiamine deficiencies can be seen in people who come under stress. Vitamin C in combination with infection will decrease blood levels and increase the urinary excretion of thiamine. It may also produce clinical scurvy. Infections also influence iron metabolism. Chronic infection may decrease iron's infection-fighting capacities, reduce iron retention, and shorten the life-span of the erythrocytes. One could call this *anemia of infection*. The relationship between infection, malnutrition, and nutrition is very complex and more information concerning the relationship is being published almost monthly.

TRAUMA AND STRESS OF PSYCHOLOGICAL ORIGIN. It has been found that stress of psychological origin increases the urinary excretion of nitrogen. This is probably due to the fact that amino acids are released from the muscle and other dispensible tissues as a result of the increased secretion of glucocorticoid hormone. Severe trauma changes the metabolic needs of the body extensively. Severe trauma might be categorized as an operation, injury, fracture, or burn. Nitrogen loss is caused partly by the increase of adrenal-stimulating hormones of the pituitary glands and increased steroid hormones of the adrenal gland. Severe trauma causes urinary losses of nitrogen, sulfur, phosphorus, potassium, and cretisin. It also increases the basal oxygen consumption and the losses of nitrogen and sulfur within the muscles. There is a decreased tolerance for glucose, and generally disturbed electrolyte balance. In moderate traumas the loss is less and can occur primarily because of food limitation, immobilization, and altered catabolism.

SURGERY, GASTROINTESTINAL DISORDERS, AND DRUGS. The nutritional need of the body when elective surgery is being contemplated will depend upon a number of factors: the extent of the surgery, previous nutritional status of the patient, the effect of the operation on the patient's ability to judge what he needs to eat, and the selection of specific operative procedures. Protein is the most important nutrient when we consider surgery; it must be used in tissue replacement. Other nutrients for nutritional consideration in wound healing include hydration of tissues and distribution of body electrolytes, Vitamin C, Vitamin K, and so forth. Postoperatively, the patient is immobilized and thus will lose nitrogen. Three to five days postoperatively there should be a great effort made to provide adequate calories to the patient to protect the dietary protein from being used up for energy. Usually supplementary thiamine is needed postoperatively because of restricted diets.

Experimenters found that the average weight loss was 6 percent within 10 days of a postoperative period, although these investigators believed that a significant portion of this weight loss was associated with preoperative procedures which included catharsis and restricted calorie intake. They found that there was a lessening of the protein loss postoperatively when protein was administered. There was a decreased destruction of muscle tissue and connective tissue with patients fed calories plus plasma or protein hydrolyse. This kind of feeding was compared with starving patients, who were supplied only with fluid electrolytes and not more than 3000 calories daily postoperatively. The aim of postoperative nutrition should be to replace the tissue loss and to enhance wound healing. Vitamin C given postoperatively will be used for collagen formation, and postoperative administration of zinc will hasten wound healing in zinc-depleted patients.

Gastrointestinal handicaps such as abnormalities occurring in the gastrointestinal tract and the organs leading to it (e.g., pancreas and liver) lead to faulty digestion and absorption of nutrients. This usually leads to malnutrition. You may recall that iron is absorbed in the upper jejunum; glucose, electrolytes, and water-soluble vitamins are also absorbed in the upper jejunum; calcium, protein, fat, and fat-soluble vitamins are absorbed in the small intestine; and Vitamin B_{12} is synthesized in the terminal ileum.

These facts should also be kept in mind after bowel surgery. The nurse should definitely watch for clinical secondary deficiencies of the above-mentioned nutrients in patients who have had bowel surgery and gastrointestinal abnormalities or diseases. We should not minimize any disorders of the gastrointestinal tract. This is the primary system through which our life-giving nutrients are absorbed from the dietary nutrition ingested. Once malnutrition takes over it can also cause gastrointestinal disorders. For example, protein deficiency can damage the intestinal mucosa, causing malabsorption. Iron deficiency can cause achlorhydria. Niacin deficiency may cause diarrhea, riboflavin deficiency, and cheilosis. There are a number of other agents than can cause malnutrition because of their effect on the digestion and absorption system. Diet therapy itself can cause digestive and absorption changes. For example, a gluten-free diet can effect the gluten enterpathy causing idiopathic steatorrhea. Organ diseases, such as those affecting the liver and pancreas, can affect digestion and absorption. Enzymes may cause metabolism errors. For example, biosalts may result in malabsorption. Diarrhea caused by an intestinal parasite will affect nutrition.

Let us for a moment discuss the interrelationship drugs have to the digestion and absorption systems. Drug intolerance may be explained by differences in the metabolic system from one patient to another. These differences may be either hereditary or be caused by diet. Unfortunately, there is a limited amount of information in the whole area of nutrition, infection, and drug therapy. There are a number of animal studies which are likely to be significant when interrelationships are studied. Some factors to be considered in the area follow:

A deficiency of substrate or enzymes for drug conjugation may be due to malnutrition. Protein malnutrition may cause infiltration of the liver. This may make the liver more vulnerable to the biochemical affects of drugs because of diminished conjugation. Unfortunately the very patients who receive the full amount of any given drug are the ones who are nutritionally impaired by primary disease, which interferes with their ability to conjugate, eliminate, or use drugs normally. Drugs and disease may affect the metabolic process both independently and jointly. While drugs may act synergistically in modifying the course of a disease, the disease, drugs, and food in combination may cause a toxic reaction. Protein depletion with an inadequate intake of sulfur-containing amino acids may inhibit conjugation and elimination of certain drugs. Starvation or caloric depletion may increase the affect of drug toxification. Drug intolerance may be caused by an enzyme defect. (Watson and Lawrey, 1967; *Dairy Council Digest, September-October,* 1969; Gershoff et al., 1968; Roe, 1967; Christakes and Miridjanian, 1968; Weisberger et al., 1969; *Dairy Council Digest,* May-June, 1966).

SUMMARY

To highlight the area: there are four factors which effect the nutritional status of the ill child. First, there are nutritional effects because of the use of therapeutic diets. For example, low-sodium diets decrease palatability of food along with the decrease in edema; high-polyunsaturated diets decrease serum cholesterol and increase depot linoleate, but may increase Vitamin E requirements in infants. Although fat diets will decrease the absorption of creatine, a high-fat diet will increase the serum cholesterol and triglycerides. High-protein diets will increase the requirement for Vitamin B_6. High-carbohydrate diets will increase serum triglycerides and thiamine requirements. Secondly, some diseases affect the nutritional status. For example, acute gastrointestinal disorders affect nutrition by causing anorexia, electrolyte, and protein losses from the symptoms of vomiting and diarrhea. These in turn cause hypermotility and malabsorption. Third, various types of drugs affect the nutritional status of the individual. For example, antacids tend to destruct thiamine; mineral oil decreases the absorption of creatine and Vitamin A. Chelating agents decrease the absorption of metals. Cation exchange resins decrease sodium, potassium, and calcium absorption. The antimetabolytes affect folic acid by reacting as antivitamin agents, barbituates and anticonvulsive drugs are also antivitamin agents and affect folic acid. Corticosteroids decrease glucose tolerance, decrease muscle protein, and increase liver fat. Fourth, drugs affect the nutritional status. For example, drugs may increase or decrease the appetite; they may increase nausea, vomiting, and diarrhea; they may change the intestinal flora; and they may have a pharmaceutical effect on the gastrointestinal tract. I think we must also watch for what current investigators call *secondary deficiencies*—those deficiencies that have come about because of disease trauma or stress. It seems to me most urgent that we begin to notice these nutrient deficiencies, whether primary or secondary, if we are adequately to manipulate the internal environment of the child (Christakis and Miridjanian, 1968).

Some Major Nutritional Concerns of Childhood

Today's American has exhibited an almost overwhelming concern for food. Nearly everyone has considered his diet for one reason or another. We have people on special diets because they are underweight or overweight, have a family history of heart attacks or diabetes, have inborn metabolic errors, and so forth. Vitamin supplements have become part of our daily nutrient intake. (There are, of course, some people in America who are concerned just with getting enough to eat.)

All this is not to say anything negative but only to point out our great concern with food. Because of this concern I should like to discuss four of the numerous areas of concern to us as modern-day Americans and as modern-day workers in the area of child health. There are many other areas which could be covered; I chose these because they included a large segment of the population or were new and had a large potential. The first three problems are of major concern: obesity, anemia, and malnutrition. While the last, malnutrition, is not usually seen in America it is of major concern in our world and we have recently been recognizing more malnutrition in this country. I will also include some current information on atherosclerosis in childhood, an area of great potential concern to us as nurses.

When we consider the problem of obesity the first question which arises is cause. Barnes (1968) maintains that the delivery of nutritional services in the United States and the nutritional education of the population could not be blamed for obesity; the cause may stem from our need to understand the total individual's behavior more clearly. For example, obesity may be *caused* by excess calorie intake, but the solution, according to Barnes, does not lie in the area of decreased calories but in how we influence man's food choices in order to improve his health—or what kind of food choices are suitable for the individual's own body chemistry.

Let us remember that the role of food includes its social function in our society. It is closely interwoven with ethnic, religious, and family customs. Food provides satisfaction and relief from stress—which, for some people, can be obtained no other way. Statistically obesity is largely found in persons of lower socioeconomic status. For example, 30 percent of lower-economic-group females were found to be obese. Stunkard (1968) ran an experiment and found that obese persons who were given a free food access in privacy ate considerably more than obese persons who had a free food access not in a private setting. This suggests that part of the problem with obesity is general lack of body control. In other words: How well disciplined is the individual? There is some reason to believe from the literature that a great deal of the problems of obese people is their inability to control themselves, not only in the area of food but also in other areas of activity. It is thought that because obesity sets up a physiological chain of events it tends to be self-perpetuating. In addition to this, there are some irreversible physiological changes which make weight gain more efficient than weight loss after the person has once become obese. Obese people have an obsessive concern with weight which often leads to passivity, expectation of rejection, and greater inactivity. Unfortunately, the basic habits of childhood are hard to change in the adult and if the child has been overweight there will be a greater tendency to continue overweightness in adulthood.

A very interesting, although devastating, side-effect of obesity is distortion of body image. Obese people exhibit many forms of neurotic behavior, although there are only two that seem to be related to their obesity. The first is overeating and the second is distortion of body image. The distortion of body image often takes the form of overwhelming negative preoccupation with obesity, so that weight and sometimes weight control becomes a paramount concern of the person. Such a person often sees his own body in grotesque form and believes that others view his body with contempt. Stunkard (1968) believes that there are three developments which predispose obese people to distort body image. First: the age of onset of the obesity; second: the presence of neurosis of one kind or another; and third: perpetual evaluation of the obesity. He found that if obesity occurred during adolescence or during childhood there was a greater tendency to have distortion of body image than obesity which occurred during adulthood. How the family felt about the child himself and about his obesity was important. For example, some families might view being large in a positive light and connect it with strength, healthiness, and manliness in boys. Other families might feel that even being a little overweight was very negative and the child who exhibited these features might become a focal point of the family's hostility and contempt. So it seems that the adolescence, preadolescence, and childhood periods are critical points at which children should attempt to control their weight.

Unfortunately, one of the growth characteristics of the adolescent is change in body fat content. We see girls getting heavy, fatty deposits in the hips and so forth. These changes probably reflect alterations in the hormonal, biochemical, and other systems rather than any overeating or decreased activity. There are sex differences in fat deposits all the way from infancy. For example, infant girls have more subcutaneous fat than infant boys, and this persists all the way through childhood and adolescence. Around 8 to 12 years, the preadolescent period, children of both sexes increase their accumulation of fat tissue. Then, around 13, boys begin to decrease fat deposits as part of their growth spurt. At 13 girls have a tendency to increase their fattiness. What happens to the biochemistry of the adolescent that increases the incidence of obesity? Heald (1969) found that there are clear-cut and different changes in two areas: (1) glucose metabolism and (2) energy metabolism. Glucose metabolism is definitely different in an obese human. Obese individuals respond to glucose tolerance tests with hyperglycemic reaction very much like diabetics, although they are not diabetic. Investigators have also found that there is hypertrophy of the pancreatic eyelet cells in the obese adolescent. There seems to be an inverse relationship between the amount of fat in the body and the increase resistance of the transfer of glucose into the muscles. In other words, obese people have a tendency to turn their glucose into fat rather than muscle. About 20 percent of all adolescents and adult obese persons show changes or differences in glucose tolerance. There is some question as to whether this is an inborn kind of deviation or whether it represents the body's adapting itself to a changed internal environment originally caused by overeating.

DIETS.   Thus we come to the dilemma of the diet. The amount of literature in this area is fantastic. Obviously I am not going to cover it in this chapter, but there are a couple of things I found interesting and which might interest you in delving more deeply into the problem of obesity. There are a great many diets which bring about rather serious fasting on the part of the person. We find these fad diets being used in large numbers by adolescents, particularly adolescent girls. There are serious risks involved, particularly with people who have any kind of infection, diabetes, liver disease, ulcers, or who are pregnant. There are many complications to serious fasting which we certainly can call starvation. For example, there can be severe orthostatic hypotension, nonochromic anemia, and so forth. People who use diets which include fasting should be made aware of the fact that this amounts to starvation as far as the body is concerned. Of the weight lost during fasting, 60 percent will probably be in muscle tissue and only 35 percent in adipose tissue. Thus the weight loss becomes the result of catabolism of tissue. There is also considerable water loss. It appears as though the last kind of tissue to be decreased is that of adipose tissue. We do not destroy the number of adipose tissue cells. There is an interesting phenomenon in that once the body has laid down the amount of fat cells that the individual is going to have (this takes place during infancy), the body will have a tendency to fill these fat cells up whenever it can. The fat cells will not be destroyed by losing weight; they will only be emaciated. Once the infant sets down the number of fat cells he is going to have, this number will be with him throughout his life. One wonders from this information if perhaps an infant who is very fat may have an abnormally large amount of adipose tissue cells. If this is true it follows that this infant as an adult will either have to be in a semi-starved state his entire life to be thin, or express his tendency to be overweight. The research on the area is not clear as yet, but it does make for a rather interesting conjecture.

When we think of reducing diets we should think of diets which contain sufficient protein to maintain the body structures, particularly during adolescence when children are growing. Children also need carbohydrates so they do not have to use protein for energy. We must remember that using protein for energy is very hard on the kidneys. It also should be mentioned that following fasting, when the person goes back on a normal diet, they will begin to increase weight even if the caloric intake is at equilibrium for their height and weight. This continued weight gain is caused because the body is restoring the protein lost during the fasting. When protein and caloric intake is resumed after fasting, the body will begin to start to gain weight again. As a matter of fact, for every pound of protein replenished the body will gain four pounds in body weight.

Exercise is another aspect of obesity. There is a great deal of literature on the subject of obesity and exercise. Obviously, this is one way to expend energy. Researchers have found that obese children do not exercise as much as normal children. The whole problem of weight control can be best summed up by something we could call preventive weight control. The population should be educated to the fact that the way to counteract obesity in families is never to have overfed the child, beginning with his infancy. There are a number of subcultures in the United States in which people really feel that if the child is of normal weight during infancy there must be something wrong with him—that is, that it is really the fat, chunky little babies that are the healthiest. Unfortunately, many things point to the fact that if the infant is a chunky little baby he probably is going to be a chunky adolescent and fat, chunky adult. It is important that health workers begin to advertise the fact that moderate eating habits from birth is the road to optimum health. It appears as though the numerous diets that are floating around our society are not working. In some way special diets appear not to be the problem. The solution appears not to be a quickie diet here and there. It is the problem of changing food intake, changing exercise habits, and, to some extent, changing how we feel about ourselves. It appears that most obese people need a total change of life-style, and we know that this does not take place very readily in adults or even in late adolescence (Stunkard, 1968; Heald, 1967, Barnes, 1968).

ANEMIA.   Anemia is prevalent not only in the United States but also throughout the world. (Anemia caused by iron deficiency has been discussed earlier in this chapter.) Anemia is most often seen during growth spurts and as a secondary deficiency during illness. Thus we often see children in hospitals or children who are chronically ill suffering from anemia due to increased malabsorption. The child is able to maintain adequate iron until a tissue overload occurs during illness.

There is a high incidence of anemia during all of the growth spurts, so that iron deficiencies should be watched for in infancy and during the preadolescent growth spurt. How can we prevent anemia? It has been suggested that there should be increased food fortification and mothers should be educated to use these fortified foods particularly during the child's infancy and preschool stage. There should be careful observation in the hospital for children who have shown any amount of blood loss. Infants of low birth weight should be checked frequently since they may need two times the amount of iron than the normal infant needs. Infants with reduced iron endowment should also be watched closely.

In summary, anemia is caused by a deficiency in iron or folic acid or Vitamin B_{12} or protein. It may also be caused by poor absorption, excessive demands upon the iron, or through blood loss or any of the disturbances in the red blood cell cycle (Kimber and Weintraub, 1968; McNeil, 1968; *Dairy Council Digest*, July-August, 1969; Flock, 1969; Patwardhan, 1966; and Brown, 1963).

Malnutrition

Within the last three or four years malnutrition has been brought to the foreground through the medium of television. We have become aware, within our country, that malnutrition in a sense encircles our affluent society. It varies from severe malnutrition in infants to undernutrition in large percentages of population. In fact, undernutrition may not express the situation accurately enough.

In a country as wealthy and as able to feed its population as the United States, it seems hard to believe that we are so poorly nourished. We have discussed poor nutrition throughout this chapter when we talked about poor nutrition in obese people and we discussed the different nutrient deficiencies. Woodruff (1966) defines nutrition as ". . . the sum of all factors in metabolism necessary for growth as well as the maintenance and repair of all body tissues." He holds that malnutrition is a disturbance of (1) neural processes; (2) the body's inability to maintain normal nutrient composition; and (3) the body's inability to respond to disease and stress. All of these factors cause malnutrition. I think we can safely say that malnutrition is commonly found throughout the world; sometimes it is found in normal children in the United States and it is commonly found in American children who are ill.

The causes of malnutrition within the United States and the world run all the way from congenital abnormalities and metabolic derangement to the secondary malnutrition of acquired disease. According to Girdwood (1969), twelve million American citizens living in poverty are subjected to primary and/or secondary malnutrition. The White House Conference in 1968 exposed some startling findings about malnutrition in this country. The Conference stated that malnutrition resulted in learning deficiencies, productivity loss, and in increased cost of care for diet related illnesses.

Malnutrition has its most severe effects upon the very young. During infant growth spurts, it interferes with both physical and mental growth. For example, at birth the infant's length is 30 percent of his adult height; at one year of age it is 44.5 percent of his adult height. At birth the infant's head circumference is 63 percent of the adult circumference. Unfortunately after the age of 6 months, when breast milk is no longer sufficient and weaning is beginning, many children do not have their nutritional requirements. Protein deficiency becomes particularly common at this time. It results in slower head growth after one year of age, which becomes progressive throughout the preschool period. Children who have suffered decreased head growth will *not* recover the growth loss when the child is again well-fed. Thus there is a permanent decrease in head circumference which equals a permanent defect. If the malnourishment is of short duration, regardless of the severity, permanent-damage defects may be prevented. If the child is older or out of infancy when the malnourishment begins, he may make up his deficits later and probably will not have permanent stunting. Thus, decreased dietary intake will cause malnutrition and decreased physical growth. The opposite does not bring about physical growth increases above what is genetically programmed. Graham (1967) stated that "when a diet with an adequate calorie intake, a generous supply of high quality protein and a sufficient amount of micronutrients is consumed with good healthy care the prognosis for growth and body length is seemingly better but not strikingly so than when the very adequate usual diet is provided over long periods so that there is chronic malnutrition this deficit will probably not be made up by further increasing the amount of food." Thus overeating or overnutrition will not produce the same kind of bodily changes that undernutrition will. There are striking differences between average nutrition and undernutrition in resulting height, weight, and head circumference that are not seen between average nutrition and overabundant nutrition. Graham did maintain that following a malnourished time in the child's life, unless it has been for a long period of time, optimal care has definite advantages over average care in making up deficiencies particularly in head size.

Scrimshaw (1967) wrote that the nutritional disease characterized by food restriction—marasmus—was common during the first year of life when postnatal brain growth was at its peak. Food restrictions were frequently found in the populations of mushrooming cities and stemmed largely from early weaning practices of low-income groups, which are patterned after middle- and upper-class behavior but are done without providing proper dietary substitutes. When protein was inadequate the disease which may follow after drastic protein inadequacy is kwashiorkor. It is generally a fatal disease and produces pronounced central nervous system damage. Scrimshaw, in reviewing animal studies, concluded that marasmus produced some behavior changes in the child; for example, they could still solve some problems. With kwashiorkor the behavior changes impair the capacity to perform tests which require learning from trials. Also growth characteristics are retarded. Retardation begins after the first four to six months of life and becomes progressively worse until the child passes the critical weaning period and succumbs to the disease or to another infectious disease. Scrimshaw also found a difference in children of industrialized countries and nonindustrialized countries in the average height and weight of the children. As far as the United States or other industrialized countries go, it is very difficult to separate nutritional aspects from psychological and social aspects of deprivation. For example, in industrialized countries children exhibit intellectual deficiencies which are also similar to children who are malnourished. Scrimshaw hypothesized that in industrialized countries it may be something other than malnourishment that causes intellectual deficiencies. He also held that current programs such as the Head Start preschool programs for underprivileged children come a little late for children who are already suffering from malnutrition—that is, by this age there is already permanent physical and psychological damage. But how much could be attributed to malnutrition and how much could be attributed to cultural deprivation, Scrimshaw was not willing to say. We know, for example, that adaptive capacity depends on the development of interrelations among separate senses, and there have been some current studies in this area of intersensory relationship. Cravioto et al. (1966) studied the relationship of intersensory development in Guatemala, with some urban middle- and upper-class children and rural children. They found that the physical structure of rural children who were less well-nourished fell behind those of the urban and upper-class children. They also found that intersensory relationships of rural children, although they improved with age, still lagged behind. Another finding was that when the children more nearly realize their *genetic potential* for growth differences in height, then nutritional and social aspects of development tend to lose significance (see also Scrimshaw, 1968; Graham, 1967; Woodruff, 1966; Calahan, 1967; Sebrell, 1967; Girdwood, 1969).

How does most deficiency come about? Usually very slowly. Heald (1969), in his article on biochemical nutritional status, lists three stages of deficiency. The first stage is characterized by depleted body storage, decreased nutrient concentration in the blood and other tissues, and depressed urinary excretion of nutrients and other metabolics; the second by manifestations of functional impairment; and the third by anatomical reflections of clinical disorders which are caused by (1) deficient diet, which is primary deficiency and (2) poor absorption because of transportation decrease and utilization (secondary deficiency). Heald concluded that undernourishment in early life retarded growth rate more than it retarded the expression of availability of nutrients, protein in particular, thus giving the body a false impression of nourishment.

Heald also believes that the *hemoglobin level* is the best available single biochemical index of general health. He found that iron deficiency anemia was very common within the United States. For example, 42 percent of females from 13 to 20 years of age had intakes two-thirds of the recommended daily allowances in 1958. (The recommended allowance is even higher now.) Heald found that Vitamin A deficiency in the United States was usually found in persons with fat absorption defects such as infectious hepatitis, wasting disease, scarlet fever, pneumonia, and rheumatic fever. He found scurvy to be prevalent in the United States in the very young and very old patients, with clinical signs appearing as early as four to six months after deprivation started (Heald, 1968).

Cravioto et al. (1966) reported on a number of experiments and also studied the ecology of malnutrition. They coined a phrase for the phenomenon which they called the spiral effect: "a low level of adaptive capacity, ignorance, social custom, infection or environmental paucity of foodstuffs appeared to result in malnutrition which may produce a large pool of individuals who come to function in sub-optimal ways." The investigators saw this spiral effect as starting with parents who were themselves victims of ignorance, using less efficient ways to adapt socially. These parents in turn reared their children under the same conditions and produced a new generation of malnourished people. Cravioto et al., maintained that serious degrees of malnourishment are caused primarily from an inadequate source of foodstuffs and secondly from infection and the like.

Not too many years ago, professional child health workers believed that malnourished children would make up for their lost growth and development as soon as their nutrition again became adequate. Cravioto et al. (1966) found that there is an initial growth recovery spurt when the child resumes adequate nutrition but that this recovery rate is the same rate as would be seen in a child of a younger age who is the same size as the malnourished child. Because of this, children who have been malnourished for a long time will end up with lower overall growth, particularly lower head circumference and shorter heights than their peers. For example, infants who are malnourished grow up to be adolescents that are shorter than their peers. Length and skeletal development remain reduced and retarded after this infantile malnutrition. They do not recover at an accelerated rate so they will not catch up with their peers. Therefore, we should not satisfy ourselves with the idea that such a child will make up such losses. There is much to indicate that he will not make up the losses and he will continue to be behind his peer group, although growing at the same rate as a child who is much younger in age but similar in size.

Cravioto et al. (1966) pointed out that not only was size affected but that there was also some indication of arrested biochemical maturation producing "retrogressions to earlier age specific patterns of functioning." The malnourished child may function immunologically at a younger age level. For example, protein metabolism is modified following malnutrition—showing high ratios of phenylalanine to tyrosine. This suggests that deprivation results in a defective enzyme system which causes an inadequate conversion of phenylalanine to tyrosine. This is what we see in newborn infants with PKU, which reinforces the idea that the malnourished child is functioning at an age level much younger than his own age (i.e., more in keeping with his metabolic or physiological age).

Cravioto et al. (1966) also cited some Russian studies in the area of essential nutrients. These workers found changes in the conditioned reflex in children even before clinical signs of malnutrition occur. Malnutrition modifies the acquisition of rate, maintenance, and extinction of conditioned reflex. The Russian investigators also found that there are marked disturbances in cortical functions, decreased capacity to elaborate new conditioned reflexes, and, if a malnourished state continued, previously well-established responses may be depressed or abolished. As the children recovered, through adequate nutrition, there was also a very slow reflex recovery.

This analysis (Cravioto et al., 1966) of exhibited psychological disturbances seems to be most important for those professionals working with children with long-term diseases. For example, a prominent feature of clinical findings of a protein-calorie malnutrition syndrome is apathy. There was a decrease in normal curiosity and desire to explore on the part of the child. Of course, apathy may have multiple causes—such as emotional deprivation or separation, which usually accompanies hospitalization. Interestingly enough, recovery among those infants whose mothers showed the greatest interest in them during hospitalization exhibited a more rapid recovery than infants whose mothers showed no interest or little interest during hospitalization. Cravioto et al. (1966) maintained that the behavior of malnourished infants resembled infants who were abruptly separated from their mothers by hospitalization. They also noted that children who remained at home and were in the affectionate care of devoted but nutritionally misguided mothers also have psychological disturbances which resemble children who have been hospitalized. In conclusion, the investigators noted that children with mild to moderate and severe malnutrition failed to respond and showed signs of progressive withdrawal or progressive behavior regression.

Heretofore in the chapter I have discussed the physical signs of malnutrition. There are also psychological changes during malnutrition which can be determined by observation. Psychological changes that will cause the course of the child's cognitive development to change. It does make one wonder how much the apathy we see in the hospital among children is a sign not so much of psychological changes caused by social external environment but of pure undernutrition or malnutrition from lack of the ingestion of recommended nutrients.

Cravioto et al. (1966) also studied the effects of malnutrition on the results of psychological testing. He found that the average IQ was more stable in well-nourished children than in malnourished children. In fact, one group of malnourished children's IQs rose 18 percent following an improvement of their nutrition. A number of studies have been done in this area. A well-known one is the study done in Africa (Cravioto et al., 1966). Children from the same background were studied. One group was undernourished and the other one well nourished. The malnourished children showed lower values for height, weight, and head circumference, and their mean IQ was well below that of the better-nourished children. In this study it was found that children developed well during the first month of life. Even those children who later developed kwashiorkor or severe protein calorie malnutrition developed well during the first month. But the children who later developed kwashiorkor showed signs of slowed motor development and particularly severe retardation of language development following the first month.

Another study conducted in Latin America (Cravioto et al., 1966). brought some interesting results. It was found that infants who were undernourished from four to six months of age had weight gains similar to the normal full-term infant in a highly industrialized society. But from 6 to 18 months the weight gain was progressively smaller than that of their peer group. At about 24 months there was a slow but steady gain. Following this there was a return to incremental values normal for the chronological age, but the children never regained the weight loss that transpired during the earlier period of malnutrition. The investigators also found that psychological deficits were most profound if distress took place during the first period (four to six months). These infants showed no signs of catching up, and increased developmental age only equaled the number of months the children remained hospitalized.

Garn and Rohmann (1966) found that protein-calorie malnutrition caused children to be progressively retarded in behavior following weaning. They evaluated this retardation by measuring manipulative gross motor skills and perceptual and linguistic development: ". . . the more the child falls behind in somatic growth, the more retarded he appears to become in such motor activities as block piling, in linguistic activities such as namings, in visual-perceptual activities such as formboard behavior, and the like." They also found that children with *secondary malnutrition* were behind in motor coordination. What is happening to the ill child is explained rather clearly by the statement: "A child who had dumped protein and lost bone is in no physical condition to improve his block piling activities nor in a mood to point out and name parts of his body" (Garn and Rohmann, 1966). We must include in our role of child health nursing the child's play. It is obvious that we can use the area of play to increase the children's development. But we must not forget that the child may not feel like participating in the activities we have planned. We must realize that this does not necessarily mean the child is being negative or is rejecting our planned activities. It may mean that the child is not absorbing or getting the amount of nutrients that will give him the energy or the physical stamina to participate in the play activity. I think we should look to inadequate nutrition for solutions to some of the problems in the child-nurse interrelationship.

As we have suggested, malnutrition not only affects the physical growth, height, weight, and head circumference but it also affects the development of the nervous system. Central nervous system development and performance basically come from the chemistry of the nerve cells; its metabolism, its cell structure, its energy kinetics, and the integrity of function. Nutrition is fundamentally related to nerve development over the time continuum.

Ninety percent of the brain growth takes place by the fourth year. The period from infancy to preschool is highly critical. It is extremely important that the preschool child is well-nourished. There is some indication from Waterlow, (1968) that the body does not just "sit still" during protein deprivation. The protein-depleted body makes some attempt to adapt to the low protein intakes. Waterlow found that the body responded to low protein intake by lowering the rate of growth with protein synthesis used to maintain some organs while sacrificing other organs. For example, there might be a decrease excretion of nitrogen due to a reduced proportion of nitrogen being excreted as urea, rather than reduced protein synthesis. Waterlow found that the general protein synthesis may decline, particularly muscle protein synthesis, suggesting an adaption to low protein intake and accompanied by changes in patterns of endocrine and enzyme activity. With low protein intake, we see changing patterns of protein metabolism which are vital to body function (Barnes et al. 1967; Caldwell and Churchwell, 1967; Frankova and Barnes, 1968; Waterlow, 1968).

In summary, it may be said that poor nutrition in early life adversely affects mental development. Unfortunately, not much is known of the effects of undernutrition over a long duration, partly because of the inability of current experimenters to ferret out environmental factors such as social stimulation from their studies. Much has been surmised from animal experiments in the area, but there is still a great deal of speculation about the interrelatedness of malnutrition and learning behavior. This lack of information is unfortunate as it is critical to the lives of the next generation, whose members are being molded now with a lack of protein and nutrients. Thus it seems better to err in the side of assuming that malnutrition is causing some of the symptoms we see and proceed to decrease the malnutrition in young children, whether it be primary malnutrition which must be dealt with through public health, or secondary malnutrition which must be dealt with by the worker in child health in the hospital setting. We must also increase our ability to observe malnutrition and nutritional deficiencies in the children with whom we work. Otherwise, it seems that our efforts in the other areas of nursing care will be futile if the child loses his ability to develop into an interrelated, thinking human being (*Dairy Council Digest*, March-April, 1969).

Atherosclerosis during Growth

Another interesting long-term disease which we are finding increased evidence of in younger persons is atherosclerosis. Heald (1969) discussed this at great length in his book *Adolescent Nutrition and Growth*. Apparently there are signs of early stages of atherosclerosis as early as infancy. Fatty tissue deposits are found in some of the arteries. There is also rupture, degeneration, and regeneration of elastic membranes in the coronary arteries. The laying-down of fatty deposit was found to be most prominent in infants of three and four months of age. Following this age it leveled off sharply and began to decrease. Whether the early fatty streaks that were found in the arteries of infants is the precursor to heart disease is not known at this time. There are definitely increases in lipids in the coronary arteries and the aorta during infancy. But we don't see mineral deposits in large amounts until the fifth decade of life. Almost all infants have these fatty deposits and it is not until 20 years of age that there became significant differences among peoples, individuals, and races.

Researchers also found that in adolescents the atherosclerotic patients showed signs of a prediabetic glucose tolerance level. In fact, there was some speculation that atherosclerosis may be an expression of a glucose metabolic defect. We see, of course, a full-fledged glucose metabolic defect in diabetes. Recent literature gives one the impression that perhaps diabetes and atherosclerosis have an original origin in glucose metabolism, but this has not been substantiated as yet. However, it is certainly something we should perhaps keep in mind. There is also some question as to whether these fatty lesions during growth are primarily related to nutrition or are merely a natural biochemistry defect of human beings. Heald (1969) concluded that nutritional factors may indeed play a more significant role in the complications which develop from these primary lesions of the arteries.

Concluding Statement

The foregoing only highlights the current concerns of modern-day nutrition of children. Researchers and professional workers in the area of child health have been concerned with the nutrition of children for decades. But only recently have we had enough technical knowledge really to see the true scope of the problem. The individual is indeed what he eats and to a great extent his body reflects the nutrition of his mother and her mother. This makes the analysis of normal individual nutritional needs highly complex. Illness further complicates the picture and long-term illness makes the constant evaluation of nutritional needs imperative. It is a critical area of health and one that warrants constant and detailed observation from the health workers who are constantly interrelating with the child.

References

Andelman, M. B., and Sered, B. R. Utilization of dietary iron by term infants. Amer. J. Dis. Child., 3:45–55, Jan. 1966.

Atkinson, H. Care of the child with cleft lip and palate. Amer. J. Nurs. 67(9):1889–1892, Sept. 1967.

Barnes, R. H. The inseparability of nutrition from the social and biological sciences. Nutr. Diet, 10:1–8, 1968.

———, Moor, A. W., Reid, I. M., and Pond, W. G. Learning behavior following nutritional deprivations in early life. J. Amer. Diet. Assn., 51:34, July 1967.

Beal, V. A. Calcium and phosphorus in infancy. J. Amer. Diet. Assn., 53:450–459, 1968.

Blumberg, R. W., Farbes, G. B., Fraser, D., Hansen, A. E., May, C. D., Smith, C. A., Sweeney, M. J., and Forman, S. J. Report of committee on nutrition: vitamin K compounds and the water-soluble analogues, use in therapy and prophylaxis in pediatrics. Pediat., 28(3):501–507, Sept. 1961.

———, Farbes, G. B., Fraser, D., Hansen, A. E., Lowe, C. U., Smith, N. J., Sweeney, M. J., and Formon, S. J. Report of the committee on nutrition: vitamin E in human nutrition. Pediat., 31(2):324–328, Feb. 1963.

Bordier, P. H., Matrajh, H., Hioco, G. W., Hepner, G. R., Thompson and Booth, C. C., Clinical vitamin D deficiency following gastric surgery. Lancet, 1:439, 1968.

Braux, E. B. The absorption of iron. Amer. J. Clin. Nutr. 12:205–209, March 1963.

Brown, R. E. A standard for childhood malnutrition? Clinical Pediat., 4(10): 565–568, Oct. 1965.

Caldwell, D. F., and Churchill, J. A. Learning ability in the progeny of rats administered a protein-deficient diet during the second half of gestation. Neurology, 17:95, Jan. 1967.

Callahan, C. L. A special report on the White House conference on food, nutrition and health. Nursing Outlook, Jan. 1970.

Cheek, D. B., Graystone, J., and Reba, R. Human growth and body composition. In Heald, F. P., ed. Adolescent Nutrition and Growth. New York, Appleton-Century-Crofts, 1969.

Cherry, F. F., Cooper, Stewart, R. A., and Platow. R. V. Call versus say formulas. Amer. J. Dis. Child., 115:677–692, 1968.

Christakis, G., and Miridjanian, A. Diets, drugs and their interrelationships: a brief appraisal. J. Amer. Diet Assn., 52:21–24, 1968.

Christakis, G., Sojecki, S., Hillman, R. W., Miller, E., Blumenthal, S., and Archer, M. Effect of a combined nutrition education and physical fitness program on the weight status of obese high school boys. Fed. Proc., 25:15–19, 1966.

Committee on Iron Deficiency, Council on Food and Nutrition, American Medical Association. Iron deficiency in the United States. J. Amer. Med. Assn., 203:119, Feb. 5, 1968.

Consolozio, C. F., Matousk, L. O., Johnson, H. L., Nelson, R. A. and Krzyivicki, H. J. Metabolic aspects of acute starvation in normal humans (10 days). Amer. J. Clin. Nutr., 20:672–683, 1967.

Cravioto, J., De Licardie, E. R., and Birch, H. G. Nutrition, growth and neurointegrative development: an experimental and ecologic study. Pediat., 38:319–330, 1966.

Current Aspects of Infant Nutrition in Daily Practice. Mead Johnson and Company, 1962.

Dairy Council Digest. Nutrition and common stresses. 37(3):May–June, 1966.

———— Nutritional implications of some problems of adolescents. 38(5): Sept.–Oct., 1967.

———— Relative nutritional value of filled and imitation milks. 39(2): March–April, 1968.

———— Malnutrition in early life and subsequent mental performance. 39(3):May–June, 1968.

———— Essential inorganic elements in nutrition: function and interrelationships. 39(5):Sept.–Oct., 1968.

———— Recommended dietary allowances, revised 1968. 39(6):Nov.–Dec., 1968.

———— Nutritional anemias. 40(4):July–Aug., 1969.

———— Current developments in childhood nutrition. 40(2): March–April, 1969.

———— Nutrition in illness. 40(5):Sept.–Oct., 1969.

Dayton, D. H. Early malnutrition and human development. Children, 16:211–217, Nov.–Dec., 1969.

Dickerson, J. W. T., and Walmsley, A. L. The effect of undernutrition and subsequent rehabilitation on the growth and composition of the central nervous system of the rat. Brain, 90:897, 1967.

di Sant'Agnese, P. A., and Jones, W. O. The celiac (metabsorption) in pediatrics. J. Amer. Med. Assn, 180:308–316, April 28, 1962.

Engle, M. A. Cardiac failure in infancy: recognition and management. Amer. Heart Assn., 32:825–830, Dec. 1963.

Famon, S. J., Blumberg, R. W., Coursin, D. B., Farbes, G. B., Fraser, D., Kaye, R., Lowe, C. U., and Sweeney, M. J. Committee on nutrition: factors affecting food intake. Pediat., 33:Jan. 1964.

Flock, M. H. Recent contributions in intestinal absorption and malabsorption. Amer. J. Clin. Nutr., 22:327–336, 1967.

Ford, J. E. and Scott, K. J. The folic acid activity of some milk foods for babies. Dairy Res., 35:85–89, 1968.

Frankova, S., and Barnes, R. J. Effect of malnutrition in early learning on avoidance conditioning and behavior of adult rats. J. Nutr., 96:485–493, 1968.

Garn, S. M., and Rohmann, C. G. Interaction of nutrition and genetics in the timing of growth and development. Pediat. Clinics No. Amer., 13:353, 1966.

———— and Wagner, B. The adolescent growth of the skeletal mass and its implications to mineral requirements. In Heald, F. P., ed. Adolescent Nutrition and Growth. New York, Appleton-Century-Crofts, 1969, pp. 139–161.

Gershoff, S. N., Gill, T. J., III, Simonian, S. J., and Steinberg, A. I. Some effects of amino acid deficiencies on antibody formation in the rat. J. Nutr., 95:184–190, 1968.

Girdwood, R. H. Folate depletion in old age, Amer. J. Clin. Nutr., 22:234, 1969.

Graham, G. G. Effect of infantile malnutrition on growth. Fed. Proc., 26:139–143, 1967.

Graham, G. G., Baertle, J. N., and Cardano, A. Studies in infantile malnutrition: IV. the effect of protein and calorie intake on serum proteins; V. the effect of dietary protein source on serum proteins. Amer. J. Clin. Nutr., 18:11–19, 1966.

Grossfeld. M. D. Club 15. Campbell Soup Company, 1965.

Heald, F. P. Atherosclerosis during growth. In Heald, F. P. ed. Adolescent Nutrition and Growth. New York, Appleton-Century-Crofts, 1969, pp. 119–128.

———— Some biochemical aspects of obesity in adolescents. In Heald, F. P., ed. Adolescent Nutrition and Growth, New York: Appleton-Century-Crofts, 1969, pp. 37–41.

———— Daugela, M., and Brunschuyler, P. Physiology of adolescence. New Eng. J. Med., 268:243–252, Jan., 1963.

———— Mayer, J., and Remmell, P. S. Calorie, protein and fat intake in children and adolescents. In Heald, F. P., ed. Adolescent Nutrition and Growth. New York, Appleton-Century-Crofts, 1969, pp. 17–35.

Herbert, V. Megaloblastic anemia as a problem in world health. Amer. J. Clin. Nutr., 21:1115, 1968.

Hill, L. F., Lowe, C. U., Smith, C. A., Smyth, F. S., Waisman, H. A., Wakeman, E. T., Wilson, J. R., and May, C. D. Committee on nutrition: appraisal of the use of vitamins B_1 and B_{12} as supplements promoted for the stimulation of growth and appetite in children. Pediat., 21:860–964, May, 1958.

———— Committee on nutrition: on the feeding of solid food to infants. Pediat., 21:685–692, April, 1958.

Janowsky, M., Martinik, J., and Slechtova. The effect of different diets on the economy of water and electrolytes during restricted water intakes in human infants. Physiologia Bohemoslovaca, 17:143–151, 1968.

Kimber, C., and Weintraub, L. W. Malabsorption of iron secondary to iron deficiency. New Eng. J. Med., 279:453–459, 1968.

Krehl, W. A. Nutrition of the low-socioeconomic class adolescents. In Heald,

F. P., ed. Adolescent Nutrition and Growth. New York, Appleton-Century-Crofts, 1969. pp. 95–99.

Leverton, R. M. A Girl and Her Figure. National Dairy Council, 1970.

Liang, P. H., Hie, T. T., Jan, O. H., and Giok, L. T. Evaluation of mental development in relation to early malnutrition. Amer. J. Clin. Nutr., 20:1290, 1967.

Lowe, C. U., Clement, D. H., Fomon, S. J., Farbes, G. B., Fraser, D., May, C. D., Smith, C. A., and Waisman, H. A. Estrogenic and anrogenic agents in meats and poultry. Pediat., 25:896–898, May, 1960.

McNeil, J. R. Iron deficiency in children. Blood, 31:641, 1968.

McWilliams, M. Milk for the infant. In McWilliams, M., ed. Nutrition for the Growing Years. New York: Wiley, 1967, pp. 28–36.

———— The first year. In McWilliams, M., ed. Nutrition for the Growing Years. New York, Wiley, 1967, p. 59.

———— Elementary School. In McWilliams, M., ed. Nutrition for the Growing Years. New York, Wiley, 1967, pp. 136–138.

———— Challenges of adolescence. In McWilliams, M., ed. Nutrition for the Growing Years, New York, Wiley, 1967, pp. 156–179.

Maxwell, P., Linss, M., McDonnough, P., and Kinder, J. Routine on the burn ward. Amer. J. Nursing, 66:522–527, March, 1966.

Myers, M. L., O'Brien, S. C., Mabel, J. H., and Store, F. J. A nutrition study of school children in a depressed urban district. J. Amer. Diet. Assn., 53:226–233, 1968.

The National Association for Mental Health, Inc. Eating Problems of Children: A Guide for Parents. Mental Health Materials Center (104 East 25 Street), New York, N.Y.

Nutrition Reviews. Gastrointestinal milk allergy in infants. 27:7–9, Jan. 1969.

———— Glyceride structure and fat absorption. 27:18–20, Jan. 1966.

———— Nutrients and genes: interactions in development. 27:1, Jan. 1969.

Ohlson, M. A., and Hart, B. P. Influence of breakfast on total day's food intake. J. Amer. Diet. Assn., 47:282–286, 1965.

Owen, G. M., and Kram, K. M. Nutritional status of preschool children in Mississippi: food sources of nutrients in the diet. J. Amer. Diet. Assn., 54:490–494, 1969.

Patwardhan, V. N. Nutritional anemias: W.H.O. research program: early developments and progress report of collaborative studies. Amer. J. Clin. Nutr., 19:63–70, July 1966.

Pearson, W. N. The biochemical appraisal of nutritional status. In Heald, F. P., ed. Adolescent Nutrition and Growth. New York, Appleton-Century-Crofts, 1969, pp. 73–94.

Pearson, W. N. The biochemical appraisal of nutritional status. In Heald, protein on serum amino acids. Amer. J. Clin. Nutr., 21:167–172, 1968.

Pfieffer, C. J. Absorption of calcium. Postgrad. Med., 43:199, Jan. 1968.

Pidgeon, V. The infant with congenital heart disease. Amer. J. Nursing, 67:290–293, Feb. 1967.

Press, E., Adams, W. C., Chittenden, R. F., Christian, J. R., Grayson, R., Stewart, C. C., and Everist, B. W. Report of subcommittee on accidental poisoning: statement on diagnosis and treatment of lead poisoning in childhood. Pediat., 27:676–680, April 1961.

Proudfit, F. T., and Robinson, C. Nutrition during infancy. In Proudfit, F. T., and Robinson, C., eds. Normal and Therapeutic Nutrition. New York, Macmillan, 1967, pp. 241–258.

Ritchie, J. H., Fisk, M. D., McMasters, V., and Grossman, M. Edema and hemalytic anemia in premature infants: a vitamin E deficiency syndrome. New Eng. J. Med. 279:1185–1190, 1968.

Roe, D. A. Diet, drugs and detoxication. N.Y. State J. Med., 67:1189, July 1, 1967.

Rubin, M. Balm for burned children. Amer. J. Nursing, 66:296–302, Feb. 1966.

Schwab, L., Callison, C. B., and Frank, M. P. Cystic fibrosis. Amer. J. Nursing, 63:62–69, Feb. 1963.

Scrimshaw, N. S. Malnutrition, learning and behavior. Amer. J. Clin. Nutr., 20:493, May 1967.

———— Infant malnutrition and adult learning. Saturday Review, March 16, 1968, pp. 64, 66, 84.

———— and Gordon, J. E. Malnutrition, Learning and Behavior. Cambridge, M.I.T. Press, 1968.

Sebrell, W. H., Jr. Changing concept of malnutrition. Amer. J. Clin. Nutr., 20:653–658, 1967.

Sherwin, R. W., and Chir, B. Perinatal nutrition as a developmental determinant. Nutr. News, 30(4): Dec. 1967.

Shulman, I. Iron requirements in infancy. J. Amer. Med. Assn., 175:118–123, Jan. 14, 1961.

Steele, M. S., and Boegli, E. H. Scoliosis. Amer. J. Nursing, 68: 2399–2403, Nov. 1968.

Stock, M. B., and Smythe, P. M. The effect of undernutrition during infancy on subsequent brain growth and intellectual development. S. African Med. J., pp. 1027–1030, Oct. 28, 1967.

Stunkard, A. J. Body Image Disturbance in Obesity. A Ross Timesaver, 10(1): Jan.–Feb. 1968.

———— Environment and obesity: recent advances in our understanding of regulation of food intake in man. Fed. Proc., 27:1367–1373, 1968.

Waterlow, J. C. Observations on the mechanisms of adaptation to low protein intakes. Lancet. 2:1091–1097, 1968.

Watson, E. H., and Laurey, G. H. Growth and Development of Children, 5th ed. Chicago, Year Book Medical Publishers, 1967.

Weisberger, A. S., Wessler, S., and Aveoli, L. V. Mechanisms of action of chloramphenical. J. Amer. Med. Assn., 209:97–98, July 7, 1969.

Welbourn, R. B., and Spencer, J. Nutritional aspects of gastric surgery. Rev. Surg., 24:233, 1967.

White, P. L. Nutrition, Today and Tomorrow. Address, 54th Annual Meeting of the National Dairy Council at Cleveland, Ohio, Jan. 27, 1969 (reprint).

Widdowson, E. M. Absorption and excretion of fat, nitrogen, and minerals from "filled" milks by babies one week old. Lancet, 2:1099–1105, 1965.

Witkop, C. J. Genetic and nutrition. Fed. Proc. 26:148, Jan.–Feb. 1967.

Woodruff, C. J. Nutritional aspects of metabolism of growth and development. J. Amer. Med. Assn., 196:214, 1966.

Zickefoose, M. Feeding problems of children with cleft palate. Children, 4:225–228, Nov.–Dec., 1957.

PART II
SPECIFIC
LONG-TERM ILLNESS
AND NURSING CARE

6 SHIRLEY STEELE

Nursing Care of the Child with Kidney Problems

Renal function impairment is attributed to illnesses that are either etiologically obscure or identifiable. In addition, symptomatology can be minimal or variable to the degree that a diagnosis is not achieved or the distinguishing cause remains an unknown because of existent advanced involvement. Many of the children we see today with complicated genitourinary problems had early presenting signs that went unnoticed or were insufficiently treated. To prevent complications associated with urinary tract illnesses and to prevent their occurrence because of complicated preceding infections, more and more emphasis is placed upon early detection and aggressive treatment.

Infections of the urinary tract are quite common in children. They are especially frequent in infants because of self-contamination directly associated with wet or soiled diapers. The occurrence of pyelonephritis, which is the most common renal disease of children, is six times as prevalent in females as opposed to males. An exception exists during the neonatal period, when there is about equal incidence. The anatomical difference probably accounts for the higher incidence in females. The short urethra in girls permits easy access for bacteria to ascend to the ureters and travel to the kidneys. Vesicoureteral reflux and posture both at night and during micturition are probably important and closely interrelated (Smallpiece, 1969). Vesicoureteral reflux has been found responsible for a large percentage of the urinary tract infections in children. Girls with thin-walled bladders or congenitally deficient ureterovesical junction mechanisms are particularly prone to reflux.

Evidence exists which demonstrates a close relationship between urinary tract infections and structural or functional defects of the urinary tract. This factor may be responsible for the higher incidence of urinary tract infections in males during the neonatal period. According

213

to Williams (1968), congenital abnormalities of the male urinary tract often cause more serious secondary effects than in females, and the secondary effects present at an earlier age. Therefore, it is essential that congenital malformations are diagnosed and treated to decrease the possibility of serious early infection and subsequent renal damage.

Additional factors which predispose the neonate to urinary tract infections are the possibility of contamination through the cord, the poor resistance of neonates to gram-negative organisms, the risk of epidemic infections in the nursery, and the adverse influence of dehydration (Smallpiece, 1969).

The circulatory system is another route for transport of infection to the urinary tract. There is considerable disagreement as to the most common route but some think that the blood route is responsible when the causative organism is a streptococcus or staphlococcus. It is generally thought that there must be some interference with the urinary flow before infection can be caused by the blood route. In addition, direct spread from a localized inflammation in the pelvis of the kidney and infection of the kidney by way of the lymphatics have both been thought to be possible sources, but are considered less seriously in the recent literature.

Establishment of a diagnosis and possible cause begins with routine and extended urinalyses.

Urinalysis

GENERAL CONSIDERATIONS

The kidney function of the newborn infant is not completely developed, despite the fact that urinary excretion begins about the ninth week of fetal life. The infant's kidneys have a limited ability to concentrate urine and therefore they need a larger amount of liquid to excrete a particular amount of solute. The infant also has difficulty in conserving body water when it is needed and in excreting excess fluid. The child's urine is usually a paler yellow than the adult's and is odorless unless highly colored. Urine excretion is greater throughout childhood than it is in adulthood. It is influenced by the fluid intake of the child, the digestive and nervous systems, and the environmental temperature. After bladder control is established, the normal child will void six to eight times every 24 hr.

URINE COLLECTION

Some general principles to keep in mind when one is collecting urine specimens are:

1. The specimen should be recently voided.
2. Use a clean container—specimen bottle with an appropriate top.

3. Be sure the container is dry; water will dilute the urine.
4. Avoid contamination; no feces or toilet paper should be in the bedpan.
5. If it is necessary to measure the urine, use a dry container and be sure to empty complete specimen into the graduate.
6. If urine sample must be retained, refrigerate to delay decomposition.

The time for collection of a single specimen is usually in the morning. A 24-hr quantitative specimen is obtained by discarding the first specimen and then collecting all urine for a 24-hr period.

A urine culture is obtained by collecting a clean-catch urine or a catheterized specimen. Each agency has its own procedure for cleansing the child with use of a variety of agents such as pHisoHex, Zephirin, and sterile distilled water. The procedure, if done correctly, frees the area of bacteria and the collected urine specimen is sent for analysis in a sterile container. If the child is not toilet-trained, after the cleansing, a sterile urine collector is applied to the perineal area to obtain the collection.

Plastic urine collectors have lessened the difficulties nurses previously had in collecting urine specimens from children. Single-specimen collectors are marked "sterile" if they are sterilized. Otherwise, the collectors are clean. There are also 24-hr collectors with tube attachments for continuous flow. The collectors have a sticky substance for easy application, but painting around the area with tincture of benzoin aids with adherence and serves to protect vulnerable skin. For best results, the collector should be applied before the benzoin dries. Adhesive tape is cruel to children's tender skin and should be used sparingly. If its use is required, the nonallergic type is best. With girls it is crucial to check carefully to see that the collector is appropriately placed on the perineum to prevent the loss of the specimen.

After the collector is applied, a loosely fitted diaper may help to prevent the child from pulling at the collector. If the child is on bedrest, elevating the head of the bed may help to prevent seepage from around the collector. Some nurses have found it helpful to place a cotton ball inside the collector to "weight it down." This practice is not completely beneficial as the cotton ball usually needs to be squeezed out to get enough urine for the specimen and, too, it interferes with laboratory results. If the child can be out of bed, it is usually easier to collect the specimen without spillage—providing the collector has been correctly applied.

Collection of the specimen is usually enhanced by giving the child fluid approximately 10 min before the collector is applied, and continuing to give fluids until the specimen is collected. Fluid intake, however, is determined by the fluids allowed for the child. (Fluid intake will be discussed in greater detail later in the chapter.)

Fortunately, the glass collectors previously used for collecting urine specimens from children are becoming obsolete. If they are used, adhesive should be put around the edges in case there are any small chips or slight irregularities in the glass. Much closer observations must be made to guarantee that the container does not get broken.

Regardless of the method utilized for obtaining the specimen, the nurse should check the child frequently so the specimen to be obtained is not lost. After removing the collector, the child should be washed and dried in case urine has come in contact with his skin.

In some agencies more elaborate methods may be available for collecting specimens from infants and toddlers. These methods usually involve specially designed beds and sheeting which provide for drainage of urine into a collecting receptacle. The advantages include freedom from contamination by feces, fewer restraints, freedom from skin irritation due to strapping or adhesive tape, and greater temperature control if the child is in an isolette.

With children who will be having numerous experiences with urine collections, it is especially important to give them good, simple explanations and preparations. It is imperative that a positive response is set for the initial collection as well as for future collections. Therefore, restraints should be used only as a last resort for getting the child's cooperation. If restraints are applied, it is necessary to help the child and parents to understand that their use is for the child's protection, not as a form of punishment. If restraints are used to obtain a continuous collection such as a 12- or 24-hr specimen, the nurse must free the restraints and turn the child periodically. She must also observe the restrained areas frequently to be sure there is no circulatory constriction. In addition, the areas should be properly padded and the restraints loose enough to allow some motion without interfering with the urine collection. It is also possible to restrain children in the sitting position so that they can be taken to the play area while the collection is in progress.

Other methods for collecting urine specimens from children include catheterization and suprapubic aspiration. Catheterization is difficult to do in children and also has been considered to produce a high incidence of urinary tract infection. If it is utilized, every measure should be taken to make the external area as clean as possible and to maintain sterility of the catheter. Bacteriostatic agents are sometimes instilled during the catheterization. Suprapubic aspiration has been suggested by Goldberg (1967) as a method rapidly becoming popular for obtaining urine specimens in children, especially under the age of two years. He suggests the method as safe and effective when there is urine in the child's bladder. It is a procedure usually reserved for the physician.

The presence of pus or bacteria in the urine does not establish urinary infection. Therefore, clean-catch urine samples are a necessary aid to the establishment of a diagnosis. Organisms can enter the sterile urine from external areas such as the prepuce in boys or the vulva in girls. Proper cleansing techniques will decrease this possibility and give a more accurate picture of the urinary constituents. Urine is a good culture medium and any organisms which enter it during voiding multiply rapidly and increase in number with time. For this reason, specimens should be sent to the laboratory immediately and marked sufficiently so they receive proper attention. If the specimen has been obtained on nights and the laboratory is not open, the specimen should be refrigerated to delay the growth of bacteria. When the urine is examined, it is the number of organisms present which is significant, so it is important to guard against contaminants being counted in the process. A variety of bacteria infects the urinary tract, but the colon bacillus is responsible in approximately 80 percent of the cases (Rubin, 1964).

Laboratory examination frequently includes antibiotic sensitivity testing in addition to counting the organisms present. This information will be utilized in treating the child and combating the causative agent. In recent years, more virulent organisms are being found responsible for urinary tract infections (Burko and Rhamy, 1970) and organisms such as Klebsiella, Pseudomonas, and Proteus are being reported. These organisms are generally less responsive to antibiotic therapy than *E. coli* and demand more vigorous therapeutic regimes.

In addition to collecting urine specimens, it is important for the nurse to make observations and recordings about the color, odor, amount, and frequency or urgency of urination. Very often children with urinary problems are placed on routine intake and output recordings. If this is not the case, the nurse should take independent action and establish the child's pattern before assuming that the relationship ratio is unimportant. In addition, she must ascertain if the child is having any difficulty or pain on voiding. These symptoms may precede, coincide, or follow voiding, and they should be charted appropriately (see Table 1).

If the child has an ileal conduit, the following method is used to obtain a urine culture. The stoma area is prepared by using specific bacteriostatic agents such as those already mentioned. A sterile catheter (a rubber No. 14, 16, or 18 straight variety) is then inserted into the

TABLE 1
NURSES NOTES

John—age 3½ years.

TIME	OBSERVATION AND ACTION
1:00 P.M.	Requested urinal—tried unsuccessfully to void.
1:15 P.M.	Requested urinal—cringed with pain as he intermittently voided 15 cc's pink-tinged concentrated urine. Stream weak, time needed for voiding: 5 min. No pain after voiding. No abdominal distention noted.
3:30 P.M.	Requested urinal—voided 10 cc's pink-tinged urine—5 min. voiding, weak stream—no pain—urine odorless—specific gravity 1.020. Specimen sent to lab for routine examination. No abdominal distention noted.

stoma under sterile conditions. The urine is aspirated by using a disposable 10-cc syringe and adapter. The urine is put directly into a sterile urine bottle to be sent to the laboratory.

The following example will illustrate what transpires after the specimen is requested.

Mary is four years old and has a history of frequency and burning on urination for the past two days. She is seen in the out-patient department for evaluation. She is prepared for a urine culture collection and the nurse collects the specimen as previously described. The urine culture is sent to the laboratory for analysis. If the culture contains more organisms than 10,000/ml the child will be started on therapy. The agents ordinarily used will be Gantricin (sulfisoxazole) or Furadantin (nitrofurantoin). These medications will be continued unless the sensitivity testing indicates resistance or the child's clinical response is unfavorable. A repeat culture will be taken one to two weeks after treatment is completed, and then every four to six weeks until the patient has been abacteriuric and off therapy for six months. If any of these cultures return positive (10,000 or more organisms) the treatment is reinstituted and the cycle reestablished.

In children who are not toilet-trained, it is necessary to estimate the urinary output by examining the diaper. Urine spreads quickly in diapers and there is a tendency to overestimate the output. Consequently, it is sometimes necessary to weigh the diaper before and after voidings to get a more accurate estimate of the output.

It is also common for children to go long periods of times without voiding before they have obvious signs of bladder distention. When checking a child for distention, have him place his hands under his head or on top of your hands. Having him keep his hands occupied will help to decrease the sequelae caused by the "ticklish sensation." The child will also be more cooperative if your hands are warm and applied gently.

Diagnostic tests and examinations

There are numerous diagnostic tests, in addition to urine examinations, done to determine the type and extent of urinary tract involvement (Table 2).

Preparation of the child and family for any of these procedures should include an explanation of the routine outlined in the particular agency. Factors relating to the time the test is scheduled, the number of trips off the unit, and restriction of fluids or food should be included in the explanation.

An example of preparation of a 13-year-old for a PSP test follows.

"George, you are having a test today that will help your doctor know more about your kidneys and how they work under certain conditions. This test is called a PSP test, which is a simple way of saying

TABLE 2
DIAGNOSTIC TESTS AND RATIONALE

EXAMPLES OF COMMON TESTS OR EXAMINATIONS	EXPLANATION
Intravenous pyelogram (IVP)	Dye is injected into the vein and excreted through the kidneys into the urine. Films are taken as dye passes through kidneys, ureters, bladder, and urethra.
Retrograde pyelogram	Dye is injected directly into the ureters by way of a catheter passed through the bladder. This test is done in conjunction with cystoscopy.
Excretory cystourethrogram	A film visualization of the bladder after intravenous injection of contrast material such as sodium or meglumine diatrizoate.
Cystoscopy	Visualization of the interior of the bladder by cystoscope. Ureteral catheters and bougies can be passed through the cystoscope into the kidney pelvis for urine specimen. Stones can also be removed or biopsy taken.
Cinecystourethrogram	X-ray motion picture of voiding and bladder function.
Renal biopsy	Operation done if direct visualization preferred. Otherwise closed procedure using percutaneous needle. Used to identify an underlying renal parenchymal disorder.
Blood urea nitrogen (BUN)	Blood determination of amount of urea and waste product accumulation.
Phenolsulfonphthalein (PSP)	Kidney function test. Dye injected intravenously. Urine specimens collected after ½ hr, 1 hr and 2 hr to determine amount of dye excreted.
Addis count	Determines type of kidney disease; 6–8 hr urine collection to determine number of cells and casts in sediment.

phenosulfonphthalein. The doctor will inject PSP dye into one of the veins in your arm. Before he does this you will be asked to drink at least a quart of water. By doing this you will help to guarantee a successful completion of the test. Your other task will be to void at certain times into these urine bottles which are already labeled for your convenience. I will come in to remind you when a specimen is due. The doctor has requested three specimens. One is due 30 min after the dye is injected, one is due at an hour after the injection, and the other 2 hr after the injection. While the test is being done it is important that you drink a glass of water every half hour. This will help you be able to void at the appropriate times. Sometimes it is difficult to void when you are asked, but please try to void each time a specimen is due. Also, the dye may change your urine to a pink color; don't be alarmed—this will disappear when all the dye is excreted. Do you have any questions?"

Specific Conditions

EXCRETION PROBLEMS

A decrease in urinary output may result from a lack of fluid intake, a decrease in the formation of urine, or an inability to excrete urine from the bladder. Urinary output may decrease in amount or it may be temporarily nonexistent. The length of time the urinary excretion problem exists is of utmost importance. For instance, the child may be playing actively on a hot day and not yield to his physiological request for fluids. He becomes moderately dehydrated and as a result his urinary output is decreased. This is a simple excretory problem which can easily be corrected by the child's taking oral fluids. In contrast is the child with impending uremia. He is temporarily not excreting urine and fluid intake will not result in a correction of the problem.

Another excretory problem common in children is frequency of urination. The exception to this fact is in the case of infants, as it is normal for them to experience frequency. This is one of the contributing factors in not trying to toilet-train infants at a very early age. However, after two years of age, frequency may be a sign of overhydration or a urinary problem such as cystitis. Frequency may be due to nervous excitement in young children and therefore it is necessary to get a good intake history regarding the relationship of the frequency to the everyday activities of the child. Other causes of frequency are a highly concentrated acid urine, which has an irritating effect that results in frequent trips to the lavatory, and renal calculi, which cause a reflex action, or polyuria. It is clear that these conditions will have differing signs which will help the physician to make a diagnosis. For example, with polyuria, the specific gravity will be lower, the urine will most likely be paler in color, and the amount will be larger than expected for a child of a particular age.

URINARY INCONTINENCE

Urinary incontinence may result when the bladder becomes over-distended with urine, causing an overflow. The overflow may be constant dribbling or it may be an intermittent urinary flow resulting without the child's knowledge. Incontinence in children may be due to congenital malformations such as exstrophy of the bladder or myelo-meningocele which are obvious and serious conditions of childhood, or it may be due to less obvious conditions such as an abnormal opening of the ureters into the vagina. The psychological—as well as the physical—implications of incontinence to children need considerable attention. A school-age child finds it extremely embarrassing not to be able to control his elimination.

ENURESIS

A form of urinary incontinence which is fairly common in child-hood is enuresis, more commonly referred to as "bed-wetting." Children differ widely in their age for completing toilet training. Frequently, a child is toilet-trained for urine during the day earlier than during the night. The wide range in establishing urinary control makes it difficult to state when a child should be free from enuresis. Each child's developmental achievements should be evaluated to decide if enuresis at a particular age is abnormal for him. A clue to abnormality can be gained by evaluating accompanying symptoms such as unexplained fevers, inability to establish a constant urinary stream when voiding, or pain during voiding which awakens the child from his sleep. The history should include details in relation to whether the child is completely wet or whether he seems to "leak" urine. The time of wetting should be established. Does he wet soon after retiring, closer to the morning hours, or on frequent occasions during the night? Does he wet every night or is the wetting sporadic? When he spends a night away from home, does he have enuresis there, too? The history should also include the fluid intake of the child for at least a day, including the times that fluids are taken. Many children develop a habit of requesting cold fluids at bedtime and it must be established if this late fluid intake is merely resulting in an expected physiological response.

PYELONEPHRITIS

In the introductory paragraphs reference was made to the relatively high incidence of pyelonephritis in childhood. The pathological process is usually more extensive than the term implies. An infection rarely is limited to a single portion of the urinary tract. This explains the use of the encompassing term rather than the specific anatomical segments. In the milder cases there is congestion and leukocytic infiltration into the renal pelvis. Throughout the interstitial spaces there are collections of bacteria and polymorphonuclear cells. It is possible to have hemorrhages throughout the interstitial tissue and the tubules. There may be extensive scarring with loss of functional renal parenchyma when the infection has been prolonged. The end result may be a small shrunken kidney (Rubin, 1964). Both congenital and acquired factors predispose the kidney to infection and should be considered in prevention. The growing kidney is more susceptible to infection than is the adult kidney.

The symptoms which frequently accompany pyelonephritis are chills, flank pain, frequency, malaise, and hematuria. The child may have any combination of these symptoms. The onset is usually abrupt and the child may spike an extremely high temperature. The temperature usually spikes intermittently over a period of a week to 10 days.

The urinary symptoms of frequency, urgency, and dysuria, if present, usually last for a period of about three weeks. Due to the debilitated condition, anemia, anorexia or failure to thrive are other symptoms that may be present for weeks following the resolution of the urinary symptoms.

The diagnosis of pyelonephritis is substantiated by the identification of bacteria and pus in the urine along with an elevated white blood count. In addition, the urine may contain red blood cells, and in severe cases, granular and hyaline casts. The child who has persistent pus in the urine should have further evaluation to establish a definite kidney involvement as pus can be a contaminant.

To further complicate the process of correctly diagnosing pyelonephritis, some children do not have any of the specific symptoms ordinarily considered pathognomonic of urinary infection. This is especially true in children under two years of age. They may merely present with a change in personality. The mother describes the child as fussy or irritable and lacking a desire to eat. The child may also have periods of vomiting which makes the infection seem related to the gastrointestinal tract. If the child's urine is not examined, he may lose weight and develop a chronic infection before the correct diagnosis is made.

With repeated attacks of pyelonephritis, it becomes increasingly difficult to make the diagnosis. Symptoms are generally lacking and the child can have a recurrent infection without having any overt difficulty. The unfortunate part is that renal damage may result without any warning. For this reason, children who have a history of urinary tract infection should be followed with routine urine examinations on a regularly scheduled basis. If pus is discovered in the routine urine, it should be followed by a urine culture.

The treatment of an acute urinary infection usually consists of a combination of antibacterial drugs; such as Furadantin, Gantricin, thiosulfil, or penicillin, as well as bed-rest (which may be enhanced by sedation), analgesics for the temperature elevation, and increased amounts of fluid intake. At times it is beneficial to manipulate the acidity of the urine through medication in order to control infection. An example of a medication used in this way is Mandelamine. This procedure is undertaken to reduce the possibility of survival of organisms by decreasing the conditions under which they survive and grow. It is used less frequently in today's therapy as currently available agents have more favorable results than earlier antibacterial drugs.

Recurrence of infection may be due to the same organism or infection by a different organism. If it is the same organism, it is usually because the organism becomes resistant to the antibiotic or chemotherapeutic agent being administered. If it is a new organism, the relapse usually occurs after a significant time period (approximately 6 months) when the urine has been clear. The child is considered more vulnerable to urinary infections once he has had one. This vulnerability may be related to host resistance or it may be due to a condition caused by the original infection, whereby the defense mechanism of the urinary tract is weakened.

When there is a structural or functional defect which predisposes the child to pyelonephritis, surgical correction is indicated. An example would be exstrophy of the bladder or a bladder neck obstruction. Even after correction, it is imperative that the child be followed medically since predisposition to urinary infections has already been established.

The school nurse has an important role to play in follow-up for these children. She is also responsible for seeing that the child is receiving his medication. The usual length of time on medication is 6 months (Williams, 1968). The nurse is also aware of the current minor illnesses, including rashes and respiratory conditions, which the child should avoid. If the child is inadvertently exposed, the nurse can call the parents so they can seek medical advice.

PREVENTIVE INTERVENTION.   The nurse in the child health conference can be instrumental in helping parents to realize that children tend to delay coming into the house to void because it interferes with their play. This delay may cause overdistention of the bladder and lead to changes which may predispose the child to urinary tract infections. The parent should be encouraged to call the preschool child into the house every 3 or 4 hr to encourage him to empty his bladder. Children should be encouraged to respond to the urge to void and thereby establish a normal voiding pattern. As children get older, they may have a tendency to be embarrassed by the need to void. To avoid embarrassment, they retain the urine and eventually the bladder may adapt itself to a position in which it can ignore the normal stimulus to empty (Smallpiece, 1969).

Preventive intervention should focus on establishing an atmosphere whereby micturition is considered a normal and necessary process unrelated to filth and free from disgrace. Even in today's modern society, there are still parents who teach their children that this normal physiological response is dirty or unacceptable. They may not intentionally teach this but their own reactions to wet diapers speak louder than words. Another aspect of intervention should focus on teaching parents that children are curious and may tend to explore their own anatomy by handling the genitalia or by inserting foreign objects which may predispose the child to urinary tract infections.

Parents should also be encouraged to periodically check the urine output of their children. This can easily be done by a quick check to see if the urine is cloudy or if the urine has an unusual smell. A "fishy" smell is sometimes associated with pus in the urine. Parents are quick to respond to blood-tinged urine but this symptom is not readily present in pyelonephritis.

In infants and young children, emphasis should be placed on changing them soon after the child has urinated or defecated rather than basing changes on the mother's busy schedule. Despite the high incidence of pyelonephritis in the diapered population, there is not strong evidence to support the fact that there is a direct cause and relationship to the disease process (Smallpiece, 1969). Evidence to the contrary is also lacking. Therefore, good hygienic practices should continue to be included in the nurse's teaching plan for the parent.

ACUTE GLOMERULONEPHRITIS

Acute glomerulonephritis has its highest incidence in children three to twelve years of age. It affects males with twice the frequency of females. It is generally considered to be an "allergic response" or an antigen-antibody reaction to a particular organism. The response usually follows an acute infection by one to three weeks, with the most common causative agent being the streptococcus. By the time the renal involvement makes its appearance, the preceding infection may be completely forgotten.

A good reason to treat comparatively benign infections such as pharyngitis, tonsillitis, and sinusitis is to prevent secondary glomerulonephritis. In a small number of cases, however, there is no history of previous infection.

There is in the literature some indication that acute nephritis may have a viral causation (Rusnac et al., 1967; Jensen, 1967). However, a viral etiology will only be responsible for a small number of the actual cases which will be seen in the hospital. The nursing care of children with viral etiology will be essentially the same, so the controversy over etiology is more significant, at this time, to the physician than to the nurse.

The onset of acute glomerulonephritis may be sudden or insidious. The child may complain of weakness, anorexia, or headache. There may be accompanying pallor and edema which is not readily recognized. The edema may merely be a slight puffiness of the eyes or feet. A good clue is the child's complaining of tight-fitting shoes. The child may appear more overtired than acutely ill. In other instances, the symptoms may be more obvious—with hematuria, nausea and vomiting, and elevated temperature. On closer inspection the child may show an elevated blood pressure and have visual disturbances.

In this disease process there is usually bilateral renal inflammation and the kidneys are slightly enlarged. There is capillary damage which permits blood cells and protein to pass into the glomerular filtrate. This property is responsible for the appearance of red blood cells, granular and hyaline cells, and albumin in the urine. In some children hematuria is not always obvious to the naked eye, but is usually present on microscopic examination. However, other children may have gross hematuria for the first few days. After the bright red appearance, the urine changes to a dark brown color before returning to amber and pale yellow.

Children who have gross hematuria are readily brought to the attention of medical personnel. The hematuria may turn the urine brown because hemoglobin is liberated by hemolysis in the urine and transformed into brown hematin by the acidity of the child's urine (Hamburger et al., 1969). However, despite their concern, the severity of the child's condition is seldom evident to the parent or child.

The child is usually hospitalized and placed on bed-rest. The diagnosis is enhanced by a thorough history. If the parent has "played down" or ignored the previous infection, they may be reluctant to tell the doctor about it. The nurse can frequently elicit this information as the parent does not always feel so guilty when talking with the nurse. Infections are often ignored if they interfere with everyday routines. For instance, if both parents work, it is difficult to keep the child home from school. This might necessitate the mother's missing time from work or an additional financial burden of hiring a baby sitter. Most parents learn that mild infections run their course and have no untoward reactions. They may have had experience with similar infections which responded well to their trusted home remedy of fluids, aspirin, and early-to-bed. They are shocked to learn that on this occasion a mild infection has resulted in a serious disease process necessitating hospitalization of the child.

In addition to the urinary findings, the child may have an elevated antistreptolysin titer, an elevated sedimentation rate (refer to Chapter 13 for more detail on these tests), a decrease in the serum albumin, and a mild anemia. The serum albumin is decreased as a result of the losses of protein in the urine. The child may have a decrease in urinary output with an elevated specific gravity.

There are occasionally changes on the electrocardiogram, which may be related to the changes in electrolytes. According to Rubin (1964), the heart may be enlarged and this is associated with pulmonary congestion evidenced by x-ray and pulmonary roles. According to Paul (1967), abnormalities of the chest were found in 90 percent of the children with acute glomerulonephritis in Singapore, where the condition is common. He suggests that the pulmonary vessels are affected in the same way as the renal vessels in this disease, and recommends that more emphasis be placed on the pulmonary changes associated with the disease process.

Hypertension may also be present and usually subsides after approximately a week of treatment. The child more than likely has had experience with having his blood pressure taken, but the superimposed trauma of hospitalization may make him leery of this procedure. (See Chapter 13 for suggestions regarding this procedure.) The elevated blood pressure usually responds well to the patient's bed-rest, but one must be careful to check it closely as activity is initiated. Occasionally the blood pressure does not decrease and this is associated with cerebral edema and cardiac involvement. Under these conditions, the child must be observed closely for convulsions and cardiac failure. Frequently there is improvement of these symtoms when the child begins to diurese.

WEIGHTS. The child is weighed on admission to establish his base weight for this illness and to prescribe medication and fluid requirements. The child's weight prior to illness is also significant. The parent may be able to give you this weight during the nursing intake history. The child should be undressed for this procedure and guaranteed privacy during the weighing. Each day the child should be weighed on the same scale, at the same time, and in the exact dress. (Some agencies permit the child to wear his underpants while being weighed.) Accurate weights are especially important as the edema may not be so easily detected in these children. With bed-rest, even before medication is started, the child may begin to experience diuresis. Weight loss can also result from the child's elevated temperature and the resultant increase in body metabolism.

Daily weights are usually taken before breakfast and after the child has attempted to void as it is fairly easy to keep a consistent pattern at this time. If weights are ordered every 8 hr, as is sometimes the case when severe edema is present, a convenient pattern must be established and adhered to. The more frequent weighings will help to establish when the child is retaining most of his fluids and will help the physician regulate medication, fluid intake, and ambulation. It is also a second check if a urine specimen accidently gets discarded. The additional weights are not a substitute for output measurement but rather a system of checks and balances.

If the child is unable to stand while being weighed, a bed scale, baby scale, or metabolic scale may be used. As with any balanced scale, it is necessary to check that the scale is accurately balanced before the child is placed on it. In addition, the scale should be balanced with the covering used for protecting the child's skin. Depending on the size of the child, coverings which may be utilized are diapers, scale paper, draw sheets, or pillow cases. Some agencies may have pads or old sheets mended for this use.

GENERAL CONSIDERATIONS. The fluid intake of the child with pyelonephritis and acute glomerulonephritis is usually increased (restriction of fluids will be discussed with nephrosis). It is easier to get the child to accept increases in fluids if they are prescribed and distributed reasonably. The age and size of the child are essential to good planning. As a natural pattern, smaller children drink lesser amounts more frequently. This concept should be utilized in planning for their increased fluid intake. The fluids should be spaced throughout the 24-hr period in order to maintain normal body fluid levels and to make allowances for fluids lost during periods when the temperature is elevated. Insensible fluid loss (the invisible loss of water without solute) is also a consideration in children, as perspiration is not always so obvious in children. Fluids are also dispersed throughout the 24-hr period so they can act as a normal irrigating system for the urinary tract. So as to allow adequate rest, they should be given during the night at the same time the child is awakened for other therapy. The increased fluids will help to prevent waste materials from passing through the urinary system in a concentrated form. One additional consideration in fluid therapy is not to overhydrate the child at any one point in time. Careful spacing of fluids will guarantee this.

Children with urinary tract involvement may have considerable difficulty voiding. To enhance voiding, stimulating fluids such as cola, tea, or coffee can be given. In addition, after approximately 30 min the child can be placed on the bedpan or toilet and Credé's method be tried. The other time-honored adjuncts to voiding—such as running water within the hearing distance of the child, providing privacy, and having the child place his fingers in water—should also be used freely.

The amount of fluid needed to provide an excess of fluid intake must take into account the solid foods consumed, the weather conditions, any losses due to vomiting or diarrhea, as well as the things already mentioned.

MEDICATION THERAPY FOR NEPHRITIS. The medication therapy in nephritis is based upon the individual child's clinical profile. More acute symptoms will, of course, need more vigorous and complicated therapy.

Penicillin is usually prescribed to combat the streptococcal infection. When an elevated blood pressure persists, Reserpine and Apresoline may be added to the regimen. When there is cardiac involvement it is common for the physician to digitalize the child and place him on a maintenance dose of Digoxin. He frequently adds a sedative to the plan when Digoxin is necessary to assure rest. There may be a trial of diuretics when edema is present and pulmonary congestion ensues. The results of the diuretic regimen are not always successful. In very advanced cases, there may be acidosis and sodium lactate may be given to correct this situation before it advances to a serious state that requires a 10% glucose solution for correction.

With the addition, subtraction, or reduction in any of these drugs, close observation of the child is essential. For instance, a child placed on Apresoline may have a rapid decrease in blood pressure necessitating a decrease or omission of the next dose of the drug. A child receiving Digoxin may have a decrease in pulse rate, below 60, which again necessitates a decrease or omission of the next dosage of the drug.

With the addition of the pharmacist to the health team providing direct care to the patient, the administration of drugs may be deleted from the list of nursing functions. This health team member may assume the responsibility for the patient's drug profile, or divided doses of medications, and probably for direct administration. Therefore, the nursing responsibilities should strongly be in favor of recognizing and reporting findings in relation to the patient's clinical picture which in turn will influence the pharmacist's and physician's drug plan. She will still need to be aware of the drugs and their expected actions and side-effects, but she will probably be freed of the responsibility of delivering the pills and carrying the keys to the medicine cabinet. In agencies where this change in health service can be instituted, the nurse will then have more time to make the essential observations which are her expertise and highly significant contributions to the health team.

NEPHROSIS

Nephrosis has its peak incidence in children under six years of age. Boys are more frequently affected than girls. The causative agent in primary nephrosis is unknown. Initially, edema is present in the child's face in the morning and in the lower extremities after a day at play. The edema is painless and does not cause functional disturbance; therefore, it may go unnoticed at first. Eventually, the edema increases and affects the entire body, being most noticeable around the eyes, abdomen, and feet. In boys, the scrotal area is also markedly edematous. If a tap is performed the fluid obtained is generally clear but occasionally milky.

A less common symptom is voice changes due to laryngeal edema. During the period when edema is increasing, the child's urinary output is decreasing and the appearance is opalescent and frothy. During diuresis, the urine increases in amount and is clear in appearance.

The pathophysiology of nephrosis centers on the increased permeability of the glomerular capillary basement membrane to protein.[1] This increased permeability is responsible for the large amount of protein excreted in the urine. Under ordinary circumstances, the kidney is able to filter out waste products and retain the protein necessary for normal body functioning. The change in kidney function results in a lowering of the serum albumin with a resultant decrease in the oncotic pressure of the plasma. This leads to a loss of water and sodium into the interstitial space, causing edema of the tissues.

Because of this loss of protein in the urine, there is a decrease in the serum proteins and reversal of the albumin-globulin ratio (A/G ratio). In addition, there is frequently a hyperlipemia and hypercholesterolemia present which is also secondary to the depletion of albumin. Hypocalcemia is common but there is rarely tetany associated with it. In addition, nephrotic urine also contains increased amounts of copper and iron (Hamburger et al., 1969) with a corresponding decrease in the serum levels.

There is a substantial amount of literature in which authors have expressed their views concerning nephrotic classification and accompanying clinical findings. To avoid confusion, the minute categorizations associated with the varying types of nephrosis will be excluded. However, clinical considerations will be incorporated in broad categories.

Congenital Nephrotic Syndrome. The first variation in this disease entity is congenital nephrotic syndrome or infantile nephrosis.

[1] Management of the nephrotic syndrome due to primary renal disease. Canad. Med. Assoc. J., 96:52, January 7, 1967.

This disease is especially important to nurses in newborn nurseries and in well-baby screening clinics. It is known that children susceptible to this disease are born before term and are usually small in comparison to their actual length of gestation. In the case of such babies, the placenta is large and frequently weighs the same as the child. The real significance of the placenta is its apparent inability to nourish the infant adequately, despite its unusually large size. These babies, according to Hallman et al. (1967) are likely to have polycythemia and advanced erythrocytosis secondary to the impaired function of the edematous placenta. Other stigmata seen in these babies include a distended abdomen, proteinuria, wide cranial sutures, low-set ears, and small snub noses and talipes. As in all diseases, not all of the signs are present in every child. It is possible that the condition is caused by an immune response between the fetus and the mother (Hamburger et al., 1969).

What is the significance of congenital nephrotic syndrome to nurses? First, nurses must be astute case finders in the delivery room and newborn services. Accurate recordings must be made of all associated aspects of the delivery and newborn period. It is no longer appropriate to chart "normal delivery" if both the mother and infant survived. The placenta must be weighed and the length of gestation clearly identified. It is unfair to jump to the conclusion that the mother calculated her expected date of delivery incorrectly. Much more emphasis needs to be placed on the child who is not up to expected standards at birth. Nursing has a major role to play in collecting data on this group of "high-risk" children.

After the newborn period, careful screening and developmental assessment will help to identify other clues to diagnosis. One frequently found symptom is the child's failure to thrive. These babies gain poorly despite the most conscientious feeding techniques. They are also frequently members of a family known to have kidney problems. It is believed (Hallman et al., 1967); that the condition is probably transmitted by an autosomal recessive gene. The nursing intake may help to identify other members of the family with "little-known" kidney problems. In addition, the nurse can observe the child in a lying position. The position which seems most comfortable to a baby with an edematous abdomen is frequently one described as opisthotonus (an arched-back appearance). The ankles of the baby are often in a flexed position (Hallman et al., 1967) and this can be a significant clue that the child has had interference with osseous growth in utero.

One of the most significant aspects of casefinding is bringing the child to adequate medical supervision immediately. These children, at this particular time, do not respond to the therapy given the child with acquired nephrosis and their life expectancy is very poor. Perhaps earlier diagnosis will result in more adequate control.

Acquired Nephrosis. After six months of age, the child is considered to have the acquired type rather than the congenital form. This group includes the children categorized as having lipid nephrosis or nephrotic syndrome. In these conditions, the therapeutic regimen has resulted in prolongation of life or even complete recovery.

In order to appreciate the extensive care plan needed to meet this child's needs, it is necessary to look at the many areas involved as a result of the disease process.

EYES. The soft tissue of the eyelids and below the eyes are common sites for edema. The classical picture of a child with nephrosis is one with slits for eye openings and swelling which causes a transparent appearance of the eyelids. The child is seen with his head tilted back in an attempt to utilize his narrow visual contact with his environment. He may benefit from soothing eye irrigations and occasionally from the use of eye ointments. The edema is transient and elevating his head may help to reduce the edema in this area. The child who sleeps without a pillow may accumulate a large amount of fluid overnight and awaken in the morning to total darkness. This can be an extremely frightening experience for the child. It is especially frightening to the preschooler, who is most prone to the disease.

In addition to the edema, the child may develop xanthomatous lesions on the eyelids which are uncomfortable and may cause the child to rub his eyes and further irritate the area. The xanthomatous lesions are thought to be associated with the high lipid levels in the blood.

SKIN. Nursing measures are intimately involved with preventing excoriation and breakdown of the overstretched skin. Careful cleansing and attention to skin areas which meet one another is paramount. Support of edematous areas by pillows may help to lessen tension on the skin and make the child more comfortable. Scrotal supports are used effectively. Creases of the groin may need to be padded with soft flannel or other cloth to prevent breakdown. During the hot weather, the child will perspire in these areas and need frequent washing, drying, and changing of the padding. The padding will also have to be checked for dribbling urine which will foster the growth of bacteria in this warm, dark area.

The child's finger nails should be kept short and clean to discourage scratching. The fingernails are frequently brittle and striated (Hamburger et al., 1969). The child's skin is dry and is prone to erysipeloid lesions which consist of red, blotching, tender patches and add an additional annoyance to the child. The skin is susceptible to bacterial and fungal infections. Bathing the child in the bathtub may be extremely soothing. The nurse should get help in transferring the child. It is essential to use good body mechanics to prevent strain to herself in lifting the child whose weight will be greatly increased by edema and whose body does not have the usual contours.

It is difficult to keep the child comfortable during the acute stages of the disease. Frequent changes of position will decrease the amount of whining, which signals discomfort. When the child is turned, the areas exposed should be gently rubbed to decrease the "wrinkle marks" which result from the contact of the edematous tissues with the bed clothing.

In hot weather, the child may get relief from using a bed cradle to support the bed linen and allow for better air circulation. The child should not be exposed to drafts or placed in direct exposure to an electric fan. He is very susceptible to infection and any predisposing factors should be avoided.

After the acute stages of the disorder, skin irritation is less common and the child will be allowed out of bed. The shifting in edema, due to the upright position, will focus concern on the child's feet. It will be necessary to check his footwear and remove constricting items. The skin areas between the toes will need to be cleansed individually and observed for excoriation. A soothing foot powder may be sparingly applied.

The child's teeth should be brushed frequently as there is an increased possibility of dental caries. Dental enamel is altered in the permanent teeth (Hamburger et al., 1969).

Hamburger et al. (1969) also mention the diminished elasticity of the external ear and also the tip of the nose after the diuresis is completed.

NUTRITION.   Underneath the edema, there may be extreme wasting of tissue and malnutrition and anemia. These factors are extremely relevant to nursing care. The nurse must utilize every possible method to get the child interested in eating. The anorexia which accompanies acute infection, an acute disease process, elevated temperatures, physical discomfort, and separation from home and family makes it essential for the nurse to be creative and patient in her approach to feeding the child.

Occasionally children are also placed on salt-poor diets or diets with elevated or decreased protein content. These moderations in the expected taste of food may further discourage the child from eating.

There may also be the added stress provided by limitation or restriction of fluids which may be necessary when the child is excreting only scant amounts of urine or having diarrhea which may result from an edematous bowel. During these periods, the child may be allowed sour balls to suck to decrease his thirst.

In the course of limited fluid intake it is extremely important to space the fluids throughout the 24-hr period. A common plan for establishing fluid intake is to base it on the previous day's urinary output. Therefore the doctor's order may read: Oral fluids 100 cc's plus the previous day's output (which provides only a minimal increase in the total fluid allotment). To make the child feel he is getting more fluid, a small glass should be utilized so the fluid can be easily seen in the glass. If a plastic medicine glass is used, be sure the child is aware that it is not medication.

URINARY OUTPUT.   The urinary output of the child with nephrosis is usually scant or nonexistent during the acute stages. It is impossible to emphasize how important it is to keep an accurate account of every voiding. As previously indicated, the daily fluid allotment may depend on it, the child's response to corticosteroid therapy will be monitored by it, and the appearance will give clues to decreasing or persistent hematuria which may indicate a nephrotic syndrome which is a combination of nephrosis and acute glomerulonephritis.

Collection of specimens, needed to follow the albumin excretion, may be difficult due to the extreme amount of edema and the decrease in urinary sensation due to the small amounts of urine reaching the bladder. The child should be tried on the bedpan or given the urinal rather than relying on his urge to void. Care should be taken not to unduly alarm the child by continually focusing on your desire to have the child void. Statements such as, "Haven't you voided today?" are taboo and should be replaced by a statement such as "It is time to try using the urinal now." The emphasis is thereby placed on the *attempt* to void rather than on the success of voiding. It must be understood that the preschooler wants to please adults and he will be disappointed if he is unable to do so by not voiding. He begins to get the impression that if he voids he will be rewarded and if he does not he will be punished. Continual failure to void results in increased frustration. This frustration added to his irritability and mood swings caused by corticosteroids can make the staff classify him as a "crabby" little boy.

CHANGES IN BODY IMAGE.   Boys need reassurance that their penis has not been removed despite its less prominent position. A statement of reassurance that the penis is still there and that you can see it from your position should precede the voiding request. This statement should be followed by one that shows the child you appreciate his concern for the changes in his body and that you know with time he will again return to his normal appearance.

The child should be provided with opportunities to express his fears regarding the changes in his body. In nephrosis, this is especially frightening because the child has to adapt rapidly to an increasing body size and then to adapt to a change in size, on almost a daily basis, when diuresis occurs. In addition, due to the intermittent nature of the disease, he may have to make this adjustment on numerous occasions.

The degree of stress caused by such changes should not be underestimated. Take for example, the preschooler who delighted in removing his socks and shoes and now cannot reach his toes; or the preschooler who was toilet-trained in a potty chair and now cannot free himself if he sits on the potty. These changes make it extremely difficult for the child to identify his immediate environment and his relative position in relation to it. His increasing size takes up more of his immediate environment and may cause him to bump into doors or fall over the side of the bed. The real significance of this information relates not only to his preservation of a healthy mental outlook but also to provision of safety. Even the young school-age child may need siderails to prevent him from falling out of bed. The siderails will also help to guarantee that a nurse is available to assist the child getting out of bed until he is aware of the changes needed to remain upright when his center of gravity is changed due to his large abdomen.

SUSCEPTIBILITY TO INFECTION.   Prevention of infection is directly related to the child's care. Children with nephrosis have a lowered resistance to infection and frequently seem to develop acute infections superimposed on chronic ones. The child may seem to have a "stuffy" nose a great deal of the time. This is probably related to swelling of the mucous membranes of the sinuses and nasal passages. Care must be taken when cleansing the nose with cotton tip applicators not to irritate these edematous linings. The same care must be taken when doing nose and throat cultures ordered to detect early signs of bacterial infection.

Antibiotics are usually administered during acute infections or exposure to known infections, but rarely prophylactically. During acute infections, antibiotics may be administered intravenously due to the decreased ability of the edematous intestine to absorb adequate amounts administered by oral or intramuscular routes. If intramuscular administration is utilized, it is especially important to insure that the medication reaches muscular tissue since the edematous tissue is prone to develop subcutaneous abscesses. Therefore, palpation for abscess formation and rotation of sites is paramount prior to giving injections.

There have been reported cases of complete remission resulting from a case of measles or chickenpox in a child with nephrosis. Prior to the good results now possible to obtain with use of corticosteroids, it was fairly common practice to try to find a child sick with one of these communicable diseases to provide exposure and cross-infection. This procedure is now less frequently used as it does not guarantee success and the child can suffer the ill effects of the communicable disease and be prone to complications without obtaining a remission. This risk was considered worthwhile when early treatment was not too successful and the disease proceeded to a higher fatal outcome.

The nurse should be aware that the child may not be immunized until he has been completely free of proteinuria and off steroids for at least a year (Soyka, 1967). This delay in immunizing is based on the assumption that there may be an association between an immune process in nephrosis and delayed hypersensitivity. These factors are thought to be responsible for exacerbations of nephrotic symptoms following routine immunizations. This factor is especially significant if the child receives his immunizations at a clinic or immunization center in which the staff is not familiar with the child's entire health and illness profile. It is a good idea to explain to the mother any proposed delay in immunizations to cut down on the possibility of error.

The placement of the child on the clinical unit should be based on decreasing the amount of contact with children with infections. Otherwise the child should not be limited in his associations with other children and adults.

The same principle should guide the mother when the child is discharged. The child should be allowed freedom of activity but should avoid other children and adults with infectious processes. Exacerbations of nephrosis can be directly related to infection.

OBTAINING BLOOD SPECIMENS.   During the acute stages of illness it is necessary to obtain frequent blood specimens for analysis. This creates a problem which can be a real frustration to the nurse and person trying to get the specimen. The preschooler's veins are difficult to locate under normal conditions. With the addition of edema, they are even more difficult to locate.

The child should be brought to the treatment room for the procedure. He should be prepared simply and honestly. Even the application of the tourniquet to his edematous limbs can be extremely uncomfortable. It is often necessary to release it and reapply it several times before an adequate vein can be identified. This action increases the child's time to fear the procedure and provides him with additional frustration.

The child is usually in a supine position for this procedure. Care must be taken to watch the child's respirations, as he has decreased respiratory functions; ascites causes pressure on the diaphragm which may be further aggravated by anxiety and crying. If there is a long delay in obtaining the specimen, the child may benefit by a rest period in the upright position.

At one time it was common practice to place the child's legs in a froglike position and draw blood samples from the femoral arteries which were easier to locate. There is now evidence (from Montreal and New York) which indicates that arterial thrombosis can result from using this site, resulting in circulatory failure and eventual amputation. This outcome may have been partly due to the steroid therapy, which is known to cause hypercoagulability, but the serious nature of the complications has significantly decreased the use of the area. If this route is necessary, the nurse must be sure to apply pressure after the sample is obtained to stop the bleeding. A small dressing is then applied with nonallergic tape. The site must be checked periodically to be sure bleeding does not reoccur after the child is moved back to his room.

MEDICATION THERAPY.   As already alluded to in the foregoing sections, a common therapy is to administer one of the forms of corticosteroid presently available. The dosage and schedule for this drug varies according to the child's age and weight, and the physician's choice. It is generally accepted that long-term therapy assures longer remission than short-term therapy.

The child may or may not be receiving diuretics. Diuretics seem to have limited value but are sometimes tried in an attempt to decrease the edema and make the child more comfortable.

During the period when rapid diuresis takes place, it may be necessary to place the child on potassium therapy because the rapid loss of sodium causes the potassium to leave the cell; it enters the circulation and is lost by excretion. Replacement may be achieved by potassium medication or by providing more potassium in the diet. A common dietary supplement is orange juice or cranberry juice which children usually accept readily. If the potassium remains in the circulatory system, the nurse should be alert for signs of hyperkalemia and refrain from offering high potassium fluids.

Newer additions to the drugs prescribed for children with nephrosis include the immunosuppressive agents. Presently the alkalizing agents and purine antimetabolites (referred to in the therapy of children with cancer) are being tried in some agencies. This more dramatic therapy is generally reserved for children who seem resistant to steroid therapy. The principles involved are similar to earlier attempts at using nitrogen mustard in treatment of children with nephrosis.

Other therapies such as the administration of salt-poor albumin and the use of exchange resins seem to be used with decreasing frequency due to the high costs of the therapy and the lack of long-lasting effects.

Antihypertensive drugs are included when the blood pressure is elevated. Antibiotic therapy has already been explained. Anemia may be treated by iron supplements or, if severe, a transfusion of packed cells.

Other medications will depend on the individual child's symptomatology. The nursing intervention again plays a big role in helping the child to accept and tolerate large and frequent doses of medication. The follow-up care is dependent on the mother and child fully understanding and appreciating the value of the medication. One older child stated that the nurse only said to take the pills. He could not appreciate the value of the medication based on such a limited explanation. It was not until he refused to take the medication, resulting in an exacerbation, that he could appreciate the true value of the medicine. Children and parents should not need to go through this biological and financial crisis to appreciate prescriped therapy. Prior to discharge, the action and reasons for medication should be explained to the family. The use of a diagram of the kidney may help in this explanation. An explanation of medications will also provide them with an opportunity again to discuss and clarify their feelings and knowledge about the disease.

UREMIA OR RENAL FAILURE

Uremia or renal failure is a very serious sequela of kidney conditions. It may result after a long series of infections or diseases processes such as chronic pyelonephritis or intermittent nephrotic syndrome, or it may be the result of an acute condition such as a traumatic injury or toxic ingestion.

The uremia may be poorly tolerated by the child if it is sudden and grave, or it may seem to be better tolerated if it develops over a slow gradual course.

Uremia results when the kidney is no longer able to excrete end products of metabolism. The most notable of which are urea and creatinine (by-products of protein). In addition, the kidney may not be able to free the bloodstream of other organic acids such as indoles, phenols, and similar toxic substances.

The symptoms exhibited by the child will not be solely attributed to nitrogen retention. They are most likely the result of a combination of nitrogen retention and fluid and electrolyte imbalances. For example, if a child has frequent bleeding gums or epistaxis it may not be merely the result of nitrogen retention. This hemorrhagic tendency is probably linked to a coagulation problem, a prolonged bleeding time, changes in capillary resistance, or it may be related to starvation. Proper attention to the child's dietary intake may lessen or correct the condition.

Other symptoms which are attributed to nitrogen retention and/or fluid and electrolyte changes include gastrointestinal symptoms: anorexia, vomiting, intermittent diarrhea, and abdominal pain. The mouth may have a "urinary odor," there may be increased salivation, and stomatitis or parotitis may develop. In advanced stages, the skin may have "uremic frost"—white crystal accumulation around the face, forehead, base of the hair, neck, and chest. Or the skin may just be "itchy." The child may be cold due to direct action of the nitrogenous wastes on his nervous system, which interferes with temperature control. The color of the skin is usually sallow, with the face and palms of the hands sometimes appearing darker. This sallowness is probably related to the anemia which is usually present in uremia.

Nursing measures will be directed at making the child as comfortable as possible during the time close medical supervision is being carried out. Depending on the medical regimen, the child may have to tolerate periods with very little fluid intake or diets restricted in protein. He may have numerous blood tests as it is imperative to monitor his electrolytes carefully, especially if exchange resins are being utilized, or there is a period of oliguria, or rapid diuresis. Intake and output, skin care, and mouth care have already been discussed in the chapter and are again mentioned because of their importance to this acutely ill child's comfort.

Two of the major electrolytes involved in kidney failure are sodium and potassium. As the kidney becomes unable to retain sodium it is excreted in serious proportions causing a *hyponatremia*. The kidney develops an inability to excrete potassium and this results in an increase in potassium in the circulatory system (*hyperkalemia*). An increase of circulating potassium can cause irritability to the myocardium which is easily monitored by an electrocardiograph tracing (see Chapter 13 for more details on EKG).

In addition, acidosis can result as the renal tubules fail to excrete hydrogen ions (H +) and regenerate bicarbonate ions (HCO_3-). This is further hindered by impairment of nitrogen secretion, which reduces the buffer capacity of the urine and further limits the secretion of hydrogen ions. Phosphate filtration is also reduced further, minimizing the buffer capacity of the tubular fluid. The resulting acidosis is reflected in a lowering of the blood carbon dioxide combining power (CO_2) and the blood pH (Creditor and Statland, 1963).

The phosphate elevation causes a reciprocal reduction in blood calcium by urinary excretion. This reduced blood calcium is responsible for the related symptoms of muscular twitching and weakness.

TREATMENT. Treatment of uremia or kidney failure must include consideration of the causation as well as the uremia itself. If the uremia was sudden, an attempt may first be made to establish urinary flow by administering a large amount of intravenous fluid in a comparatively short amount of time. The nurse must observe the child closely for signs of fluid overload during this procedure. If urinary flow is not established, then a more serious condition exists and fluids will be given with great caution. It is very important not to overload the child's circulatory system with fluids (*hypervolemia*). Consideration is given for insensible fluid loss via the skin and respiratory routes and modifications made when other fluid losses result from vomiting or diarrhea. However, the major way a child regulates his fluid is by way of the kidneys, and when there is impairment in kidney function the child can easily become seriously edematous. This edema can result in pulmonary edema and death if the necessary precautions are not taken.

An attempt might also be made to have some of the electrolyte changes altered by the use of exchange resins. These agents can be administered orally or rectally. The resins attempt to exchange potassium ions for ammonium or sodium ions. If the resins are successful there will be a decrease in the hyperkalemia. This decrease will be noted in a slowing of the pulse and a return to a regular beat.

The rectal instillation of resins is similar to any rectal instillation. The resins are mixed with a specific amount of water and instilled by gravity using a rectal tube and funnel or cannister attachment. The child is encouraged to breathe deeply through his mouth during the instillation and the fluid is administered slowly so that it does not stimulate a quick evacuation. To be most effective, the solution must be retained a sufficient amount of time for the potassium exchange to take place. If the solution is not expelled after 2 hr, a rectal tube may be inserted or a small enema administered to start the evacuation. The fluid returned should be subtracted from the original amount of the instillation to determine the amount of fluid retained, if any. This retained fluid will be used by the physician in adjusting the child's intake. This is the safest method of dialysis in present use.

DIET. The dietary regimen for children with renal failure is a controversial area. The opinions vary from little restriction in diet because it interferes with the child's growth (Edelmann and Bunstein, 1968) to ones that recommend very specific and stringent dietary restrictions by using a carbohydrate-fat diet (high caloric) with restriction of proteins and potassium (Hamburger et al., 1969). The amount of restriction depends on the degree of renal insufficiency present. In addition to protein restrictions, water and sodium are also prescribed cautiously. Water is usually given in sufficient amounts to achieve adequate urinary output. Care must be taken not to cause excessive excretions which will force sodium excretion in large amounts. Salt may need to be added to the diet but with cardiac involvement salt will be restricted.

The child on a restricted diet is usually given supplementary vitamins as a protein-free or restricted diet is poor in vitamins.

With these general ideas as to dietary treatment, the nurse can readily see that her role in the care of these children will be intertwined with the role of the dietician. Working effectively together they may help to prevent refusal of food, dehydration, or the necessity for alternate routes of intake such as tube feedings or intravenous therapy.

PERITONEAL DIALYSIS. Peritoneal dialysis is a procedure utilized in children with severe kidney damage or impending renal failure. In this procedure, dialysis is performed by using the peritoneum as the dialyzing membrane. In exchange resins the intestine was used as the

FIG. 1A.   Equipment for peritoneal dialysis.

dialyzing membrane. The principle is the same: a sterile solution of electrolytes is introduced into the abdominal cavity and waste products are removed from the body by osmosis. The peritoneum acts as a semipermeable membrane similar to the nephrons in a normal kidney. Approximately a liter of fluid is introduced through a catheter inserted into the child's abdomen. The solution utilized is similar to extracellular fluid but it lacks potassium and it contains dextrose. Potassium and other waste products diffuse through the peritoneum in an attempt to equalize the solution on both sides of the membrane. The dextrose makes the solution of sufficient osmolarity to prevent absorption of the dialyzing fluid into the blood. After the solution is introduced it is allowed to remain in the abdomen for a period of approximately 30 min. The fluid is then allowed to drain out by gravity into a sterile bottle (see Fig. 1A & B).

While the procedure seems very simple, it is not without dangers. It has certainly made dialysis available to more persons than was possible when only the artificial kidney (hemodialysis) was available.

According to Boen (1964, pp. 69–71), the following are some of the major advantages of peritoneal dialysis compared with the artificial kidney.

FIG. 1B.   Schematic drawing to illustrate intermittent peritoneal dialysis in use.

1. Simpler equipment makes it available in nearly every hospital.
2. Abrupt changes in blood volume can be avoided.
3. There is ample opportunity to change the composition of the irrigating fluid. It is therefore possible to avoid an insufficient or excessive correction of disturbances in electrolyte or water balance.
4. Can be used after surgery or with patients with bleeding tendency.
5. When increased protein breakdown is evident, peritoneal dialysis can be used longer.

Major disadvantages to peritoneal dialysis include the following (Boen, 1964, pp. 69–71).

1. Water is removed more slowly by this procedure.
2. Infection is a possibility.
3. Intestine can be perforated during introduction of trocar.
4. A loss of about 40 gm of protein may occur.
5. Abdominal pain and discomfort may occur.
6. Not able to use where abdominal injury is present or with severe peritonitis.
7. Sterile irrigation fluids necessary with peritoneal dialysis but not with the artificial kidney.

Since hemodialysis is used less frequently with children, it will not be further discussed in this chapter.

A closer look is now needed at some of the disadvantages and their implications for nursing. The first disadvantage relates to water excretion. The nurse must remember that the child can have respiratory distress due to the pressure of the solution on the diaphragm. She must also help the child to relax so this increase in fluid does not cause undue abdominal discomfort. Preparation for the "full feeling" will help the child understand what is happening and lessen his fears.

The second disadvantage is danger of infection. This danger can be minimized by keeping the dressing and area around the catheter as clean and dry as possible. Periodic cleansing with antiseptic solution and application of sterile dressings under aseptic technique will lessen the possibility of infection. When new solutions are added, they must be done under aseptic conditions and any medications, such as heparin or antibiotics, must be added with care.

The child should also be kept away from other children or adults with infections, as their resistance to infection is poor. If members of the health team or family are not feeling so well as usual, they should not visit the child until all doubt of illness is erased.

The disadvantage of loss of protein is especially significant as it further adds to the malnutrition and wasting prevalent in these children. As the child's anorexia improves due to the removal of waste products, it is especially important to use this time to have the child eat. It is also common to have the child's disposition improve with dialysis and he may be more eager to choose foods and liquids which he has refused on other occasions.

PREPARATION OF THE CHILD FOR DIALYSIS. The child is prepared for peritoneal dialysis either before he is taken to the treatment or minor surgery area, or in the area before the procedure is started. He is asked to void to deflate the bladder. A sketch of the dialysis set-up is useful in preparation as the child may get very confused by just an explanation (see Fig. 1A). The child is asked to lie in a recumbent position with his pajama bottoms removed and his pajama top pulled up above the nipple line. The child is asked to lie with his arms up under his head or tucked under his buttocks on each side. This will help to keep his hands restrained without too much adult help. (The child is usually premedicated before coming to the area and this aids in limiting discomfort.)

The child is then told about the abdominal preparation, the cool antiseptic solution, and the sterile drape. He is told he will feel a prick of a needle which is special medicine for putting the skin to sleep so it will not feel any more pain. The nurse offers her hand for the child to squeeze and indicates it is OK to cry if he wants to. He is encouraged not to move as the covers will slip off and wiggling also interferes with the doctor's work. His cooperation is stressed as being a real asset to completing the procedure.

The physician then injects the xylocaine (or similar substance) and prepares the area for the incision and introduction of the trocar. The child is then told he will feel pressure on his "tummy" or abdomen but it will not hurt. During the insertion the conversation can center on topics of interest to the child, as he is prepared for the immediate procedure. If he cringes or wiggles, refocus on the procedure and make a supporting statement such as "You are doing nicely, try to lie still, the doctor is almost through with this part."

After the catheter is inserted, a trial for proper functioning, considering patient comfort, is done by using 200–300 cc's of fluid. The child is prepared for the "full feeling" and observed for any overt or covert signs of discomfort. The catheter is either sutured or taped in place and a dressing applied. The child is told the procedure is just about over and he will be returned to his room as soon as the drape is taken off and he is moved from the table to his bed or a stretcher.

The child is then told that periodically the fluid will be exchanged and each time he will be told about it. He will not feel any different than when the doctor did it this time.

The nurse is then responsible for explaining that his vital signs will be taken frequently during the dialysis so he will not be alarmed. It is necessary to keep a close check as there will be a quick change in the electrolyte composition and too rapid fluid exchange can result in shock.

Nursing responsibilities will also include warming the solution before hanging a new bottle. A solution at body temperature is less likely to cause discomfort than a cold solution. She will also keep a very accurate intake and output (see Table 3). If the child retains the fluid he may be turned carefully to aid the gravity drainage (the child

TABLE 3
RECORD OF PERITONEAL DIALYSIS THERAPY

JOHN JONES	AGE 12	AUG. 31, 1970						Differential
Solution	Medications	Solution In			Solution Out			
Inpersol 1.5%	Added	Start	End	Volume	Start	End	Volume	
	Heparin 0.5 cc	12:00	12:20	300	1:20	1:40	275	+25

is usually in a supine position with his head elevated approximately 45° during the dialysis). Care is also needed to prevent breakdown of debilitated skin (as was discussed earlier in this chapter). The tubing must also be kept free of kinks to provide adequate drainage and it must be observed for small clots or waste material which may interfere with flow. If flow cannot be reestablished by "milking the tube gently," the doctor should be notified. Heparin is sometimes ordered to decrease the clot formation or the physician may need to move the catheter to a better position. Coughing and deep breathing should be encouraged to decrease the possibility of pneumonia developing.

There are several signs which signal distress. Increased respirations may indicate that too much fluid is being administered for this particular child. Occasionally a child complains of shoulder pain, which is probably due to the same cause. Abdominal pain may be a sign of peritonitis or infection. Diarrhea is a common side effect of dialysis. A deterioration in the child's mental state may be related to the electrolyte exchange. All of these signs should be reported to the physician and recorded accurately.

After the dialysis is completed the catheter is removed and a small sterile dressing is applied over the incision. Intermittent dialysis is usually done by a new paracentesis puncture and new catheter. Using a new set-up each time seems to cut down the risk of infection. It does present a new stress situation to the child each time, however. Usually the child cries when he knows it must be done again, but that is the extent of his resistance. He seems quickly to equate the dialysis with an increase in well-being.

MEDICATIONS.   When a child is in renal failure it is necessary to monitor medication therapy much more cautiously. Many drugs are normally excreted by the kidneys and without normal renal function there may be toxic levels built up in the blood. A drug which is greatly affected is digitalis. Both digitalization and maintenance requirements are decreased when kidney failure is present. Several of the antibiotics also fall into this grouping; examples are streptomycin, kanamycin, and tetracycline (Schwartz and Dunea, 1967).

Some agencies do cultures on the first and last solution of the child's dialysis and order antibiotics if indicated. These antibiotics are sometimes added to the dialysis solution.

Medication given the child in renal failure is principally concerned with the underlying cause or with symptomatology. Therefore, if the child has tetany, calcium may be given; if there is cardiac involvement, digitalis derivatives and barbiturates; and if there is pneumonia, antibiotics. At present there is no drug which can satisfactorily treat nitrogen retention (Hamburger et al., 1969).

Kidney Transplantation

The use of transplanted kidneys in the human is generally reserved for patients with irreversible renal damage. Successful transplants were first done between identical twins and are now successful between less closely related individuals because of tissue cross-catching and the use of immunosuppressive drugs. Early transplants used total body irradiation prior to surgery to decrease the possibility of rejection. This procedure is used less now as drugs such as imuron have proved effective. Total body irradiation is especially serious to children as it will interfere with future growth.

Obtaining satisfactory kidneys for transplantation is not a simple process. A living donor has to undergo major surgery without being promised any definite results for the recipient. A kidney from a cadaver must be selected very carefully to be sure it is a healthy kidney, and obtaining kidneys must be done after the person is officially pronounced dead. Then the kidney must be removed and preserved while being cross-matched. In this instance the kidney must be given to a compatible candidate rather than one specific person waiting for a transplant. Obtaining kidneys leaves open many moral issues and makes it more difficult to provide the organ necessary to try to prolong another's life.

While the child is waiting for a compatible kidney, he is maintained on intermittent peritoneal dialysis. Between dialysis, the child is usually permitted to be discharged.

When a living donor is found, the child and donor are admitted to the hospital for more extensive blood work and kidney function tests, including arteriograms. If the donor is found compatible, both the donor and child are scheduled for major surgery. The child is started on chemotherapy approximately a week before surgery. The donor may be discharged until the day before surgery. If the child is severely debilitated transfusions may be indicated preoperatively. On the day of surgery, each patient will have his own surgical team responsible for his care. The donor kidney is removed and refrigerated (cooling to 4°C is achieved by immersing the kidney in cold saline solution for 5 min or direct perfusion of the kidney with a special solution cooled to 4°C). The cooling process prepares the kidney for prolonged ischemia without causing functional defects. The recipient is prepared to receive the donor kidney. The usual site for the kidney is the right iliac fossa (see Fig. 2). The kidney is turned over so that its posterior side is anterior to make it easier to anastomose the renal vein to the external iliac vein and the renal artery to the hypogastric artery. The ureter is either anastomosed to the recipient's ureter at the kidney pelvis or directly into his bladder.

FIG. 2. *Kidney transplant* (A). The new kidney is placed into recipient's iliac fossa opposite the side from which it is taken. (B) Incision site.

In some instances, the kidneys (bilateral nephrectomies) are removed approximately a month prior to surgery and the child is maintained on dialysis. This gives the child an opportunity to recover from major surgery before being subjected to the transplant.

In other instances, the surgeons prefer to remove the recipient's diseased kidney(s) and/or spleen at the time of transplantation. Mention is also being made of correction of urinary tract defects in combination with transplants. An example of such a repair would be a YV plasty. If these procedures are done, the child will probably have a more difficult postoperative course due to the more extensive surgery involved.

The spleen is considered to play a role in the rejection process, but many surgeons now believe its removal has not significantly reduced the possibilities of rejection and are not routinely removing the organ. The removal of the kidney(s) is based on the theory that the diseased kidneys can play a major role in postoperative infection.

Each child will be considered individually for the best possible course of action.

It is also important to keep in mind that as the recipient surgical team is preparing the child to receive the kidney, they may decide that the child's possibilities of accepting the donor kidney are too slim and the surgery will not proceed. In this case, the donor surgical team is notified not to proceed with removal of the kidney. A reason for cancellation of the surgery would be severe cardiac failure in the child. Frequent communication takes place between the two surgical teams during the procedure to insure both patients the best possible care and consideration.

POSTOPERATIVE CARE.   The child will be placed on reverse isolation because his resistance to infection is very low due to the immunosuppressive drug therapy. It is best if one nurse cares for the child during the early postoperative period. This will help to cut down on infection and also guarantee continual monitoring of the child's condition.

Immediately postoperatively, the kidney usually excretes adequate to large amounts of urine. This can make the family extremely optimistic, even if they have been told this is the expected outcome. The urine excretion has its darker side also; it is a hazard because with the excretion come resultant fluid and electrolyte changes. These changes pose a threat to the child's life and must be watched carefully. Vital signs are taken every 15 min. during this early stage; the temperature is taken at least hourly. The child usually has a nasogastric tube which is connected to gentle intermittent suction. If a catheter or catheters are in place they are connected to drainage. Urine is checked frequently for specific gravity, sugar and acetone, protein and color. The doctor will usually leave specific directions for calling him regarding the results. For instance, if urine has +2 acetone, notify M.D. In addition, there will be specific orders regarding regulation of intravenous fluids. They will be given in accordance with the previous hour's urine output. In addition, intravenous flow is regulated to take into consideration nasogastric drainage, usually every 4 hr. Weights are also taken and may influence the intravenous intake.

After the period of diuresis the child's urine output will stabilize and a period of good renal function will exist. This quiescent period is usually followed by a period termed "rejection crisis." This attempt at rejection is signaled by scanty output, proteinuria, elevated temperature, weight gain, hypertension, or uremia. Immunosuppressive drugs are given to counteract the rejection; commonly used agents are imuran, prednisone, actinonycin C, and anti-lymphocytic globulin (ALG). In addition, local irradiation to the site may be tried. Peritoneal dialysis may be instituted if anuria persists or the electrolyte imbalance is severe. The large doses of steroids may cause gastric irritation (ulcers) and an antacid may be given to counteract this response. Stools may be tested for guiac as a precautionary measure.

During this postoperative period, the child may feel increasingly better than he has felt in a long time. This improvement in affect is very encouraging to the parents as they breathlessly await the outcome of the transplant.

As soon as the nasogastric tube is taken out, usually on the first postoperative day if bowel sounds are present, the child is started on oral fluids. If these are tolerated he is progressed to a soft diet. Any diet restrictions will be based on symptoms, but generally the diet will be fairly free to encourage the child to eat and begin to rehabilitate himself.

During the entire time the child is hospitalized, his decreased ability to fight infection must be kept uppermost in mind. If isolation is discontinued, the child should be kept away from obvious sources of infection. The parents should be made aware that they will need to take the same precautions when the child is discharged. Some agencies keep the child on strict isolation prior to surgery and until discharge, but this practice is decreasing in frequency as bacterial studies have shown that most of the bacteria present are actually related to the patient rather than to the clinical areas. Bacteria are most often found in the patient's mouth, nose, feces, or on the skin and can be treated effectively.

The child will continue taking medications after discharge so the parents must have explicit directions regarding them. Refer to Table 4 for side-effects of particular drugs to include in the parent teaching.

In addition, the parents must be aware of signs and symptoms which necessitate medical intervention. Refer to Table 5. Late rejection crisis usually occurs between the third and twenty-sixth month after surgery. This wide variation in time makes it difficult to prepare the family for the situation.

After discharge, the child will be followed very closely on an out-patient basis. The parents must understand the value and rationale for this continued close supervision. In addition, they must be helped to begin to let the child develop independence so that his additional years will be well spent.

While many cases have successful outcomes, it must be kept in mind that death is a very real threat postoperatively. Transplantation of kidneys has resulted in improved techniques but success can not be guaranteed.

PSYCHOLOGICAL IMPLICATIONS. The chance that a child facing imminent death might survive almost seems to make any risk worth taking, at first glance. However, kidney transplant is still a big risk, as already explained. In addition, another healthy person may be taking a risk by donating his healthy kidney based on his present excellent health. Today's good health does not guarantee tomorrow's good health, as is well known. If a parent donates a kidney to his child, is it unreasonable for him to feel he has made a real sacrifice and expect a return for this sacrifice? If a relative donates the kidney is it unusual for the parents to feel they owe him something? These

TABLE 4

IMMUNOSUPPRESSIVE MEDICATIONS[1]

NAME	SIDE EFFECTS
Imuran (azathioprine)	Bone marrow depression (leukopenia)

Prednisone	Rapid withdrawal may cause severe rejection in addition to adrenal insufficiency.
	Transient retention of salt and water
	Increased blood pressure
	May raise BUN
	Euphoria or emotional instability
	Increased appetite
	Diabetes mellitus
	Cushnoid conditions:
	  a. purplish or reddish striae of skin
	  b. development of supraclavicular fat pads
	  c. abnormal growth of hair
	  d. rounded contour of face
	Delayed healing
	Masking effect on infections

Actinomysin C	Irritations of mucus membranes
ALG (Anti-lymphocytic globulin)	Severe pain, fever, edema, and swelling at injection site Chest pain Muscle cramping Shortness of breath Flushing or cyanosis Nausea and vomiting

[1] Adapted from Bois, M.S., et al. Nursing care of patients having kidney transplants. Amer. J. Nurs., 68:1245, June 1968.

are the very questions that make the psychological implications of kidney transplant almost as great as the surgical ones. Let me illustrate by a clinical example. Susan was five years old when first brought to the hospital with severe kidney damage. Her mother also had kidney damage and even with this history, she did not seek medical attention for Susan until the child's disease was too far advanced.

Susan was treated with intermittent peritoneal dialysis but her condition continued to deteriorate. The parents were informed that Susan's only chance for survival was a kidney transplant and this held only a slim margin of hope. Mrs. G. convinced her husband he should donate a kidney, if he was compatible. Mr. G. was not enthusiastic about the surgery but agreed after many conferences with the physician and social worker.

Postoperatively, Mr. G. was a model patient. It was difficult to believe he had major surgery. His recovery period was uneventful and he was discharged after a week. But, Susan's body did not accept the

TABLE 5
SIGNS AND SYMPTOMS HERALDING COMPLICATIONS IN
KIDNEY TRANSPLANT PATIENTS[1]

SIGNS AND SYMPTOMS	CAUSES
Skin infections ("herpes")	Lower resistance of the body
Dysuria, frequency, or burning on urination	Urinary tract infection
Hematuria	Urinary tract infection or homograft rejection
Oliguria or anuria	Inadequate fluid intake or homograft rejection (urinary tract obstruction)
Pain in the kidney site, or any abdominal pain	Homograft rejection or gastrointestinal complications
Lethargy	Homograft medication side-effects, rejection, or electrolyte imbalance
Elevated temperature	Homograft rejection or infection
Joint pain	Medication side-effect (steroids)
Rapid increase in weight	Excessive fluid or food intake, or decreased renal function
Nausea or vomiting	Infections, gastrointestinal complications
Vertigo; postural hypotension	Antihypertensive medications or electrolyte imbalance
Headache	Hypertension, medication side-effects, excessive sodium in diet, central nervous system infections
Chest pains and respiratory difficulty	Pulmonary embolism, pneumonia. atelectasis, or cardiac complications
Change in bowel habits and in color or consistency of stools	Hepatitis, ulcers, hemorrhoids, fecal impaction, or bowel obstruction
Visual disturbances (blurring, dizziness)	Medication side-effects (anthihypertensives, steroids) glaucoma, cataract

[1] From Bois, M. S., et al. Nursing care of patients having kidney transplants. Amer. J. Nurs. 68: 1243, June 1968.

kidney and after a period of peritoneal dialysis and conscientious care, she died.

During Susan's hospitalization Mrs. G. derived a great deal of satisfaction from the nursing staff. She did not seem close to Mr. G. or able to communicate readily with him. She spent very little time visiting him after his surgery. The relationship seemed strained and one wonders about the implications of the child's death to this marriage. If the child had survived would the mother be closer to the father for his role in the recovery? With the death will she blame her husband because it was his kidney the child's body rejected? Did the mother have such extensive guilt for not seeking medical attention that she had to offer the child everything possible before she could face the child's death?

This situation illustrates the magnitude of the psychological aspects related to kidney transplants and especially in relation to decisions which must be made for the child by an adult.

With adult patients, some agencies use psychological testing to help in determining whether a patient should be considered for a transplant. It is not this simple with young children as they seldom understand what is truly involved. Perhaps with further advancements in the field, the problems will be eased and the decisions easier to make.

Case Presentation and Study Questions

Kevin is a 6-year-old white male with a history of nephrosis probably beginning at seven months of age when his mother noticed intermittent puffy eyes and rhinorrhea. He was treated for allergy until a routine urinalysis (at 2 years of age) disclosed proteinuria. The patient is now admitted with 4+ protein and a sed rate of 103.

1. The +4 protein and sed rate of 103 are significant. Explain.
2. Is there any connection between the "allergy" and the disease process nephrosis?
3. What other laboratory determinations will be done?
4. How will you prepare Kevin for these tests?

After a more extensive work-up Kevin was given a trial of steroids and diuretics.

5. Why were these drugs chosen and what is the expected outcome?
6. What are the side-effects of these medications?
7. As a nurse, what are your responsibilities in relation to medications both while the child is hospitalized and in relation to home care?

Kevin does not respond to therapy and a renal biopsy is done. It shows proliferate glomerulonephritis with sclerosis of the vessels. It is decided to start Kevin on intermittent peritoneal dialysis.

8. How will you prepare Kevin and his family for this procedure?
9. What are the expected outcomes from the dialysis?
10. After dialysis is started, what are essential nursing functions?

You are responsible for making a nursing referral to the community health nurse.

11. What information will you include?
12. What feedback can you expect from the community health nurse to be used by the health team in the hospital?

References

Boen, S. T. Peritoneal Dialysis in Clinical Medicine. Springfield, Ill., Charles C Thomas, 1964.

Bois, M. S., et al., Nursing care of patients having kidney transplants. Amer. J. Nurs., 68:1238–1247, June 1968.

Chisholm, C. D. Dialysis for renal failure in children. S.A. Med. J., December 1967, p. 1169–1172.

Creditor, M. C., and Statland, H. Kidney diseases. In Statland, H., ed. Fluid and Electrolytes in Practice, 3rd ed. Philadelphia, Lippincott, 1963 (Chapter 16).

Daeschner, C. W., Jr. Evaluations of the child with hematuria. Hosp. Med., September 1967, p. 59–74.

Downing, S. R. Nursing support in early renal failure. Amer. J. Nurs., 69:1212–1216, June 1969.

Eckstein, H. Enuresis. In Williams, D. I., ed. Paediatric Urology. New York, Appleton-Century-Crofts, 1968.

Edelman, C. M., and Bernstein, J. The kidneys and urinary tracts. In Barnett, H., ed. Pediatrics, 14th ed. New York, Appleton-Century-Crofts, 1968 (Chapter 24).

Feldman, W., et al. Intermittent peritoneal dialysis in the management of chronic renal failure in children. Amer. J. Dis. Child., 116:30–36, July 1968.

Goldberg, I. The diagnosis of pyelonephritis in childhood. Manitoba Med. Rev., January 1967.

Hallman, N., et al. Main features of the congenital nephrotic syndrome. Act. Paediat. Scand. Supplement 172, 1967.

Hamburger, J., et al. Nephrology. Philadelphia, Saunders, 1969 (Chapters 6, 7, 18, 58).

Jensen, M. Viruses and kidney disease. Amer. J. Med., Vol. 43, Dec. 1967.

Juzwiak, M. Nursing the kidney-transplant patient. RN, p. 34–41, May 1968.

Kanter, A., et al. Peritoneal dialysis: indications and technique in the surgical patient. Surg. Clin. N.A., 48:47–55, February 1968.

Kaye, M., and Conty, C. Nutritional repletion during dialysis. Amer. J. Clin. Nut. 21:583–589, June 1968.

Keuhnelian, J., and Sanders, V. Urologic Nursing. London, Macmillan, 1970.

Kreider, N., and Curtiss, J. A case study of a chronic, progressive physical disability. J. Rehab., November–December 1968.

Krupp, M. A. Diagnosis of medial renal diseases. In Smith, D., ed. General Urology. California, Lange Medical Publications, 1966.

MacGregor, M., and Freeman, P. Subclassification of childhood urinary tract infections as an aid to prognosis. In O'Grady, F., and Brumfitt, W., eds. Urinary Tract Infection. New York, Oxford University Press, 1968.

Martin, A. J., Jr. Renal transplantation: surgical technique and complications. Amer. J. Nurs. 68:1240–1241, June 1968.

O'Doherty, N. Urinary tract infection in the neonatal period and later infancy. In O'Grady, F., and Brumfitt, W. eds. Urinary Tract Infection. New York, Oxford University Press, 1968.

Pande, S. R., et al. Electrophoretic studies of the serum and urinary proteins in nephrotic syndrome. Indian J. Med. Sci., 1967 (reprint).

Paul, F. M. The roentgenographic changes of the lung in acute nephritis in Singapore children. J. Singapore Paediatric Society, Vol. 9 No. 2, October 1967.

Rubin, M. Disturbances of the kidney. In Nelson, W., ed. Textbook of Pediatrics, Philadelphia, Saunders, 1964.

Rusnac, C., et al. Contributions to the problem of the viral aetiology of certain acute nephrites in children. Pediatria Vol. XIV, No. 4, 1967 (reprint).

Samler, L. P. Clinical and immunological aspects of glomerular disease in children. J.A.M.W.A., Vol. 22, Oct. 1967.

Sato, F. F. New devices for continuous urine collection in pediatrics. Amer. J. Nurs. 69:804–805, April 1969.

Scott, J. E. Urinary infection. In Williams, D. I., ed., Paediatric Urology. New York, Appleton-Century-Crofts, 1968.

Smallpiece, V. Urinary Tract Infection in Childhood and its Relevance to Disease in Adult Life. St. Louis, Mosby, 1968.

Soyka, L. F. The nephrotic syndrome: current concepts in diagnosis and therapy advantages of alternate day steroid regimen. Clinical Pediat., Vol. 6, Feb. 1967.

Swartz, F. D., and Dunea, G. Acute renal failure. Med. Times 95:1287–1294, December 1967.

Watkins, F. L. The patient who has peritoneal dialysis. Amer. J. Nurs., 66:1572–1577, July 1966.

Williams, D. I. Paediatric Urology. New York, Appleton-Century-Crofts, 1968.

Winter, C., and Roehm, M. Sawyer's Nursing Care of Patients with Urologic Diseases. St. Louis, Mosby, 1968.

Winter, C. Practical Urology. St. Louis, Mosby, 1969.

7 MARY NORMA O'HARA

Nursing Care of the Child with Long-Term Respiratory Problems

The respiratory problems described in this chapter were selected because of the long-term nature of the entity and the implications for nursing management. Allergy, with special emphasis on asthma, as well as bronchiolitis, tuberculosis, and cystic fibrosis are included.

The majority of these disorders will most likely require hospitalization at least once during the course of the disease. Some will require frequent visits to the clinic or physician's office. Regardless of the setting, all of these illnesses will require knowledge on the part of the nurse in relation to the disease process, significant observations for assessment and planning of care, instruction for the child and family, and evaluation of the plan for management.

In the mid 1960s, one of the major causes of early infant death was the respiratory distress syndrome. Respiratory disease was not a common cause of mortality in preschool and school age children. Accurate statistics on morbidity are more difficult to find. The National Institutes of Health provides a picture of those illnesses which are more common in childhood and which tend to interfere with the child's normal activities. The majority of these conditions are a result of injuries or acute infectious diseases and respond to appropriate medical treatment. A significant number, on the other hand, are chronic in nature and require highly specialized care.

It is imperative from our knowledge of the effect of hospitalization on the child and family, as well as from an economic standpoint, that every effort be made to prevent complications when possible and to provide intensive care measures so that early discharge is possible.

The average number of days a child is hospitalized has declined rapidly in the past several years, but the number of children receiving care on an ambulatory basis has rapidly increased. It is vital that planning for discharge as well as patient-family teaching begin early in the hospitalization so that early discharge does not require readmission due to poor preparation.

In discussing long-term or chronic illness, the fact that they persist may be the only commonality. Some disorders are irreversible while others may be transitory and respond to a therapeutic regimen. Some of these conditions may have their onset in infancy, while others appear in early or late childhood. For example, cystic fibrosis, which causes severe respiratory problems in many instances, may be diagnosed in the newborn period through meconium ileus. Asthma may have its onset in infancy or in childhood.

Cultural and social factors must be considered. We should also examine attitudes of nursing personnel toward children with chronic disease. Caring for children with long-term problems can contribute to professional development not only in terms of learning nursing care but also in increasing knowledge and skills. The goals for treatment are different in a long-term respiratory problem from those in acute illness. Rewards are not attained so readily. The nurse must realize her limitation—as should other members of the health team. The combined efforts of the physician, nurse, physical therapist, occupational therapist, and social worker in complex cases will be necessary to attain the goals established.

Bronchiolitis

One of the early respiratory problems in infancy may be bronchiolitis. The symptoms are similar to those of asthmatic bronchitis, i.e., wheezing, dyspnea, cough, and fever. In addition, lethargy, cyanosis, and sternal retractions are present. There is no definitive evidence to date that the infant with bronchiolitis will or will not develop asthma in later years.

The concern in dealing with respiratory problems in infants is related to the size of various tubular structures of respiratory passages. The small bronchioles in the infant are vulnerable to obstruction due to inflammation of mucosa and tenacious mucus within the lumen.

If alveolar ventilation is inhibited, hospitalization will be required. On admission, the patient's major problem is with the egress of air. The inflow of air is delayed when air is sucked through obstructing exudate. Upon expiration, air remains trapped in alveoli, resulting in emphysema. The chest appears barrel-shaped and the chest wall and diaphragm are forced into a position of full expiration (Fig. 1).

CLINICAL EXAMPLE.   John G. was a five-month-old who was admitted to the division with rapid, shallow respirations. During inspiration the suprasternal notch and intercostal spaces and ribs retracted. A "hacky" cough could be heard frequently. He was cyanotic while coughing or crying. He appeared to devote all his energy to breathing. Only a feeble attempt was made to play when a toy was presented to him. Rest-

FIG. 1. Normal bronchiole and constriction of air passages during bronchospasm.

lessness was noted due to the respiratory effort, and caloric and fluid intake were deficient. His mother stated that cough and lack of sleep had been problems. Anoxia and exhaustion were evident.

Therapeutic measures—which were intensive and life-saving—included administration of antibiotics and oxygen, the use of high humidity, and adequate fluid intake. The infant's response to a croupette, which provided high humidity and oxygen, was dramatic. Close observation and surveillance of the infant was most important.

When abdominal distention is present, elevation of the head of the infant or placement in a portable infant recliner may be beneficial. The shirt should be loose so that the chest can easily be exposed to evaluate respiratory difficulty. Since oxygen and humidity are indicated, the nurse must assess the device's effectiveness. If the croupette is functioning improperly, the increased restlessness observed may occur because of the lack of oxygen and/or increased temperature within the tent due to lack of ice in the chamber rather than a progression of the child's condition. Parenteral fluids may be instituted until adequate oral intake is possible. If a restraint is indicated for any reason, care should be taken to avoid any pressure on the chest or abdomen that will aggravate respiratory effort.

Small frequent amounts of fluids, when tolerated, are indicated.

Personnel should be encouraged to plan administration of medications, fluids, and comforting measures, during the acute stage, in such a way that exhaustion is not promoted.

Asthma

Allergy is listed as one of the major chronic illnesses experienced by children today. It has been stated that over five million Americans suffer from asthma and approximately three-fifths of these people are children. Many children are often susceptible to infections. Absence from school may occur in the first or second week of the new term due to sudden exposure to nose and throat infections of classmates. In surveys which include chronic conditions causing days lost from school, asthma is often the single chronic condition causing the highest percentage of days lost. Since asthma is a long-term problem, the importance of early diagnosis and effective management is important in order to avoid complications of this chronic disease. Fontana (1969, pp. 29–30) believes that "the term asthma should only be applied to allergic reaction producing dyspnea, wheezing, and coughing and not for the non-allergic bronchial lesions producing similar respiratory symptoms. . . . Asthma is a disease entity with known etiological factors that can become complex with chronicity and lead to death." (p. 3). This allergic disease involves the bronchi and bronchioles with an increased production of tenacious mucus, edema of the mucosa, and bronchospasm. Therefore, the airway is reduced. Since there is a combination of large and small airway obstruction, air is trapped and hyperinflation of the lungs occurs. The lungs become larger and the vital capacity decreases; breathing becomes more difficult. Alveolar ventilation is decreased as well as arterial oxygen tension with an increase in arterial carbon dioxide tension. Early treatment is essential (Figs. 2 and 3).

Bronchial asthma may be due to extrinsic causes such as inhalants, foods, or drugs. In some instances, it is associated with bacterial or viral infection. At times, there is a combination of an extrinsic cause, such as food, and an intrinsic cause, such as infection.

In the acute asthmatic attack, the severity of symptoms depends on the inflammatory reaction of mucosa, the amount of bronchospasm, and the degree of obstruction of airways and distended alveoli.

When proper allergic management is provided, the effects are often reversible. In the long-term cases, response to medication may be poor due to changes that have taken place in the bronchi and alveoli resulting in lowered vital capacity and deformity of chest cavity.

ASTHMA IN INFANCY

The infant may fail to thrive or have vomiting, diarrhea, excessive mucus, or other respiratory manifestations. When asthma is diagnosed

FIG. 2.   (Top) Longitudinal section of bronchiolar obstruction.
FIG. 3.   (Bottom) Enlarged cross-section of obstructed bronchiole.

in infancy, the condition is often the result of food sensitivity. This is one reason why it is important to teach mothers to introduce one new food at a time, especially when there is a history of allergy in the family, so that reactions can be evaluated over a two- to three-day period. A skin rash may be observed rather than respiratory symptoms. In reviewing charts of older children with asthma, it can be seen that infantile eczema was often recorded in the history.

Although there is considerable difference of opinion among physicians as to which foods tend to cause allergic reactions, milk, wheat, eggs, and citrus juices are usually among those listed to be eliminated. Peanut butter is often also listed as an offender in preschool or school-age children.

When foods are being eliminated, usually a hypoallergenic diet is instituted. Milk is usually replaced by a soybean preparation; rice, oats, or barley cereal and specific vegetables; fruits; meat (such as lamb), and synthetic vitamins. After a week on a regimen, one new food may be added at a time and the infant observed for any reaction. A simple log should be kept by the mother with comments relating to tolerance of foods or symptoms noted. Later the physician may add milk, wheat, and eggs. A written diet, clearly stated—including foods to avoid—is important for the mother. For example, although milk was not given, a cube of cheese containing milk might have been offered. Reading of labels for content should be stressed.

This regimen may seem difficult for a mother to accept. She may become discouraged when the infant refuses foods allowed. This reaction should be anticipated and ways suggested to modify the diet within the restrictions. The refusal of food may also be due to deceleration of the growth rate. Force-feeding should be avoided and there should be acceptance of the fact that appetite will vary from one meal to the next.

Role of the Nurse. As the child grows, inhalants take on a more prominent role and may be responsible for respiratory symptoms, although dust can still be a problem in the infant age group.

The allergic history will be the initial step in diagnosis. The nurse in the clinic or office may observe that on the visit following the initial workup, the mother may share additional important information that she did not recall on the first visit.

Explanation of what to expect should be made as to the physical examination, laboratory tests, or special pulmonary function tests. With a young child, the mother can play an important role. Tricks for examining tots, such as having the mother urge the child to puff on her hand or a plastic windmill may permit auscultation. Children often panic when undressed completely, even with the mother present. Removal of clothes from the upper half and replacement after head, neck, and chest examination may avoid this reaction. Enlistment of the aid of an older sibling helps on occasion to serve as a model of what to expect. Distraction is often effective in dealing with toddlers. For example, a toddler, clothed in pajamas, resisted standing still on the scale. He clung to the shaft and screamed loudly. His pajama bottoms began to slip. The nurse suggested he hold his pajamas up. He removed his hands and held onto his pants. His weight was secured with no further resistance.

Environmental contacts that may need to be eliminated to study the effect are often dust, flowers, animal dander, and feathers, to mention a few. Although this may seem like a reasonably simple request, assistance may be needed through a home visit. Sleeping arrangements should be explored. Usually dust should be kept to a minimum in the house as a whole. Realistically, it is the child's bedroom in which special emphasis is placed. The removal of a favorite pet from the household can become a tragic request in the eyes of the entire family. Resentment could be directed toward the allergic child by other siblings. A free guide distributed by A. H. Robins is available in many physician's offices or upon request. Considerations are included which assist the family in controlling dust and other allergenic articles (Fig. 4).

When certain articles must be replaced, such as feather pillows for kapok and mattress covers, or the use of a special air cleaner, air conditioner, or humidifier is suggested, the present family budget may not stretch. The problem may require assistance from the welfare worker in some instances or substitutions may be made. Articles used by other family members, such as powders, perfumes, and scented tissues, may be offending substances.

Emotional Aspects of the Disease. Psychiatric studies of children with asthma have indicated that the onset may follow the death of a close member such as a grandparent or parent. In some children emotional upsets may play a major role in onset of symptoms. Although these situations do not cause the asthma, they do aggravate it.

The child's liabilities should be assessed to determine what action can be taken to reduce the child's disability. The nurse should observe the child's behavior as to how he approaches living with a disability and how he cooperates with those offering treatments or other help. Failure to cope with the disease may lead to inappropriate psychological defenses. The goal of treatment should be shared with the child and involve him in the plan of care.

The values held by the child will likely determine his attitude toward his disability. For example, a five-year-old will view limitation of motor activity very differently than will an adolescent. On the other hand, to an adolescent, one's cosmetic effect assumes central importance, and motor limitation may not be so significant to such a person as to the younger child. The mother's acceptance of the illness may affect the extent to which the child will accept it. In pediatrics, it will often be observed that children who seem to adjust to their illness frequently tend to be more dependent on adult relationships and especially on those caring for them during convalescence. A school-age child may identify with one particular staff member and make many requests that normally he could handle himself in order to prolong his stay in his unit. Most of the children on a pediatric unit find a certain amount of solace in the attention of the staff. However, a few may appear to need and enjoy dependency and exaggerate helplessness. The nurse should be alert to this and a team conference may be indicated to help the child become more independent. Chronic or severely handicapped children are unable to express aggressive impulses through physical activity used by healthy children in acts of play. Competitive sports are often out of the question for the child with a pulmonary disease problem, and this may affect self-esteem. Other types of activities should be identified that will still involve the child with his peers, such as serving as score keeper, being the assistant in charge of checking equipment, or engaging in a similar activity that is an important contribution to the school or team effort. In general, children are permitted to participate in activities according to their capability.

Hospitalization. Many acute attacks of asthma can be managed at home, but admission may be necessary when the child has failed to respond and respiratory insufficiency continues. In some instances, there is an inability of the family to cope with the illness; hospitalization may be required to provide an opportunity for diagnosis or may be an emergency admission with status asthmaticus. The child's response to admission must be considered and reassurance may be needed by the parents. Their main concern is often that the nurse will not be with the child if and when another attack occurs, or that the patient will not make his needs known. The attitude of the nurse on admission can indicate an understanding of their concern and a beginning sense of trust can develop. Encouraging the parents to call later in the evening means a great deal when they wish to return home but are reluctant to leave.

Some hospitals have considered development of a special unit for allergy in their construction programs. Air conditioning and hypoallergenic bedding and furnishings are provided. For those not acutely ill, kitchen facilities and a dining room are available as well as a play area. Oxygen and resuscitation equipment is built into the walls. Children wear their own clothes, and the staff—made up of pediatric allergist, nurse, nutritionist, medical social worker, and psychologist—utilizes the team approach. The team is highly skilled in the art of observation and assessment, which includes home visit as well as understanding the relationship of wheezing to factors such as parental visit, activity, timing of medications, and response.

Residential centers for asthmatic children are available in at least 10 states. Some children seem to improve after separation from family and environment. Some physicians prefer partial separation and select an installation fairly close to the child's home.

The Nurse in the Out-Patient Clinic. Since the incidence of allergy is high in the pediatric population and the number of allergists limited, the clinic is usually one of the busiest. Following the precise history, physical examination, and laboratory tests and/or x-rays, the patient is skin tested. These tests are done by a scratch or intradermal, usually on the upper arm. To complete the series, depending on the number ordered, may take three or four visits. The approach of the staff is important initially, so that anxiety and fear of "shots" can be alleviated. Some allergists do not order skin tests to determine food allergens since they believe the best way to avoid food phobias and to detect reaction due to foods is to put the child on a strict elimination diet and have the mother keep an accurate diet chart.

CLINICAL EXAMPLE. I should like to describe an allergy clinic I observed in a large medical center. When the clinic was first instituted, the house officers in the pediatric clinic interviewed the patient and family, wrote the orders, and administered the injections. Because of their rotations through the service, changes were frequent. Therefore, the child was relating to several physicians.

It was decided to assign one nurse to the allergy clinic and she gave the injections on written order of the house staff. During "hay fever" season, over 100 children, averaging three injections each were seen on some days.

The next change that was instituted was to assign half of the allergy clinic population to the nurse who had been giving injections only, so that more responsibility was assumed for interviews, injections, and follow-up. A guide provided by the physician was used to determine dose of injections. A house officer and staff nurse continued to be assigned to the other half of the patients, which I'll refer to as Clinic B. It was observed that the children assigned to the nurse, Clinic A, looked forward to greeting her and to observing the preparation of their injection. Children assigned to Clinic B were unhappy because a new person was assigned to give their injections. They resented this at first; but adjusted to the change. They still returned to visit the nurse in Clinic A, who had previously been their nurse. What was it that appeared to make the difference in attitude of the children in the two clinics?

Mrs. S., in Clinic A, consulted the allergist in the clinic when necessary and referred patients to be seen by him. She tried to recall something special about each child, jotting down personal notes on a small slip of paper on the chart. Upon the return visit to the clinic, it was not unusual to hear her say, "How did you make out in the school play?", "You decided on long hair!"; "Who won the game?".

When a new child or one who becomes upset over injections has an appointment, his injections are prepared prior to entering the room to avoid waiting, watching, and worrying. Soon the child adjusts and he is able to watch preparations as well as other youngsters receiving their injections. By the third or fourth visit, there are no more tears.

Now that the role of the nurse is being extended to make better use of her educational preparation toward improved patient care, she reviews with the parents the list of allergens, goods, and other factors that should be eliminated and discusses the plan that has been identified for management.

School problems and requests for excusal from gym are not uncommon. One 10-year-old wanted to be excused from school in order to be at the clinic at 1:00 in the afternoon rather than 3:00 in order to meet his friends. Some preadolescent girls wanted excuses from gym for various reasons. The philosophy of the clinic's staff in relation to activity is that children are allowed to participate according to their individual capability and individuals are not excused unless their physical condition warrants it. Most excuses are written "to participate as tolerated."

Use of oxygen.   Anticipation of respiratory emergency and knowledge of location of emergency equipment cannot be overemphasized regardless of the respiratory condition. An important consideration in administration of oxygen is a low flow rate. The reports of the blood gases are evaluated. Careful observations of the patient's response to oxygen by the staff, are vital, since severe respiratory acidosis may develop in patients with severe asthma who receive high inspired oxygen concentrations. This results from continued airway resistance and not because of poor ventilation. If oxygen is administered at higher levels, hypoxia results due to the rise in alveolar carbon dioxide tension.

When oxygen is ordered by croupette or tent, it is the responsibility of the personnel (including physicians) when opening the tent to do something for the patient, to leave the patient with the canopy tucked in and the oxygen and motor turned on before leaving the bedside; otherwise the patient is without therapy. In high-humidity tents, 70 to 100 percent humidity can be provided. The child who cannot see through the fog of the tent or whose clothes are supersaturated may resist the tent and need more frequent attention.

As the infant or child responds to therapy, one of the early indications that the tent may no longer be required may be determined by observing the behavior of the child. A toddler may be observed sitting at the foot of the bed breathing "normally." Nurses must utilize judgment in carrying out their responsibilities. Evaluation of color, cough, and respiratory effort during the bath or at feeding time should be carried out. A trial period without the croupette or tent may be indicated to determine progress. On the other hand, a tent that has been discontinued may need to be reordered.

Parents are often concerned that the child will be afraid in the tent. It is helpful for the admission nurse to remain at the bedside until the patient is settled in the tent. It has been my experience that the child experiences some relief almost immediately and will begin to settle down. Parents should be permitted to remain. It is important to stress to the staff the importance of a light by the bed of any child in oxygen or special tents. There is a need to assess respirations and color frequently, and there is an apparent distortion which the patient perceives looking through plastic. This is particularly true for toddlers.

Medications. Medications play an important role in relief in asthmatic symptoms. It is important for the nurse to know the nature of drugs, such as bronchodilators, aerosol sprays, expectorants, or tranquilizers, in order to assess symptoms and take appropriate action. Self-medication should be discouraged. Most intractability is caused by medications and not by psychological or environmental factors. Some consideration is being given to recommending the prescription basis for buying hand nebulizers. The patient's chart should be properly tagged or flagged, if there is a history of specific drug sensitivity. Strong sedation is usually avoided. Pediatric doses of tranquilizers have been used. Antibiotic therapy is usually ordered when an infection is present.

Epinephrine is a most effective drug in treatment of allergic conditions. Proper dosage and discretion is vital so that effective response will occur when most necessary in a severe asthmatic attack. Many physicians will be very specific in instructions to the parents and may not teach or permit parents to administer this drug in the home. Their rationale is related to concern over leading to an adrenalin-fast patient and belief that the patient should be seen by the physician to evaluate management. Overdosage is noted by increased pulse, elevated blood pressure, headache, and increased apprehension.

Aminophylline suppositories are effective when proper dosage is used; 5 mg/kg of body weight is listed as an effective dosage. The parents should be instructed that suppositories have been ordered and how and where to insert them. This may seem obvious; however, one mother who was told that the nasal symptoms her child was experiencing would improve after this medication, returned to the clinic to report that "the medicine was too big to put in Johnny's nose." If vomiting or restlessness occurs, the drug should be stopped. When half of a suppository is ordered, it should be sliced longitudinally so that the medicine is equally distributed.

Bronchodilator aerosols contain agents to relieve bronchospasm. Some incorporate isoproterenol with corticosteroid. This type of therapy is preferred by some authorities for chronic adult asthmatics for relief of bronchospasm rather than for children. Several reasons are given for this stand: (1) the side-effects, such as dependency or addiction, result from increased use, as well as toxic symptoms; (2) they lead to intolerance to other medications used in the treatment of asthma; (3) pulmonary complications; and (4) sudden or unexpected death may result.

According to Fontana (1969, p. 57), "in the asthmatic child with uncontrollable chronic disease or life-threatening, acute respiratory failure, the steroid drugs are most useful in conjunction with, but not as a replacement for the standard allergic management procedures. The general management procedures including: hydration, expectoration, tranquillization should certainly be tried for a period of time before steroids are prescribed." Steroids are usually continued for a seriously ill child who has already been treated with them. Saturated solution of potassium iodine may be used to activate proteolytic enzyme, which acts on secretions. Administration with fruit juice or milk with each dose lessens gastric irritation.

Aerosol therapy may be ordered for a young child or infant to decrease mucosal edema and to relieve bronchospasm. This therapy may be in the form of cold steam, mucolytic agents, antibiotics, enzymes, or oxygen. Some ultrasonic equipment provides much finer particles with dense concentrations. When the small infant is treated with aerosol therapy that utilizes ultrasonic equipment, daily weight should be taken to evaluate water retention. The effects of excess water include convulsions, edema, and circulatory failure. Bronchospasm seems to develop more readily in dehydrated patients from any agent that might irritate the bronchial tree. Therefore, hydration is very important before aerosol agents are instituted.

Tuberculosis

In reviewing statistics related to tuberculosis in children, it is evident that the disease is still an important health problem. Tuberculosis control programs attempt to prevent the spread to the pediatric population. Casefinding to prevent contact of infected individuals with those who are healthy is important. It is estimated that approximately 50,000 new cases are discovered in the United States each year. Certain segments of the population have a higher incidence. Social and environmental stress play a significant role. There is a greater susceptibility to tuberculosis during infancy and puberty.

Since few patients with tuberculosis are hospitalized today, one might question including this condition in discussing implications of long-term respiratory problems for nursing. However, child health nursing is no longer confined to the hospital but extends into homes, schools, and clinics. It is often through health supervision or the ambulatory service that the condition is found.

Tuberculosis is highly contagious and is usually spread by droplets containing the viable tubercle bacilli. When children are in contact with an individual with the active disease, they are very susceptible. Often it is difficult to trace the contact that is the host for the infection. The infection usually occurs as a result of inhalation of droplets of sputum sprayed by coughing, sneezing, or talking. Discussion will be confined to primary pulmonary tuberculosis, although extrapulmonary tuberculosis occurs.

The pulmonary lesions in children may be seen in any part of the lung, with some tendency to be localized near the periphery. The site is more likely to be in the lower part of the lungs. At the site of the initial focus, there is an accumulation of polymorphonuclear leukocytes followed by proliferation of epithelioid cells which surround the tubercle bacilli, creating the typical tubercle formation. Lymph nodes are usually involved at the time of the initial parenchymal lesion in children. There is a strong tendency in children for these lesions to heal by calcification.

Since more individuals reach maturity today without having acquired the disease, there is an increase in the primary infection in adults. Primary tuberculosis infection has been referred to as the childhood type of tuberculosis. The course of primary tuberculosis is benign in the majority of cases. Most complications such as tuberculosis meningitis result from hematogenous spread from the primary focus. Chronic tuberculosis is usually referred to as "adult" or reinfection type. It is seldom seen before 10 years of age and is more frequent after puberty.

Tuberculin tests play an important role in the diagnosis and are recommended by several authors for children to begin at 6 to 12 months of age and be administered at school entry and at 14 years of age. The purpose of the test, how it is administered, and the significance of the reaction should be explained to parents in the clinic. There are certain limitations to the test, but a positive reaction in the tuberculin test indicates the presence of tuberculosis infection and is allergic or hypersensitive to its protein. Although the degree of activity cannot be determined, further procedures, such as chest x-ray and examination of gastric contents, may be ordered. False-positive and false-negative tests can occur for various reasons. Mantoux test is considered an accurate reliable skin test. Old Tuberculin (OT) solution or Purified Protein Derivative (PPD) solution can be utilized.

A new stabilized Tuberculin PPD Solution is now commercially available for the intracutaneous Mantoux Test.[2] It is no longer necessary to use the tablet form and dilutent. The potency of this new form has been extended, and it is stable up to 12 months when stored between 35° to 46°F. The skin of the forearm is cleansed with alcohol or acetone and allowed to dry. The initial test dose consists of 0.1 ml of First Strength PPD injected intracutaneously on the flexor surface of the arm about 4 inches below the bend of the elbow. The PPD test is read 48 to 72 hr after administration of the tuberculin. The widest diameter of distinctly palpable induration should be recorded. Presence of redness, edema, or necrosis should also be recorded. A positive reac-

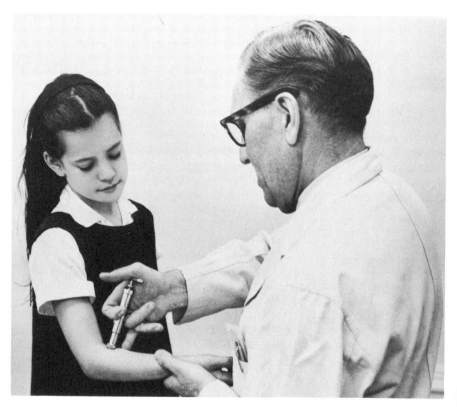

FIG. 5. Physician administers the Heaf Test to Adrian. (Courtesy of Panray-Parlam Corp., Englewood, N.J.)

[2] Manufactured by Connaught Medical Research Laboratories, University of Toronto, Ontario, Canada. U.S. Distributor: Panray Division, Ormont Drug and Chemical Company, Englewood, New Jersey.

tion indicates a sensitivity to tuberculin, which may be the result of a previous infection with mycobacteria. This infection, likely due to mycobacterium tuberculosis, may have occurred years ago or may be of recent origin.

Clear instructions should be given to the parents when the test is administered on an out-patient basis. A small drawing or picture is helpful to give parents, and the parent is either contacted or requested to call the clinic for the report. It may be necessary to repeat the test.

There are two multiple puncture tests: the Heaf test and the Tine test. The Heaf test is administered with a Heaf gun with disposable cartridges making multiple simultaneous punctures of the skin through a layer of concentrated PPD (Figs. 5 and 6). Three to seven days later, the test is read. A positive reaction is indicated if four or more papules appear. The tuberculin Tine test is an inexpensive, newer test and consists of a sterilized disposable unit with four tines which have been predipped in Old Tuberculin concentrate (Fig. 7). Two millimeters or more of palpable induration around one or more puncture sites is equivalent to five millimeters or more by the standard intradermal Mantoux Test. This may be considered positive.

Regardless of which type of test is used, the child may express fear or apprehension because a puncture of the skin is involved. When the test is administered to a young child, the child should be held on the lap, holding the arm gently and distracting the child with a conversation to allay fear. The wheal on the skin can be compared to a mosquito bite to a preschooler. A child who knows how to count can be encour-

FIG. 6. A closeup view of the Heaf gun with disposable cartridges. (Courtesy of Panray-Parlam Corp., Englewood, N.J.)

FIG. 7. Administration of the Tine Test used in tuberculosis detection. (Courtesy of Lederle Laboratories, Division of American Cyanamid Co., Pearl River, N.Y.)

aged to count with the nurse to see how long it takes for the test. This technique is quite effective.

GASTRIC LAVAGE

It is difficult to obtain a specimen of sputum to recover the tubercle baccilli from children because organisms from lung lesions reaching the pharynx are swallowed. Therefore, a gastric lavage may be ordered. Yet the number of bacilli and the frequency of positive cultures recovered by gastric lavage is small, and it is therefore recommended that the procedure be carried out each day for three successive days. Gastric lavage should be performed early in the morning after an overnight fast. The contents of the stomach are aspirated and placed in a sterile container. This may be followed with 60 ml of sterile water, and this is aspirated and added to material in the container (Kendig, 1968). This procedure may be carried out by the nurse or physician. The specimen should be sent directly to the laboratory for culture.

It is not my intent to describe the complete procedure for lavage but to comment on a few important aspects. In infants and young children, proper restraint is necessary. A mummy restraint is usually most effective so that the procedure can be carried out safely but as quickly as feasible. The attitude of the nurse and the manner in which the restraint is applied makes a difference. For example, "I am doing this to make it easier" rather than an attitude such as "I'll wrap up you so you can't move." Nonverbal communication speaks louder than words. When a catheter is inserted, coughing, difficult breathing, or cyanosis may indicate insertion into the larynx. If such a reaction occurs, remove the catheter at once. For confirmation of proper placement of the catheter in the stomach, gastric contents can be aspirated. The size of the catheter is determined by the child's age. As with any pediatric procedure which is uncomfortable, the nurse should hold the infant, or in the case of an older child spend a few minutes with him, for reassurance after the procedure.

TREATMENT

With the advent of antimicrobial drugs, such as para-aminosalicylic acid, isoniazid, and streptomycin, mortality rates in tuberculosis were greatly reduced. Therapy is initiated as soon as a diagnosis of tuberculosis is made.

Isoniazid is given usually orally by tablet or syrup. Side-effects to be watched for include neuritis and convulsions. These are more common in the adult or adolescent than in younger children. When this drug is given to young children, it should be crushed and the taste disguised through the use of puréed fruit or preserves. It is usually ordered in divided doses at the morning and evening meals. Pyridoxine is administered in association with INH to prevent peripheral neuritis.

PAS (para-aminosalicylic) is sometimes administered with isoniazid to provide a higher blood level, since PAS competes with isoniazid for acetylation in the liver. Gastrointestinal symptom may be a sign of toxicity.

Dihydrostreptomycin is more likely to produce eighth cranial nerve deafness. Streptomycin sulphate is given intramuscularly. Toxic symptoms include: disturbances of vestibular function, fever, vomiting, and a variety of skin eruptions. Personnel as well as parents should be alert to the problem of deafness. Observe how the child responds when his name is spoken or to conversation, as well as the degree of loudness of the radio or television.

Unless there is some specific reason, children are usually checked by the physician monthly while on medication. Periodic x-rays are ordered. Annual check-up should be stressed after therapy is completed.

Children, and adolescents in particular, cannot appreciate the importance and effectiveness of the antimicrobial drugs. These drugs may be given over a long period of time. Charts, logs, or any other creative methods may act as a necessary stimulus to assist the child in taking his medication. Protection should be provided to prevent intercurrent infections so as to avoid lowered resistance. Exposure to communicable diseases should be reported at once to the physician. Household contacts of a reported case of tuberculosis are skin tested and chemoprophylaxsis is advised. Other methods used to prevent tuberculosis include: isolation of those adults with infectious tuberculosis and use of BCG vaccine (used mainly for children exposed to an individual in a home or in a high-incidence population).

Older individuals can appreciate the changes that have been brought about in the therapy for tuberculosis. Years ago there was considerable stigma attached to tuberculosis. Parents or grandparents of the child involved may still recall the sanitarium, the mountain climate, and the elaborate isolation technique carried out. These attitudes could be easily transmitted to the adolescent. Members of the health team should be sensitive to the concerns and attitudes of the family toward the disease. Whichever member is in the best position at the time to handle these concerns should do so. It may be the nurse, physician, or social worker. What is important is that they be handled.

A diet high in protein, with adequate calories to promote growth, is furnished. If the child is asymptomatic, limitation of activity is not required. In those children who are symptomatic, prolonged bedrest is rarely used after therapy has been instituted. Prolonged bedrest may lead to further complications. The guide generally used for activity is the comfort of the patient, but excessive sunlight should be avoided. Bedrest should not be used as a threat.

Suitable toys and activities should be provided to amuse preschool children when activity is limited. School-age children may be more restless. Painting, books, crafts, felt boards, puzzles, and records may help to pass the time. New hobbies should be promoted. The school-age child or adolescent should be encouraged to talk about his concerns related to the illness so that guidance can be provided. He should understand the goals of treatment and be involved in the plan for his care when possible. Contact should be maintained with peers through letters and phone calls until visitors are permitted, or he returns to school. Children with primary tuberculosis return to school when they are asymptomatic. A conference with the teacher in the school may be indicated to clarify any questions she may have about the child's ability to attend school and engage in activities permitted.

Cystic fibrosis

Cystic fibrosis was selected for inclusion in the chapter on nursing care in long-term respiratory problems of children because it is recognized as one of the more common chronic diseases in children today and represents the most serious lung problem. It is an inherited disease of children in which there is a dysfunction of all or most of the exocrine glands. The incidence is thought to be 1 in 1000 or 1 in 2000 live births. This condition can range from a very mild form of the disease, with good nutrition and no respiratory involvement, to the severe form with extensive pulmonary obstruction and marked malnutrition that imposes very limited activity.

Dramatic changes have been brought about in the past 15 years through study and research resulting in improved management of the disease. The prognosis is often dependent upon the degree of pulmonary involvement.

Early diagnosis and aggressive therapy have been responsible for survival of infants and younger children into adolescence or adulthood. Presently more children are surviving to later years. More deaths occur between the third and ninth month of life.

Patients who manifest symptoms of the disease are homozygotous. Some authorities feel that if heterozygotes for the mutant gene could be detected, counseling these individuals against marrying each other could play an important role in future prevention in the high incidence areas.

Characteristic symptoms in children with all the clinical manifestations of this disease are due to involvement of three areas: the pancreas and other abdominal organs, lungs, and exocrine sweat glands. Most of the clinical manifestations are secondary to obstruction of some of the organ structures due to secretions which behave abnormally. Bronchial obstruction leads to bronchopneumonia. Pancreatic duct obstruction leads to pancreatic insufficiency. Intestinal obstruction leads to meconium ileus in newborns. In hot weather or in febrile episodes, excessive lose of sodium chloride in sweat leads to dehydration, reduction of extracellular fluid volume, and then cardiovascular collapse. Hyperthermia, coma, and death may follow rapidly. When one reviews charts of patients with diagnosis of cystic fibrosis, it is usually found that repeated respiratory symptoms were reported in infancy and early childhood. Rectal prolapse and nasal polyps occur and are difficult to explain. Frequent bulky, foul, fatty stools arouse suspicion of the disease, as well as failure to gain weight without anorexia.

Diagnosis is usually made from the family history and after the following tests: (1) sweat test to determine electrolyte content (in cystic fibrosis there is a marked elevation of sodium and chloride levels, two to five times above normal); (2) test for absence of pancreatic enzymes by aspiration of duodenal secretions (the viscosity of pancreatic fluid is increased and there is an absence or deficiency in pancreatic enzymes—namely, trypsin, lipase, and amylase); and (3) pulmonary function tests (the degree of pulmonary involvement is important in determining the severity of the disease and the prognosis).

The child may be already hospitalized for respiratory symptoms and the disease suspected, or the tests may be ordered on an out-patient

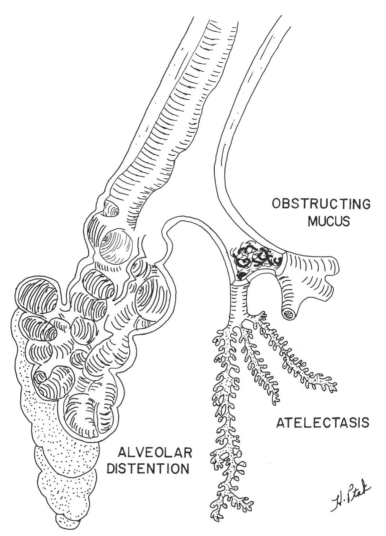

FIG. 8. Schematic representation showing pathology resulting from accumulation and obstruction.

basis. In either case, the nurse has an important role in explaining the tests and supporting the child during the tests, carrying them out skillfully, comforting the child after the tests, and providing adequate responses to parents' questions or concerns.

When meconium ileus occurs in the newborn, surgery is usually required to relieve the intestinal obstruction. The lumen of the small intestine is plugged with puttylike meconium near the ileocecal valve, which is inspissated. Abdominal distention and vomiting occurs.

Postoperatively, a high protein formula is offered and pancreatin is initiated. A work-up for cystic fibrosis is performed after the infant has recovered from surgery.

The discovery of increased sodium chloride in the sweat of children with cystic fibrosis was of real value in the advent of improved diagnosis of cystic fibrosis. Several methods have been used for the sweat test. The "bag method" was used extensively until the last few years. This method was not the safest. The skin was washed to remove surface chloride and a plastic bag was used to wrap the child and additional blankets used to stimulate sweating. The temperature was recorded rectally before the test and at least every 30 min by the axillary method during the procedures, as well as after the test was completed. At least 0.5 ml of sweat was required.

The most reliable and safest method today to collect sweat for chemical analysis is the pilocarpine iontophoresis technique, which can be used even on newborns. A dilute solution of pilocarpine is introduced into a small area of skin on the forearm, with a weak direct electric current, to stimulate local sweating. The sweat, collected on a small gauze pad, is analyzed for sodium and chloride concentration. This test is much easier for the child to accept and is less traumatic.

Duodenal intubation is a direct approach to examine enzymes. The procedure should follow at least a 6-hr fast. Some sedation may be ordered about ½ hr before the test. The nasogastric tube is inserted, and if secretions are tested with litmus paper, the paper should indicate an alkaline reaction, which confirms the presence of pancreatic juices. Secretions aspirated must be kept cold and analyzed without delay in the laboratory.

Insertion of any tube is an uncomfortable, frightening experience for the child. In the case of an infant or toddler, restraint will be required. Sometimes the procedure is lengthy. Distraction, such as reading a story or using an animated toy, will help. A preschool child will often offer resistance when the tube is inserted, but once the test is under way he may relax. A nurse should remain with the child. After the removal of the tube, the patient may be fed, and special attention for a few minutes will help the child regain his composure.

It is important to know what pulmonary function tests will be carried out so that explanations can be provided as to what to expect and how to cooperate, if the child is old enough. Pulmonary function in children over five years of age can be more completely evaluated than in younger children. No single, simple pulmonary function test accurately depicts pulmonary function in cystic fibrosis patients. Personnel who assist with these tests require special training, and must be selected for their ability to work with children.

Treatment of bronchial obstruction, when it occurs, is considered of vital importance. A great deal of the team effort is devoted to this aspect of care. The abnormal viscid secretions in the lungs of these children are a continual process which results in bronchial obstruction and requires vigorous measures. Normal cleaning mechanism by which dust and bacteria are removed is impaired. Accumulation and stagnation of secretions results in chronic bronchial and bronchiolar infection; partial bronchial obstruction, producing patchy emphysema; and complete bronchial obstruction, producing atelectasis (Fig. 8 and 9).

As a result of infection, pulmonary obstruction is increased and further impairs the normal cleansing mechanism. This creates a vicious circle (Fig. 10). The purpose of therapy is to liquify the secretions and to promote and maintain pulmonary drainage. Methods which will be discussed include: aerosal treatment, mist tents, postural drainage, and breathing exercises.

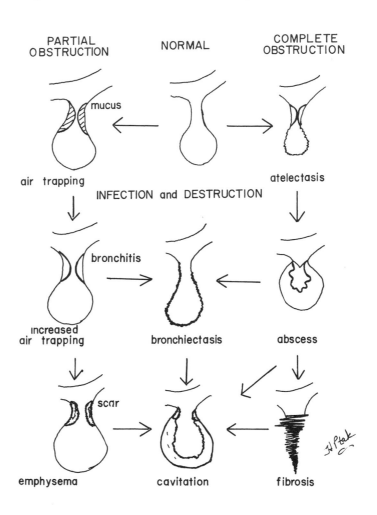

FIG. 9.   Pathologic physiology of cystic fibrosis.

THE VICIOUS CIRCLE OF CYSTIC FIBROSIS

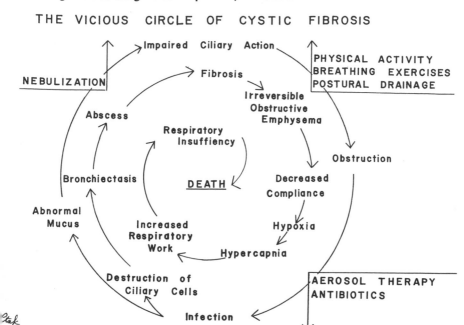

IT CAN BE BROKEN

FIG. 10. Infection creates further pulmonary obstruction (a vicious cycle).

THERAPEUTIC MEASURES

BRONCHOPULMONARY HYGIENE. Nebulization therapy is utilized to wet and thin respiratory mucous secretions and to disperse the appropriate agent, such as bronchodilators, antibiotics, or mucolytic agents onto the mucous membranes of the tracheobronchial tree. The aim of nebulization therapy is the provision of particles of water, or of water-containing medication, for deposition in the respiratory tract at the site of the disease process. The size of the particles deposited is determined by the nebulizer used as well as the solution and humidity of the air used for nebulization to provide the mist. In order to produce very fine particles for the smaller bronchioles, 10% propylene glycol may be used in order to reduce vapor tension of the nebulized solution. It is important that an adequate amount of water or medication is inhaled and deposited for the treatment to be effective. The child should be encouraged to breathe slower and deeper so more deposition can take place. Compressed air rather than oxygen is usually used with a croupette or standard oxygen tent. Cooling measures assist in maintaining the tent temperature under 80°.

MIST TENT. Mist tent therapy is used to provide longer periods to thin tracheobronchial secretions. Many physicians who have had considerable experience with treatment of patients with cystic fibrosis, now begin mist therapy as early as possible, regardless of absence of pulmonary symptoms, for prophylactic reasons. The tent is utilized during sleeping hours. This applies to the adult as well as the infant or child.

Equipment consists of a croupette or regular oxygen tent and nebulizers powered with compressed, filtered air from a portable compressor or from a cylinder of oxygen. The mist should be dense so that it is difficult to see the individual in the tent. The ultrasonic type nebulizer is used for the child when the solution must be provided to the periphery of the lungs (Fig. 11). The type of solution used will depend on the type of nebulizer and the patient.

When the mist tent is used therapeutically rather than prophylactically, it is ordered during the initial hospitalization to provide intensive therapy or for subsequent acute flare-ups. The patient will remain in the tent for the majority of the 24-hr period (Fig. 12).

When the therapy is first instituted, the nurse must remember that large amounts of thinned secretions may be evident and intense bronchial drainage must be provided. Careful and frequent observation should be provided by the nursing staff. Suction may be required. The length of continuous therapy will depend on signs of response to treatment. It may be as long as 10 to 14 days.

INTERMITTENT AEROSOL THERAPY. A face mask or plastic mouthpiece is the type of equipment used with a nebulizer for intermittent aerosol therapy. It provides administration of small quantities of prescribed solution than the mist tent. Some children will use intermittent therapy in the day time and the mist tent at night.

For the infant or young child, holding the child on your lap with the face mask held near the face provides for an effective treatment. Distractions through use of a toy or making a game of applying the mask gains the cooperation of the toddler. The acutely ill child may remain in bed with the use of the nebulizer attached to the croupette or tent. Positioning of the infant is most important. He should be placed on his side as well as alternating elevating and lowering the head of the crib.

POSTURAL DRAINAGE. Postural drainage is utilized with inhalation therapy to promote hygiene for tracheobronchial tree. Techniques used are not complicated and should be learned by the nursing staff, whether hospital- or community-based, and the family. The physical therapist, today, is usually responsible for this function and he is an important member of the health team. The staff nurse may need to provide therapy during part of the 24-hr period when the therapist is not available. The community health nurse will need to evaluate the program in the home. A referral may be indicated to the physical therapist upon return to the clinic.

The various positions utilized will be determined by the area of the lung involved (Fig. 13). One particular lobe is drained at a time. Clapping or vibration of the chest wall is carried out during expiration,

FIG. 11. DeVilbiss ultrasonic nebulizer designed specifically for home mist tent therapy. (Courtesy of DeVilbiss Co., Somerset, Pa.)

while in the postural drainage position. The best time is usually before breakfast and before retiring. Each position is assumed for at least 2 min.

Rapid clapping is best carried out with cupped hands on the uppermost area. Air is trapped between the hand and the chest wall. At the same time, the patient is urged to exhale and cough to raise sputum.

FIG. 12.   DeVilbiss ultrasonic nebulizer with frame and canopy. (Courtesy of DeVilbiss Co., Somerset, Pa.)

Vibration through the hands follows this by tensing the upper area and shoulder muscles. Vibration is applied during slow exhalation with slight pressure over the area to be drained. Coughing and expectoration is again urged.

Practice in each of these techniques will provide skill. The therapist usually demonstrates it and the mother participates over a period of time until she feels comfortable in her performance. It is helpful if another member of the family can also be trained (Fig. 14).

The physical therapist will also teach the child and parent breathing exercises in order to increase expiration and strengthen the diaphragm for improved ventilation.

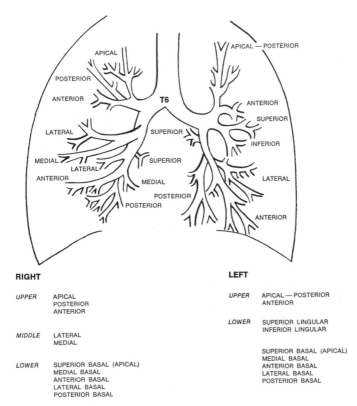

RIGHT

UPPER	APICAL
	POSTERIOR
	ANTERIOR
MIDDLE	LATERAL
	MEDIAL
LOWER	SUPERIOR BASAL (APICAL)
	MEDIAL BASAL
	ANTERIOR BASAL
	LATERAL BASAL
	POSTERIOR BASAL

LEFT

UPPER	APICAL — POSTERIOR
	ANTERIOR
LOWER	SUPERIOR LINGULAR
	INFERIOR LINGULAR
	SUPERIOR BASAL (APICAL)
	MEDIAL BASAL
	ANTERIOR BASAL
	LATERAL BASAL
	POSTERIOR BASAL

FIG. 13. Segments of the bronchial tree. (Courtesy of The Children's Orthopedic Hospital and Medical Center, Seattle, Washington.)

GENERAL MANAGEMENT. Infants receive low-fat, high-protein formulas. Soybean protein is not absorbed so well as protein in cow's milk and is not used in cystic fibrosis. The dietary management for older children includes high-protein diet, high-caloric snacks, and moderate restriction of fatty foods. Although undigested fat and proteins as well as calcium and fat-soluble vitamins are lost with the stool, the voracious appetite of these patients lends to a large intake of food, so that absorption of as little as 50 percent of the ingested material may be adequate for satisfactory nutrition.

When enzyme preparations are instituted, the voracious appetite declines. During respiratory infections, anorexia is often present. Pancreatic extract is administered in granular or tablet form when the food is eaten. The dosage is adjusted according to the appearance of the stools; for example, unformed bulky, floating stools indicate more pancreatin is necessary. If excessive pancreatin is administered, anorexia and constipation may result. Skim milk is often advised until later childhood. Adolescents require less dietary restrictions as a whole.

FIG. 14. Instruction sheets provide aid in teaching parents procedures to be done at home. Part 1. (Courtesy of the Children's Orthopedic Hospital and Medical Center, Seattle, Washington); Part II, [Lower Lobes]. (Adapted from design and material by Eloise Draper, LPT., available from Pediatric Department of University of Louisville Medical School, Louisville, Kentucky.)

Fat-soluble vitamins in water-miscible base are required so that absorption can take place.

In hot weather it may be necessary to add extra salt to the diet. In emergency, saline solution may need to be administered intravenously.

Antibiotics are ordered by some physicians for treatment of a specific organism involved in an infection. Some authorities prefer intermittent intensive therapy. There is agreement that respiratory infections should be treated adequately and long enough to be effective.

An expectorant, such as saturated solution of potassium iodide,

LOWER LOBES

SUPERIOR SEGMENTS

LEFT LOWER
LOBE

RIGHT LOWER
LOBE

BED LEVEL, LYING FACE DOWN WITH PILLOW UNDER STOMACH, CLAP
AND VIBRATE JUST BELOW THE SHOULDER BLADES.

BASAL SEGMENTS

ANTERIOR
RIGHT AND LEFT LOWER LOBES

POSTERIOR
RIGHT AND LEFT LOWER LOBES

LYING ON BACK WITH PILLOW UNDER
KNEES, CLAP AND VIBRATE OVER LOWER
RIBS.

LYING FACE DOWN, CLAP AND VIBRATE
OVER LOWER RIBS.

LATERAL

LEFT LOWER
LOBE

RIGHT LOWER
LOBE

LYING ON RIGHT SIDE, CLAP AND VIBRATE
OVER LOWER RIBS.

LYING ON LEFT SIDE, CLAP AND VIBRATE
OVER LOWER RIBS.

PLACE ARMS AND LEGS IN COMFORTABLE POSITIONS.

PROCEDURE FOR POSTURAL DRAINAGE

1. CLAP ABOUT A MINUTE IN EACH POSITION
2. VIBRATE DURING 5 EXHALATIONS; REST ON INHALATIONS
3. COUGH
4. REPEAT PROCEDURE IF SO ADVISED BY DOCTOR
5. DO 3 TIMES A DAY (UNLESS OTHERWISE ORDERED BY DOCTOR)
   A. MORNING — BEFORE BREAKFAST — DO UPPER, RIGHT, MIDDLE,
      AND LEFT LINGULA LOBES.
   B. MID-DAY — BEFORE LUNCH OR AFTER SCHOOL — DO RIGHT MIDDLE,
      LEFT LINGULA, AND LOWER LOBES.
   C. EVENING — BEFORE DINNER OR BEFORE BED — DO UPPER AND LOWER LOBES.

FIG. 14 (cont.). Instruction sheets provide aid in teaching parents procedures to be done at home. Part II. (Adapted from design and material by Eloise Draper, LPT.; available from Pediatrics Department, University of Louisville Medical School, Louisville, Kentucky.)

may be ordered. Codeine and similar cough suppressants are counter-indicated.

Oxygen therapy is used with discretion. It may be required for hypoxia. If used with mist tent, concentration should be less than 40 percent and blood gases monitored.

PROBLEMS FOR THE FAMILY

What does the diagnosis of cystic fibrosis mean to the family? In the family in which this is the first case, it may be overwhelming or it may mean very little at first. The reaction will be dependent on their exposure to information through television, radio, newspapers, magazines, yearly drives to assist handicapped children, or experience with a child of a neighbor, friend, or relative with the disease.

For the family who does not realize the impact of the disease, the nurse will need to expect questions and concerns after the physician has talked with the family and after they have read about the disease or talked with relatives or friends.

For the nurse to appreciate the meaning of this illness to the family, one would have to consider the following:

1. *Present mortality statistics.* If this child is diagnosed early and medical care and a health team are available for supervision and management, the outlook is brighter.

2. *Effect of child's therapy on routine of the household.* Learning what is involved in the treatments and acquiring skill in preventing or treating bronchopulmonary obstruction is necessary. Clapping and vibration is usually carried out four times a day before each meal and at bed time. For a mother with other children this is very demanding on her time and it affects household routine. This is only one aspect of the therapy that is time-consuming for her; it requires a great deal of energy and patience.

3. *Need for special or improvised equipment in the home.* The family must know how to maintain it and where to have it repaired.

4. *Effect on sleeping arrangements.* If space is limited, the mist tent and compressor may present special problems.

5. *Sleep disturbance for other family members.* This may particularly affect the mother who may listen for the cough or sleep lightly in order to hear the child if he calls.

6. *Effect on visitors in the home.* Whether it is relatives, neighbors, peers of the other siblings, or friends of the child involved, concern will be present in relation to problem of infection. Respiratory infections, pertussis, and measles in particular can prove very serious for the child with cystic fibrosis. The mother may need assistance so that visitors are not eliminated entirely. Stools are foul-smelling and incontinence may occur. Suggestions which will assist in control of odor of stools include: changing the infant's or toddler's diaper as soon after defecation as feasible; the use of a product available on the market for deodorizing the bathroom. Solutions are available to use in the water tank of the toilet which are automatically dispensed after flushing, for control of odor.

7. *Effect on family outings.* This may involve visiting relatives, weekend excursions, or yearly vacation plans. Now special equipment may need to be transported or planning ahead to know which city has a pediatrician or facilities available if needed in an emergency. In many instances, the family may eliminate these trips due to expense.

8. *Effect on husband-wife relations.* Concern over hereditary

aspects, possible future pregnancies, as well as family budget may occur.

9. *Willingness to accept financial assistance.* Assistance may be necessary from welfare or state aid, if necessary, for special diet, cost of medicines, and equipment. One should consider the family's ability to accept services from the local chapter of the Cystic Fibrosis Research Foundation, if available in their community, or to acquire such services if in a small town.

10. *Problem of travel.* If medical facilities and special clinic are at a long distance from home, travel for the parents and obtaining a babysitter for other siblings can impose additional burdens.

11. *Problem of finding a babysitter.* They will need a babysitter who can manage the child and be trusted to make the right judgment so that parents can have an evening out together.

Perhaps this is only the beginning of the list, and you could add many more items.

Some points to remember in assisting the family from the beginning to begin to cope with these factors:

1. *Each member of the health team has a contribution to make.* Each should be alert for cues about denial or acceptance of the disease. The clergyman may have an important role in assisting the family in terms of concern over mortality or guilt in relation to heredity.

2. *Education and preparation for discharge begins early after admission.* Begin slowly, provide demonstration and repetition. Continue presence of a skillful person at hand to take over in the beginning when necessary until parents are confident that they understand the regimen. The personality of each parent may determine the best approach.

3. *A home visit by the nurse from the clinic or the community health nurse to assist in transition from hospital to home.* It is becoming a more frequent practice for the community health nurse to come to the hospital prior to home visit to meet the child and to review the needs of the child and plan of care. Information should be shared with her to assist in planning.

4. *Listening carefully to the parents to identify cues that will furnish insight to areas that need further discussion.* For example, if the mother will tend to be oversolicitous, or if concern over the acquisition of infection is going to create a crisis in the household.

5. *Knowledge of community facilities and services available to family.* The nurse may need to refer the parents to the social worker or may acquire information needed from the social service agency and handle the problem herself. Another example is knowledge of some babysitting service often provided by nursing students or college students so that parents may have an evening out.

6. *Keep channels of communication open between members of the health team.* This is necessary so that needs of the child and family

are being met to the extent possible. Parents may need assistance with other siblings. It has been observed that parents often are unwilling or unable to discuss the implications of cystic fibrosis or the disease itself with other children. Behavior problems can result due to emphasis on needs of the affected child.

PROBLEMS FOR THE CHILD

The age of onset as well as the degree of pulmonary involvement will affect the problems for the child and his ability to cope with this chronic disease.

Considerations and activities that should be included in nursing care plan in the hospital or the home are:

1. *Provision of good oral hygiene.* Saliva is more salty. With expectoration after postural drainage, oral care will provide comfort. Teeth may also become discolored from antibiotics and current studies on this matter are being carried out in dental schools.

2. *Help the child accept the need for medications.* Make them palatable when possible. Explain the purpose of each, if the child can understand. Use dolls for demonstration of the injection or the use of the space mask for inhalation if he is a preschooler. Iodides are more palatable if administered in grape or orange juice or a cola drink.

3. *Sites for injections are always rotated.* This is most important due to wasted gluteal muscles and decreased amount of adipose tissue.

4. *Anorexia may be a sign of depression.* This should be assessed carefully. History of likes and dislikes can provide some choice within the limitations of the diet. Eating with a group in the playroom may aid appetite. Effect of medications on appetite may need to be evaluated.

5. *Weight loss.* Weight loss and increased anterior-posterior diameter of the chest is a clue to progress of the disease.

6. *Odor of stools.* This should be combatted so that patients or other visitors do not make comments that would offend or embarrass the child and his family. Staff should air the room and request housekeeping to provide a deodorizer. Aerosols or special deodorant products are available on the market that are effective for the household. In case of an infant or toddler, change the diaper as soon after the stool as possible. Care of the skin in the diaper area is important. Ointments should be applied as indicated. Bony prominences may need protection.

7. *Temperature.* If the temperature of the room is lower at night, the mist tent is more comfortable. Hyperthermia can result from the use of a mist tent in a hot room.

8. *Shampoo is required frequently due to mist tent.* The hair becomes sticky from various aerosols.

9. *Increased oral fluid intake.* This acts as an expectorant and should be included in the plan as a very simple tool to improve respiratory problem.

10. *Repeating instructions.* When instructing the child, keep in mind the short attention span of the younger age group. Repeat instructions to the child about breathing and coughing with a rhythmic approach.

11. *Use of word games or funny stories.* This makes the time seem shorter for the child during therapy for bronchopulmonary hygiene. Games for two, such as Old Maid or Parcheesi, are fun. Laughter helps the child breathe more deeply. Wind instruments are also effective.

12. *Sommersaults, hand stands, tumbling.* These activities are appropriate to provide pulmonary drainage and are more attractive to the young child. In the hospital, a bicycle or work-out on a mat in the playroom or in physical therapy will provide needed activity for the child. Running and swimming are allowed as tolerated.

When the child returns to school, the teacher will need to understand the nature of the child's problem, the reason for his cough, and the problem of exposure to infections. If the cough is severe in the morning at home, the child may be absent until noon. Chill should be avoided. If there is a fire drill, a coat should be available. Outdoor clothing should be put on just prior to leaving school to prevent overheating and perspiration. The nurse in the school or community can serve as liaison between home and school.

It should be pointed out to the teacher that physical activity is an important aid to preventing the accumulation of secretions in the lungs. Running and active play are more effective in raising sputum than any other form of therapy. Activity should be encouraged during recess period. If a large amount of mucus is present and coughing is severe, the child can be positioned on a straight chair which has been turned upside down and padded so that the child's head is lowered. A tilt board in the gymnasium is also effective. A supply of tissues and paper cups for expectoration of sputum should be available. The child should remain at home when coughing is excessive so that therapy can be evaluated.

The developmental needs of the child should be considered whether one is dealing with an infant, toddler, school-ager, or adolescent. Physical, mental, emotional, and social needs must be considered. Hobbies that will promote satisfaction within the limitations imposed by the disease will meet an important need. Music through use of records provides pleasure for many age groups.

Information about the Cystic Fibrosis Foundation should be provided. Through the local chapter of the Foundation, parents will have an opportunity to meet with parents of children with the same problem as well as to receive information about the disease and research being conducted.

A mother at one of the local meetings suggested that percussion and postural drainage be accompanied by music from a record player or radio. The rhythmic beat made the activity less tiring. Another suggestion for the older girl who is embarrassed when her friends ask her about the mist tent consists of using a four-poster bed with a canopy and draping long sheets of plastic to provide a tent.

Follow-up clinics for patients with cystic fibrosis provide the family with an opportunity to discuss problems with members of the health team as well as the reassessment of the therapy.

These clinics also provide a source for teaching for students in the health field.

Treatment continues over an indefinite period and encouragement and support must be provided.

A Home Care Evaluation sheet (See Appendix IV) provides a method of recording pertinent information so that the therapeutic plan can be studied and modified if necessary at the next clinic visit. This would be used after return to home after the first hospitalization or it may also be requested if the child was having recurring respiratory and gastrointestinal problems. There is hope for even greater improvement in the outlook for cystic fibrosis patients as the diagnosis is made earlier and effective treatment instituted. Continued research may also furnish new information for more effective management.

Case Presentation and Study Questions

Barbara, 10 years old, was admitted with status asthmaticus. Dyspnea, coughing, and wheezing were evident. Her orders included: arterial blood gases, correction of acid-base balance, steroid therapy, oxygen, and Isuprel by nebulizer.

Barbara has been hospitalized previously on this same unit.

Consider the following questions in providing nursing care for Barbara:

1. What are some of the immediate actions of the nurse upon Barbara's admission?
2. What considerations should be given the immediate environment in Barbara's hospital room?
3. What types of play activity would be appropriate to provide after recovery from the acute stage?
4. What might the psychological effects be of prolonged steroid therapy on a 10-year-old?

References

Ad Hoc Committee on Chemoprophylaxsis. Amer. Rev. Resp. Dis., 96:31, 1967.

Anderson, C. M. Long term study of patients with cystic fibrosis. Mod. Probl. Pediat., 10:344, 1967.

Barnett, H. L. Pediatrics, 14th ed. New York, Appleton-Century-Crofts, 1968.

Caplin, I. The Allergic Asthmatic. Springfield, Charles C Thomas, 1968.
Di Sant' Agnese, P. A. Clinical findings and research in cystic fibrosis. Mod. Probl. Pediat., 10:10, 1967.
Falliers, C. When to hospitalize the child with asthma. Hosp. Pract., 3:24, June 1968.
Fontana, V. J. Practical Management of the Allergic Child. New York, Appleton-Century-Crofts, 1969.
Gallagher, J. R. Medical Care of the Adolescent, 2nd ed. New York, Appleton-Century-Crofts, 1966.
Holschaw, D. S. Common pulmonary complications of cystic fibrosis. Clin. Pediat., 9:346, 1970.
Horesh, A. J. Allergy and infection. J. Asthma Res., 6:147, 1969.
Horowitz, L. Chronic obstructive bronchopulmonary disease in children with asthma. J. Asthma Res., 6: 211, 1969.
Johnson, M. E., and Fassett, B. A. Bronchopulmonary hygiene in cystic fibrosis. Amer. J. Nurs., 69:320, 1969.
Kendig, E. L. Disorders of the Respiratory Tract in Children. Philadelphia, Saunders, 1968.
Kershaw, J. Handicapped Children. Birkenhead, Willmer Brothers Limited, 1966.
Matthews, L. W., and Doershuk, C. F. Inhalation therapy and postural drainage for the treatment of cystic fibrosis. Mod. Probl. Pediat., 10:297, 1967.
National Research Foundation, Professional Education Committee. Guide to Diagnosis and Management of Cystic Fibrosis. (A Syllabus for Physicians.) New York, The Foundation, 1963.
Nelson, W. E. Textbook of Pediatrics, 8th ed. Philadelphia, Saunders, 1964.
Tempel, C. W. Tuberculosis prevention: the child-centered program. Amer. Family Physician, 14:69, 1968.
Rapaport, H. G. An allergist looks at chronic disease. J. Asthma Res., 7:3, 1969.
Wohl, T. Current concepts of the asthmatic child's adjustment and adaptation to institutional care. J. Asthma Res. 7:41, 1969.
Young, W. F., and Jackson, A. D. M. The prognosis of cystic fibrosis. Mod. Probl. Pediat., 10:350, 1967.

8 DOROTHY HOEHNE

The Child with Scoliosis: Nursing Intervention

Scoliosis is a complex deformity for which there is a considerable diversity of opinion about applicable terminology, associated descriptive classifications, and methods for therapy.

Although scoliosis is defined as a lateral curvature of the spine, the deviation is identified in relation to the side of the convexity and in accordance with the spinal segments involved. Curval divergence from the midline may be localized to short segments or it may involve the entire spine. Abnormal increase in the anterior-posterior spinal curves is termed either kyphotic or lordotic, depending upon the direction of the convexity (Fig. 1A and B). A variety of patterns exists and the curvature is usually accompanied by vertebral rotation toward the convexity. There are two main classifications—functional and structural—each with a number of broad differentiating categories. For the sake of continuity, specifics will be identified for each differentiated category. However, the primary emphasis of this presentation will be related to the idiopathic form of structural scoliosis.

Functional Scoliosis

In functional scoliosis, also known as nonstructural, postural, or nonprogressive, "there is no underlying organic disease within the spine itself and characteristically it is actively correctable by the individual who has it" (Lowell et al., 1965). Conditions outside the spine which cause temporary vertebral malalignment are abnormalities of the lower extremities with resultant inequality of leg length, as well as muscular tension, ocular defects, and faulty posture. The curve takes the form of the letter "C" and is described by some as compensatory

FIG. 1A. Anterior convexity, cervical and lumbar areas—*lordosis* Posterior convexity, thoracic and sacral areas—*kyphosis*. B. Normal spine—posterior. C. Functional scoliosis "C" curve seconday to a short left leg and pelvic tilt D. Structural scoliosis; "S" curve.

(James, 1967) or secondary (Morgan, 1967a) functional scoliosis (Fig. 1C).

Shortening of an extremity creates a pelvic tilt that usually involves the entire mobile portion of the spine in a gently curving arc as the individual attempts to maintain head and trunk balance. With the individual standing, lifts placed under the affected extremity will cause the curve to disappear. Disappearance is also noted when the individual sits or is supine. Treatment consists of constructing special shoes to increase the height of the affected limb. In gross discrepancies, surgical correction may be indicated.

Since the iliopsoas muscle is affixed to the spine, pelvis, and femur, it not only serves to maintain upright stabilization but it also provides for movement associated with pelvic flexion and femoral flexion, external rotation, and adduction. A unilaterally short, tense, or contracted iliopsoas causes abnormal tension and the compensatory lumbar curve results in an altered gait and faulty posture (Fig. 2A and 2B). Range-of-motion examinations reveal limitation of movement and associated patient discomfort. X-ray film comparisons depict the

FIG. 2A. Psoatic limp, external rotation, flexion, and adduction of hip on affected side. B. Psoatic gait, unilateral to indicate external rotation.

A

B

decrease in curvature that occurs when the child or adolescent transfers from the erect to the supine with thighs-flexed position. Treatment consists of exercises that stretch the involved muscles.

Keiser (1967) includes ocular defects in his categorization of nonstructural etiologies, but further information is lacking. Orthopedic surgeons have mentioned that a "blind spot" will cause an individual to tilt or lean to avoid this disturbance in visual acuity. As a consequence, the assumed posture leads to spinal deviation.

Retention of faulty posture assumed in utero infrequently contributes to the presence of a congenital "C" curve. Compensatory curves are nonexistent at this point since developmentally the individual has not attained the sitting or erect position. The normal structures are flexible and thus overcorrection is the method for resumption of normal alignment.

In relation to faulty posture, there is a difference of opinion regarding the approach for management. The slouching or slumping seen primarily in female adolescents, usually resulting in a mild left convexity, is considered correctable by conscious control and improvement of posture and body mechanics. Morgan (1967b) advocates the use of physiotherapy with emphasis on posterior spinal exercises until adequate muscle tonicity is attained for the maintenance of correct posture. Although James (1967), Morgan (1967a), and Lowell et al. (1965) agree that there is no evidence to support or suggest that the curvature resulting from faculty posture does not develop into a structural deformity, James (1967) indicates that the transitory condition disappears with or without treatment. Until such time as structural changes are detected, it is unjust to restrict a child's activity and create undue parental anxiety. The child would suffer from unwarranted restriction and the parents would endure added expense.

Another category is reflex or sciatic scoliosis that most commonly involves the lumbar area, when an individual attempts to avoid the pain associated with forward slipping of all or part of one vertebra on another, or "spondylolisthesis." Although the cause and natural history of this condition in children is not clearly defined, it appears that spondylolisthesis is an inherited predisposition to a developmental vertebral dysplasia. This can be attributed to the condition's tendency to occur in families and the correspondent progressive increase in incidence with age until late adolescence.

An occasional condition in childhood, it is characteristically without symptoms. But there are definite physical signs, since the child eases the pressure on the nerve root by leaning over to the extent that all or almost all pain is alleviated. Limitation of straight leg raising and forward spinal flexion point to the lesion in the lumbar area. Lateral x-rays will show the lumbar abnormality. Early surgical exploration and stabilization is advocated.

It would be misleading to confine spondylolisthesis to one category because it is associated with structural deformation and can be found under several classifications depending upon the author's placing it with associated contributing conditions. Wiltse (1969) provides the reader with an inclusive compilation of the various types, classified in accordance with the etiology. Although the causes serve as a base, Wiltse explains the possible reasons for elusive etiologies.

The characteristic posture ascribed to sciatic scoliosis is also noted in persons with lumbosacral or sacroiliac joint inflammation or a prolapsed disc. Although orthopedic physicians disagree with James (1967) when he indicates that the latter is not an uncommon condition in childhood, the possibility of its presence should not be overlooked. Another point here is that incidence figures vary in accordance with geographical location. This frequency differential between North America and Great Britain remains unexplained. In any event, treatment is directed at the primary cause.

Structural Scoliosis

As mentioned previously, the second main classification is structural scoliosis. It is frequently referred to as progressive or fixed because voluntary correction is impossible and the condition leads to permanent anatomic changes unless preventive measures are taken. Generally, the deformity assumes the shape of the letter "S" (Fig. 1D) as compensatory or secondary curves develop above and below the primary curve in the individual's attempt to maintain balance. If these secondary curves neutralize the lateral displacement caused by the primary curve, compensation is achieved because the occiput remains in a line directly over the sacrum and an erect posture is maintained. On the other hand, if curval compensation is inadequate, decompensation exists when the head is no longer centered over the sacrum. If the secondary curves are more than sufficient, the primary curve is overcompensated. With lateral progression, there is vertebral wedging, angulation, rotation, and thoracic cage deformity. Rib protrusion on the convex side is the most deforming component of thoracic curves. As lumbar curves lack rib involvement, they are less deforming.

Associated changes resulting from scoliotic deformities are reflected in anatomical alterations which affect the individual's vital functions and appearance. In analyses of the established curval patterns, progression has been attributed to gravitational activity and secondary growth disturbances. The curval deviations alter normal muscular action to the extent that reciprocal muscular and/or gravitational opposition is lacking. An altered center of gravity contributes to excessive pressure exerted upon the curval concavity with a consequent diminution of vertebral growth in this area. The time element is crucial, since these forces influence developing curvatures until maturity.

Structural scoliosis occurs as a result of congenital spinal defects and as a manifestation of an established pathological condition. In addition, the etiology associated with the greatest number of structural deformities—idiopathic—remains obscure.

CONGENITAL FACTORS

Anomalous spinal development results from congenital vertebral wedging, vertebral fusion, vertebral absence, and most frequently hemivertebral formations, occasionally compensated by the existence of other hemivertebra facing in the opposite direction. (Fig. 3A, B, C, and D). These deformities can occur alone or in combination to the extent that a single outstanding defect is unidentifiable. As growth progresses, the deformity may become more prominent. Since there are no set surve patterns (Goldstein, 1964), irregularities are identified and categorized in accordance with the extent and level of involved segments, with or without fixed pelvic obliquity. This approach aids in therapeutic evaluation and provides for greater prognostic value.

Early surgical intervention is necessary to prevent disabling deformity associated with an undifferentiated vertebral fusion and pelvic obliquity. Vertebral fusion may be symmetrical (Fig. 3B), but when it is asymmetrical, it is referred to as an unsegmented, unilateral, or bony bar (Fig. 3E). This includes several vertebrae, and involves the

FIG. 3. Vertebral bony anomalies. A. Vertebral wedging—partial unilateral failure; B. Vertebral fusion—symmetrical failure; C. Hemivertebra—complete unilateral failure; D. Double hemivertebra—balanced; E and F. Unsegmented bar—asymmetrical fusion failure; posterior spinal
elements only; G. Unsegmented bar; asymmetrical fusion failure; disc area and posterior spinal
elements.

posterior spinal elements, the disc area, or both (Fig. 3F and G).
As this posterolateral bar replaces the normal pedicle and the laminar
structures (Goldstein, 1964), the area lacks growth potential and
rapidly creates a severe lateral angulation and/or increased anterior-
posterior curve in which the convexity is directed anteriorly. There is
a literal "backward bend," and rapid progression is noted—particularly
during the growth spurts. Roentgenographic oblique views often intensify the appearance of the bar, but laminography is superior in
determining the structural defects.

On the other hand, anterior vertebral fusions or absent vertebrae
usually create angular deviations and/or exaggerate the normal anterior-
posterior curves in which the convexity is directed posteriorly (kyphosis).

When the convexity increases in severity, the cord can become stretched over its apex and paresis results. Fortunately, this grave complication is an uncommon occurrence. This can be attributed to early recognition and correction with the consequent avoidance of serious difficulties.

Pelvic obliquity may be fixed or nonfixed. Fixed pelvic obliquity, with elevation of the pelvis into the curve concavity, occurs because of sacral or lower lumbar vertical involvement with rigidity or an insufficient number of vertebrae involved to provide for compensation. Since the obliquity is an integral part of the scoliotic deformity, simultaneous correction via fusion to include the sacrum is accomplished to prevent recurrence. With this type of correction, the individual is taught hip motion and the squatting position to maintain fusion integrity and spinal alignment. The nonfixed type may be secondary to a hip flexion contraction, which may be treated separately. It is important to note at this point that there is a difference between pelvic "obliquity" and pelvic "tilt." The former term refers to the presence of a fixed deformity while the latter serves to describe nonstructural involvement.

Rib deformities, rib absence, rib excess, or rib fusion almost always accompany the dorsal vertebral anomalies. These defects are usually on the curval concavity. If fusion occurs, its location is of significance if it is next to and continuous with the vertebrae. The osseous mass is usually associated with an unsegmented bar (Lowell et al., 1965; MacEwen et al., 1968). It has been reported that congenitally rare rib fusion creates a scoliotic deformity by acting as a restraint or "tether" (MacEwen et al., 1967) during the growth process. However, contrary to the advised method for correction, excision of the fused area does not arrest curval deterioration and it may only minutely contribute to the corrective procedure (James, 1967). Therefore, further measures for therapy are indicated.

Congenital spinal and rib abnormalities are frequently associated with other anomalies involving the head, trunk, gastrointestinal or genitourinary systems, and extremities. Treatment is concurrent as warranted because required therapy for many of these associated defects does not interfere with the method for spinal defect correction.

As long as there is spinal growth, curve progression is anticipated. Problematic complexity exists because attention is directed at treating the present deformity as well as preventing further developmental disability. Since congenital curves are unpredictable as to progression, regardless of their apparent severity, close observation and follow-up is required to determine not only the appropriate measures for treatment but also the most suitable time for intervention. Roaf (1966, p. 53) indicates that "many curves remain comparatively mild up to the time of the pre-adolescent growth spurt and then become rapidly worse." Morgan (1967b) points to the increased need for recognizing curves that will lead to ultimate deformity as opposed to those that will remain benign. Prognostic variables are not only associated with curval patterns and rate of progression but also with the age at which deterioration starts and the specific etiology involved.

PATHOLOGICAL FACTORS

Causation has been linked to numerous pathological entities that also contribute to the secondary development of the scoliotic type deformities. Secondary occurrence is attributed to conditions within as well as outside the vertebral column. Although presentations by authorities varied concerning these illnesses, frequency was labeled as either occasional or rare because the disorders comprise a minute percentage of the structural curves. Therefore, adaptation of a practical etiological outline (as follows) best illustrates their presence.

> Neuropathic: Paralytic—post poliomyelitis
>   Syringomyelia
>   Neuofibromatosis (von Recklinghausen's disease)
>   Friedreich's ataxia
>   Cerebral palsy
>   Myelomeningocele
>   Charcot-Marie-Tooth neuropathy
>   Congenital absence of pain
>   Diastematomyelia
>   Spina bifida
>   Hysteria
>   Other nerve pathology
> Myopathic: Muscular dystrophies
>   Amyotonia congenita
>   Arthrogryposis multiplex congenita
>   Other muscle pathology
> Osteopathic: Osteogenesis imperfecta (fragilitas ossium)
>   Scheuermann's osteochondritis (adolescent kyphosis)
>   Eccentro-osteochondrodysplasia (Morquio's disease)
>   Thoracogenic
>   Postthoracoplasty
>   Postempyema
>   Other bone pathology
> Extrinsic: Marfan's syndrome (arachnodactyly)
>   Frame scoliosis
>   Postirradiation growth disturbances
>   Tumors
>   Congenital heart disease
>   Other pathological conditions

In the neuropathic group, consequent spinal deformation is principally associated with the neurological lesions seen in syringomyelia, neurofibromatosis, and Friedreich's ataxia. Paralytic curval development is influenced by the location of muscular imbalance and contractural asymmetry. Fixed pelvic obliquity due to myofascial contracture sometimes accompanies and accentuates these spinal deviations. The difficulty noted with paralytic scoliosis is that curval patterns can increase even after bony maturity is attained. The paralytic category was treated separately by some because production of trunkal muscular imbalance in most spinal deformities was a sequel to poliomyelitis. With the advent of immunological agents, the decreased appearance of residual deformities associated with polio, and the decline in incidence, the condition can be placed along with the other neuropathies.

In the rare myopathic group, scoliosis is usually due to the pseudohypertrophic form of muscular dystrophy. It is assumed that the defect is paralytic in origin and surgical intervention is considered when the breathing capacity becomes impaired. For further information regarding these illnesses and those in the aforementioned group, the reader is referred to Thomas (1968) and Cooke (1968).

In the osteopathic group, congenital vertebral bony anomalies were excluded because of previous consideration. Spinal deviations resulting from chest wall and pleuritic alterations have become a rarity since the introduction of antibiotic therapy and associated decrease in thoracic disease.

In the extrinsic group, James (1967) discusses most of the illnesses, but Marfan's syndrome appears under the heading of metabolic etiologies. However, discussion of the condition can be found in texts concerned with connective tissue disorders. Scoliosis occurs not only secondarily to tumor activity but also as a consequence of radical surgical intervention. In both situations, progressive spastic paraplegia can appear—in the former, as a result of cord compression from within and in the latter, being due to stretching of the cord over the apex of the developing curve.

The term "other" appears in each group; the etiological listing is by no means complete. However, it does demonstrate the enormity of the situation. In addition, recent evidence (James, 1967; Farkas, 1967; Thomas, 1968) indicates that scoliosis can occur in the adult; thus, these entities were excluded.

IDIOPATHIC SCOLIOSIS

The largest group, idiopathic, constitutes approximately 85 to 90 percent of the structural curves. Although the cause is unknown, as the name implies, proposed etiological theories include intrinsic as well as extrinsic possibilities. There is no doubt that idiopathic scoliosis is a familial condition (Wynne-Davies, 1968). Recent evidence (Cowell, 1970) indicates that the mode of inheritance is sex-linked dominant. To date, however, the research remains speculative since there is no conclusive evidence to support causation in an otherwise apparently healthy child.

Since the underlying cause remains obscure, analysis has led to the identification of single or double primary curval deformations that involve the thoracic and lumbar vertebrae. Identification is in relation to the anatomical location of the curval apex.

1. Thoracic—curve restricted to dorsal area.
2. Combined thoracic and lumbar—curves appear simul-

taneously and progress in a similar manner. There are
two forms:
(a) right thoracic—left lumbar
(b) right thoracic—left thoracolumbar.
3. Lumbar—curve restricted to lumbar area.

As previously indicated, compensatory balancing curves form after
the primary curve. These curves usually remain flexible, but they may
acquire structural characteristics to the extent that primary curve
identification becomes extremely difficult or impossible. When this
situation arises, the curves are termed major regardless of their
questionable sequential appearance and, thus, they require surgical
correction. However, surgical intervention is not required if secondary
curves retain their flexibility and/or involve little structural change,
since sufficient straightening with balance will occur after the primary
curve has been surgically corrected.

The coexistence of primary and secondary curves explains the
citations regarding three and four curve patterns. "A common primary
curve of the three-curve pattern is the right thoracic or the left thoracolumbar curvature. The classic four-curve pattern is the combined
thoracic and lumbar curve with equal angular deformities and structural
changes in both curves" (Goldstein, 1964). Each pattern exhibits varied
signs and has a tendency to arise during specific growth periods.

Since all age groups are involved, the growth periods have been
arbitrarily divided to indicate peak periods. The infantile period extends
from birth to the age of three, and the juvenile period has an onset
between the ages of five and eight but extends from age three to ten.
The adolescent period has an onset after the eleventh year and extends
to the end of skeletal growth.

Infantile Idiopathic Scoliosis. James (1967) describes two forms
of infantile idiopathic scoliosis, one benign and the other progressive.
The first resolves without treatment, while the second deteriorates and
requires immediate, aggressive therapy because the thorax can become
grossly deformed, with a consequent reduction in vital capacity.
Initially, it is difficult to differentiate between the two types. However,
time and close observation reveal that the benign thoracic curve exists
without compensation, and resolution occurs before the age of two with
complete disappearance before age five. The sequential change is that
the lateral deviation disappears first with a year or two passing before
complete rotational resolution. This possibly explains why, in some
children, there is the simultaneous occurrence of a minute lateral
curvature and persistent clinical and radiological rotation.

Both conditions have as a common feature a molding (plagio-
cephaly) of the head that spontaneously returns to normal. The face
looks smaller on the involved side and, although the child appears to
have torticollis, the muscle is normal. The disorder's presence is infrequent at birth and varies in severity, thus calling for astute observation for its appearance and the accompanying curve. Rib bulging on

the curval convexity indicating vertebral rotation is the first sign of the deformity. If the curvature remains evident when the infant is suspended by the arms, that position is used for anteroposterior roentgenograms for diagnostic confirmation.

On the average, the diagnosis is established at fifteen months; but a notable feature of the progressive form, and no other idiopathic curve, is the probable simultaneous occurrence of kyphosis with the scoliotic deformity. Kyphosis is difficult to evaluate owing to the extreme vertebral rotation noted on x-ray, for the anterior-posterior film frequently depicts a lateral vertebral view.

Roaf (1966) indicates that both forms are abiotrophic since it is thought that an intrinsic tissue weakness or defect is responsible, but growth brings about its appearance. He considers their differentiation largely artificial because many infants with the progressive form fail to thrive—having poor appetites, and in general, poor muscular and skeletal development. Other characteristic features that may accompany the progressive thoracic curve are a poorly developed mandible, small-lobed ears, and a small, sharp, poorly developed nose.

Transition from Infancy to Adolescence. In infantile idiopathic scoliosis, curval deterioration onset is related to the growth increments associated with sitting height and the middle years. As a result, anticipated progression includes ages ranging from two to four years and again between six and ten. In relation to the rest of the body, thoracic disproportion may be accompanied by a generalized failure of growth and development. Because there is a delay between the diagnosis and curval deterioration onset (five to six years) the outcome for some children with thoracic curves is less grave. The key factor here is time—time provided for thoracic development with the possible chance for little functional impairment at maturity in the presence of a severe curve. The juvenile group is considered small because nearly all the children have undergone corrective measures or have been receiving therapy from an earlier age. Since comparatively few curves occur during the middle growth period and most are considered extensions of the infantile group, some authorities view idiopathic scoliosis as having two periods: the infantile, with the predominant one occurring in adolescents.

Although Goldstein (1964) and James (1967) emphasize that infantile and juvenile curves have the worst prognosis because they are exposed to the total effects of growth, James specifies that the fixed curval location is the primary prognostic determinant. Fortunately, these curval patterns are relatively uncommon and comprise a small percentage of the idiopathic group.

A curious phenomenon exists in that infantile scoliosis, resulting in a left thoracic convexity, is found primarily in boys while the adolescent form produces a right thoracic convexity and has a predilection for girls. There is a gradual transition in sexual dominance with a slight peak change occurring during the juvenile period beyond the age of seven and a marked increase during adolescence. In a sense, the same holds true for the curval pattern. Delay of age of onset is accompanied by an increased frequency of right-sided thoracic curves. Since idiopathic scoliosis has a predominant onset during early adolescence, attention will be focused upon this age group.

Anatomical Alterations. Anatomical alterations call attention to the presence of idiopathic curval deformations. Pain is an unusual symptom, and its presence strongly suggests spinal tumor formation and/or a coexistent condition. Consequently, the unexpected and unexplained curval patterns are discovered during various rates of progression; the overt physical changes serving as a cause for referral.

Physical alterations are not always detected because the child and his parents become accustomed to his appearance. In addition, the subtleties associated with developing spinal deformations go unnoticed since teenagers are not inclined to disrobe before their elders. Usually, changes are brought to the family's attention by a friend or relative who has not seen the child for a period of time, or frequently the deformity is discovered during a routine physical examination by the family and/or school physician. Sometimes routine chest x-rays depict a curvature and this results in referral. Occasionally, curves are noticed during gymnasium classes or during beach outings.

If parents notice a physical change, it is in relation to alteration of attire. During shopping sprees they may note absence of uniformity due to uneven shoulder or hip levels, and/or a disparity in sleeve and trouser length or hem line. The mother may experience difficulty in making clothes or altering clothes for the same reasons. In some instances, the child or a dressmaker calls the condition to the parents' attention—the child out of frustration in trying to deal with the situation and a dressmaker in making an alteration to conform with the youngster's stature. A mother who assists her daughter with buttoning or zipping a dress or blouse may detect a prominent scapula and experience difficulty with closure. On rare occasions, a mother notices that one breast appears larger, indicating the presence of a forward rib rotation on the concave and involved side. Or when laundering, she observes the unequal length in brassiere straps. At times, a parent may notice a physical deviation when his child is bathing.

Consultation. Observations and/or referrals lead to orthopedic consultation either at the physician's office or an out-patient facility. The diagnosis is made after careful scrutiny and elimination of possible other causes. Physical alterations are more noticeable in thin youngsters as opposed to those who are well-endowed. The deformity arises at a crucial time in life when an individual is self-conscious and becomes increasingly aware of the need to be attractive. It is quite disheartening to know that medical science does not have the answer. Therefore, as with any childhood illness, we should extend ourselves and truly indicate sincere assistance.

A complete and thorough history is invaluable in ascertaining the patient's life style and health status. When one talks with parents and/or teenagers, reference is sometimes made to parents' and/or relatives' disability and/or previous illness. Spinal deformation in family members has relevance for evaluating inheritance factors, but this requires careful scrutiny because the incidence of other back deformities may serve to confuse the family. Also, motility contributes to the dearth or lack of knowledge concerning conditions in distant but related people. Also, previous illnesses may have no association with the present need for consultation.

On the other hand, records may reveal the presence of a condition that secondarily contributes to the development of a scoliotic deformity, particularly if the family cannot recall the specific condition. Former x-ray examinations, if any, will serve as determinants in evaluation. Sickness immediately preceding the physical changes should also be ascertained. Pinpointing the time of onset not only serves as a clue to a possible congenital defect or coexistent contributing condition, but it also provides the physician with information concerning the possible length of exposure and curval progression. More often than not, the youngster's history is negative, with no evidence of previous infectious processes or neuromuscular diseases.

In observing and talking with the youngster, the nurse can ascertain his growth and developmental level and discover his interests and concerns in relation to daily activities, as well as his view regarding the required referral. Knowledge regarding exposure to prolonged periods of sitting or standing suggests a change to relieve the stress imposed upon the spine. Habits of exercise and rest are reflected in participation in sports or more sedentary activities. These youngsters are noted for feeling chronically tired or experiencing periodic fatigue. However, it is only upon close questioning that they admit to decreased activity tolerance in comparison with their peers. Learning about the patient's activity level has implications for immediate guidance and future plans for meeting medical as well as individual needs.

The child's growth rate and general health is investigated. Some parents report that their child has progressed normally, while others indicate that growth has been rapidly excessive or delayed. Comments concerning their child's physical stature center upon his tendency to be thin, anemic, or obese. The stage of secondary sexual developmental characteristics serve as a rough guide in relation to skeletal maturity. After menarche, the age at which menstruation began, its regularity, and span should also be ascertained. "Occasionally, one fact of note is that the patient may have been somewhat late in menarche, and irregular menses are a relatively frequent finding" (Nelson and Harrington, 1967). The physician utilizes this information for diagnostic inclusion and may diagramatically plot the individual's height and weight on a predetermined scale to confirm developmental expectations and identify deviations from the norm.

Harrington (1968) strongly recommends that the wearing of glasses be noted, as he observed that visual impairment arose six months to one year before the onset of idiopathic involvement that proved to be quite severe. How visual acuity relates to the total situation remains obscure, but Harrington thinks it may conceivably serve as a significant determinant for future involvement.

Dietary intake is not to be overlooked for indiscretions take place during this time in the teenager's attempt to meet society's emphasis on physical appearance and peer acceptance. Not all teenagers are guilty in this respect, but listening to their dietary pattern gives the nurse an idea of their understanding of nutrition and possible lack of proper intake. Remember, it is quality, not quantity. A mother, guardian, and in some instances a father, will supply information concerning the child's eating habits by specifying likes or dislikes and/or by describing extremes in appetite. Family meals will reveal cultural patterns and possibly a need for parental assistance in planning. Planning may be related not only to ingredients but also to economics. Mothers frequently allude to this need, thus the nurse must be attuned to such verbal clues.

Parental-child interaction serves as a guide for establishing anticipated participation, but the first meeting is by no means conclusive. Reservation in judgment is called for and extenuating circumstances as well as fear may have influenced all those concerned. Peer relationships serve as another factor for immediate and future consideration, but this is often revealed during talks with the child and observation of his response to others.

Much of the information obtained can be explored and/or judgments substantiated at a later time, but the nurse can be selective regarding initial data that will aid the physician in establishing a diagnosis. A general "feel" of the situation is called for and conversation, although directed, should proceed in accordance with the parents' and/or child's pace. During visits, constructive use of time is not put to full advantage if other health-team members are not contacted at appropriate times regarding information obtained, established patient and family needs, and accomplished plans. Effective communication cannot be overemphasized.

THE ORTHOPEDIC EXAMINATION

When you are preparing the child and family for the orthopedic physical examination, include the fact that routine roentgenograms follow it to verify the physician's findings, to depict coexistent contributing conditions, and to determine the degree of curvature. Photographs are also taken to provide an objective record for the described alterations and for comparative evaluation with photos taken during and after treatment. It is important to indicate that the child will have to disrobe, with the exception of briefs, because complete visualization is necessary for accurate evaluation of curval presence and accompanying anatomic alterations. Consideration for patient privacy preceding, during (via proper gowning and draping), and following the examination is important because extreme sensitivity characterizes this age group.

GENERAL ASPECTS

Initially the examination is general, consisting of recorded and described observations related to postural alignment and asymmetry during weight bearing (Fig. 4A, B, C, and D). In some instances, a vertical (plumb) line from the patient's occiput or seventh cervical or first thoracic vertebra is extended to lie between the internal maleoli through the buttocks cleft to reveal the amount and location of lateral deviation. A plumb line may be used in a side view, extending full length from the shoulder apex to determine body weight distribution. The lateral view reveals any forward thrust of the head, as well as accentuation of normal spinal curves, rib deformations, and abdominal protrusion. An anterior view discloses chest and rib changes and any difference in breast position and size, while the posterior view reveals anatomical displacement and winging of the scapulae. Both views exhibit pelvic and shoulder girdle asymmetry along with alterations in

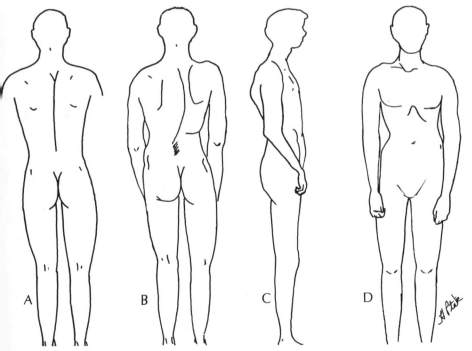

FIG. 4. Postural alterations in scoliosis. A. Normal posterior view; B. Scoliosis posterior view; C. Scoliosis lateral view; D. Scoliosis anterior view.

stance. Spatial discrepancies between the hanging arms and the body are noted, along with any disparity in the lower extremities. A valuable physical sign and diagnostic aid is the placement of the elbow in relation to the iliac crest. Normally the elbow lies slightly above the iliac crest, but with scoliotic deformation it is found to lie at or even below the crest level.

Further evaluation entails recorded measurements of the individual's height, both sitting and standing. This is accomplished not only by determining the total height but by determining the anatomical proportions that comprise it. The distance from the vertex to the pubis (upper segment) and the distance from the pubis to the sole (lower segment) are appraised and related to the total. These values are utilized periodically during comparative follow-up examinations to determine if the total height changes can be attributed to lower extremity growth or trunkal alterations. Decrease in height is attributed to curval progression and discal system compression. It is pleasing to note that an increase in sitting height reflects growth when x-ray analysis discloses no increase in the scoliotic deformity.

With the person in a recumbent position, leg measurements disclose any shortening—either true or apparent. The anterior superior spine of the ilium is the beginning point for measuring a true discrepancy, while the umbilicus serves as the departure point for an apparent discrepancy. Both measures terminate at the lower margin of the medial malleolus. While the true and apparent discrepancies produce a spinal curve convex to the short side, elevation of the short extremity to level the pelvis will cause disappearance of the evident rotation on forward bend. When this occurs, the erroneous diagnosis of structural scoliosis is avoided and the primary cause is treated accordingly (James, 1967).

Unusual sitting and walking postures are noted. A change in gait results from the altered center of gravity. The findings depend upon the curval pattern, its severity, and the degree of compensatory changes.

SPECIFICS

Differentiation between flexible and structural curval components as demonstrated via spinal range of motion signals the specific aspects of the examination. "The forward bending position is of exceptional diagnostic assistance. This position calls for the patient to stand with legs straight and bend forward from the waist, leading with the head and allowing both arms to dangle at the sides" (Harrington, 1968). Forward flexion not only eliminates functional deformities but it also accentuates structural components present in primary and associated compensatory curves. Persistence of fixed rotation aids in identifying primary curval direction and location.

"If on forward bending visible vertebral and rib rotation exists only in one site, there is but one primary curve. If there are two areas of fixed rotation (they will be on opposite sides of one another), there is a double primary curve scoliosis" (James, 1967, p. 3).

> In many patients with right thoracic primary curves, the lumbar secondary or compensatory curve has become highly structural and therefore both curves have become major. If these curves are added to the combined thoracic and lumbar primary pattern and to the combined thoracic and thoracolumbar pattern, the total pattern becomes quite common. James does place them into one group and indicates that they constitute a very frequent pattern (Moe, 1969, p. 212).

This point of fact is to be kept in mind when one reads articles or texts, because incidence reports will vary in accordance with the author's categorization and identification of idiopathic curval patterns.

When the patient leans forward, the pelvis is held stationary and passive lateral postures indicate the extent of spinal flexibility. The degree of flexibility aids in the physician's prediction of curval correction from conservative or surgical measures. The degree of fixation is also determined when the individual is asked to stand as tall as possible by reaching for the examiner's hand when it is placed slightly above his head. Another possible method is the application of head traction. The examiner gently holds the youngster's head and chin and, with distraction, notes the extent of receding correction.

In thoracic curves, the severity of rib protrusion on the side of the curval apex is directly related to the aggregate of vertebral rotation. When the individual bends forward, its presence is more obvious. With posterior rotational progression, the ribs acquire a sharp angle producing a "razorback," "keel-shaped," or "rib hump" deformity (Fig. 5A, B, C, and D). Dorsal surface rib protrusion produces a pseudokyphoscoliosis when in actuality the curval deformation is lordo-scoliotic (James, 1967; Roaf, 1967).

With thoracic involvement, the cardiorespiratory function is carefully evaluated as structural changes may produce restrictive ventilatory abnormalities that lead to reductions in the total lung capacity and the vital capacity. In addition, pulmonary vascular bed restriction leads to pulmonic hypertension and eventually to right-sided heart failure. The pathogenicity of cardiorespiratory decompensation occurs primarily in persons during the third decade of life or beyond. However, excluding primary neuromuscular diseases with secondary structural deformation, there are exceptions. Therefore, treatment is directed at early detection and the prevention of severe thoracic cage deformation with a view toward maintaining cardiorespiratory integrity.

While some patients have a surprising degree of effort tolerance in the presence of a severe curve, others experience gross restriction of effort with relatively mild scoliotic deformation (Zorab, 1967). In addition, Inkley (1969) indicates that extremes in postoperative complications have occurred in relation to resultant preoperative lung function studies.

FIG. 5. Keel-shaped or razor-back deformity. A. Normal posterior view; B. Razor-back posterior view; C. Normal anterior view; D. Razor-back posterior view.

Postoperative complications were minimal in patients with extreme pulmonary malfunction, while some patients with modest abnormalities experienced marked difficulties. Because of this, it is difficult and probably unreliable to stipulate an end point for pulmonary function techniques. The tests' greatest value lies in the identification of patients who may present a hazardous postoperative course.

At the same time, a careful history may reveal the presence of an obstructive lesion as occurs with asthma and chronic bronchitis. In some instances, then, a patient may have ventilatory restriction due to deformation in addition to obstruction of air flow because of a clinical entity. The nature of these obstructive illnesses and the patient's response is also determined. In addition, the frequency of susceptibility to upper respiratory infections serves as a guide for future therapy. Medical treatment, if any, is continued or initiated as deemed necessary.

Indication of the individual's vital capacity as related to the rigidity and rib deformation is obtained by measuring chest dimensions during full respiratory exchange. Specific orders to detect physiological changes may include spirometric or pneumotochogram readings, blood gas studies, an electrocardiogram, and a chest x-ray. A chest x-ray reveals not only the degree and rotation of a thoracic curve but also the heart's size, position, and shape, as well as useful information concerning lung field vascularity. The same considerations are accorded to persons requiring surgical intervention, particularly those with a poor respiratory reserve.

Other aspects of the examination concern features associated with conditions contributing to the secondary development of structural deformation. This includes checking for neuromuscular deficits, particularly lower extremity sensory loss and muscular atonicity. Decreased muscle tone in the presence of a tendency toward tall stature in a person with long slim limbs and sparse subcutaneous fat may indicate Marfan's syndrome. A skin survey not only discloses hygienic practices (including the existence of acne) but also the presence of scars indicating previous chest or spinal surgery, and the presence of skin aberrations such as the pigmentary (café au lait) spots associated with neurofibromatosis. In some instances, the status of dental alignment serves as a future referent with regard to chosen therapeutic measures.

As previously indicated, clinical findings are substantiated via x-ray. Roentgenographic analysis is the method utilized for documenting spinal deviation, but evaluative accuracy is dependent upon radiological consistency. This explains the adherence to standardization in film size and the preference for roentgenograms that distinctly visualize the entire spine and pelvis. Since patient size governs the ordered film size, adolescents require 36-inch cassettes at a distance of 6 feet. In instances in which this larger equipment is not available, two 14 by 17 inch films are taken and pieced together to achieve the desired view. This knowledge may be conveyed in response to the youngster's inquiry, or incorporated into explanations concerning the need and procedure for required examinations.

Additional information is obtained about patient maturation, spinal segment variation, gravitational centricity, spinal length, and the degree and extent of primary and secondary curval deformation. This information is ascertained from the usual routine anteroposterior and lateral views. However, the number of views requested varies with the physician's preference, the patient's age, and the clinical results.

Anteroposterior exposures without postural exaggeration are aimed at including the entire spine with the desired incorporation of the iliac crest to depict the apophysis (Fig. 6). The extent of apophyseal ossification excursion along the top of the iliac crest from lateral to medial

FIG. 6. The iliac apophysis has completed its excursion along the top of the iliac crest. Starting near the anterior superior spine it has grown round to reach and dip down towards the posterior superior iliac spine. This is known as Risser's sign and indicates the end of

reflects vertebral growth and thus serves as a guide for spinal growth completion and possible length of exposure to progressive deformation. Significant progression is not expected beyond this point, but this practical biological standard is not absolute. It has been found that curval progression ceased not only prior to and during excursion but also after apophyseal completion (James, 1967). For the possible few who might progress beyond the post state, patients are followed for two years to assure curval arrest (MacEwen et al., 1967). Careful follow-up continues beyond completion until the apophyses have fused to the iliac crests (James, 1967).

Asymmetrical development of the iliac apophyses is noted on occasion. (Fig. 7). When this occurs, the immature apophysis is considered the prognostic determinant. The average age for completed excursion is 14 years in girls and 16 years in boys (Wilson, 1967). With apophyseal excursion determination, wrist and hand films—which are required for younger children, for skeletal age—are excluded and not considered routine. Their request is individual.

Sometimes recumbent anteroposterior films are ordered along with those taken in the erect position to determine flexible and structural components because resultant comparative differences in primary curval measurements provide the physician with a view toward correction potential. Supine or erect side-bending films are advocated for the same reason. However, their value is open to question. Because interpretive accuracy cannot be attained, the afforded impressions do not contribute concretely to the total picture (Harrington, March 1968). What was once considered an essential exposure has been discontinued by James and abandoned by others because great variation in mobility

FIG. 7. Risser's sign. Asymmetrical development of the iliac apophyses.

resulted postcorrection as opposed to anticipated computations made before correction (James, 1967).

Since transfer from the erect to the supine position influences curval measurement, reliance upon the latter exposure may result in a missed minimal curve. If an author confines his discussion to supine or sitting positions, chances are he is referring to those patients who are incapable of maintaining an erect position and, hence, have an illness that contributes to secondary structural deformation. For these patients, the sitting film is preferred. While the supine exposure supplies quality bone detail, it does not depict the true amount of curvature (Moe, 1969). Although erect roentgenograms are preferred, James (1967) indicates that whatever the routine for radiography, consistency should prevail because of position variability.

Moe (1969) and Roaf (1967) indicate that forceful distraction films are of value in determining large, major curve correctability. With the patient lying supine, simultaneous strong exertion is applied to the head with a halter or to the shoulders and pelvis or legs. Maximal tolerated distraction is not necessary for small curves. While forcible side-bending films serve to confuse the evaluation, the value concerning forceful distraction does not receive further elaboration.

Additional roentgenographic analysis concerns the rated extent of vertebral rotation, the severity ranging from a neutral position to that of a 4+ displacement. Cobb originated this technique by using the spinous process tip position as a base for rotational migration in relation to the vertebra situated beneath it. By dividing the vertebral body into six segments, progressive severity is rated from the body vertex to the body concavity in accordance with the segmental base location. In using the same values, Moe (1969) and his colleagues have altered the approach by replacing the spinous processes with the vertex pedicle shadows to permit easier visualization. The rate of displacement was transcribed to represent degrees of vertebral body rotation (Nash et al., 1969). Since it is difficult to ascertain changes due to deformation or rotation, both techniques lack precision. However, they have merit and Nash and Moe (1969) express their reason for choice.

Other films may be related to close-up views of the primary curve or curves. Because a lumbar curve may be associated with a spondylolisthesis, a lumbosacral exposure is considered routine or imperative. If any abnormality remains in question, additional films follow. Depending upon clinical results, specific examinations such as tomograms may be requested.

X-ray technique determination of curval magnitude is not precise because structural deformation is accompanied by vertebral rotation and a scoliotic curve is not a true arc (Moe, 1969). However, in measuring the primary curval angle(s), the Cobb and the Ferguson methods are the two most widely used on erect anteroposterior exposures. Although both techniques are similar in locating and identifying end vertebrae, the remaining sequential steps are fundamentally different and provide divergent values. Thus they cannot be used interchangeably and consistency with each is a key note. To avoid confusion or a possible interchange, Moe (1969) indicates that the Cobb method may be adopted as the standard and favors this trend for evaluative accuracy. This trend is quite evident in the readings because most authors specified their use of the Cobb method without mentioning the Ferguson technique or stated their favor for choice. While Moe (1969) and Campbell (1963) provide descriptions for each technique, Moe (1969) also discusses the advantages and disadvantages for each.

The differences of opinion and/or apparent controversy regarding the number of initial roentgenograms and those required during follow-up are also reflected in the concern for overirradiation. Because growth potential remains, the idiopathic structural deformation requires close supervision and therapy that extends over a period of years. Objective evaluative measurement regarding curval evolution requires serial x-ray examinations. Comparative analysis for comprehensive review occurs on the average of from four to six months, and it is thought that the erect anteroposterior exposure suffices. Deviation from this approach is in relation to a change in the course of events.

Harrington (1968) states:

> There are many variations from one spine to another, but the common denominator may lie in each vertebral segment as an entity within itself. The forces over time to which each vertebra is subject in the acts of daily living may provide a factor in the mechanics alone. [This factor is calculated after the degree of deformity is ascertained via the Cobb method.] The number of vertebrae in the curve are then counted, and the degree measurement is divided by the number of vertebrae. The resultant quotient represents the factor.
> . . . the mechanical stability of the spine is lost when the factor exceeds five and that when the factor is three or higher, the reciprocal ability of the spine in function is jeopardized. Therefore when a factor of three is reached the spine is vulnerable to progression; but when a factor of five is found in the growing scoliotic spine, progression is inevitable. The rate of progression is usually relative to the amount of involvement and to whatever treatment may have been initiated, though the actual rate is unknown.

SPECIFIC GUIDELINES

Although definitive information is lacking regarding the point at which mechanical instability occurs and about the inevitability of curval progression, the nurse—via astute observation for subtle postural alterations—can contribute to the early detection and thus early therapeutic intervention of spinal deformation. Casefinding need not be confined to health facility activities, but is an ongoing process regardless of the setting. With a view toward casefinding as a form of prevention, school and camp nurses can play a large part by adopting a simple method for disclosure that requires little time but accomplishes early review with a possibility for close follow-up through to maturity.

Having the child bend over, and dotting the bony spinal processes with either a magic marker, skin pencil, or pen facilitates the identification of any lateral deviation when the child stands erect. In addition, detection concerning discrepancies in shoulder and hip heights can be accomplished with the use of a wall chart or area of a wall that has been painted with alternating horizontally parallel colored lines. The use of colored masking tape strips will accomplish the need for visual accentuation provided the tapes are applied with accuracy on a straight wall.

Information concerning desired body mechanics and problems encountered with or resulting from poor postural habits can be incorporated in health education courses. Practical approaches for parental participation may be imparted during a scheduled Parent Teacher Association meeting. The nurse can contribute to parents' and teachers' knowledge and concern for child health by describing the aforementioned physical alteration and demonstrating with the use of a model or visual aids the manner in which detection can be accomplished. Providing people with a system for communicating their concerns for suspected difficulties sets the stage for interschool communications as well as a step toward meeting health care needs. Since idiopathic scoliosis has been linked with heredity, the nurse can utilize this knowledge in her teaching approach concerning modality. Screening with requests for further evaluation coincides with the old adage: "an ounce of prevention is worth a pound of cure."

If the diagnosis is confirmed, the physician outlines his plan for treatment which incorporates conservative corrective measures, surgical intervention, or both. Much depends upon the youngster's age (the time remaining until maturity) and the extent of present curval deformation. However, the physician is honest and forthright regarding estimated curval correction and emphasizes the fact that 100 percent return is never attained.

With a view toward long-term involvement and the essentials for care, cost represents a considerable financial burden. Parental concern is frequently expressed in relation to direct inquiries regarding the cost of therapy or indirectly in comments associated with postponement or elimination of familial plans and needs. Not infrequently, it is the youngster who expresses worry regarding impingement upon family desires and the anticipated cost.

Whether this concern is expressed or not, the nurse can explain that financial assistance is available. Although this opportunity is open to the family, it should be conveyed that the suggestion by no means implies that they are incapable of meeting their child's health needs or that it represents an insult to their integrity. It is imparted with the full realization that their child's diagnosis and required therapeutic regimen impose a financial strain and that money is available for such a purpose. If the nurse is unsure of what is available in the patient's community, resources to consult are the Health Department and/or the Department of Social Services.

Naturally, the procedure for obtaining funds will vary from one geographical area to another, but a description related to the method for application will give the family an idea of what is involved. Usually, the hospital business office personnel or the physician's secretary or office nurse files an application with the county health department where the family resides. The form contains the parents' names, occupation(s), address, type of insurance (if any), the child's diagnosis, and the physician's prescription regarding needs for correction. In turn, a mutually agreeable appointment is arranged between the family and a health-team member from the contacted agency. Family financial responsibilities are reviewed since income is not the sole consideration, and it is from this information that full payment is excluded or the family contributes in part via scheduled installments. Concomitant with the agency referral, the prescription and patient diagnosis are sent to the bracemaker, who contacts the family about an appointment for brace-fitting.

While awaiting the appropriate time for treatment, the individual can assume changes in posture that will relieve the stress imposed upon the spine while he is in the erect position. Giving consideration to the patient's daily-life activities, the nurse, in exploration with the individual involved, can suggest ways in which stress can be alleviated and fatigue avoided. Since mechanical forces have been implicated as part contributors to increased spinal deformation, recumbency wherever and whenever possible is the desired position. Because the standing position already causes stress, fatigue superimposes further stress upon an already-malforming condition. One can naturally assume that restrictions will be imposed upon the individual's life-style as a consequence of therapy. Therefore, prior preparation with a view toward the specific therapeutic treatment is recommended. An important consideration is that, even though one assumes or knows that restrictions will be imposed, suggestions for change cannot be given without the individual's life pattern and needs being taken into account. Directions in preparing the individual to become acclimated to these upcoming therapeutically imposed conditions and the exploration of his life-style will not only reflect your concern for him as an individual but is also the appropriate approach to a gradual introduction of what is to come. Do not overburden the youngster with an elaborate detailed plan, but be realistic in suggesting approaches for counteracting situations that would add further insult and thus increase the chance for progression.

Remember, progression is likely so long as there is growth remaining. Consequently, alterations in life-style are necessary, but suggestions should be without loss in peer identification and activities of the adolescent age group.

An important area of concern is that of the individual's posture. Adolescents are not exactly known for elegant posture; therefore, suggested guidance with regard to posture improvement will take time and patience. Emphasis should be placed on proper sitting posture to enhance the avoidance of fatigue. Also, as a means of improving posture, the individual should be advised to stand in a doorway or against a wall and straighten up as tall as possible by tilting his pelvis under and pushing his head back against the partition.

Rest and relaxation are important elements in the therapeutic process, but due thought should be given to the individual life-style of the adolescent involved. One suggestion deals with the time-honored tradition of phone calls. The individual should be advised to recline on the floor or couch with his knees flexed and feet flat. This procedure leads to maximum comfort and probably longer phone conversations, which will most likely leave the individual's mother overjoyed at the prospect of her child's total monopoly of the telephone. Reclining on the floor or couch should be suggested for other sedentary activities, such as reading or watching television. If the individual lies on his side, he should be advised to lie on the side of the concavity or the hollow side of the curve. That is, if the primary curval apex is on the right, the individual should lie on the left. These suggestions can also be applied to reclining at a beach or at the side of a pool.

In this respect, swimming is a fine, and, in fact, a desirable activity—with care being taken to avoid fatigue. Swimming requires stretching and reaching motions which enhance muscular range of motion, muscular development, and tonicity. Swimming can be included within the context of exercises that can be accomplished while one awaits specific forms of therapy, and which provide the individual with the best possible chance for functional alignment. The hyperextension required for swimming aids in strengthening back muscles and the activity increases deeper respirations. Ventilatory exercises with a focus upon inspiratory capacity is also incorporated to enhance chest mobility.

Chinning is an exercise which incorporates forces for straightening and strengthening with minimal vertical load. This suggestion is particularly appropriate for boys, as they are proud of their physical prowess. They can utilize this exercise as a means for muscle building, but at the same time it serves to strengthen back and abdominal musculature. Although girls have also enjoyed this practice, it is not usually recommended because they generally do not have the muscular strength required for accurate execution. Chinning bars can be positioned between the posts of the doorway to a bedroom or can be part of a recreation area in the family room.

Another exercise that achieves the same goal as chin-ups is push-ups. This exercise can be utilized by both boys and girls with the modification that girls push up with their knees on the ground. Sit-ups can be utilized by both sexes in strengthening the abdominal muscles and increasing abdominal muscle tone. This exercise is recommended in considering the use of the abdominal muscles in the elimination process during required recumbency in the course of therapy.

A difficult but not insurmountable consideration is the amount of time spent in the sitting position during school hours. Transference to the erect position for change of classes provides some relief, but it does not meet the need for the alleviation of mechanical stress. However, proper sitting positions can be demonstrated that will provide for proper alignment and thus impose the least amount of stress. An introduction to and consultation with the physical therapist ensures the accurate and appropriate use of active exercises. These exercises may be included, eliminated, or modified in later therapy.

The physical education instructor should be informed of the individual's condition in order that time be provided for rest during periods of exercise to eliminate the possibility of developing fatigue. Actually, the individual will set his own limitations, but if the instructor is aware of the situation, he will not reprimand him for not keeping up with the group. Consideration for this need should be a casual accomplishment so that the individual's need is not consistently brought to the attention of the group. Again, this is an age group in which peer acceptance and group belonging provide the need for identification; but, at the same time, the fact that the individual is unique in his life pattern and functioning within the group should be recognized. If the individual receives an honest, direct explanation concerning the needs for medical supervision, he in turn can assume the desired responsibility for his own care and impart the knowledge to his peers when deemed necessary.

A primary consideration, in addition to the explanation of alterations to the individual, is the explanation of these same alterations to his parents. This is done not because the adolescent is incapable of comprehending, but because the parents have a need and, in fact, a right to know the rationale for care prior to chosen therapy.

Successful therapy relies not only upon patient cooperation and effort but also upon family participation as well. Children are not to be typified in accordance with growth and developmental expectations nor should explanations be given solely upon the knowledge of parental culture or occupation. Remember, explanations should be within the child's and parents' realm of understanding.

In providing optimal care, close coordination of effort calls for the continuous communicative interchange between and among health team members. Conveying accomplished plans and initiating necessary referrals and instituted methods for therapy provides the team with a total regimen and thus keeps to a minimum the number of persons in contact with the patient and family. Duplication of services and unnecessary exposure to numbers of people is overwhelming, taxing, confusing, and reflects poor planning. Since treatment is continued until and beyond maturity, efficiency of service is mandatory.

Therapeutic Measures

In focusing upon the adolescent, the diagnosis and the required care and confinement (home and hospital) can be viewed as a crisis imposed upon a developmental crisis. Recognition of the implications for nursing intervention does not suffice. It is the action taken with

FIG. 8. The localizer cast completed and with a "V" cut over the trachea. There is a plaster collar which extends up on the occiput behind and the mandible in front.

recognition that provides for effective assistance in crisis situations. Do not underestimate the person's ability to withstand stress, but work toward utilizing his identified strengths in meeting or coping with the problems encountered. This requires skill and is by no means simple, but it will contribute to reciprocal growth. There may be questions along the way to which there are no ready answers, but there is no harm in asking. The harm results from not asking! Honesty, accuracy of information, and a search for understanding with realistic considerations in the provision for care cannot be overemphasized.

When hospitalization is required, a greeting and exchange of names sets the stage for providing an environment conducive to the establishment of a constructive nurse-patient relationship. This may sound insultingly elementary, but too frequently we are guilty of identifying an individual not by name but by his probable diagnosis, his room assignment, or his private physician. The degree of anxiety may or may not be overt and thus some degree of familiarity must be established before formal admission occurs. A brief orientation to the surroundings and explanations concerning specific hospital policies reflects your concern for their anticipated needs and acclimation to the situation. Patient and parent teaching continues and/or commences upon formal admission in association with reasons for routine examinations.

Although there are a variety of therapeutic measures, and methods for correction vary, treatment is accomplished via mechanical means and force, internal splinting, or both. Essentially treatment falls into two broad categories: either conservative (or nonoperative) and surgical (or operative). While the basis for therapy is individualized in accordance with the patient's general condition, the curval deformation, and the patient's personality, the overall aim of therapy is to prevent further negative progression and to regain and maintain spinal stability and alignment.

CONSERVATIVE MANAGEMENT

Nonoperative devices are numerous but the two most widely used methods of approach are the Risser localizer or semibent cast and the Milwaukee brace (Fig. 8; 9A and B). Criteria for their selection is based upon the patient's age and degree of curval involvement with a view toward anticipated progression and the time remaining until maturity (Keiser, 1967; Harrington, 1968). Although both are accompanied by specific exercises and are successful nonoperative methods, they serve to attain maximum curval correction prior to surgical intervention and are also used postoperatively for maintenance of fusion integrity. While both methods achieve the desired goal, that favored for effecting mechanical curval prevention or correction via distraction is the Milwaukee brace. The reverse appears to hold true for the postoperative period, but to a much greater extent. The localizer cast is preferred for postsurgical recumbency and ambulation. Supplemental use of the brace is an exception. Since support is simultaneous with correction and the brace provides for greater chest mobility, its use is with paralytic deformation or ventilatory impairment.

Depending upon the patient's age and curval severity, both nonoperative methods involve relatively lengthy time periods. Although the cast exerts more static corrective force (Keiser, 1967), positive curval changes and patient growth result in periodic reapplications. Because it is worn continuously and is frequently uncomfortably warm and odorous, its disadvantage lies in the fact that it cannot be removed for hygienic measures. On the other hand, bathing can be accomplished with the continuous use of a brace. It also provides for greater freedom of movement in association with exercises and depth of respiration; parts can be replaced separately and the pelvic girdle is renewed with

FIG. 9. A standard Milwaukee brace showing the detail of the occipital pad (O) that is notched to avoid pressure on the occipital protuberance; the neck ring (R) which is hinged in front and fastened behind by a knurled nut (K); the neck pad (N) is to cushion the holding force against the neck as the patient is shifted to the left by the thoracic pad (T); the posterior uprights (U) are twisted 90° at the cephalad ends and attached to the lateral sides of the neck ring. The twist makes them slightly flexible in two directions.

The strap (B) that tightens the pelvic girdle (G) is fastened by a buckle; a frame work of Monel metal (M) reinforces the pelvic girdle. It must be formed into half of a narrow cyclinder in the waistline where the cowhide of the girdle is molded deeply.

The lumbar pad (L) may be slipped under the girdle, or outside of the leather as correction is obtained. The pad is floated on a nylon strap which is secured at both ends by truss studs. A similar stud (X) secures the strap for the thoracic pad. The pad is effective at first in reducing the rib hump. Later, to avoid exaggeration of the thoracic lordosis, the strap may be curled around the nearest bar (S′, insert) and held with the truss stud. As the girdle is tightened, the nylon belt may be shifted to the posterior bars. Note the detail of the narrowly molded Monel metal (M′) at the waist. B. The chin support must have a thin firm pad (P). The anterior bar (A) is made of duralumin to permit some x-ray penetration. It must be far enough from the chest to permit deep inspiration. It gives some support to the leather apron of the girdle (G). The anterior end of the strap for the lumbar pad (S) is shown as it comes forward to be secured to a truss stud on half of the hinge (H). The latter permits easy opening of the girdle. There are two hinges for the neck ring, one in each anterior corner. The ring flange (F) for the right shoulder is provided with a small extension to prevent cutting into the shoulder anteriorly. When the patient tilts his pelvis and moves the torso away from the left lumbar pad (exercise 7), the ring flange presents elevation of the right shoulder and an increase in the right thoracic curve. (From Blount and Bolinske. Phys. Ther. 47:919–925, 1967.)

growth. Its use is gradually withdrawn as the individual approaches maturity and correction is attained and retained. In addition, the brace is more comfortable, and advocates stress that its use eliminates complications related to cast applications.

Milwaukee Brace. A complication that has been overemphasized (Blount, 1969) but may be encountered with prolonged use of the brace is mandibular recession and malocclusion. Since the vertical force applied superiorly to the mandibulo-occipital assembly resolves in an arc surrounding the lower cranium and mandible, it disseminates via multiple bone growth centers—the total effect being one of compression. This complication is particularly applicable to the younger age group. However, changes vary with age and depend upon the extent and duration of compression. It is for this reason that an orthodontist is consulted prior to brace procurement to ascertain dental and jaw alignment. Upper and lower dental impressions are taken for comparative bite analysis after therapy. In addition, a cephalometric roentgenogram and a lateral facial photograph may be taken.

A recent precautionary measure has been to supply the youngster with a night retainer, but its value in limiting dental deformation has not been indicated (James, 1967; Blount, 1969). Serious displacement is uncommon, while minor protrusion is common (James, 1967). Goldstein (1964) points to the fact that specific remedial therapy is required for those patients known to have malocclusion prior to use of the brace because progression can be expected with its use. Blount (1969) indicates that significant changes will not occur in patients with good dentition, but he emphasizes the proper maintenance of appropriate support. In some instances, the orthodontist will prescribe specific active exercises to curtail and/or prevent changes. However, with brace removal, there is a tendency toward spontaneous reconstruction (James, 1967).

The orthopedist reflects his regard for the psychosocial impact when he provides the adolescent with an honest and intelligent rationale concerning the goals for therapy, associated regulations, and imposed restrictions that accompany brace prescription. He uses a photograph or an illustration of the brace to complement his description of its function and forewarns the youngster that exerted pressure will be felt under the chin and over the iliac crests. The physician also indicates that surgical intervention may be required for stabilization following the onset of maturation. In this manner, the patient and parents are informed as to the approximate length of therapy and an operative procedure is not a sudden suggestion at the end of a trial with a brace. Much time is taken to impart the reasons for compliance with imposed restrictions and to ascertain their understanding of required therapy.

Often it is the nurse who anticipates or conveys patient and family concerns to initiate the need for self-expression and further inquiry. Listening to what is said and how it is said serves as a guide to feelings and possible needs. However, do not rely solely upon the spoken word. Observed responses speak louder than words and are crucial clues as to how the person really thinks or feels in the situation. Sighs of relief or expressed acknowledgment frequently follows what was hesitatingly withheld. Reiteration of information is necessary because there is much to assimilate. Therefore, patience is required in supplementing or clarifying previous information.

When a Milwaukee brace is chosen, the individual may be scheduled for an approximate two- to three-week hospital stay that entails the application of traction to attain the best possible fit for a brace (Fig. 10). This practice is analogous to dressmaking in that the desired weight loss should precede the measurements for the design chosen. In other words, dimensions taken prior to the weight loss will result in an improperly fitted piece of apparel. The time interval represents inclusion for patient preparation and reflects the two weeks required for attaining practically maximum angular correction. Preliminary

FIG. 10. One type of head and pelvic harness (Cotrel's) that can be used to provide for continuous distraction of the spine. The doctor may prescribe that this be worn continuously for several weeks prior to surgery or to the application of a scoliotic brace. By elevation of the head pulley, traction is applied primarily to the occipital bone. The patient is encouraged to actively stretch her trunk, insofar as possible, by reaching and holding to the head of the bed. The pelvic straps maintain her pelvis in a fixed position. (From Larson and Gould. *Orthopedic Nursing*, 7th ed, 1970. Courtesy of The C. V. Mosby Co.)

traction prior to brace application may also be used in situations in which the patients and parents feel unusually insecure. This approach provides for gradual adaptation to the brace under direct team supervision.

When the patient is being prepared for the brace fitting, he should be told that the orthotist will measure physical proportions, such as the distance from the chin to the chest after the application of a plaster mold (negative), the dimensions of which serve as a guide for making a positive model. The brace is then built over the positive model and the orthotist diligently checks his computations to afford the best possible fit. It is at this point that the patient is told that he will have to disrobe and wear a form-fitting stockinette or undershirt for skin protection prior to the negative cast application. It should be explained that he will stand between a metal frame as if in a doorway and will grasp the poles on each side, but the bracemaker will direct and prepare him for the correct position. A head halter is applied for suspension and the cast will extend from the upper part of the thighs to the costal margin (Fig. 11). In addition, the plaster is molded to body contour as it is applied with accentuation of the full width and extent of the iliac crests so that when the pelvic girdle is applied the pressure is disseminated over a wide skin area. Diagrams or a demonstration can accompany explanations to provide for clarity. The patient is forewarned that

FIG. 11. Preparing the cast for making the Milwaukee brace. The groove above the iliac crest is accentuated in the way shown.

the plaster sets rapidly and this process is accompanied by a feeling of warmth or heat as if one were wrapped in a thermal blanket.

Meantime, the physical therapist and nurse work closely together with the patient and parents in establishing a prescribed exercise program (Table 1, 1-6). The physical therapist teaches the patient via

TABLE 1. EXERCISES TO BE PERFORMED IN THE MILWAUKEE BRACE

OBJECTIVE	EXERCISES AND DESCRIPTION

To strengthen thoracic muscles and improve posture. Each exercise is held to the count of five and done ten times once or twice daily.	1. Pelvic tilt, supine (on back) with the knees flexed.
	  a. Tighten the buttock muscles.
	  b. Expand the chest but breathe regularly.
	  c. Force the small of the back into the floor by tightening the abdominal muscles and pushing backward. (When there is difficulty in learning the mechanics of the pelvic tilt, it is well to execute it first with the patient in the quadruped position.)

	2. Pelvic tilt, supine with the knees straight. Repeat a, b, and c under 1.

	3. "Sit up" with pelvic tilt.
	  a. With the knees extended and held firmly, tilt the pelvis.
	  b. Come to a sitting position. With the elbows straight, reach for the knees. When this is easily accomplished, do the exercise with the knees flexed; later with the elbows flexed on the chest. (In the brace, the patient cannot "roll up" in the proper manner and needs assistance when he first tries to come to the sitting position.)

	4. Pelvic tilt standing.
	  a. Relax the knees, tilt the pelvis.
	  b. Elevate the chest slightly but breathe regularly.
	  c. Walk, holding the tilt. Make this posture a habit. (The corrected posture is most easily retained by having the patient hold his abdomen away from the support of the girdle most of the time.)

	5. Hyperextension while lying prone (face down).
	  a. With the knees held down, tilt the pelvis.
	  b. Raise the head and shoulders against resistance.

	6. Push-ups with the pelvis tilted. (If girls have difficulty supporting themselves on their toes, they may rest on their knees at first.)

To reduce the deformity.	7. Active correction of the major curve.
	  a. Tilt the pelvis.
	  b. "Pull away" from the pad. Avoid sway-back.
	  c. Walk habitually in this corrected position. (It is important that the shift away from the major pad not be anterior, to increase the lordosis. The shift must be toward midline and backward. In the correction of a

Table 1 (*cont.*)

OBJECTIVE   EXERCISES AND DESCRIPTION

primary right thoracic curve, the lumbar pad prevents the exaggeration of a left lumbar compensatory curve.)

8. Chest expansion for correction of lordosis, rib hump, and thoracic valley.
   a. Tilt the pelvis in the standing position.
   b. Inhale deeply and press backward toward the posterior bars with the chest wall. The thoracic pad will engage the rib hump and rotate the spine. The thoracic valley will fill out.

   (This can be most easily taught if the therapist places his hand over the thoracic valley and then has the patient attempt to "squeeze" it against the bar by breathing deeply and arching his back like a cat.

   A stubborn thoracic lordosis is best overcome when the posterior end of the strap for the thoracic pad is secured to the first upright bar (Fig. 9A[S]) so that the holding force of the pad has no anteriorly directed component that would increase the thoracic lordosis. If the lumbar pad is removed and the pelvic girdle tightened so that the upper rounded edge of the girdle on the left side has the holding force of a low lumbar pad, all external obstruction to correction of lordosis is removed.)

Adapted from Blount, W. P., and Bolinske J. *Physical Therapy*, 47: 919–925, 1967 (October).

demonstration and passively guides the patient during the learning process to assure that he performs the exercises correctly and gets a feel of proper positioning. A full-length mirror aids in visualization of anatomical placement. Although exercises are taught by the physical therapist in most instances, it is the nurse who supervises the activity— particularly in the home situation after the patient has received his brace. Therefore, proper supervision requires that the nurse be proficient in this area. Realistically speaking, there are also many regions where physical therapists are in short supply and maintenance programs are a large part of the nurse's responsibility. Home visits by a physical therapist are not economically feasible for some patients and are considered by some to be an unnecessary burden. When one considers the effects of immobility—not only during ambulatory therapy but during required nonoperative and operative recumbency—nursing intervention comprises a large part of the plan. A few essentials for care include the maintenance of proper position and alignment, prevention of contractures, and exercises to maintain healthy tissue and to prevent disuse atrophy.

Getting Used to the Brace. When the brace arrives, patient-parent teaching continues with introductory directions concerning the technique for its application with the least amount of patient discomfort (see Fig. 9A, B). The patient is instructed to position the brace around

him and to fasten the neck ring securely. While he lifts the anterior
uprights and stands as straight and as tall as possible, his parent lifts
the posterior uprights. With the brace in this position, the pelvic girdle
is snugly tightened for comfort and rests within the soft waist area.
This position is the proper locale; thus the pelvic girdle should lie between the patient's last rib and well above the pelvic bones. A trim fit
is mandatory for proper brace function. Directional failure and lack of a
secure fit can result in irritation and tissue breakdown over bony prominences. Therefore, should the patient experience discomfort, he is advised against loosening this component because it will increase his
discomfort and possibly lead to further tissue damage. The last adjustment has to do with the fastening of holding pads that are placed at and
below the apex of primary curve(s). There are five in number but their
use depends upon the extent of deformation and the need for obtaining
maximum correction. Specific directions and return demonstrations are
repeated as necessary to assure ease and comprehension of the application technique. This is one reason for frequent initial visits.

With proper application, the patient may also experience discomfort because initial adjustments are necessary and spinal derotation is
sometimes rapid during this period. This results in a sudden increase
in height, a change to which the patient must rapidly become accustomed. Although he must be assured that adjustments are expected
and are no cause for alarm, it must be explained that temporary visual
problems might accompany this height change. Experienced visual difficulties are in association with depth perception and distance. Some
patients comment that they have to duck obstacles that were not a
previous problem or that they misjudge entrance ways. The orthotist
will make the necessary adjustments and mark the straps during the
initial visits to indicate the desired fastening point. Written instructions reinforce previous learning and serve as a guide regarding brace
technique and care.

Written instructions are also provided in association with prescribed exercises. The exercises taught during the prebrace period represent the first group of two types that comprise the program (Table 1).

The first group (Nos. 1–6) is a standard conditioning routine,
done both in and out of the brace to maintain the strength of
the trunk muscles that are mechanically restricted by the brace.
These exercises prepare the patient to keep his good posture
without the abdominal support and holding action of the brace.

In addition the activity associated with games and ordinary
daily living is highly desirable while the patient wears the brace.
Vigorous exercise includes incidental movements that are translated to active correction of the major curve. The holding forces
of the brace prevent the torso from lapsing into deformity.
When the patient is lazy and cannot, or will not, engage in some
recreational exercise, supervised physical therapy is intensified
to maintain the strength of the muscle groups of the torso that
promote good posture.

The second group of exercises (Nos. 7 and 8) of the series
are specific movements in the brace designed to diminish the

major curve, decrease the lordosis, reduce the rib hump and force out the thoracic valley on the other side. They consist of these two routines: pelvic tilt and then without increasing the lordosis, an active shift away from the check pad for the major curve; pelvic tilt followed by deep inspiration and vigorous rounding of the back posteriorly in an attempt to reach the posterior bars. With this movement the rib hump impinges on the thoracic pad and is effectively checked. The spine rotates and the thoracic valley is filled out. At the same time the thoracic lordosis is greatly reduced. In a flexible patient the improvement is dramatic. When these two movements are repeated in the brace many times a day, the permanent gains are gratifying (Blount and Bounske, 1967*).

Although exercises are an important aspect of the program, it would be misleading and, in fact, erroneous to think that they are a cure-all for structural deformation. While they serve their purpose, an overvaluation and an intricate plan only serve to bore the patient and impose unwarranted restrictions.

The brace is not removed during the exercise program as it guides the corrective movements by preventing gross substitutions.

In the attempt to correct scoliosis, asymmetric exercise without the brace is dangerous because the movement which corrects one curve will aggravate the compensatory curves. This over-correction is desirable only when it is needed to improve trunk balance.

When asymmetric exercise is performed in the Milwaukee brace, unwanted motions are checked before their amplitude is sufficient to produce an undesirable effect. The two specific exercises mentioned above cannot be done well without the brace. In it they are productive of rapid improvement unless the curve is rigid (Blount and Bounske, 1967*).

While some asymmetric programs are helpful (Blount, 1967), the point here is to exercise caution with their use and patient choice by checking for their desirability and effectiveness. This holds true for any form of exercise not instituted by the physical therapist. Planning a schedule with the patient provides him with the choice for electing the most suitable times for accomplishing the exercise program. At the same time, flexibility is built into his daily routine.

Since the patient lives in the brace 24 hr a day, seven days a week, there are some helpful guidelines that will aid him during the adjustment period and the time required for its use. The brace is always worn over a cotton T-shirt or undershirt which will absorb body perspiration, protect vulnerable areas, and aid in maintaining the condition of leather brace parts. Since the brace is more comfortable in the recumbent position, chosen time for rest in the prone, side-lying, or supine position aids in muscle relaxation and torso elongation. When sleeping, it is best to lie on the side of the primary curval concavity.

Because the horizontal lateral position creates pressure on the shoulder, torso, and greater trochanter, skin care is crucial for the pre-

* Courtesy *Physical Therapy* (47:919–925, 1967, October).

vention of tissue irritation and breakdown. The chin support area is also one that deserves attention. Discomfort from pressure is experienced during the initial adjustment period, but this is relieved with rest.

At first the brace feels excessively long, not only when the patient stands, but particularly when he assumes the sitting posture. This feeling decreases with time, but there are accommodations to make life simpler. The height of a table or desk can be raised for eating or study periods. Strategic stacking of books to the desired height is another approach. A portable tilt table can be used for study during school and at home. In science classes, microscopes can be placed at a higher level and/or at a slant for easier visualization and use. Selection of a low chair, kneeling on protective pads or pillows, or standing at a counter are other methods for meeting dining needs. In situations in which these adaptations are not possible, prism glasses may be used. If sitting does not permit bending beyond a right angle, the placement of wedge-shaped pillows on slanting cushions will furnish the leverage required for sitting comfort. Not all patients experience the same difficulties, but for those who require assistance, the previous examples serve as possible suggestions to anticipated needs.

Tending to hygienic needs takes time and patience because they are accomplished with the brace intact. However, the brace may be removed once or twice a week or for a 2-hr interval per week for a bath and shampoo. Massaging pressure points is soothing and preserves tissue integrity. This aspect for care can be demonstrated along with helpful hints for bathing with the brace intact. The use of body oils and powder is discouraged because of surface friction rub and caking with moisture. Covering the chin piece with a stretch sock or soft fabric will serve to keep this area dry. At the same time, it provides a barrier to possible allergic responses. In some instances the chin support is made of plastic, but proper skin care and cleansing still applies.

Some teenagers require assistance with treatment for acne that is not necessarily confined to the face. There are a variety of products on the market that aid in curtailing pustule formation and/or healing surface areas without scar formation, providing the individual properly cleanses involved skin areas and refrains from the temptation of picking or expelling pus via pressure with the thought that this will hasten the healing process. It does not, and actually adds insult to injury, with possible consequent infection and scarring. If necessary, exploration for a change in hair style in keeping with patient satisfaction and peer standards accomplishes the desired omission of bacterial and hair oil contamination of skin blemishes. In some instances specific dermatological treatments are necessary. This aspect of care may appear as a departure from specifics associated with nonoperative intervention but it is a vital consideration to adolescents and coincides with the need for a desirable appearance.

Although the Milwaukee brace is a successful nonoperative method, it can cause much wear and tear on the teenager's wardrobe. The truss studs and projecting brace parts can be covered with teflon pads or plastic tubing acquired from the orthotist. The use of adhesive bandage for clothing protection is discouraged. Today's fashions offer a wide selection of attire that will fit loosely over the brace. Suggestions for purchase can be made with a view toward cost and consideration for family economics. In addition, mothers can alter their daughter's underpants by creating a slit that facilitates elimination. Many teenagers design and make their own clothes.

Another consideration is the life of the brace. Changes are made in relation to replacement of the leather girdle lining and brace parts damaged by normal wear and growth. The individual and his parents are shown how to check for and keep the metal screws and rivets in place to assure proper maintenance and function. Mild soap and water is used for cleaning leather or plastic parts; the use of cleaning fluids and alcohol is drying to leather and thus their use should be avoided. If saddle soap is used, it should be sparingly applied with a damp cloth. During therapeutic withdrawal, the brace should be stored in an upright position in the corner or convenient section of the room—never under the bed or behind furniture where lint, dust, animal hairs, and so forth can contribute to unnecessary wear. Some parents or patients devise a storage bag made from denim to preserve the life of the brace.

Although contact-competitive sports are not permitted, activity is encouraged. Consequently, brace breakage or malalignment can occur and this impairs brace function. Patients and parents are encouraged to visit their orthotist for immediate repairs. Patient safety and the safety of others is a prime consideration. Prohibition avoids exposure to exhaustive participation in lengthy practice periods and forceful activity under fatigue conditions. Competitive athletic programs require too much exertion and are considered detrimental to health (Harrington, 1968).

Although active position change is accomplished in a relatively short time period, the patient may experience an aching sensation in his jaw during the initial adjustment period. This is due to his reliance upon the chin support as a chin rest. Its purpose is to serve as a reminder to extend his spine to effect derotation. Chewing sugarless gum relieves the discomfort and also stimulates muscular growth with the hope that malocclusion is avoided. Such muscular activity is also encouraged by daily snacks of raw fruits (apples) or vegetables (carrots). The physical therapist (or in some instances the orthodontist) may provide instruction in jaw exercises.

Prescribed exercises are altered in accordance with the patient's progress and alacrity. Initally, they are difficult for all, but each person differs in his response to brace adaptation and therapy. Alterations are made to increase the difficulty and thus increase the patient's strength. Changes provide for diversity and flexibility, but also curtail the boredom that can occur with repetitious routine.

Patient Follow-Up. Since the frequency for corrective adjustments diminishes after the required initial changes, the interval between clinical follow-up visits increases with time. The patient and
parents are taught the proper method for adjusting brace length during
the introductory period following proper application, but periodic check-
ups occur at a minimum of three months and at a maximum of four
months per year. Therefore, home visits are necessary to provide for
continued assistance not only for mechanical application and extension but also for the time usually required to assist the teenager with
the stress and conflicts experienced as a result of chosen therapy and/or
the deformity. Initially, it may be easier if the patient lies in the prone
position for brace application while his parent fastens the appliance.
After a few weeks, it can be accomplished in the erect position to the
extent that the patient applies it without assistance.

The correction rate varies with age and curval flexibility, but the
need for mechanical extension is determined by asking the patient to
extend his spine and to lift his chin and head out of the brace. Another
approach is one in which the patient exerts downward pressure upon
the hip areas as he attempts to pull his head out of the brace while
grasping the side of the neck piece. In either case, if this action is
nearly accomplished, the brace is extended to take up the slack. The
occiput pad should fit snugly while the chin piece should not be too
high. The correct chin height is determined in several ways, but Blount
(1969) reports the best results when the patient was able to raise his
chin 3 to 4 centimeters from the pad. The chosen method for adjustment calls for direct observation and is conveyed to the visiting nurse
for appropriate follow-through. In turn, a resumé is included in the
patient's record concerning his progress and the team has an up-to-
date report.

An erect anteroposterior evaluative roentgenogram that incorporates the entire spine is taken at each quarter and compared with the
results of one taken 24 hr after brace application. The dimensions
obtained from the initial examination and those that follow are transferred to a single document for a chronological record that provides
the physician with a quick view of patient progress. While some
physicians order examinations with the patient out of the brace as well,
Harrington (1968) indicates that this approach exposes the individual
to excessive irradiation; the film taken in the brace is sufficient. Parents
will express the same concern when they consider x-ray requests unreasonable. However, confinement to single exposures with an explanation as to their purpose is acceptable and not an objectionable request.

During revisits, the team confers regarding suggested changes
for brace components to effect the desired anatomical correction and
to provide for patient comfort. Exercises are reviewed and changes are
instituted accordingly. The patient recognizes that mechanical extension will not be so frequent as in the beginning of therapy, for this
fact is imparted with the full recognition that changes may or may

not be slight during treatment; thus the patient might meet with disappointment should correction not progress to his liking. The length of therapy does depend upon patient age and skeletal maturation, but it is only human to anticipate positive alterations with strict adherence to imposed restrictions. Therefore, though patients are delighted with total improvement, compassionate and sincere understanding of his expressed impatience or depression is called for. This approach also holds true for those patients who have digressed from the appointed regimen. The reason for this very human response must be sought before one considers a reprimand. One has to be gentle but firm in supplying reminders for the necessary therapy. Obviously there are limitations to this form of behavior, but recognition of level of competence is necessary, and perhaps consultation with or referral to the psychologist or other qualified team member is required.

Much parental support is needed here also, because parents exert influence upon their child's behavior and desire for freedom from restriction. It is not easy for parents to adhere to a plan when pleas from their youngster are to the contrary. Consistent responses concerning disciplinary action are a keynote as with any child, but parents think they are "mean" and express feelings of guilt when restrictive measures are called for. Consequently, listening to and providing time for parents' expressed concerns in addition to suggesting alternative constructive approaches is an activity that deserves attention and contributes to the welfare of all concerned.

Gradual Withdrawal of the Brace. If treatment is effective, the brace is worn throughout the growth period and usually six months beyond maturity, which is confirmed via apophyseal x-ray. With the cessation of bone growth, the individual is gradually weaned from the brace—first during the daytime hours to the extent that by the sixth month the brace is worn at night only. Graduated periods vary, but whatever the chosen method of approach, the patient is followed closely for any sign of curval progression. When the patient has reached a stage at which eight or nine hours per day are spent without the brace, follow-up erect roentgenograms are then taken without external support.

During the weaning process, rest periods may be abandoned or taken at the patient's discretion. Exercises continue and are performed both in and out of the brace until this procedure is accomplished on alternate days. Eventually, all exercises are executed without the brace. This approach provides for the gradual reestablishment of trunkal muscular tonicity because degeneration and partial atrophy is one undesirable effect that accompanies external immobilization.

Another undesirable effect is that of vertebral bone structure demineralization, but graduated withdrawal provides the time required for rectifying this deficit, a distinct advantage that does not accompany cast usage. The normal stress that accompanies ambulation and muscular activity without external support restores the reciprocation of bone deposition and absorption resulting in recalcification and structural firmness. Youth is a decided advantage because reciprocal osteoclastic and osteoblastic activity is more rapid in the young.

Therefore, the weaning process not only serves to restore calcium and muscular integrity but it also points to the need for optimum patient activity to achieve the desired outcome. In addition, the effects of immobility during therapy signifies the valued recognition for active participation in self-care and mobility commensurate with imposed limitations and patient capabilities. This holds true for the greater degree of immobility incurred during methods prior to and following surgical intervention.

Assessment of Therapy. Surgery is required if the curve progresses despite conservative management with the Milwaukee brace. Although this nonoperative measure may suffice with a consequent avoidance of surgical manipulation, it also serves as a holding maneuver to curtail progression until age reflects a suitable time for surgical correction and stabilization. It is thought that there is a definite relationship between the end results of surgical correction and skeletal maturation. Operative procedures afford better terminal results when the patient has nearly attained or, in particular, has reached maturity (Keiser, 1967). Harrington (1968) indicates that conservative therapy with effective brace application yields successful results in curval deformations ranging from 20 to 45 degrees. Nelson et al. (1967) stipulate curval measurements as being between 30 and 50 degrees. Keiser (1967) and MacEwen et al. (1967) state that surgical management is utilized in curves 50 degrees and above. Nelson et at. (1967) agrees and indicates that with successful holding maneuvers and patient maturation, surgical intervention is required to maintain stability. James (1967) explains that a satisfactory situation is one in which deterioration is prevented in curves of 20 or 30 degrees, but that surgical intervention is indicated beyond these figures to assure significant correction. Blount (1969) specifies that in situations in which patient-parent enthusiasm falters with conservative therapy, the only alternative is spinal fusion. Other criteria concerning the need for operative intervention are related to identified conditions that contribute to the secondary development of scoliotic deformation.

As to the type of deformity, primary thoracic and thoracolumbar curves are those that respond to effective brace application (Campbell, 1963; Swenson, 1969). Swenson includes high dorsal curves but also indicates that the brace is ineffective in low lumbar curves that involve the sacrum or pelvis. A generally accepted view is that late adolescent double primary curval patterns are best treated via brace application without sequential surgery. Existent deformation is trunkal shortness, which is noted on forward flexion because the curves opposite to one another balance each other. Fusion offers little advantage and is considered ineffective because it arrests growth and exposes the individual to lengthy surgical procedures (James, 1967).

OPERATIVE MANAGEMENT

Operative management consists of attaining and maintaining as much correction as is feasible via a variety of external methods of force and support (Keiser, 1967; Riseborough, 1967; Goldstein, 1969; James, 1967; and Evarts, 1969) that can be used alone or combined with a variety of surgical techniques (Goldstein, 1969a; Schmidt, 1969) that serve to correct cosmetic alterations, but principally to supply internal fixation and correction (Nelson, 1967; Wilson, 1967; Goldstein, 1969b; Roaf, 1969; and Dwyer et al., 1969). Internal fixation is accomplished via different fusion techniques (Campbell, 1963) but primarily through Harrington instrumentation simultaneous with fusion (Wilson, 1967; Goldstein, 1969). Postsurgical methods for immobilization differ also, but external support is required to provide time for consolidation and to maintain fusion integrity. These internal methods render the spine inflexible and thus corrected areas are transformed into solid bone columns (Keiser, 1967). Resulting spinal rigidity prevents movements associated with the normal flexible column, a change that requires consideration in an individual's choice of occupation and daily activities.

The methods for choice depend upon the curval severity, clinical findings, and physician preference. As previously indicated, there are a variety of preoperative appliances, but this presentation will be confined to those that are in common use namely, the Risser localizer cast (Fig. 8) and Halo-femoral or Cotrel traction (Fig. 10) (Keiser, 1967; Goldstein, 1969). Surgical intervention will be limited to the Harrington instrumentation technique.

The Risser localizer cast is included to the purposeful exclusion of its antecedent, the Risser-Ferguson turnbuckle cast (Fig. 12) because its advantages have practically eliminated choice for the latter technique (Riseborough, 1967; James, 1967).

> The localizer cast has in great part replaced the turnbuckle cast for correction of scoliosis. The localizer cast is different from the turnbuckle cast in that the corrective forces are applied by head and pelvic distraction along with lateral pressure just prior to and during application of the plaster cast so that at completion of the cast the correction has been accomplished. It is also useful for preliminary correction either prior to instrumentation or preliminary to further correction to be obtained by the wedging principle (Goldstein, 1969).

If further correction is desired, another approach is serial cast applications (Riseborough, 1967; and May et al., 1967).

The localizer yields greater success in correcting rib angulation. (Campbell, 1963). Although its predecessor, the turnbuckle, is an effective technique for correcting curves associated with pelvic obliquity

FIG. 12. Risser-Ferguson Turnbuckle Cast used for forcible correction of scoliosis. The turn-buckle and hinges are incorporated into the plaster. Each time the turnbuckle is adjusted new points of pressure tend to appear. Prevention of pressure areas and skin breakdown may be difficult. (From Larson and Gould. *Orthopedic Nursing*, 7th ed., 1970. p. 371. Courtesy of the C. V. Mosby Co.)

and for reducing rigid deformations, its application is inappropriate for combined thoracic and lumbar patterns or simultaneous primary and major thoracic curves. While the turnbuckle can be used in single primary curves, the localizer can be applied in both single and combined curval patterns (Goldstein, 1969).

Advocates of the localizer stress that it is less time consuming and more easily applied than the turnbuckle (Evarts, 1969; Riseborough, 1967). The turnbuckle involves lengthy hospital confinement and recumbancy (Wilson, 1967) that reduces freedom of movement and increases patient exposure to the undesirable effects of immobility. In addition, its use carries with it the danger of overcorrection (Wilson, 1967; Goldstein, 1969).

Risser Localizer Cast. Perhaps the localizer's greatest advantage lies in the fact that it permits earlier postoperative patient ambulation (Riseborough, 1967; Evarts, 1969). Discussion of the Risser localizer cast was reserved for this section because the device is perhaps the most widely used technique prior to surgical intervention (Keiser, 1967; May et al., 1967). It is not only a successful nonoperative method but its use is also prevalent during postsurgical therapy. Therefore, the points for patient care can be incorporated into one area of this presentation.

When casting is required as a nonoperative measure or preliminary to operative intervention, it is helpful to provide the patient with a picture or model simultaneous with explanations concerning cast application and care. Patients dread the prospect of having to be "encased" in such a device and imaginative inquiries primarily reflect the need for assurance that their growth will not be hampered during required therapy. Often times they have seen others on the unit or in the clinic receiving this form of therapy but casts vary with associated patient diagnoses and physician choice. Therefore, clarification regarding associated patient contact is called for and reference should be made to a specific example to assure correct patient knowledge. Peer companionship is of inestimable value and conversations reflect sincere concern for one another's welfare. Shared experiences point to the fact that he will survive cast application, for self-endangerment is a very real concern.

Although application techniques vary, it should be explained that he will be placed on a special frame lying on his back as if reclining in a bed (Fig. 13). A form-fitting stockinette or other fabric will cover his torso and felt strips or other padding will be placed over areas that require protection and coverage for proper body cast application. These areas usually include the back of the head, the occipital region, the neck front, jaw, and chin, the shoulder girdle, the sacrum, and the iliac crests. After longitudinal traction is accomplished, pressure will be applied upon the curval apex(es) and at opposite ends as counter pressure to obtain optimum correction with a minimum amount of patient discomfort, allowing soft tissues to adjust to the position change. Posterolateral forces directed against the lateral deviation(s) also aid in correcting rotary deformation as well (Evarts, 1969; Riseborough, 1967). Since distraction is dependent upon precise application, the plaster is well-molded in the soft waist region above the iliac crests and in and about the occipital and mandibular areas (James, 1967; Goldstein, 1969). With established distraction and lateral force, the application of plaster is completed, and once set, the temporary traction devices are removed. The cast is beveled and trimmed and dependent areas are checked. Particular attention is given to the mandibular margins and inner aspect of the occipital area. A roentgenogram depicts the amount of correction attained.

When a cast application is scheduled, comparative dental impressions and facial photographs precede and follow its application, since malocclusion can accompany its use (Goldstein, 1964). This is particularly applicable to nonoperative therapy, but pressure points must be

FIG. 13. Localizer cast application. Patient is in position on Risser localizer table for application of a localizer cast. The pelvic girdle between two layers of waxpaper is applied over
padding and can be easily withdrawn after the cast is completed. Increasing head halter and
pelvic traction is applied to patient tolerance. The localizer is adjusted below the apex of the
rib cage deformity for correction of a right thoracic curve. The plaster is applied with the
patient under the influence of the distraction and lateral pressure forces. (From Goldstein.
American Academy of Orthopaedic Surgeons: Symposium on the Spine, 1969. Courtesy of The
C. V. Mosby Co.)

ascertained and examined during nonoperative and preliminary
therapy.

SOME NURSING FUNCTIONS IN CAST APPLICATION. With the
knowledge that plaster radiates heat during the hardening process,
this action should be explained to the patient prior to and gently
reiterated during cast application. Beads of perspiration will form on
the patient's forehead and trickle alongside his face. Therefore, tissue
wipes should be available. Although manipulation is accomplished in
accordance with patient tolerance, he will experience discomfort during
the maneuver. A gentle touch and/or a squeeze of the hand conveys
acknowledgment of his experienced discomfort. Human concern is
priceless. This procedure is extremely exhausting and several days are
required for patient adjustment.

Upon transfer to the stretcher and back to his bed, an explanation
should be given as to how this will be accomplished for immobility and
a cumbersome cast can contribute to an overwhelming feeling of helplessness. The bed should be equipped with a bedboard to provide a firm
foundation for cast support. However, the wet cast is vulnerable to

pressure points from the patient's body weight. Therefore, pliable pillows with protective covers should be placed across the bed to afford support during the crystallization process and changed accordingly. Since the patient lies supine, this critical aspect for care will prevent flattening of the cast over the sacrum and buttocks, common sites for tissue damage.

Proper support during transfer should be provided not only to assure cast integrity by avoiding indentations from mishandling, but also to provide for patient security and proper alignment. Once the patient is in bed, a recheck should be made to insure proper alignment and to note if any part of the cast is impinging upon skin surfaces. Naturally, other pillows are supplied for patient comfort. Excess plaster should be removed from skin tissues with a damp cloth.

The cast should be exposed during the evaporation (drying process) but care must be taken to provide for patient privacy and comfort with coverage of exposed anatomical areas. Drying is best accomplished via natural means, but sometimes artificial presentation of heat is employed. This is usually accomplished with the use of heat cradles or incandescent lighting. However, caution must be exercised with their use once the plaster has set because intense heat can interfere with crystallization and cause tissue damage in the form of burns. Heat should not be applied in the immediate postoperative period because it may dilate blood vessels and cause hemorrhage. If lighting is used, it should be placed at least a foot or a foot and a half distance from the patient and enclosed for safety. If the cradle is used, it should not be covered because the trapped moisture that occurs with condensation is detrimental to the course of drying. Another method is the use of electric fan(s), but the patient should be protected via adequate covering because accelerated evaporation and the body's response to radiated cast heat causes chilling. *This is not a popular method* because uniformity in crystallization is lacking.

Frequent position change with maintenance of alignment is necessary to achieve cast solidification, but it is also a necessary approach for preventing pressure necrosis. The physician will indicate the desired time for the first alteration because several hours are required to provide for initial drying and patient rest. Assistance is necessary to furnish adequate support with turning, and explanations should precede and accompany each planned position change. The approach for care should be organized with the necessary equipment in readiness to efficiently accomplish the nursing goal and preserve patient strength. Patient turning should be accomplished in unison so that the body cast and extremities move in one plane. This is commonly known as "log-rolling." Care must be taken to avoid turning the patient upon his upper extremity. Careful placement of extremities should precede the slow but deliberate movement into the new position. Once the desired change is reached, the patient should be moved to the center of the bed to avoid a possible precarious situation and to provide for patient security with the felt and needed surrounding support. This is an opportune time to replace moist or dampened linens, to straighten wrinkled linens, and to check for possible cast difficulties.

As previously indicated, the sacral region can be a problem but other significant areas of concern are the mandibular margins, the occiput, the iliac crests, the lateral pressure points, and the cast edges. Tissue pressure against the cast can result in serious nerve and circulatory impairment. Detection is crucial because tissue trauma from pressure can result in edema, paralysis, or necrosis.

Palpable examination will reveal any rough edges that may serve to irritate dependent areas. The mandibulo-occipital areas can also be felt and visually examined for any signs of pressure, irritation, or skin breakdown. If the cast is still wet, rough edges can be rectified without adverse effects. When the cast is dry, the stockinette can be pulled out and over the cast edges and application of circular or pointed adhesive strips (petals) will serve to furnish a smooth undersurface and maintain the cast ridges, thus protecting vulnerable skin surfaces. In instances in which another protective fabric is used, fabric extension may not be possible but described adherence of adhesive will accomplish the same aims.

Skin color will serve as a clue to any possible circulatory alteration, particularly in nonoperative casts that include the thighs (Goldstein, 1969) to obtain better pelvic girdle distraction. If this situation exists, the extremities should be felt for any indication of a temperature differential in addition to notations for swelling or irritation. Slight pressure exerted upon the nail-bed tip (blanching sign) with a rapid release will disclose possible circulatory impairment; the change from white to pink should be immediate. A sluggish return indicates possible difficulty. If the thighs are not included, as is frequently the case for operative intervention, the groin area should be examined for circulatory (femoral pulse) and tissue integrity.

With consideration given to cast length (extending from chin and occiput to hips or thighs), the patient's mobile capacity via range of motion will serve to reveal the possible presence of nerve impairment. Concomitant with casting is the need for patient activity with a view toward prevention of contractures and concern for the undesirable effects of immobility. Therefore, primary measures that accompany cast therapy are proper anatomical alignment and remedial exercises. It is important to remember that malalignment can contribute to constriction, possible consequent anesthesia with nerval deterioration, and pressure necrosis. If observed edema is not relieved with a change in position or, if position is accurate and not a contributor to its formation, then immediate physician notification is appropriate. Jaw exercises also aid in reducing the initial discomforts associated with the distracting force.

After the initial cast application, the patient will experience an aching sensation from the enforced distraction. Medication is usually ordered to alleviate the discomfort or what is commonly known as the "cast syndrome." In the latter, the patient may have an elevated temperature, complain of nausea, or experience episodes of diarrhea or vomiting. This is due to cast constriction. Other factors that may contribute to this situation are the lack of intake prior to casting, patient anxiety, or experienced heat radiation during cast solidification.

An additional concern that accompanies crucial nursing responsibilities is the detection of tissue trauma or possible ulceration beneath the cast. Expressed feelings of numbness or a burning pain, tingling or throbbing exemplify tissue trauma with swelling and probable nerve involvement. Loss of sensation is indicative of nerve compression. This points to the need for not only explaining and conscientiously adhering to activities concerning disclosure, but also to the need for detecting a possible odor that would reveal necrotic activity. This scent is best detected during removal of bed covers because of the odorous buildup in an enclosed area. Detection for ulceration can be accomplished via touch by slowly moving the fingers over the suspected pressure area; a change in cast temperature (increased) can be felt. A check for drainage or cast stains and discoloration will reveal possible necrotic activity. An increase in the patient's temperature and pulse may also indicate infection. Reported areas of impingement may result in further cast trimming, padding, or the removal of a cast section that overlies the tissue area in question. Removed cast sections(s) are saved for reapplication and secured with tape after examination and/or required treatment. Tissue bulging may be observed with uncovered area(s), particularly if there is a long delay in cast section replacement. In extreme instances, the cast is laterally bivalved for inspection and subsequent therapy.

Astute and frequent observation for signs of pressure includes not only the cardinal indications but also patient complaints or remarks and nonverbal behavior such as a change in facial expression that reveals discomfort. Often a patient will endure the discomforts experienced with cast application and complications and remain silent rather than "disturb" the busy health team. Not infrequently, this reticence is associated with the fear of relief from distress via injected medication. It is helpful to convey acceptance of this fear by verbal acknowledgment with an explanation concerning the availability of oral medication, providing oral intake is permissible. Age has no barrier when it comes to fear of medication injections. Therefore, explanations should accompany all nursing measures regarding the concern for cast management and patient comfort. However, caution should precede the natural impulse to provide medication for relief without first exploring with the patient the "type" of experienced discomfort. Exploration with the patient should reveal genuine concern—verbal and nonverbal—and time should be taken to pinpoint the probable difficulty. In this manner, personal interest is shown, while at the same time, an accurate description is obtained for report and notification.

In addition, if the nurse assigned to care for the patient does not

know the exact lateral pressure areas, the descriptive applicable notations will serve to fulfill the guidance needed. Change of shift reports
should contain this information in addition to patient progress. If a
nursing team member is new to the situation, nursing activities should
be explained, explored, and demonstrated. This provides for accurate
nursing care and enhances a nurse's self-growth.

If further correction is desired, the physician may choose to reapply (serial) casts (Riseborough, 1967) or wedge the original cast
(Goldstein, 1969). Wedging is accomplished by transversely slitting
the cast on the curval concavity with simultaneous removal of an
angular (pie) slice at the curval convexity. With the use of a cast
spreader, the transverse slit is expanded to increase correction. The
cast is then reinforced and plaster is applied to fill the initial openings.
In both situations, the areas for pressure change and consequent observations are directed to these new locations.

In providing for daily patient needs, equipment should be assembled at the patient's bedside in an orderly fashion to provide for
efficient service. This approach provides for continuity, because care is
accomplished without repeated interruptions for omitted articles, an
exasperating and tiring experience for the patient and the nurse.
Economy of effort results in more time spent with the patient, goals
being accomplished in less time, and more available time to tend to
other patients' needs.

During the daily bath, the patient should participate as much as
possible to meet the need for self-help and to accomplish desired
mobility within the confines of cast restriction and patient status. The
bedside table can be turned within easy reach of articles for dental
hygiene or grooming, which can be placed in a tray directly on the
bed or on a chair while the patient is in a side-lying position. The
adolescent should not be placed in an awkward dependent position by
having to ask for these articles. It should be remembered that the
"little things" are those that count. It is also a way of showing individual care.

While bathing the parts that are impossible for the patient to
reach, an inspection should be made of the cast edges for crack-
ing/crumbling, of internal structure by feeling for a wrinkled or loose
lining, or skin underneath and distal to the cast edges for irritation
and pressure, and for the hidden possibility of broken plaster pieces.
It is wise to check under the patient's arms to be sure that the cast
is not impeding movement or creating difficulties with pressure. Another area of concern is the buttocks, since additional cast trimming
may be necessary to provide for adequate elimination and to decrease
possible points of pressure. Petal adhesive strips may suffice, but repair
may require additional application of plaster.

Skin surfaces that surround the cast trim should be clean and dry.
These areas may be massaged where appropriate to enhance circulation
and to maintain tissue health. All exposed bony prominences should

receive proper meticulous attention for the same reasons. Painful irritation can accompany the frequent position changes. This fact also points to the need for proper support and alignment. The insertion of foreign bodies to alleviate the itching that accompanies cast usage can contribute to skin irritation and breakdown. Air blown down the cast with an asepto syringe or other acceptable device will provide the necessary relief.

CAST MAINTENANCE. Occasional cleansing with a *damp* sponge or squeezed-out cloth will aid in cast maintenance, but caution is a watchword. Cleansing materials saturated with water serve to soften the plaster and shorten cast life. Dampness resulting from repeated scrubbing leads to mold formation. If accidental wetting occurs, the use of a hair dryer over the area will hasten drying. Waterproofing with the use of lacquers or shellac should take place after the cast has dried. Otherwise, their application will interfere with the crystallization process. In addition, soiling can occur during elimination in instances in which required recumbency is a part of therapy. The strategic placement of pillows to create an incline may avoid soiling while the fracture pan is in use. Insertion of a plastic disposable covering under and over the cast edge will provide for added protection. It is easier to turn the patient on his side and then roll him back onto the pan; many patients prefer this approach. Patient privacy should be assured and toiletry articles placed within easy reach. The urinal should be replaced as necessary.

If the patient requires a shampoo, this can be accomplished by positioning the patient's head as close to the bed edge as possible. The cast can be protected with plastic that is tucked in and around the back of the neck. The plastic is converted into a trough that extends into a receptacle. A towel may be placed underneath for added protection and absorption of water should it escape through the plastic edging. It is best to use a glass for pouring water, but when a sink is in the patient's room, hosed rubber devices with a gentle spray have come in handy for this purpose.

PATIENT-PARENTAL TEACHING. Concurrent with the preceding activities are patient and parental instruction regarding the necessary precautions and associated needs for cast maintenance and personal hygiene. This can take place not only during the initiation of non-operative therapy for home care, but also preliminary to or following surgical correction. Much depends upon the individual situation. Information, resubstantiation, and demonstrations with return demonstrations take time and should be imparted in accordance with the individual's readiness and pace. During nonoperative and postoperative home care, visits are necessary to assure continuity and to provide any additional necessary assistance. Prepared written instructions will supplement oral and demonstrated activity and also serve as a ready reference for those responsible for patient care. Necessities for home care, particularly during recumbency, are: a bed board; fracture pan and urinal for male patients; prism glasses and mirrors that reflect print; and other objects to aid in daily activities. Referral to a health agency should be made and assistance for obtaining articles for home use. Return visits to the physician's office or an out-patient facility are necessary for follow-up, and for both conservative and operative correction. It is also at this time that previous hospital and/or home teaching is reinforced and patient-parent concerns ascertained or explored.

The Halo Apparatus. Another therapeutic approach is the halo apparatus with femoral Steinmann pin or skeletal cast countertraction (Fig. 14) (Roberts, 1967). Its use is with severe deformities requiring prolonged therapy, particularly those in which ventilatory restriction has resulted in a respiratory deficit (Evarts, 1969). This technique combined with a portable volume control respirator has enabled patients with severe or paralytic involvement to withstand the stresses of major corrective surgery. The portable respirator permits easy patient access

FIG. 14. The Halo Traction Apparatus. (Courtesy of Vernon L. Nickel, M.D. Rancho Los Amigos Hospital, Downey, California.)

in the provision for care and is equipped with an alarm system to alert staff to impending patient difficulties.

Although very severe idiopathic thoracic deformation may now be an exception, it is necessary to reiterate that surgical intervention is preceded by numerous cardiopulmonary examinations.

> A thorough evaluation of pulmonary function is mandatory in the determination of surgical risk. The 50° or 60° curves seldom show any marked reduction in pulmonary function, and the blood gases will be normal, but this is not true of curves of 100° or more, where chest distortion is very severe. These patients usually will show a marked reduction in their vital capacity, their maximum breathing capacity and their oxygen tension blood analysis. Elevation of the carbon dioxide tension is found frequently in the severe curves (Moe, 1967).

In addition, respiratory deficits as high as 40 percent have occurred in curval deformities ranging between 75° and 100° (Bame, 1969).

An advanced tracheostomy may be performed not only to provide time for patient adjustment but to assure ventilatory integrity during surgery (Moe, 1967). An elective tracheostomy in conjunction with the portable respirator affords optimal patient safety during rod insertion and arthrodesis simultaneous with respiratory augmentation. When these two measures are combined with halo traction, halo unit skull attachment pursuant to cast application and halo connection follow ventilatory teaching and adjustment. On the other hand, the tracheostomy succeeds the desired attained curval reduction and is accomplished several days prior to surgical intervention.

The halo head ring anchored to the outer table of the calvarium via four steel pins—two anterior and two posterior—may be applied while the patient is under general or, more frequently, local anesthesia. Nickel et al. (1967) indicate that the ring may be fastened while the patient is supine but it is easier to accomplish when the patient is in a semisitting position. The correct ring size is determined by measuring the patient's maximum skull diameter with a flexible wire from which a traced pattern is used to determine the individual's need. Although the halo rings come in four sizes, the desired circumference is approximately ½-inch greater than the patient's head measurement. Proper placement is evident when the frontal receptor for the vertical traction rod is in direct alignment with the patient's nose. The lower ring edge level should be situated right above the ears and a quarter inch above the eyebrows (Nickel et al., 1968).

The patient is permitted nothing by mouth prior to the procedure. An experienced surgeon can complete the ring attachment in 10 min (Nickel et al., 1968). However, it is inadvisable to quote a specific time interval because the patient can be either delighted or disappointed. Application of the remaining equipment will consume more time depending upon the type of countertraction employed. Individual circumstances determine the method of approach and timing for completion. For example, if skeletal cast countertraction is desired, it is common practice to wait one or two days before application to attain medical stability following ring attachment with general anesthesia. On the other hand, the entire suspension assembly and cast may be completed at once with local anesthesia.

A detergent or germicidal shampoo with shaving (Nickel, 1968) or clipping (Moe, 1967) and cleansing of the four pin insertion sites is the preparatory method. In this manner, disturbance of the individual's hairdo is kept to a minimum. Since there is a greater incidence among females, consideration for patient morale and pride supersedes the former often traumatic practice of shaving the entire head.

When the cast is employed in conjunction with the halo apparatus, its application is accomplished with an anterior opening to overcome the ventilatory restriction inherent with cast usage and, thus it provides for the needed chest mobility. The shoulder straps are set high to accommodate the change in anatomical alignment when the spine straightens. After two anterior main support rods are attached to the halo outrigger and mounted to the cast, the temporary traction is released. Periodic adjustments to lessen curval deformation may span several weeks preparatory to surgical stabilization. However, traction with reduced force is maintained postoperatively for approximately a month to maintain the correction. Once sufficient stabilization is achieved, the patient may ambulate in the halo body cast (Fig. 15) or external support may be maintained via a localizer cast or Milwaukee brace (Riseborough, 1967; Bame, 1969; Evarts, 1969).

If bilateral counter femoral Steinmann pin traction is used, insertion is at the distal end of each femur. Plaster strips that include the pins encircle the thighs for soft tissue immobilization and to lessen the chance for pin-tract infection. Skeletal traction is achieved during one procedure; halo attachment precedes pin insertion. This method is particularly useful when external thoracic pressure is to be avoided (Evarts, 1969; Riseborough, 1967). Usually equal amounts of traction are applied to the halo and lower extremities, but increased weight may be added to the extremity on the side of the curval concavity. To level the pelvis in obliquity, the leg on the higher side bears more weight than the leg on the lower side. Traction is gradually increased over a two- to four-week period and is maintained during and after internal fixation. Sometimes a cast is applied prior to surgery to hold the maximal correction obtained (Roberts, 1967). External fixation is achieved as described in the previous paragraph.

PATIENT PREPARATION.   Prior patient preparation includes explanations concerning the purpose for halo traction, the method of application, and approximate time required for therapy. Since the halo is quite elaborate in design, it is best to complement explanations with visual aids or introduce the teenager to a patient undergoing treatment to enhance comprehension and to allay the fear that accompanies

FIG. 15. Femoral pins removed, the patient can ambulate while in the halo body cast. (From Boone. *Amer. J. Nurs,* 69:1937, 1969.)

the patient's first exposure to the apparatus. He should be assured that the device does not penetrate the brain by receiving a diagramatic review, if necessary, to exemplify the fact that the pins are inserted into the cranial external cortex. Scalp incisions are unnecessary because the pins pierce the soft tissue and flare upon contact over a wide area with minimal skull penetration. The pins are locked into place once the desired pressure is attained. In addition, should the pin become loosened, a lock on its exterior prevents the chance for increased skull penetration. An anesthetic (local or general) is administered for the procedure and medication (analgesic) is available post application to relieve the initial discomfort.

Other patients will indicate that the device is quite comfortable, but sometimes in their earnest desire to help the youngster facing this procedure, they report that the apparatus is painless. Diplomacy should prevail when rectifying this error in patient protected reassurance for two reasons: one, because the patient will experience initial discomfort and should be prepared for its occurrence, and two, correction should be accomplished without loss of patient self-esteem.

At the same time, he will see that the hair is cut or shaved approximately 1 to 2 inches in diameter at the pin insertion sites. He will be able to have hair shampoos during therapy and the shaved or cut areas will require trimming because of regrowth. This is particularly applicable to prolonged treatment which is usually associated with other primary conditions that have contributed to secondary scoliotic deformation, or to extended therapy due to intervening complications.

AFTER-CARE. While traction is applied, its effectiveness depends upon assiduous care and astute nursing intervention. Initially, the patient will experience some discomfort in becoming accustomed to the recumbent position, to the halo apparatus, and to the countertraction employed. Headaches or pain around the pin sites occasionally follow halo application, situations in which medication is readily available. It is expected that there will be some exudate and inflammation surrounding the pin sites. Transient swelling and erythema may be noted but rapid disappearance usually occurs (Nickel et al., 1968).

However, frequent checks for pin stability and impending infection are crucial because loose screws can also create pain and clicking at the site with erythema, excessive tissue granulation, and drainage. Subtle generalized swelling can be felt, but contour asymmetry may also be noted. There may be puffiness about the eyes or the eyes may lack their usual luster. Changes in the patient's temperature or pulse may signify difficulty. Patient comments may alert the nurse to probable problems, but in any event, noted changes should be reported and recorded.

Although infection is infrequent, there are specific situations that predispose the individual to its occurrence. Patients with strong neck muscles experience pin problems. This may be attributed to a probable increase of stress at the site. Patients with oily skin or loose tissue beneath the scalp are prone to pin difficulties (Nickel et al., 1968). Therefore, daily nursing care should include attention to the hair and scalp, to note the possibility of excessive oiliness and the subsequent need for frequent shampoos.

Routine cleansing varies with regard to daily time intervals and solutions. Hydrogen peroxide is usually used to remove the crusts and exudate. Moe (1967) specifies the sequential use of alcohol, aqueous zephirin, and a gentle pHisoHex scrub for cleansing, followed by the application of Betadine. Bame (1969) indicates that hydrogen peroxide is used twice daily and the area is painted with an antiseptic. Some physicians are inclined to think that the crust formation about the pin sites is nature's way of protecting the area. While cleanliness is of great importance, disturbance because of frequent crust removal may contribute to irritation and consequent inflammatory problems.

If edema formation is evident, traction weight reduction may result in its abatement. Loose pins are gradually tightened with a torque screwdriver. This action usually relieves the symptoms and is accomplished without analgesia. The change in pressure is well tolerated. On the other hand, if tightening is met with no resistance or infection is evident, the pin is removed and a sterile pin is inserted in an adjacent aperture after the apparatus and scalp have been thoroughly cleansed. Functional disruption does not occur with pin transference. The halo is secure after this maneuver and the pins must remain tightly affixed to the skull for patient comfort and effectiveness. This holds true for its initial application when proper placement is achieved. The first day or two the screws may be slightly tightened for adjustment. However, Nickel et al. (1968) advise against routine tightening during therapy because this activity accelerates erosion through the outer skull tables.

Traction effectiveness depends upon proper alignment. When the halo is used in conjunction with femoral traction, the equipment must remain in good condition without functional impairment. The nylon ropes should remain straight, passing through the rotary bearings over the pulleys without evidence of wear, and the suspended weights should hang freely. The nylon cords are melted at their ends to prevent raveling and are a preferable substitute for the usual rope because of longer durability.

As previously indicated, weight increments are gradually applied, but the total is measured in accordance with the patient's age and body weight (Moe, 1967). With weight addition and curval derotation, there is a change in the patient's height simultaneous with the possible need for shortening rope length to maintain traction. In addition, the bows extending from the Steinmann pins must remain clear to avoid inadvertent pressure on the patient's lower extremities. Tape placed across the bow rope connection serves as a reminder to maintain clearance (Bame, 1969). This points to the need for constant vigilance to detect adverse changes in equipment due to stress and the necessary adjustments that accompany curval correction. More importantly, it is the patient's response that governs weight addition or withdrawal. The length of therapy, therefore, is determined by patient progress and curval rigidity. Bame (1969) indicates that weights attached at either end have reached as high as 40 pounds, but Moe (1967) reports that weights exceeding 30 to 35 pounds have not been useful in achieving additional correction.

During required immobilization, flotation pads, foam wedges, or synthetic or natural sheepskins may be placed on the mattress or beneath bony prominences to provide for patient comfort and inhibit skin breakdown. While patients favor the supine position, which provides for maximum effectiveness, the lateral posture can be accomplished with relative ease and patient comfort increased with the use of support pillows or sandbags. A footboard or one devised from a blanket or sheet should be used to prevent footdrop and the heels should be elevated to avoid probable breakdown. The patient is able to move or reposition his head because a plate with ball bearings is connected to the halo base. Caution should be exercised in turning the patient because the halo magnifies sound. To avoid the annoying vibrations that accompany accidental knocking, rubber corks can be attached to the screw ends. Sometimes the slippery Formica surface of a traction board is used to facilitate head movement while sustaining the head and halo in an extended position (Bame, 1969).

As the patient becomes accustomed to the apparatus, usually within two to four days, he becomes more proficient and secure in providing for self-care. Dining needs are met without aid and minimal assistance is required for turning and bathing. Hygienic measures can be accomplished with patient positioning and comfort in mind. That is, the anterior surface can be cleansed while the patient is supine and the remaining posterior can be completed after the patient is turned to the lateral position. Vulnerable skin areas such as the rib hump, sacrum, and trochanter should receive special attention with massage not only during bathing but also during alternate position changes. Hair care can be accomplished by the nurse when the patient is lateral and/or supine. It is easier for the patient to tend to dental needs while lying on his side. The fracture pan facilitates positioning because of its size and it is more comfortable than the conventional bed pan. Bed covers, the patient's accumulated articles, and other equipment should be placed so as not to interfere with functional alignment.

Proper anatomical alignment contributes to patient relaxation and decreases the possibility of muscular aches and spasms that can accompany forcible correction. Also, the nurse must be ever mindful of the internal alterations that coincide with curval derotation and the simultaneous manifestations that may reflect accommodating difficulties.

Neurological impairment may be detected by observing the patient's response or lack of it to daily care measures. Does he respond to touch or changes in temperature? Is spinal nerve pressure contributing to progressive lower extremity paresis or to the patient's inability to void? Is it also reflected in expressed complaints of upper extremity numbness or tingling? Are the pupils of the eyes equal or does he experience double vision? These are but a few examples. However, early detection may mean the difference between correction and permanent nerve damage. Frequently the situation is rectified by a temporary pause in therapy or reduction in traction weight.

Similarly, organic thoracic displacement may be detected observationally or by careful monitoring and comparison of vital signs. If a cardiac problem accompanies the spinal deformity, the patient may become cyanotic when placed in the supine position. On rare occasions, the gradual addition of weights may create a respiratory deficit and cardiac failure may ensue (Bame, 1969). In these situations, treatment is altered or discontinued.

While traction may have a positive influence upon the curval deformity, it does not necessarily alleviate the ventilatory restriction incurred with scoliosis. Therefore, progressive respiratory training accompanies therapy and culminates into one pattern. The physical therapist may initiate the regimen and external aids may be incorporated to enhance vital capacity. However, the nurse can play a large part in this area by having the patient deep breathe and cough for a few minutes with each position change or even between times. Deep breathing and coughing requires periodic encouragement particularly when the patient is in the lateral position opposite the curval apex. This posture may create breathing difficulties, and it is a natural response on the part of the patient to resist assuming it.

Other alternatives to achieving an increased capacity are methods that will visually reveal patient progress. One approach is to have the patient blow a piece of paper from his overbed table as far across the room as possible; the increase in distance and the necessary change to heavier paper revealing progress. Wind instruments and the blowing up of balloons may aid ventilatory exchange. Blow bottles in which the patient can see the transference of liquid from one to the other also accomplishes the same purpose. Ventilatory instruction preliminary to surgery also provides for a smoother postoperative course and is continued during this time period.

HALO REMOVAL. Traction is maintained until such time as roentgenographic analysis depicts the desired optimal correction. When the halo has achieved its purpose and/or it is followed by another appliance, removal is easily accomplished with little or no discomfort provided the patient's head is adequately supported. Pin site closure usually takes place within three to five days (Nickel et al., 1968). Care includes maintaining cleanliness, along with observation for prompt healing.

HALO—SKELETAL TRACTION. When the cast is coupled with halo traction, the previously described nursing responsibilities associated with both may be adapted and applied. With an anterior opening, the nurse can insert her fingers under the edges to feel for possible pressure points, particularly along the rib cage. When compared with halo-femoral traction, this method provides for greater freedom of patient movement. For the nonambulatory patient, Nickel et al. (1968) use a device with a circular frame to which the halo has been added and the cast attached (Fig. 16). The patient is suspended between two bike rims and the spokes serve as improvised supports. It rests on a bed with ample room between the patient and the mattress, and the rims set within grooved wooden blocks for stability. Nursing measures are simplified because teh patient can be turned with relative ease, and the apparatus facilitates care associated with elimination. Also, the patient can be placed in a prone position to read or write.

Cotrel Traction.   If Cotrel traction (Fig. 10) is used, the patient should receive an explanation as to how the head and pelvic halter are applied. He can see pictorially or by viewing it on another patient that the head harness fits onto the chin and reaches around to the occiput. Leather straps extend from both sides of the head and meet at the point for traction attachment. Jarring of the head is avoided by providing support during application and gently lowering the weights until they are in proper position and in direct line with the patient's spine. The two points for pressure are the chin and occiput, but the occipital area receives the greatest amount of pull because the head pulley is elevated. These two prominences along with tender facial tissues should be checked for possible irritation and breakdown. Frequent observations should include proper placement so that the chin pad is

FIG. 16. The Circle Frame simplifies nursing care of the nonambulatory patient in the Halo Traction apparatus. (From Nickel et al. *J. Bone Joint Surg.,* 520A(7)1408, 1968.)

not compressing the patient's throat and the hair remains free from entanglement. Also, the head halter should not be pinching the patient's ears or pulling upon tender skin.

While the pelvic harness straps serve to provide leverage and stability, maintenance of alignment is stressed because of the relative ease with which a patient can impede its function. The pelvic harness should fit snugly without imposing stress upon the iliac crests. Proper positioning along with associated nursing responsibilities is essential. In many instances, the patient is able to tell if he is malaligned and seeks the desired position for comfort. By being present and assisting with the initial procedure, the nurse is in a better position to note and report improper alignment.

SURGICAL INTERVENTION

If surgery is required, temporary internal fixation with Harrington instrumentation is used as either a major or a supplementary corrective technique (Fig. 17A-C) (Goldstein, 1969b). Direct force is applied to the rotational and angular spinal deformity by the insertion of a pre-stressed stainless steel distraction-compression assembly which may be used for any curve located between the first thoracic segment and the sacrum. Two rods, one on each side of the curve, are implanted through specially designed hooks that are secured to the appropriate vertebrae as determined by roentgen analysis. Distraction is exerted upon the concavity and the rod is inserted at or beyond the curval end vertebrae while the compression rod extends along the convexity between the end vertebrae (Fig. 17B) (Harrington, 1964; Riseborough, 1964; Evarts, 1969).

The instruments may be combined with a variety of techniques to achieve the desired correction (Harrington, 1964), but Riseborough (1967) indicates that the threaded compression system is not in common use. When ambulation is resumed, it does not significantly reduce the magnitude of forces exerted upon the distraction rod. Stretching of the curval concavity is accomplished in a similar manner, as seen with the use of an automobile jack. Notches at the upper end of the distraction rod provide for the gradual incrementation desired to attain correction and to allow for tissue adjustment. The corrective force is discontinued when spinal resistance is such that further attempts could exceed bone pressure endurance and result in a fracture at the purchasing sites (Harrington, 1964; Roaf, 1966).

Grafts for arthrodesis may be obtained from the tibiae, ribs, (Roaf, 1967) or iliac crests (Evarts, 1969; Riseborough, 1967; May et al., 1967), but the iliac crest is the favored donor site (Evarts, 1969). Cortical cancellous tibial grafts are not desired (Riseborough, 1967) because they leave a defect in the bone and osteoporosis from immobility may lead to a fracture when the individual introduces stress with weight-bearing (Campbell, 1963). If a tibial graft is used, careful

FIG. 17. Harrington Treatment by Instrumentation and Fusion. A, Roentgenogram of the spine of an 11 year old girl showing idiopathic scoliosis with a right dorsal primary curve of 55° and a left lumbar one of 60°. B, Roentgenogram of the spine made after the curves have been corrected to 10° each by instrumentation, and the spine has been fused by the Moe technique. C, Roentgenogram of the spine made 3 years after fusion. Note that ossification of the iliac apophyses is complete. About 5° of correction have been lost, but the spine is stable and the patient is free of discomfort. (From Harrington. In Crenshaw, ed. Campbell's Operative Ortho-

350

handling of the extremity is essential during the postoperative and convalescent periods. The ribs may be used when their resection is part of the corrective procedure (Goldstein, 1969a,b). The bone bank (May et al., 1967) and commercially processed nonantigenic bone are additional sources of supply (Keiser, 1967). Although heterogeneous, homogeneous, or ilial cancellous bone are customary alternatives for fusion reinforcement with instrumentation, the osteogenic potency of fresh autografts has no substitute (Evarts, 1969). In some instances, sufficient supplemental bone for fusion may be secured locally by crushing and imbricating the decorticated posterior vertebral elements (Keiser, 1967; Roaf, 1966). Exposure to surgical trauma is reduced and, cosmetically, the patient is spared from having another scar.

When casting is used preliminary to surgery, a posterior window is created to provide ample access to the spine and outer aspect of the ilium opposite the curval concavity for grafting during rod insertion and fusion. Precordial and abdominal windows are also devised; the former serves as a precautionary emergency measure in case of cardiac arrest, while the latter affords exposure to the least amount of pressure during surgery. (Fig. 18A, B). External pressure upon the anterior abdominal wall can cause a major increase in inferior vena caval pressure. With partial or complete vena caval obstruction, blood returning from the lower parts of the body is diverted into the valveless vertebral venous system for transport to the heart, thereby increasing the amount of blood loss experienced during surgery (Relton et al., 1967). Intraabdominal pressure is minimized while the patient is prone because lateral bolsters provide the necessary support. Most of the patient's weight is borne by the iliac spines and clavicles. The precordial segment is loosely replaced while the remaining windows are retained and reapplied postsurgery.

Some physicians laterally bivalve and remove the cast as a provisional safeguard for the anesthetized individual and retape or restrap it into place after anesthetic recovery until suture removal, at which time a new cast is applied (Larson and Gould, 1970; Campbell, 1963; May et al., 1967). This approach provides for easy patient access for examination and treatment when postoperative complications such as vomiting, distention, or chest or abdominal pain intervene. In some instances, the cast is left off completely and a new one is applied, sometimes under moderate traction, after the suture line has healed. Proponents of retention of the preoperative cast during surgery and the postoperative phase fear correction loss with its removal. Postoperative immobilization periods vary in the provision for external support while the fusion mass consolidates and matures. Required recumbency may extend over a period of three to four months while ambulation with external protection may fall between two and four months (Goldstein, 1969; James, 1967; Page et al., 1967).

With cast removal during or after therapy, the nurse should refrain from vigorously cleansing the underlying crusty dead skin cells

FIG. 18. Preoperative localizer cast. A. Large posterior window through which fusion is performed allows wide exposure of one ilium, for removal of a large amount of iliac bone graft, as well as the area of the spine to be fused.

because this activity can result in irritation and bleeding. Periodic gentle washing with warm, soapy water and the application of emollients will gradually achieve the same purpose.

In preparing the patient for cast removal, explanations should include the fact that manual or electric cutters are safe and harmless devices. The electrical tool may frighten some patients but supplied assurance dispels this fear. The new-felt freedom after removal is met with ambivalence; the relief from confinement is coupled with the odd sensation that is associated with loss in external support and muscular tonicity. Therefore, the nurse's response should reflect an understanding of the patient's reaction as well as the anticipated effects of immobility. In addition, gentle, deliberate changes in position followed by the strategic placement of pillows for support are essential. If the patient

FIG. 18B. Front of the localizer cast, showing the large abdominal window that minimizes pressure on abdominal contents when patient is prone during surgery. The chin-neck trap door allows direct laryngoscopy for intubation for anesthesia. The precordial window is also shown. (Figs. 18 A B from Goldstein. American Academy of Orthopaedic Surgeons: Symposium on the Spine, 1969. Courtesy of The C. V. Mosby Co.)

is ambulatory, he should be assured that continued activity will restore muscular tonicity.

Instrumentation with Fusion. In situations in which instrumentation with fusion is necessary, the surgeon meets with the patient and family concerning this decision, the risks involved, and the anticipated changes that accompany correction. General anesthesia is employed and the technique is accomplished under strict asepsis. The patient may have a posterior midline incision that extends from the first thoracic vertebra to the sacrum. A second incision may be described depending upon the physician's choice for supplementing the fusion mass. The necessity and method for providing external support and immobilization is also included. If patients have failed to respond to conservative therapy or surgery is required to hold the correction attained by conservative means, the same appliance may be used post-surgery or the physician may transfer to another method. When casting is used before and after surgery, the patient is familiar with the technique and this aids in his adjustment during the postoperative period.

Although instrumentation has shortened the required period of immobilization (Evarts, 1969; Wilson, 1967), the length of therapy is considered because the adolescent's education is temporarily interrupted and the family needs assistance in arranging for continued schooling and home care. Time is provided for all to adjust emotionally to the need for surgical intervention; frequently information has to be clarified and supplemented. Financial aid is another consideration because the required therapy is costly.

PREOPERATIVE PREPARATION. Preoperative preparation includes the routine measures accorded any patient undergoing major surgery. As previously indicated, additional examinations may be ordered in relation to the scoliotic deformity, but information should be provided concerning the nature of the routine examinations and procedures as well as those specific to the individual patient situation. The nurse should assist with them whenever possible, but more importantly, she should provide the necessary, often unsolicited, patient support.

If a patient has been recumbent prior to surgery, it is possible that he has become accustomed to eating while lying on his side and using the bed pan or urinal in the supine position. "Logrolling" may also be a familiar procedure. Passive-active and respiratory exercises may have been a part of previous therapy. However, it is best to review what has taken place to ascertain the patient's understanding and capabilities before initiating instruction, particularly guidance, associated with coughing and abdominal breathing techniques that serve to facilitate postsurgical recovery. Postoperatively, the nurse will have to be persistent in encouraging these patient activities. Shallow, quiet respirations, accumulated bronchial secretions without coughing, and decreased mobility connected with experienced pain and use of depressant analgesics can lead to atelectasis and pneumonitis.

With the knowledge that ventilatory restriction can accompany scoliotic deformation, respiratory aids that stimulate deep breathing are important adjuncts to avoiding post-operative pulmonary complications. One such aid is the lightweight plastic Adler rebreather (Fig. 19A-C) that adds . . . approximately one liter to the respiratory tract dead space [by producing] a hyperventilatory response roughly equivalent to that seen with the inhalation of 5 percent carbon dioxide (Adler and Brodie, 1968).

> The inside of the rebreather is compartmented by walls with openings remotely located from one another which insure thorough mixing of air during rebreathing (Fig 19C). The re-

FIG. 19 Adler Rebreather. A, Illustrated from above; B, Side view—Hyperventilation is stimulated when the patient, with nose clip in place, rebreathes her own air with its increased CO_2 for 3 to 5 minutes every hour; C, Cutaway view shows how air is mixed inside the device. (A and C from Adler and Brodie. Amer. J. Nurs, 68:1287, 1965. Courtesy of Richard H. Adler.)

breather is easy to handle and to keep by the bed off the floor. The patient experiences no resistance or discomfort while using the device. The movable plastic mouthpiece is designed for comfort and to prevent air leak around the mouth. Included with the rebreather is a plastic-covered malleable nose clip with which the patient can compress his nostrils during periods of rebreathing. Patients are instructed to use it for approximately five consecutive minutes at hourly intervals. Actually, nearly optimum effects are obtained by the end of a three-minute rebreathing period (Adler and Brody, 1968).

Instructions are imprinted on the apparatus to serve as a reminder in the event that the patient forgets (Fig. 19A). By describing the device's function and the manner in which it is used preoperatively, the patient is provided with a familiar technique during the postoperative period. Sometimes the rebreather is used in conjunction with intermittent positive pressure breathing (IPPB) therapy, particularly for patients who are known to have an obstructive condition.

Although nutrition is an important aspect of therapy, the purpose for omitting intake the evening prior to surgery and immediately following it should be explained. It should also be added that a gradual introduction to fluids with an eventual return to "normal" intake will follow. A nasogastric tube is inserted prior to surgery to avoid the accumulation of fluids which might be vomited and aspirated and to avoid the discomfort associated with distention. The patient's parents should be informed of this routine approach to lessen the anxiety that accompanies their first postoperative visit.

X-ray analysis includes the identification of the superior and inferior hook purchasing sites of the curval concavity (James, 1967). Vertebral levels for fusion are located by taking a spine-marker film. This is accomplished by injecting sterile methylene blue, under aseptic conditions, through the soft tissues and ligaments over a spinous process tip. With the needle piercing the spinous process, a roentgenogram is taken. The needle serves to identify the spinous process on film, while the dye provides for accuracy in locating the same spinous process at surgery (Goldstein, 1964, and 1969). Some physicians will remove the needle and tape a metal wire at the injection site to achieve the same purpose (Campbell, 1963). Since the medication is excreted by the urinary tract, the patient's urine will appear blue-green. In supplementing the physician's explanation, the nurse should include this anticipated response so that the patient is spared an incident of alarm from this natural occurrence. Since the examination takes place one to three days prior to surgery, its excretion may be noted prior to and/or following surgical intervention. James (1967) indicates that this technique is routine with some physicians and radiographic markers should be used in case of doubt. When the fusion is to extend across the thoracolumbar area, the ribs are used for identifying vertebral levels for arthrodesis.

Although various solutions are employed in preparing the surgical site, the area usually extends from the occiput to the gluteal folds and includes the posterior surface to the midaxillary lines. Several preparations are commonly requested 48 hr prior to surgery, but on the evening before the operation the area is shaved and cleansed. On the morning of surgery, it is wise to check that the shave has been accurate while cleansing before proceeding to the sterile orthopedic prep. Once this is accomplished, a sterile sheet is placed over the area. It is *not* wrapped around the patient, but it is secured with the use of circular gauze. Ace bandages are usually applied to both legs from toes to midthigh to maintain adequate circulation and are removed 24 hr after surgery. The preoperative medication is given at the specified time.

Since time is of the essence, the nurse should utilize it to full advantage in working closely with and providing the individual with the necessary preoperative instruction. Although she may be knowledgeable in relation to adolescent growth-developmental expectations and corrective surgical measures, she should remember that she is working with an *individual person* who requires her sincere interest and skill.

While the patient is in surgery, his unit is prepared for his return. Since the patient will not be able to assume the sitting position, a gatchless bed is preferred. However, if one is not available, the levers may be taped to serve as a reminder that they are not to be used. Signs placed at the foot and/or head of the bed may also be printed to accomplish the same aim. Many patients will design their own to alert staff members to this fact. Sometimes illustrations accompany exclamations such as, "Do not gatch bed!", "I'm to remain flat!", "Logroll me!", "Do not touch that gatch!"; or "It takes two to turn me!" This is one activity that reflects their understanding and concern for accurate care during the postoperative period, but it is also a way in which they can participate in providing for their needs.

POSTOPERATIVE CARE. A bed board should be placed under a firm mattress and an intravenous stand along with other postoperative bedside equipment should be situated in readiness for his return and smooth transfer from the stretcher to the bed. Much depends upon hospital protocol. Sometimes a patient is sent directly from the recovery room to the intensive care unit, and by the third postoperative day intravenous therapy has been discontinued. On the other hand, the patient may be transferred directly to his unit after spending several hours or a day in the recovery room. In some instances an x-ray is taken during the immediate post period to check for rod placement and degree of correction, while at other times the roentgenogram is ordered immediately preceding cast application or reapplication 10 to 14 days after surgery. Also, the patient's height may be measured and compared with the preoperative or admission results.

Postoperative care will differ according to the presence or absence of external support. If the patient returns in a body cast, then previously described nursing responsibilities associated with its use apply. The patient is turned—logrolled—approximately every hour and alternates between the supine and partial (30° is the limit) side-lying position. Although this activity extends over a possible two-week period, the patient may move his head and extremities. He should never be placed in a position that would hinder adequate support or impose stress upon the suture line.

On the other hand, if the patient returns without external support, the usual request is that he remain flat for the first 6 hr or in some instances the first 48 hr. The patient may be "logrolled" after these time periods, and the use of a small pillow is permitted after the second day. Again, proper positioning is essential, but the patient should not attempt a position change or to flex his back at any time. This holds true for all postoperative patients who have undergone instrumentation with fusion.

Because the patient cannot relieve spinal muscular tension by movement or a change in position, the need for pain medication (narcotic) may be frequent and the dosage quite high. This experienced discomfort is accompanied by the presence of severe bone pain, particularly during the first few days following surgery. The nurse should exercise judgment in providing for the necessary relief and in differentiating between possible cast complications, when it is in use, and the discomfort associated with surgical intervention. Possible neurological complications may be detected by checking for motion— ask the patient to wiggle his toes—and a change in sensation in the lower extremities. If neurological problems occur and they do not stem from possible cast compression, they are usually due to pressure phenomena secondary to bleeding or a bone fragment. The patient's level of alertness and comments are clues to the identification of possible problems. If the nurse has any question regarding patient status, immediate physician notification is appropriate.

Careful monitoring of vital signs is essential for noting probable respiratory or circulatory difficulties. With distraction rod insertion and adjustment, there is a possible shift in thoracic content along with a pressure redistribution within the vascular system. Respiratory embarrassment may ensue and the patient's blood pressure and pulse may reflect the altered pressure change.

Since multiple transfusions are administered to replace the blood lost during surgery, the patient may still be receiving a transfusion upon his arrival to the recovery room or occasionally upon return to the unit. The nurse should be alert to the possible development of a transfusion reaction and the probable endangerment of hypervolemia. In the latter, the patient's face appears lividly cyanotic, the jugular veins become prominent, the blood pressure rises, and the pulse increases in volume and rate. A hemoglobin and hematocrit may be ordered the morning of the second postoperative day.

> The adrenal cortical response to the stress of surgery usually results in retention of water and sodium and loss of potassium for the first one or two postoperative days. Another reaction which may take place at the same time is decreased or absent peristalsis, so the patient is given nothing by mouth and

nasogastric suction is continued. Fluid and electrolyte balance must, therefore, be maintained by intravenous infusions . . . [that rectify the initial alterations and maintain physiological integrity until the patient is capable of retaining oral intake]. Intake and output records are necessary to determine the amounts of fluid needed and to prevent the overhydration which predisposes to pulmonary edema (Boegli and Steele, 1968).

[The patient's age and weight are also considered in the calculation for fluid need and replacement per hour and day.]

The patient may be unable to void, for a variety of reasons: edema resulting from the surgical trauma in the area of the spinal nerve roots, sympathetic stimulation, lying in a horizontal position, muscular tension, or oliguria. If micturition has not occurred after 12 hr, catherization may be ordered (Boegli and Steele, 1968).

Sometimes a Foley catheter is inserted during surgery and connected to gravity drainage during the immediate postoperative period. The output is measured every 8 hr or oftener, and a specimen for culture is obtained prior to the catheter's removal two days postsurgery. The nurse should check to make certain that the tubing remains free from external obstruction and its patency is constant. The sedimentation rate may be a part of the nurse's responsibility in addition to the other activities that accompany elimination needs.

Meantime, the patient's lips may be moistened and ice chips offered prior to the introduction of clear fluids on the first postoperative day. A medication to combat nausea may also be ordered and given at the nurse's discretion. Resumption of peristalsis and functions of elimination usually return to normal 48 to 72 hr after surgery. It is at this time that the nasogastric tube is removed. When clear intake is tolerated, fluids and foods are encouraged.

Bowel function should be checked daily by observing for abdominal distention and listening for bowel sounds. When patients in casts fail to expel flatus and feces, the consequent discomfort experienced in a restricted apparatus can lead to autonomic shock. Sometimes a medication such as Ilopan is ordered routinely to prevent abdominal distention, paralytic ileus, and the delay in resumption of intestinal motility.

The possible development of infection is also a concern. A temperature elevation the first postoperative day may indicate the presence of a pulmonary or urinary infection (Moe, 1967). Conscientious adherence to encouraging coughing and deep breathing techniques along with the use of external respiratory aids is an essential preventative approach. Urinary frequency with little output, bladder distention, itching or burning upon micturition, or facial grimacing during elimination may signify impending difficulties. A foul odor or the specimen contents may reveal a probable infection. In any event, urine and blood cultures are ordered along with a chest x-ray. Prophylactic medication is not requested at this time.

Although the wound may be inspected when the temperature rise is reported, an elevation 48 hr after surgery signifies probable infection at the operative area, particularly if other possibilities have been eliminated (Moe, 1967). The compression dressing requires surveillance for possible drainage or oozing, but the nurse should not forget to check the donor site (if one was used) as well. A blood culture and an aspirated culture of either blood or purulent material from the fluctuant wound is sent for analysis. If an infection is present, the patient is returned to the operating room for the necessary treatment. Moe (1967) indicates that with Harrington instrumentation, an intervening infection is usually found to extend the length of the rods as opposed to confinement to one locale. The wound is cleansed, debrided, and suction-irrigation tubes are placed along the affected area. The instruments are not removed. Wide-spectrum antibiotics are administered intravenously until the results of a wound culture taken during surgery reveals the required drug alternatives. Systemic antibiotic therapy is continued for several weeks beyond the local tubular suction-irrigation treatment, which usually reveals a clear return within seven to ten days. While irrigation may be discontinued during this time, suction is maintained a few more days to assure a clear and negligible return. There will be a noted, often sudden, change in the patient's temperature toward normal and healing ensues. The patient's white blood cell count and sedimentation rate also return to normal. Although the method for intervention is explained by the physician, the nurse should prepare the patient for the additional enumerated examinations and provide the necessary support.

While wound infections have been known to occur during the immediate postoperative period (Boegli and Steele, 1968), a persistent, slight, or moderate temperature elevation may reflect the delayed type of infection which is known to make its appearance two to three months following discharge from the hospital (Moe, 1967). In contrast to the immediate postoperative infection that is red, tender, and painful, visual and palpable inspection of the incision site proves negative. There is a favorable response to the administration of antibiotics and the patient appears to have recovered prior to discharge. When this type of infection occurs, a spontaneous sinus develops and purulent drainage follows. Treatment is the same as that described for immediate postoperative infections. However, the length of external support for fusion integrity may be extended.

A subdued environment without extraneous stimuli serves to lessen the heightened sympathoadrenal medullary response that follows major surgical manipulation. The increase in epinepherine speeds up glycogenolysis, thereby increasing the blood sugar level.

Because of the marked increase in protein catabolism and the need for massive regeneration of bone tissue and wound healing, a diet high in protein, iron, vitamin C, and thiamine becomes very important. Calcium intake is somewhat restricted, however, because the patient's immobility causes a sudden release of stored calcium into the circulation. Under these circumstances, an otherwise normal calcium intake may raise the serum calcium beyond the point where it can be excreted by the kidneys. This would predispose to the development of renal calculi. Extra fluids will also help to prevent this development (Boegli and Steele, 1968).

Since predisposition to tissue irritation and necrosis accompanies the initial increased metabolic activity, frequent position changes with adequate anatomical support and strict attention to skin care are essential. While back care is an important part of maintaining tissue integrity, the nurse should refrain from vigorously massaging this area during the immediate post period to avoid disturbing the surgical wound. The region around the buttocks may be an exception, but *gentle* cleansing is the watchword. Skin care and proper alignment is continuous with careful consideration for cast care, intake and output, and passive-active exercises.

Although required recumbency fosters healing, the transition from passive to active patient exercise aids in venous return and avoids the possible development of thrombi formation. Ace bandages aid in circulatory function, but the nurse should feel the lower extremities for possible swelling and tenderness or observe for circumferential differences during the immediate post period. Early detection can alert the physician to possible impending difficulties with institution of corrective measures before more serious symptoms and signs appear.

DISCHARGE PREPARATION. After approximately one-and-a-half to two weeks, the sutures are removed and a cast is applied or reapplied in preparation for discharge and home care. Several days are allotted to provide for the necessary adjustments that accompany cast usage. The patient has reached the stage at which turning to the side position is easily accomplished and the prone posture is not permitted. As previously indicated, the nurse utilizes this time in providing the patient and family with instructions concerning cast maintenance, associated observations, positioning, and exercise. Lower- extremity abduction is avoided because the muscles for thigh abduction originate from the lower spine and pelvis. This position would exert strain upon the operative site. In addition, avenues for communication are provided should the patient experience any difficulty or the family require further assistance. Close coordination of effort in providing for patient and family needs involves contact with and/or referral to the necessary community agencies and educational institutions. Arrangements are made prior to discharge to assure continuity and immediate assistance.

RESUMPTION OF AMBULATION. Approximately three to four months postsurgery, a new cast may be applied to provide for the patient's first attempt at assuming the vertical position and gradual return to ambulation. In some instances, a cast change is not required because the cast applied prior to discharge does not impose restrictions with resumption of ambulation. Transfer from the horizontal to the upright posture is gradually achieved to provide for vascular adjustment by tilting the bed in reverse Trendelenburg position or by placing the patient on a tilt board. Daily angular incrementation is accompanied by close observation for patient tolerance to the desired position change.

When the patient first begins to assume the upright position, he may experience dizziness and loss in balance. Several attempts may be required before he succeeds in standing alone. Low-heeled shoes with a soft lining are a necessary adjunct in providing for proper support and alignment and in minimizing the sympathetic response that accompanies return to the upright posture. Vasoconstriction contributes to the patient's initial discomfort, as reflected in comments associated with muscular aches and painful sensations in the soles of the feet. Warm-water soaks will provide soothing relief. The nurse should have assistance during this maneuver to provide for patient safety and support and explanations should reflect the natural anticipated response to assauge patient anxiety. Lower-extremity exercises concurrent with increased daily eposure to ambulation continues for an approximate three-week interval.

The change in height that accompanies curval correction may impose perceptual difficulties and the patient should exercise caution when walking through passageways or downstairs. Since cast weight may add to the awkward sensation, the patient should grasp the handrail whenever possible to assure stability when moving down a flight of stairs. The nurse should accompany the patient during the first few exposures to aid in this adjustment.

Once ambulation is well established, the patient may assume the sitting position, but he is advised against jolting his spine to avoid insult to the surgical site. The use of arm chairs is demonstrated to accomplish smooth transfer from the standing to the sitting position and vice versa. If a chair without arms is used, the patient is shown how to grasp the seat to accomplish the same purpose. Circulation to the lower extremities should not be impeded by the cast and the patient is cautioned to observe for this possibility. Adjustment in cast length may be necessary.

With cast usage, the patient may require some assistance with choice in attire. Loose-fitting styles will not accentuate cast contour and outfits with high collars and straight lines will not draw attention to its presence. Durable material should be chosen since contact with the cast hastens wear.

Once full resumption of ambulation is achieved, the patient may return to school. Exercises continue with increased activity to gradually restore muscular tonicity and stability. A new cast that does not include the shoulders and neck may be applied to provide for the required external protection until it is no longer needed (Fig. 20).

Patient Followup.   Periodic visits to the physician's office or clinic for x-ray analysis is necessary to assure fusion consolidation because

FIG. 20. Post Harrington Rod full body cast—ambulatory. (From Davis. Amer. J. Nurs., 68: 2403, 1968.)

a pseudoarthrosis may contribute to a substantial loss in correction. This is an actual graft defect that may exist in one or several areas along the fused spinal segment, and careful inspection of lateral oblique and anteroposterior films is essential in diagnosing its presence. If a loss in correction occurs, surgical reconstruction is necessary.

On the other hand, a pseudoarthrosis may occur with instrumentation and not result in a loss of correction. Surgical inspection and correction is postponed, but the area is carefully observed for progressive solidification without loss. If this occurs, the patient is spared further surgical trauma. If a change is noted to the contrary, then surgical intervention is necessary (Moe, 1967).

It is too early to evaluate the long-term effects of instrumentation. The rod has been known to slip or break on occasion, but it has only been removed in instances of experienced patient discomfort. Slipping from the hinged vertebrae is viewed thus far as a natural occurrence since the spine grows away from the support it no longer needs. From all appearances, the spine remains stable. Removal techniques involve the same intricate surgery required for its installation. Therefore, surgeons are inclined to leave it in place provided the patient is without difficulty.

If all goes well, the patient is ready for cast removal—but he should be prepared for the dizziness that accompanies the sudden withdrawal of external support. This may be attributed to the neurovascular reaction that is associated with peripheral vessel dilation and consequent hypotension. As previously indicated, tender skin and its care along with associated effects of immobility should be explained. Delicate fabrics should be worn to prevent further skin irritation and breathing exercises are continued to aid in the transfer from abdominal to thoracic excursions.

Proper positioning and alignment is reviewed and stressed along with the required rest and nutrition that aids in growth and health maintenance. Since surgical intervention has imposed upon spinal mobility, this influences the patient's choice for a future occupation. Guidance and counseling services with vocational examinations may be of considerable assistance in ascertaining the patient's future role in society.

NURSING RESPONSIBILITIES APPLICABLE TO ALL SITUATIONS. Each patient requires the nurse's individual attention during the provision for required therapy, but consideration for schooling and peer group contingency with diversion is applicable to all situations.

The adolescent's education is a vital concern and any delay or postponement of this continuing process is to be avoided. Arrangements for continued schooling can be made prior to admission. If in-patient care requires a short stay, as in preparatory traction for the fitting of a Milwaukee brace, school work may be brought in via the patient's parent or a peer. On the other hand, if a lengthy stay is required, other arrangements are suggested. A two-way telephone hookup is available for a direct link between the patient and his school. A receiver-transmitter apparatus is placed in the patient's room and in his classrooms at school so that he can directly participate in classroom lectures and is also able to communicate to ask questions. Other alternatives include scheduling of surgery during summer vacation period and utilizing tutors for various subjects.

A very real and necessary consideration is that of suggesting diversions for the bed-ridden and immobilized individual. One need only imagine what it would be like to remain confined in a bed for an extended period of time in order to realize the complexity of the problem of suggesting appropriate activities. Boredom is perhaps worse than physical discomfort in a bed-ridden situation. Variety is not only the spice of life but also the key to the success for any suggested recreation.

Activities are centered upon attracting the individual's attention so that he cannot be preoccupied with his or her bed-ridden state. Therefore, they have to be based upon the individual's interests and abilities to avoid suggesting something in which an individual may be interested but perhaps has relatively little ability (for example: delicate art work) and thus produce frustration over boredom, or worse, in combination with it. This is not meant to discourage the initiation of new interests or the improving of an individual's limited ability in any area. However, care must be taken that the diversions which are suggested are geared to the specific individual with the purpose of attracting his attention and relieving idleness.

Activities may be arbitrarily classified into two categories for the sake of clarity and convenience. The first category can be termed general diversions that are of interest to both adolescent boys and girls. These include: the telephone, watching television, listening to the radio, and reading books and magazines. Prism glasses can be supplied for reading in order to insure maximum comfort. The other category can be termed specific diversions and is applicable to either boys or girls. These include: stamp or coin collections, games of all sorts, construction projects, arts and crafts, exercises (hand grips and hand bar bells for boys) and so forth. The above listing is by no means comprehensive. Much can be accomplished in this area with creativity and ingenuity on the part of the attending nurse(s).

There are some practical suggestions for the nurse concerning patient activities. Watching television can be boring in itself. Yet, if time is taken to supply the individual with advance program listings, then the individual can choose programs in which he is interested. Also, advanced listings aid in the anticipation of a desired program which can be a way of reducing disinterest since the individual has something to look forward to. A word of caution! Television should not be a replacement for human contact and communication.

The nurse can also consult with the physical or occupational therapist to discover which exercises and recreational materials can also be used as a means of occupying the individual's attention during certain times of the day. A telephone should be within easy reach since its use consumes much time and provides for communication with family and friends. Another point to remember is that whatever the individual may need is to be situated within easy reach so that dependence on the nurse is reduced and a sense of relative self-sufficiency is enhanced.

Group recreation sessions should be organized to supply much needed human contact and entertainment. These sessions can include band or combo concerts, sing-alongs, group parties, games, and so forth. The individual's bed can be wheeled into the recreation area or other acceptable means can be adapted to achieve this end. The importance again is to draw the individual's attention away from his bed-ridden situation and to relieve boredom.

Frequent visits by relatives and friends aids in his continued identification with loved ones and the outside world. In situations in which parents' working hours do not coincide with visiting times, special arrangements should be made to make visits possible. If the hours are limited, then steps should be taken for greater liberalization. When patients do not have visitors, and this does happen, volunteers should be contacted to provide for individual attention.

Finally, after the required stay in the hospital, the individual will be released to go home. While home he will still have a subdued lifestyle as the provided external support imposes immobility. Some practical suggestions for diversions would be: to put the individual's bed in the recreation area of the home to be near the family; to keep a telephone within easy reach; and to supply comparable activities to those in which the individual participated in the hospital. Another feasible activity would be to take the individual for a ride, especially if he is in a sitting cast or brace. If not, this can be accomplished by having him lie flat in the rear of a car or station wagon. Visits from friends should be encouraged and arrangements should be made to make it pleasant and convenient for the individual's friends to come and see him. The family should be encouraged to make every effort to accept the individual into their normal life pattern without excessive pampering and coddling. This will not only make it easier for the patient to adjust to his new, but temporary, life-style; it will also enhance his own self-esteem since he will not be overly conscious of his altered situation as a family member.

References

Aegerter, E., and Kirkpatrick, J. A. Orthopedic Disease, 3rd ed. Philadelphia, Saunders, 1969, Chapters 6 and 21.

Adler, R. H., and Brodie, S. L. Postoperative rebreathing aid. Amer. J. Nurs., 68:1287–9, June 1968.

Baker, E. A. and Zangger, B. School screening for idiopathic scoliosis. Amer. J. Nurs., 70:767, Apr. 1970.

Bame, K. B. Halo traction. Amer. J. Nurs., 69:1933–7, Sept. 1969.

Blake, F. Immobilized youth. A rationale for supportive nursing intervention. Amer. J. Nurs., 69:2364–9, Nov. 1969.

Blount, W. P. Nonoperative treatment of scoliosis. In American Academy of Orthopedic Surgeons: Symposium on the Spine. St. Louis, Mosby, 1969, pp. 188–95.

———— and Bolinske, J. Physical therapy in the nonoperative treatment of scoliosis. Phys. Ther., 47:919–25, Oct. 1967.

Boegli, E. H., and Steele, M. S. Scoliosis—spinal instrumentation and fusion. Amer. J. Nurs., 68:2399–403, Nov. 1968.

Carnevali, D., and Brueckner, S. Immobilization—reassessment of a concept. Amer. J. Nurs., 70:1502–7, Jul. 1970.

Cooke, R. E., ed. The Biological Basis of Pediatric Practice. New York, McGraw Hill, 1968.

Cowell, H. R. Genetic aspects of orthopedic disease. Amer. J. Nurs., 70:763–6, Apr. 1970.

Crenshaw, A. H., ed. Campbell's Operative Orthopedics, 4th ed. St. Louis, Mosby, 1963, Vol. II, pp. 859–1778.

———— Campbell's Operative Orthopedics, 5th ed. St. Louis, Mosby, 1971.

DeGeorge, F. V., and Fisher, R. L. Idiopathic scoliosis—genetic and environmental aspects. J. Med. Genet., 4:251–7, Dec. 1967.

Donnellan, W. L., Kidd, J. M., and Swenson, O. Tumors of the head and neck. In Swenson, O., ed. Pediatric Surgery, 3rd ed. New York, Appleton-Century-Crofts, 1969, Vol. 1, pp. 367–8, Chapter 24.

Dwyer, A. F., Newton, N. C., and Sherwood, A. A. An anterior approach to scoliosis: a preliminary report. Clin. Orthop., 62:192–202, Jan.–Feb. 1969.

Enneking, W. F., and Harrington, P. R. Pathological changes in scoliosis. J. Bone Joint Surg., 51:165–84, Jan. 1969.

Evarts, C. M. Trends in the management of scoliosis. Cleveland Clin. Quart., 36:23–33, Jan. 1969.

Farkas, A. Basic factors in the development of scoliosis. Bull. Hosp. Joint Dis., 28:131–49, Oct. 1967.

Gazioglu, K., and others. Pulmonary function in idiopathic scoliosis. J. Bone Joint Surg., 50:1391–9, Oct. 1968.

Goldstein, L. A. The surgical management of socliosis. Clin. Orthop., 35:95–115, July–Aug. 1964.

——— Concave rib resection and ligament release for correction of idiopathic thoracic scoliosis. In American Academy of Orthopedic Surgeons: Symposium on the Spine. St. Louis, Mosby, 1969a, pp. 254–64.

——— Treatment of idiopathic scoliosis by Harrington instrumentation and fusion with fresh autogenous iliac bone grafts. Amer. J. Bone Joint Surg., 51:209–222, Mar. 1969b.

——— Turnbuckle and Risser localizer casts in the correction of scoliosis: selection of patients and techniques. In American Academy of Orthopedic Surgeons: Symposium on the Spine. St. Louis, Mosby, 1969, pp. 241–253.

Guyton, A. C. Textbook of Medical Physiology, 3rd ed. Philadelphia, Saunders, 1966, p. 1106, Chapter 76.

Harrington, P. R. Nonoperative treatment of scoliosis. Texas Med., 64:54–65, Mar. 1968.

——— Spine Instrumentation and Fusion Technique. (Booklet) 1964. Presented to U.C.L.A. extension course in medicine in Los Angeles, California, March 14, 15, 1964.

——— and Tullos, H. S. Reduction of severe spondylolisthesis in children. Southern Med. J., 62:1–7, Jan. 1969.

Inkley, S. R. Pulmonary function in scoliosis. In American Academy of Orthopedic Surgeons: Symposium on the Spine. St. Louis, Mosby, 1969.

James, J. I. P. Scoliosis. Baltimore, Williams & Wilkins, 1967.

Johnson, J. T. H., and Robinson, R. A. Anterior strut grafts for severe kyphosis—results of 3 cases with a preceding progressive paraplegia. Clin. Orthop., 56:25–36, Jan.–Feb. 1968.

Keiser, R. P. Treatment of scoliosis. Nurs. Clin. N. Amer., 2:409–418, Sept. 1967.

Larson, C. B., and Gould, M. Orthopedic Nursing, 7th ed. St. Louis, Mosby, 1970, pp. 366–77.

Levine, D. B. The influence of spinal deformities on chest function. Phys. Ther., 48:968–72, Sept. 1968.

Lindahl, O. Resection of vertebral transverse processes in idiopathic scoliosis. Acta. Orthop. Scand., 37:342–7, 1966.

Lowe, L. W. Congenital kyphoscoliosis with paraplegia due to intradural dermoid cyst. Proc. Roy. Soc. Med., 61:668, July 1968.

Lowell, D. J., Bostic, W. C., and Connelly, J. P. Scoliosis in children. Med. Sci., Aug.:43–58, 1965.

MacEwen, G. D., Conway, J. J., and Miller, W. T. Congenital scoliosis with a unilateral bar. Radiology, 90:711–5, Apr. 1968.

——— and Shands, A. R., Jr. Scoliosis—a deforming childhood problem. Clin. Ped., 6:210–6, Apr. 1967.

Makley, J. T., and others. Pulmonary function in paralytic and non-paralytic scoliosis before and after treatment. J. Bone Joint Surg. (Amer.), 50:1379–90, Oct. 1968.

May, V. R., Jr., and Mauck, W. R. Exploration of the spine for pseudoarthrosis following spinal fusion in the treatment of scoliosis. Clin. Orthop., 53:155–22, Jul.–Aug. 1967.

Meyer, H. L. Predictable problems of hospitalized adolescents. Amer. J. Nurs., 69:525–8, Mar. 1969.

Moe, J. H. Complications of scoliosis treatments. Clin. Orthop., 53:21–30, Jul.–Aug. 1967.

——— Methods and technique of evaluating idiopathic scoliosis. In American Academy of Orthopedic Surgeons: Symposium on the Spine. St. Louis, Mosby, 1969, pp. 196–240.

Morgan, T. H. Scoliosis. Maryland Med. J., 16:71–4, Sept. 1967a.

———— Scoliosis: II. The management and treatment of scoliosis. Maryland Med. J., 16:159–61, Oct. 1967b.

Nash, C. L., Jr. and Moe, J. H. A study of vertebral rotation. J. Bone Joint Surg., 51:223–9, Mar. 1969.

Nelson, P. W., and Harrington, P. R. Decisions in scoliosis. Southern Med. J. 60:894–6, Aug. 1967

Nickel, V. L., and others. The halo. J. Bone Joint Surg., 50:1400–9, Oct. 1968.

Olsen, E. V. The hazards of immobility—effects of immobility on psychosocial equilibrium. Amer. J. Nurs., 67:794–6, Apr. 1967.

———— and Edmonds, R. E. The hazards of immobility—effects on motor function. Amer. J. Nurs., 67:788–90, Apr. 1967.

———— and Johnson, B. J. The hazards of immobility—effects on gastrointestinal function. Amer. J. Nurs., 67:785–7, Apr. 1967.

———— and McCarthy, J. A. The hazards of immobility—effects on respiratory function. Amer. J. Nurs., 67:783–4, Apr. 1967.

———— and Schroeder, L. M. The hazards of immobility—effects on urinary function. Amer. J. Nurs., 67:790–2, Apr. 1967.

———— and Thompson, L. F. The hazards of immobility—effects on cardiovascular function. Amer. J. Nurs., 67:781–2, Apr. 1967.

———— and Wade, M. The hazards of immobility—effects on metabolic equilibrium. Amer. J. Nurs., 67:793–4, Apr. 1967.

Relton, J. E., and Hall, J. E. An operation frame for spinal fusion: a new apparatus designed to reduce haemorrhage during operation. J. Bone Joint Surg. (Brit.), 49:327–32, May 1967.

Riseborough, E. J. Treatment of scoliosis. New Eng. J. Med., 276: 1429–31, 22 Jun. 1967.

Risser, J. C., Norquist, D. M., Cockrell, B. R., Jr., Tateiwa, M., and Hoppenfeld, S. The effect of posterior spine fusion on the growing spine. Clin. Orthop., 46:127–39, May–June, 1966.

Roaf, R. A new plate for correcting scoliosis. (Summary). Proc. Roy. Soc. Med., 62:272–3, 3 Mar. 1969.

———— Growth deformities of the spine. Physiotherapy, 54:7–13, Jan. 1968.

———— Scoliosis. Baltimore, Williams & Wilkins, 1966.

———— The treatment of scoliosis. Int. Surg., 47:266–75, Mar. 1967.

Roberts, J. M. New developments in orthopedic surgery. Nurs. Clin. N. Amer., 2:383–90, Sept. 1967.

Schmidt, A. C. Osteotomy of the fused scoliotic spine and use of halo traction apparatus. In American Academy of Orthopedic Surgeons: Symposium on the Spine. St. Louis, Mosby, 1969, pp. 265–282.

Smith, D. W. Recognizable patterns of human malformation. (In the series: Major Problems in Clinical Pediatrics.) Philadelphia, Saunders, 1970, Vol. VII.

Swenson, O. The chest wall. In Swenson, O., ed. Pediatric Surgery, 3rd ed. New York, Appleton-Century-Crofts, 1969, Vol. I, Chapter 26, p. 400.

Tachdjian, M. O. Musculoskeletal system. In Swenson, O., ed. Pediatric Surgery, 3rd ed. New York, Appleton-Century-Crofts, 1969, Vol. II, Chapter 79, pp. 1350–1353 and 1396–1404.

Thomas, P. K. The neuromuscular disorders in which scoliosis may occur. In Zorab, P. A., ed. Proceedings of a Second Symposium on Scoliosis: Causation. London, Vincent House, 1968, pp. 46–49.

Vallbona, C., Harrington, P. R., Harrison, G. M., Freire, R. M., and Reese, W. O. Pitfalls in the interpretation of pulmonary function studies in scoliotic patients. Arch. Phys. Med., 50:68–74, Feb. 1969.

Wilson, F. C., Jr. The treatment of scoliosis. N. Carolina Med. J., 28:139–43, Apr. 1967.

Wiltse, L. L. Spondylolisthesis: classification and etiology. In American Academy of Orthopedic Surgeons: Symposium on the Spine. St. Louis, Mosby, 1969, pp. 143–67.

Winter, R. B., and Tongen, L. A. A malignant chest wall sarcoma with bilateral pulmonary metastases—a fifteen-year survival after multiple radical local excision and resection of bilateral pulmonary metastases and a successful treatment of scoliosis secondary to tumor surgery. Surgery, 62: 374–8, Aug. 1967.

Wynne-Davies, R. Familial (idiopathic) scoliosis: A family survey. J. Bone Joint Surg. (Brit.), 50B:24–30, Feb. 1968.

Zorab, P. A. The medical aspects of scoliosis. In James, J. I. P., ed., Scoliosis. Baltimore, Williams & Wilkins, 1967, pp. 238–46.

——— (ed.) Proceedings of a Second Symposium on Scoliosis: Causation. London, Vincent House, 1968.

9 SHIRLEY STEELE

Nursing Care of the Child with Congenital Anomalies and Minimal Cerebral Dysfunction

"I got up one night and went to the bathroom. I was hemorrhaging. My husband called my doctor and he said to bring me to the hospital immediately. I was seven weeks early but I never once considered any harm would be done to my baby. I had an emergency Cesarean section. As I went to surgery I felt very secure that my fourth child, although premature, would be perfect. Two days after delivery my daughter died. To that point I never gave up hope, I wanted my baby."

The foregoing statements were made by a neighbor. I include them now to portray the optimistic outlooks mothers have for their offspring. Despite very complicated pregnancies and deliveries, mothers still anticipate the delivery of a "normal child."

"It is the mother who 'produces' the infant, it is she who 'gives' it birth. If the 'product' turns out to be defective (a term here used to include all defects in the child, whether physical or intellectual), the mother perceives this as a defect in something she has produced" (Ross, 1964, p. 56). The mother who delivers in the hospital may have her feelings of defeat reinforced by the hospital staff. The maternity unit is generally considered a "happy" unit. Fortunately, most of the events taking place here result in a new life and a fulfillment of a goal for the child's parents. The child with a defect is not an ordinary part of the unit and, therefore, the staff's care for this child is not ordinary. Joyful overtones are not appropriate at this birth. As a result, the staff frequently withdraws and does not give the mother the support she needs to cope with the birth of a child with a defect.

"The mother is thrust into the stark reality very soon after the

371

birth. The father, because of his less active role in the birth and immediate post delivery period can deny the situation longer than the mother. The father also is able to fall back on the defensive fantasy that the child is not really his own" (Ross, 1964, p. 56).

The nursing personnel in the delivery room have a vital role to play in the beginning coping process. The nurse must be especially careful of her facial expressions. Even the forehead above the surgical mask can give nonverbal clues that something is wrong. Withholding the baby from the mother's sight is another way of saying that your child is "less than expected." If the mother has actively participated in the labor and delivery process, she will be most anxious to view the child immediately after birth. It is only fair to prepare her for the child with its defect and show her the child, briefly. The silence which frequently prevails during this crisis period is most anxiety-producing to the mother. She may very well imagine a much more severely handicapped child than her baby. This needless anxiety may influence the future mother-child relationship. In addition, it may lead to the mother's distrusting the medical and nursing personnel that she will need to have confidence in during the long-term care of the child.

In some hospitals, the doctors prefer to talk with the father prior to telling the mother about the child. If this is the chosen plan, the mother must be given close nursing supervision to make her feel personally comfortable. At least, this physical comfort will help her to relax. The sooner the mother is told, the easier it will be to begin to help her plan for the child in a constructive way.

After the announcement has been made to the parents, many different defense mechanisms may be utilized by the parents. The mother is usually more subject to them than the father. Some of these defense mechanisms are described by Ross (1964) and are summarized briefly here. She may choose to *repress* the incident, trying to keep the handicapped child out of her conscious awareness. She may utilize *projection,* trying to treat the child as though it had its source outside herself. She may utilize *sublimation* whereby she represses the impulse until it can be changed from a socially objectionable to a socially valued outlet. She may use *intellectualization* whereby she controls affects and impulses through thinking about them instead of experiencing them. Another possibility is *displacement,* which can involve aggressive impulses being used against the self. Another mechanism is *controlling;* this allows her to interfere with suggestions or attempts of others, or allows her to comply without thinking. *Denial* is a very commonly utilized mechanism; it allows the mother to keep threatening perceptions from coming to the surface. *Withdrawal* is a mechanism which may occur as a temporary and immediate response to threat and usually lasts only until she is able to bring another defense mechanism into play.

An understanding of the possible mechanisms the mother can use will help us to plan nursing intervention effectively. The mechanism of *withdrawal* is frequently utilized immediately after delivery. It can be expressed by a desire to sleep. This can be very beneficial sleep for the mother. There is no need to try to talk her out of it. She needs rest following the labor and delivery. She also needs sleep to aid in developing strength to deal with the resultant stress produced by delivering a handicapped baby.

It is important to remember that the use of defense mechanisms aids our daily living and their usage is normal during crisis periods. The assistance the mother receives can turn these defense mechanisms into useful tools for coping with the unique problems she will have to face. The use of *denial*, for instance, is not abnormal at first. However, its persistence can be abnormal. How, then, can the nurse help the mother to relinquish the use of denial? One way is to show the baby to the mother early. The baby should be exposed to the mother while the nurse is available. The mother should explore the child slowly and carefully. She should be encouraged to ask questions. The nurse must watch the mother closely to interpret her tolerance level. If it is evident the mother cannot benefit from further time with the baby and nurse, then the session should be terminated. A new time should be set up for the mother to see the baby again. Perhaps viewing the child in the nursery can help to prepare the mother for the next visit. Rooming-in should not be discouraged unless the baby is severely handicapped and needs vigilant observation. The less severely handicapped baby may benefit greatly by being close to his mother's side so that when she feels the urge to see and handle the baby, she can do so. The policies governing many maternity areas sometimes interfere with the optimum times at which the mother feels ready to have her child. Rooming-in can circumvent this problem.

To help alleviate denial, the mother must learn to love the baby first and then to cope with the accompanying defect. *Acceptance* of the defect is an extremely difficult process. Therefore, to learn to *cope* with it is a more realistic goal. It normally takes a mother a period of time to adjust to the separation of the baby as a separate entity from herself. She needs a period of time to feel the baby, hear the baby, see the baby, and cuddle the baby in order to complete the separation process. The same process is necessary to the mother with a handicapped baby. After she sees the baby as a new life then she can proceed with her additional adjustment.

The more natural the periods of time the mother and baby spend together, the easier the process of adjustment will be for both mother and baby. Special care necessary for the baby should be introduced slowly. The mother cannot be expected to assume responsibility for these procedures until she has had appropriate orientation and practice. When the mother finally is able to assume the responsibility for these procedures, her denial of the baby's condition is usually lessened or alleviated.

Ross (1964) states that "religious attitudes" may offer *rationalizations* whereby the defective child comes to be viewed as a special sign of grace, for only the most worthy of mothers would be "entrusted" with the care of a handicapped child. This is but one variable that can influence the mother's reaction to her baby. The verbal responses of the mother may give clues to her real feelings regarding the baby. However, her verbal responses may be conditioned by her background or her family rather than by her true feelings. Let me illustrate by examples. The mother may have religious beliefs that all children are a gift of God. As such, she feels she must be satisfied with her baby despite her disappointment. Her statements might be, "It is God's will" or "If God has chosen me to raise this baby, I will."

Another conditioned response might be in relation to "old wives tales" such as, "I expected the child to be affected because I was scared during a thunderstorm." This comment not only indicates an attempt to find a reason for the handicap but also represents a conditioned response elicited by family and acquaintances. The mother's true feelings are not unleashed in the statements. A nurse's response might be, "It is difficult to understand the reasons for a baby being born with a handicap. It is also normal to be disappointed." It is probably not the appropriate time to deal with the misconceptions about the "old wives tales" at this moment. This can easily be handled during future conversations.

The impact of this birth is extremely personal and individualized and no set plan of care will meet the mother's needs. The nurse needs to be alert for clues and to act appropriately. For instance, the mother may ask the nurse if she has ever seen another baby with this defect. The nurse needs to show her concern for the baby and then to answer the question. An example would be, "I know you are concerned about your baby's cleft lip and I can certainly appreciate your concern." The rest of the response depends on the nurse's past experience. If the mother seems to need assurance that other babies have had the condition, the nurse can reply that she has studied the condition but has not had any personal experience with it. She can also refer the mother to someone who has had the experience.

Thus far I have related my remarks to babies that will be expected to survive the immediate postdelivery period. In keeping with this category, mention needs to be made of the guilt a parent feels for the birth of a defective child. In addition, the mother begins a mourning process for the normal child she expected to deliver. This mourning process progresses from the initial phase of numbness and disbelief, to the dawning awareness of the disappointment and feeling of loss with the accompanying affective and physical symptoms, to the last stage of the grief reaction in which intense reexperiencing of the memories and expectations gradually reduce the hypercathexis of the wish for the idealized child (Solnit and Stark, 1961).

This mourning process is a very important part of the postdelivery period. Mourning is a strenuous process and it leaves very little energy for the person to deal with other activities of daily life. The timing of this is crucial as it happens right after the stress situation of birth. The imposition of too many crisis situations at the same time makes it extremely difficult for the person to regain equilibrium. It should also be noted that this mother is now extremely vulnerable. It will take less to upset her than it would ordinarily. Her ways of handling past stress situations will also play a big part in her adjustment to this crisis situation.

The mother needs time to work through her own feelings. Frequently, a medical social worker can be instrumental in helping her with this process. The social worker will also be a welcomed member to the professional team during the period of long-term care. Caplan (1959) states that it is a very difficult thing for a family, particularly for a mother, to deal with a child who has a congenital anomaly or a birth injury. If she is left on her own she is very likely to develop a disturbed relationship with the child and so compound his difficulty. In keeping with this same concept, I believe it is extremely important to have a community health nursing referral made immediately after the birth. This will give the community health nurse the opportunity to visit the hospital, talk with the mother, and consult with the professional staff. The multidisciplinary team is needed to help the family get the very best care and guidance for the child.

Discharge

MOTHER AND BABY

The trend towards early discharge of maternity patients lessens the period available for the mother to adapt to her situation prior to discharge. This early discharge can be beneficial in reuniting her with her more normal home situation. However, it also means that responsibility for normal tasks can be added to her already overburdened backlog of emotionally charged tasks. The community health nurse can plan visits to give the mother an opportunity to talk. The visit usually provides the mother with an excuse to sit down and relax. As time passes, the mother is usually in a better position to begin to manage the problems which will result from the child's handicap. All of the information given the mother during her confinement will probably need to be reviewed. It is natural that she will be able to ask more intelligent questions as she begins the normal care of the child. She may need encouragement to bathe the child and handle him. Her normal maternal instincts to care for the child may be overshadowed by her fear of the defect. If the defect necessitates a change in bathing techniques, the nurse can demonstrate the altered bath. An example of this might be a child discharged with an untreated meningomyelocele. With her other children, the mother has used a bathinette. The baby seemed to enjoy being bathed in the shallow water. With her handicapped child, she is unable to use this comfortable method, so she does not bathe the baby. The nurse demonstrates proper handling of the child and bathing with a sponge or washcloth. A protective shield is placed below the meningomyelocele. A small piece of plastic or saran wrap can serve this purpose (see Fig. 1). During the bath demonstration the nurse emphasizes the need to prevent pressure on the sac. She tells the mother to observe for drainage and to report it to her doctor. She demonstrates the proper positioning after the bath, placing the baby on its abdomen rather than its back. If the lesion is very large the sac may need support by sandbags on each side of the baby. The baby's head should be turned to the side and the usual precautions taken to avoid suffocation. This is especially important as the baby may have a decrease in motor control. Care of the child with a myelomeningocele is covered in greater detail later in the chapter.

The reactions of others to the baby will influence the mother's reactions. It is very difficult to form positive feelings when everyone else seems repelled by the situation. The nurse is in a perfect position to provide one positive response. In order to be most effective, the nurse needs to work through her own feelings regarding the defect. There is no guarantee that she will not be repelled by the situation. The nurse should view the baby alone before viewing it with the mother present, if this is possible. Then she will have an opportunity to "see through the defect" to view the baby as an individual. This is an important part of learning to cope with the handicapped child.

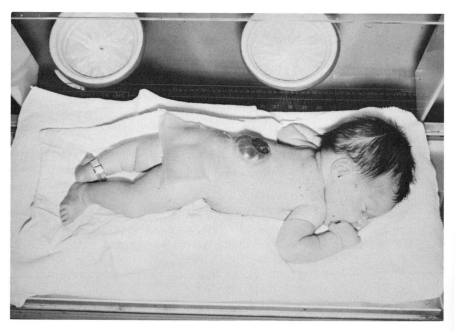

FIG. 1.   Protective shield placed below the meningomyelocele of an infant.

A situation involving the birth of a child with a cleft lip provides a good example to illustrate an appropriate positive response on the part of the nurse. When a baby is born, the cleft becomes a barrier to the normal tendency for the mother to kiss and hug the child. The nurse can demonstrate acceptance by warmly hugging the child. This close association accompanied by endearing words can be very reassuring to the mother. After cuddling the child and smiling warmly, the nurse can return the baby to the mother's arms. A statement such as, "You must be eager to know what the doctors can offer your baby" will be useful in determining the mother's readiness for information and need for support.

It is important to realize that the extent of the defect has little bearing on the response of people. Even a very small defect such as an extra digit can cause grave concern. The nurse should not attempt to predetermine the amount of concern the family will have for any defect. The impact of any defect, no matter how small or large, can be determined only by direct association with the parent. Each parent will have an individualized reaction.

MOTHER WITHOUT BABY

Early discharge of the mother often necessitates the separation of mother and baby. The baby may not be ready for discharge because of the anomaly. This presents a different set of problems. A community health nurse referral is still essential. The nurse is then able to visit the mother prior to the baby's discharge.

The nurse is able to evaluate how the mother is coping with the separation from her new offspring. She is also able to start evaluating how the mother is readjusting to her family.

The period prior to the baby's discharge can be effectively utilized to provide the mother with opportunities to grieve for the normal child she expected and to derive satisfaction from the child she delivered.

The nurse should refer to the child by name to emphasize to the mother that she has another child. The referral to the baby and the problems connected with the baby help to bring the baby into the mainstream of the family. If the baby is not included in the conversation, separation will provide the mother with an excellent opportunity to deny the existence of the problem and perhaps even the existence of the baby.

Separation can be effectively utilized to give the mother an opportunity to recover from the crisis, created by birth, prior to assuming the responsibility for the baby's care. However, the separation period should be supplemented by visits to the hospital to see the child. If possible, she should even be given the opportunity to hold and perhaps even feed the baby. In this way, she will begin to know her child while someone else is assuming the primary responsibility for the child's care. The father should be encouraged to visit the child with the mother. He is usually able to provide support for the mother. At the same time, he will also begin to appreciate the added responsibilities he will have because of the baby.

The mother discharged without her only child may feel a real emptiness. She expects a reward for her labor and delivery. Going home empty-handed does not fulfill her expectations. She may long for her baby just to talk to. The nurse can help by visiting and breaking up the long empty hours. The mother who has young children may find her days less empty, but adult companionship is very important during trying hours. The other children are too busy with their own lives and regaining their mother's attention. They do not show concern for their new brother or sister, probably because they do not really realize the child exists. Even if they do, they may not want the child and they may be secretly delighted that the child did not come home.

It is very important for the mother to receive progress reports from the hospital. These reports can be given by the doctor, the nurse, or the clergy. All are in a position to offer the mother information from their own special vantage point. The doctor is obviously the one responsible for keeping her up-to-date in relation to the medical plans and the baby's prognosis. The nurse is in the best position to keep her informed of the baby's eating, his weight gain, how he is sleeping, and any developmental milestones he surpasses. Mothers appreciate knowing that their baby yawns when he is finished eating, or he sucks on his fist, or his one lock of hair curls. These are the very personal things which help the mother identify with the baby as a person. The clergy provides a dimension that none of the previous information grants. Somehow a clergyman has an "extended power" which gives solace to a person who "believes." When he calls and just says, "I saw Danny today", it provides a source of "higher" quality. His visit and his call are an important part of the mother's readjustment to a normal routine.

If possible, a time should be arranged with the mother, by each of the professionals, so she does not get needlessly apprehensive when the phone rings. It is human nature to expect the calls from the hospital to be "bad news." If she becomes anxious by the ring she may not be able to benefit from the messages planned to reduce her anxiety.

The longer the baby remains hospitalized, the more difficult it may be to help the mother build a relationship with her baby. It is important to stress the positive aspects of the baby's being united with the family, as soon as possible. Otherwise the mother may begin to feel that the baby "would be better off in a home." This statement gives the nurse the opportunity to discuss the pros and cons of institutionalization. Depending on the seriousness of the anomaly, the nurse can discuss with the mother the benefits the baby will derive from being with his own family. She can also familiarize the mother with the agencies and institutions in the community which help with her particular problem. Parents must be the ones who decide whether the baby will be institutionalized.

Children born with congenital anomalies are born with varying degrees of handicap. The anomaly may cause severe interference with function or it may be so subtle that at first glance it seems insignificant. The handicap may be so subtle at birth that it is not recognized, such as minimal cerebral dysfunction. While the chapter dealing with general ideas regarding long-term illness applies here, there are also additional considerations when one is caring for the child born with a congenital anomaly or minimal cerebral dysfunction. Some of these factors also apply to other long-term conditions, but they are included here as they have such a vital role to play with these conditions.

Olshansky (1962) points out that parents of handicapped children have varying degrees of capability in handling the child over their lifespan. The parents' ability to handle the situation coincides with significant milestones in the child's development. The child born with cerebral palsy may be a great shock to the parents. The initial shock is cushioned when the child survives the initial critical period after delivery. The child learns to suck after practice and patience and begins to gain weight. The parents receive satisfaction from their child's physical progress. They begin to question whether the original diagnosis of cerebral palsy is legitimate. The parents have two older children and they have a fairly good memory about their development. When Barry does not sit up at six months, they relate this to his rough start. At nine months Barry still does not sit up and they become aware that he is much slower than their other children. At twelve months their disappointment is very evident. They are reminded of the diagnosis and they

FIG. 2. A typical postural stance of a child with cerebral palsy, when correct bracing is not employed.

are made painfully aware of their child's problem. At this point in time, the parents are less likely to function as effectively as when a crisis is not present. At the next major developmental milestone they may again be reminded of the diagnosis. This continues over the child's life cycle. Some of the milestones may be more "pain producing" than others. These might be the milestones of going to regular school, or late adolescence when the child should be planning marriage.

Nursing intervention in relation to feeding and positioning the child with cerebral palsy is very important. The child without appropriate supports will have little stability (see Fig. 2). In order to gain stability he will need assistance through bracing, proper seating, and use of an adjusted table (see Fig. 3A & 3B). Such a chair and table can be easily made.

FIG. 3A. A child with cerebral palsy sitting in a relaxation chair.

FIG. 3B. A cut-out table makes it easier for the child to eat. The dog is a distractor and should not be allowed near the child when he is trying to eat.

There are other factors which may interfere with the parents' ability to cope with the handicap, such as the repeated "threats" of surgery or the fear of progression of the condition.

The professional personnel should be alert to these check points and make themselves readily available to the parents. It may only take a talk with the social worker or the listening ear of the nurse to help the parents over these hurdles.

PARENT EDUCATION

Another important factor to remember in caring for children with anomalies is to be sure that the parent is considered as an integral and vital member of the team. The parent needs to know exactly what they are or are not expected to do. Frequently therapies are provided and their lack of carry-over into the home is the result of neglect on the professional personnel's part to teach the parents what to do. The young child spends the majority of the time at home. The child with a severe anomaly spends an even greater amount of time in the home. To guarantee maximum function for the child, the home must provide the milieu to learn and grow.

I am reminded of a situation in which a child with lower-extremity paralysis needed a ramp into the house to facilitate her getting in and out of the house on crutches and braces instead of being pushed in a wheelchair. When I first spoke to the mother about the ramp she said she would have to talk to her husband, as the ramp would destroy their small front lawn. I spoke with the father and his answer was, "Miss Steele, I'll build a ramp so fast your head will spin!" And the ramp was built. The parents were never asked to build the ramp, or at least they were not asked at the appropriate point in time so their child had been kept inside except when someone was available to wheel her chair down the front stairs. (This feat even challenged the muscle power of her father!)

Children with severe anomalies also need periodic reevaluation so the parents have an up-to-date report of their assets. The parents also need help in determining when to push for new developments. The child with cerebral palsy may have gross motor deficiency. The mother learns to expect the child to be slower than her other children. She continues to feed the child without reevaluating to see if the child is maturing enough to begin the developmental task of self-feeding. During the occupational therapy or nursing reevaluation, the child is fitted with a feeding device, the involuntary movements of the other extremities are controlled by especially prepared weights, the child is placed in a comfortable chair with a feeding tray, and a bib is applied. The child is given pureed food and encouraged to feed himself. His efforts are rewarded and encouraged by praise. He is allowed to continue feeding himself until he seems to be tiring or becoming too frustrated. A little frustration is healthy to encourage learning in the handicapped child as well as in the normal child.

After the reevaluation of the child, the parent is given specific realistic goals to achieve before the next clinic visit. In the interim, the mother is encouraged to telephone when she has a question.

SCHOOL: REGULAR OR SPECIAL?

The answer to the question of school for the child with an anomaly is not an easy one. Generally the child who is not too physically incapacitated will attend regular school. The teachers will need to be fully aware of any special needs of the child. The child with more severe handicaps will probably attend a special school for the handicapped. Some school systems do not have special facilities available and the children will have to be bussed long distances. The children may even have to be transported by the parents, which places an additional strain on the family.

Children who attend special schools have the benefit of competing with other handicapped children (see Fig. 4). However, this does not realistically prepare them to function in the more diversified society at large. It is true that some of the children with more severe handicaps may never be capable of competing at this level. Their potential for achievement may well be restricted to "sheltered workshops" or living within a family or in an institution. The special class may adequately prepare them for these roles.

Children who attend special classes learn to help those less capable than themselves. They develop an empathy for one another that is difficult to explain. It is common to see a child with braces pushing a paralyzed child in a wheelchair. They also help each other with items which are "out of reach" and thereby aid the teacher in teaching.

When the special classes are all located in the same building, the teachers have the benefit of sharing teaching methods with one another. When the classes are spread singly or in some clusters in several areas, the teachers may find it more difficult to share teaching ideas with other teachers of the handicapped. There is one other complicating

FIG. 4. These handicapped children enjoy the swimming pool at the Children's Rehabilitation Center in Buffalo, New York, a unit of the Children's Hospital. They are assisted by college student volunteers, all future teachers of exceptional children.

item inherent in special education; that is, when children are cast in a particular mold, their achievements are frequently based on the expectations of that mold. Frequently, this decreases the amount of stimulation the child receives.

The child who attends a regular class may be so different from the other children that he is given special privileges. Or he may be laughed at or ridiculed by the other children who do not understand the child's differences. Being an outsider can severely hamper his opportunities to learn.

Architectural barriers may determine where a child can attend regular school. A child with two lower-limb prostheses may have to attend a school for the handicapped because he cannot sufficiently negotiate the many stairs in an old school building. If the stairs were not so steep a regular school placement would have been far superior as the child would be given credit for his assets rather than focusing on his defects, which are adequately corrected.

School placement for the child with minimal cerebral dysfunction is more appropriately included in the section specifically dealing with this particular handicap.

Examples of Defects and Nursing Intervention

Other chapters in the book also deal with possible congenital or acquired defects. Therefore, the areas of heart, scoliosis, and cystic fibrosis will not be included in this chapter. The magnitude of these problems necessitates chapters dealing specifically with the topics. Further, I will not attempt to cover all the conditions which require long-term care but rather some of the more common conditions.

HYPOSPADIAS

Hypospadias is a relatively common congenital anomaly of the penis, occurring once in 2,400 live male births . . . Hypospadias is an abnormal opening of the urethra, frequently on the underside of the penis. It may vary in degree from a minor shift in the opening to such a complex malformation that the sex of the child is questionable. The penile shaft distal to the hypospadiac meatus is angulated ventrally. This aspect of the deformity is termed "chordee" (King, 1967, p. 1097).

The impact of this condition on the parents can be almost devastating. The reproductive organs of the male child are usually a highly emotionally charged area to the parents. They may possibly have some knowledge of this condition from past experience. Although the condition does not follow a strict Mendelian inheritance, it does run a familial pattern in families.

The defect makes it impractical to circumcise the infant. This may be very upsetting to the parents, especially if they belong to the Jewish faith, in which religious ritual is connected with circumcision.

The nurse in the newborn nursery can easily detect the variance in voiding pattern. It is her astute observation regarding frequency of voiding, amount of voiding, and difficulty in voiding that may alert the physician to additional defects.

Although fathers are usually able to conceal their concern for children with defects until school age, it has been my experience that they are very concerned when their son is born with a hypospadias. They frequently ask the question. "Will he be able to marry and have children?" The mother may ask more immediate type questions, such as, "Can it be repaired?" "What did I do to cause it?"

After a period of observation, the infant can be discharged home without any specialized care. The time for the surgery will vary with the physician. The surgical procedures are done to straighten the penis by release of chordee, and subsequent operations to construct a cylinder of buried skin to serve as a urethra. This may be accomplished in one or more stages (King, 1969, p. 1099). The opinion concerning optimal age of the child for repair also varies with physicians. It is usually planned to try to complete the repairs before school age. This will permit the child to void in the normal standing position, if the condition was severe enough to interfere with this normal process. If the repair is to be done in more than one stage, six months are allowed to elapse before the second stage is done. In spite of careful attention to surgical technique and postoperative care, the two-stage operation results in urethral fistulas in about 40 percent of patients so treated (King, 1969, p. 1102).

One child who had seven surgical procedures to try to repair the defect was asked why he was hospitalized. He threw back the covers from the bedcradle, exposing himself and said, "See I just wasn't put together right!" This child benefited by water play in the bathtub. Prior to putting the child in the bathtub, his Foley catheter was clamped off. He was taken twice a day to the tub by a nurse and appropriately supplied with toys. At first, he merely used the tub to bathe. Then he began to act out. His first change in attitude occurred when he splashed the nurse "accidentally." He eventually became able to ask, "Why do I need this tube?" He then teased, "I'm going to pull it out!" The soothing bath plus the close relationship of water to his problem, allowed him to express his true feelings which he was not able to do in his bed or wheelchair. The use of the bathtub varies with different physicians as some prefer not to have the child take tub baths. If this is the case, a bath basin is the second best idea. Boats and sponges can be used in a small basin. However, the child does not get the added benefit of the feel of being submerged in the water.

Immediately postoperatively the child may have a dressing. The dressing is utilized to help alleviate edema and to reduce the tension of the suture lines. This dressing should not be removed, as it is used for pressure. If there is an unusual amount of drainage—some is to be expected—the physician should be notified. The parents need to know that the dressing is a necessary part of the repair, so they will not be tempted to move it to see how the incision looks. The indwelling catheter may be a source of concern to the patients especially, if immediately postoperatively, the urine is a little pink-tinged. Any serous drainage mixed with urine looks like a larger amount than it is. The parents must be assured that the child is not hemorrhaging and that this situation will clear. They should also be told the optimal positioning of the catheter for draining. Parents frequently move it to facilitate playing games. I have seen the catheters draped up over the bed cradle by an unknowing parent.

A bed cradle is frequently utilized to keep the pressure of the bed clothes off the area. The child is also left without pajama bottoms. To guarantee privacy, the sheet must hang freely over all sides of the cradle. The school-age child is especially modest and will appreciate the excess sheeting. I do not approve of using diapers anywhere on the child's bed. A diaper is a degrading object to any child who has outgrown them. When the child's dressing is removed, anywhere from two to five days postsurgery, pajama bottoms or a sheet are usually allowed to cover him when he is up in the wheelchair. The use of the bed cradle is usually continued until the sutures are removed.

In a two-stage procedure, the second stage is frequently more anxiety-producing to the parents, as its success or failure determines whether more surgery will be indicated. If parents have prepared themselves for two stages, the addition of another may produce another crisis situation. It may decrease their hope that the child will ever have a successful repair. The child may be more concerned with the pain from the procedure rather than the results of the surgery.

I feel there are a few additional things which need to be considered by nurses. First, it is not consistent with our culture to focus as much attention on the genitals as is necessary during the postoperative period. Therefore, observations of the genitals may be deemed necessary only by the doctor. If the catheter has to be irrigated, every care should be taken to guarantee privacy. Discussion of the drainage and emptying the urinary drainage bag should not take place in the corridors, playroom, or other public areas. It is better to take the child to his room for the short time needed to complete this task. Children are frequently selfconscious of the drainage tube and bag so this material should be placed as inconspicuously as possible. The child may fear the removal of the Foley catheter as he fears voiding. After the Foley is removed, the child may need to be encouraged to void by the usual methods of increasing fluid intake, running the water in the sink, and providing privacy in the bathroom. The child may feel more comfortable with his mother present. She should be instructed to note the stream and where the voiding takes place. The child may choose to sit down on the toilet at first, as this has been the way he voided prior to surgery.

Standing is usually accomplished readily by just showing him that this is the way other boys void. The need for him to be like his peers is very great at the school-age period.

The aim of the surgical procedures should be to obtain correction with the smallest amount of emotional shock possible. The effects of hospitalization can be lessened by the parents and the medical personnel being as truthful with the child as possible. The child should be an active participant when the results of the surgery are known. If future surgical procedures are indicated, he must be helped to understand the reasons for the operation and not just made to conform.

TRACHEOESOPHAGEAL ATRESIA

In contrast to the previously discussed condition, tracheoesophageal artresia necessitates fairly immediate surgery. The long-term care begins soon after birth. The condition is rather easily diagnosed by passing a catheter through the baby's nose into the esophagus. If there is an obstruction, the catheter will coil in the pouch. It is usually routine to pass a catheter soon after the birth of the baby, while he is still in the delivery room. If this has been omitted, the nurse who feeds the baby the first time will find the baby regurgitating the formula as it cannot get past the defect. In addition, the baby may have a great deal of mucus and if this is aspirated, he will become cyanotic.

The excessive mucus is caused by the baby's inability to swallow his own saliva. Cyanosis may also result from laryngospasms due to the accumulation of saliva in the pouch. The excessive saliva spills over into the larynx and causes the laryngospasm and resultant cyanosis. It is imperative that proper suctioning be done to remove the saliva.

The size of the baby is a major factor in relation to the surgical risk. The improved techniques in surgical procedures, pediatric fluid therapy, and the use of local anesthetics have greatly increased the survival rate of babies born with this condition. A significant number of infants having tracheoesophageal anomalies are also premature. An attempt is usually made to have the baby reach 5 pounds prior to the surgical correction. However, a gastrostomy may have been done to decompress the stomach and to decrease the possibility of aspiration pneumonia prior to the time of the surgical correction.

If the baby has to be transferred to another area of the hospital or another hospital, it is imperative that the mother see the child first. The mother should even be allowed to hold the baby. This will help her to work through her grief if the baby dies. It will also decrease the fantasies she has of the handicapped child. She may even benefit from seeing the baby having slight respiratory difficulty or bubbling mucus. I vividly recall one mother whose full-term baby was having respiratory distress and was kept in an isolette. The mother had a real desire to have her baby get well. She could not imagine what was wrong with the baby. The explanations from her husband, doctors, and nurses did not provide her with a vivid picture of the baby's condition. She was finally taken to the premature-suspect nursery to view the baby. She took one look, saw the baby gasping for every breath, saw the deep retractions, and immediately knew the baby was in critical condition. Although she was upset, she now stated she understood what we were trying to tell her about her baby. The baby died and she was left with the feeling that there was nothing that could have saved the life of her baby. She experienced much relief from knowing this.

I do not mean to make the impression that I expect these babies to die. I feel that seeing the baby can also help the mother during her long separation from the child. It is at least a slight reward for her months of waiting and her labor and delivery period.

Preoperatively the baby is usually kept in an isolette to maintain body temperature. The baby is usually placed in a semisitting position to minimize the possibility of aspiration. The use of oxygen and humidity follow the suggested plan for any premature infant.

The postoperative course will depend on the type of congenital malformation. (Fig. 5).

Figure 5B illustrates the most common anomaly and therefore the postoperative nursing care described here will be based primarily on this type.

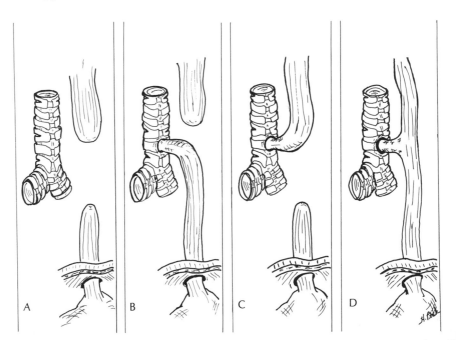

FIG. 5. View A, Esophageal atresia without tracheoesophageal fistula; View B, Esophageal atresia with tracheoesophageal fistula with distal segment; View C, Esophageal atresia with fistula between proximal segment and the trachea; View D, H-type tracheoesophageal fistula without atresia.

A gastrostomy can be done to facilitate early feeding. "Occasionally an anastomosis can be done and the gastrostomy omitted. Subsequent dilation and calibration of the anastomotic site with bougies is always helpful and sometimes mandatory" (Ferrer, 1968, p. 1520).

Immediately postoperatively the baby is returned to an isolette with humidity. The isolette does not preclude the mother from touching the baby after appropriate handwashing and gowning. Hospital policies frequently discouraged this practice. Fortunately, interest has been shown in the isolation produced by isolettes. Music via music boxes, musical toys, or commercial concerns is now being introduced into isolettes. Patterned or designed sheets are also being used and toys are no longer out of bounds.

The nurse will begin the gastrostomy feedings when ordered. They may be given by gravity with use of the glass funnel of an Asepto syringe. The tube is elevated up through the hole in the top of the isolette. After the feeding, the tube can be left open and any postfeeding vomiting will be allowed to pass freely up the tube. Care must be taken not to put tension on the gastrostomy tube when one is turning or bathing the baby. The feedings should be sterile and prepared as carefully as any newborn feeding. The gastrostomy tube is left open after the feeding so that any regurgitated fluid will pass out the tube without putting pressure on the suture line.

Despite the baby's innate desire to suck, pacifiers are frequently omitted as they increase the production of saliva. It is important to know if the surgeon allows pacifiers. If he does, a sterile nipple filled with sterile cotton should be utilized as a pacifier for the infant. This will help to satisfy the required sucking needs of the infant. It can also be used to soothe the baby who is not getting the ordinary handling and cuddling. Some surgeons prefer the baby to be moved very little immediately postoperatively and therefore nursing procedures are planned to minimize contact.

The mother needs an opportunity to learn to do the gastrostomy feedings if the device is not going to be removed before discharge. In the more involved cases, the reconstructive stage of the surgery is frequently delayed until the age of two and a half or three. In less severe cases surgery may be done in six months. Therefore, the mother needs to be very comfortable in caring for the infant with gastrostomy.

Another postoperative nursing function is the conscientious pharyngeal suctioning. This is done to prevent the baby from aspirating secretions and developing atelectasis or pneumonia. It should not be done unless indicated, as the suctioning can cause undue irritation. The suction catheter should be marked so that it is not inserted too deeply, causing pressure on the sutures. The pressure used for suctioning should be as low as possible to still adequately remove the tenacious material.

When oral feedings are started, they must be given slowly and cautiously. Difficulty with the feeding is reason to stop the feeding and notify the doctor. Continuing to feed may further complicate the situation. The most competent nurse should be assigned to this baby for his feedings.

The oral feedings are usually started between the tenth and fifteenth postoperative day. They are usually started by giving small amounts of glucose water and gradually increased to formula. The baby is usually allowed to suck for a limited period, approximately 15–20 min, and the remainder of the feeding given by the gastrostomy tube.

The baby is frequently kept in the isolette until a couple of days before discharge, to decrease the possibility of infection. The nurse should check with the physician to see when it is permissible to take the baby out of the isolette for feedings.

When the baby is able to take the whole feeding by mouth, the gastrostomy tube is clamped. If the total repair has been accomplished, x-rays are taken to be sure there is no leakage. If the results are adequate, the gastrostomy tube is removed.

Depending on the severity of the anomaly, the surgical corrections may take a long time to complete. Each surgical procedure causes a separation of the mother and infant. These separations are during the period most important for the infant to be with his mother. The severity of the condition necessitates doing surgical procedures at the poorest time, developmentally speaking, for the child. As there is no way to safely delay surgery with its long hospitalizations, other things must be done to help compensate for the surgery. These other things I have described, and strong emphasis is placed on permitting the mother as much contact with the child as is considered safe.

MENINGOMYELOCELE AND HYDROCEPHALUS

"Meningomyelocele is a nervous system anomaly of the newborn. The protruding pouch contains meninges, neural tissue, and spinal fluid. The condition is accompanied by hydrocephalus in 75% of the cases" (Amador, 1969, pp. 1206–1207).

The child born with meningomyelocele is one of the more dramatic examples of children with long-term illness. With the advent of antibiotics, infections have been amenable to control and the children frequently survive.

"The lesion may be located anywhere along the spinal cord, however, the most frequent area is the lumbar region, 40%, and then the lumbosacral region, 30%" (Amador, 1969, p. 1206).

Immediately after delivery the child is kept warm as the interference with the neural system gives the child a poorer temperature regulation mechanism than the "normal" newborn. Frequently, an isolette is utilized. It is generally accepted practice to place the baby on the abdomen with his face to the side. A plastic strip is usually applied below the meningomyelocele over the rectal area (see Figure 1). The mildest form of adhesive should be used to keep it in place. Disposable plastic urine collectors with their mild self adherent can be easily applied. Saran Wrap, which has a tendency to adhere to skin surfaces, can be tried. The shield will help to protect the lesion without the necessity of covering the area with dressings. The lesion itself usually is treated by exposure to air.

Positioning is imperative to prevent the baby from developing contractures. The baby frequently has associated bony abnormalities and every attempt should be made to prevent the development of additional ones. A physical therapist should evaluate the child early, and also a physiatrist to determine the child's muscle potential. Early surgical correction is now beginning to be more widely used. It is believed that early correction helps to prevent more serious muscle involvement and neural deterioration. The surgical correction of the lesion is frequently preceded by a shunting procedure for the hydrocephalus. The shunt is done to control the increased cerebrospinal fluid pressure which may result from repairing the sac.

There are several types of shunting procedures referred to in the literature. Three of the most common types of shunting procedures are the ventriculoauricular, ventriculovenous, and ventriculoperitoneal. The positioning of the baby postoperatively will be determined by the type of shunting procedure, the meningomyelocele, and the postoperative evaluation of the fontanelles. "Valve systems are usually inserted and they are pumped frequently post-operatively to remove small pieces of matter which may find their way into the tubing and valve systems" (Amador, 1969, p. 1220). Hospitals vary in their practice as to whether nurses and parents are taught to pump the system. However, in any event, the nurse can evaluate the child to help determine if there is an obstruction in the system. The fontanelle becomes full or tense when there is an interference with the flow of cerebrospinal fluid. The child becomes listless, may fail to feed or begin vomiting, and is irritable and fretful. He does not respond to voice or touch as quickly when there is an obstruction. If the obstruction becomes extensive, the child may develop respiratory problems and progress into coma. Early recognition of symptoms will allow the physician to investigate the obstruction and to do a revision, if necessary.

Over a long time period, the shunt will need revisions due to the growth of the child. The child may dislodge the tubing from its site as he grows. To date, no tubing has been found that can successfully "lengthen" with the child.

Following the shunting procedure, the meningomyelocele is usually corrected—although, as previously stated, some physicians prefer to close the meningomyelocele first and to insert the shunt later. Again, after closure of the sac the positioning of the baby depends on all the contributing factors. A general rule is to keep the baby off the operative sites. Changing of position is especially important to prevent respiratory complications. Feeding the baby is usually done in the crib or isolette until healing begins to take place. The best position is usually to place the baby on the side opposite the shunt. Burping must be done cautiously depending on the location of the meningomyelocele lesion.

As soon as the baby's condition is stabilized the mother should begin to feed the child. She should be taught the signs to note in relation to the shunting procedure. She should be given explicit directions for bathing the baby with special emphasis on the operative sites. She should be given directions for passive exercises to the lower extremities, if indicated. The parents need to become aware of the necessity and value of close medical follow-up for their child. The parents should also be aware of the complications which might result from the decrease in circulation to the lower extremities, including such factors as keeping the baby dressed warmer and preventing pressure. Decubitus can develop from bed clothes which are tucked in too tightly. The baby's limited ability to turn himself should be explained so the parents will turn the child periodically.

The urinary system also needs close supervision. The paralysis caused by the neural damage frequently results in urinary dribbling. The use of Credé is usually indicated in order to manually express the urine.

Credé is the application of pressure over the bladder area. It is easily accomplished by gentle pressure of the palms of the hands. The mother is taught to express the urine manually at definite intervals to help empty the bladder. As the child gets older, he can be taught to do the Credé himself. The process can be facilitated by using toys to help the child put pressure on the bladder. Such toys as balloons, horns, bugles, or plastic bubbles can all be utilized when the child is sitting on the potty chair or toilet. The older child, who has outgrown these toys, can be taught to pucker up his cheeks with air and then blow slowly through his closed lips. Additional pressure can be made by using the hand to cover the lips and therefore create more resistance. This procedure may also depend on the preference of the physician. Even when it is utilized, the baby is usually wet more frequently than the noninvolved newborn. The skin of the child is especially prone to breakdown as it has poorer nourishment and less adequate temperature control. Frequent diaper changing and cleansing of the area is necessary. If a rash begins, exposure to the air should be tried. Occasionally it is necessary to apply an ointment, such as A&D or Desitin, to help alleviate the rash. If skin breakdown occurs, the mother should be cautioned to call the doctor for directions.

The severity of the kidney involvement usually increases with time. It is one of the most challenging aspects of the long-term case. The child is prone to frequent urinary infections and they are usually difficult to control with medications, as the child develops resistance to them. The child who dribbles all the time is usually diapered to keep her[1] outer clothing dry. This diapering provides an excellent media for

---

[1] Here I use the pronouns "her" and "she" because the urinary problem is more difficult to control in girls. In boys, there are urinary appliances which are fairly successful. However, boys should also be given time to go to the bathroom. They must empty the appliance and wash and dry the penis to protect it from excoriation due to continual contact with the urine.

bacteria to multiply when it is wet for long periods. The diaper is usually covered with a plastic panty that further adds to the warmth, and the warmth contributes further to the bacteria formation. When the child is old enough to enter school, it is important to plan times for her to go to the bathroom or nurse's office to change the diapering. If there is a space available, diapering can be brought in once a week and stored. If there is not a space available, the child should bring adequate daily supplies. Bringing the supplies in a child's lunch box or small doll suitcase will lessen the child's resistance to taking the supply.

A definite time should be established for the child to go to the bathroom. She cannot feel wetness and frequently the odor of urine is more noticeable to others than the child herself.

Depending on the severity of the accompanying handicaps and the facilities available, the children may need help to complete their personal care. Handrails help a great deal especially if one is placed near the toilet and another near the sink. It is also convenient to have a table available near the sink so they can place their supplies on it.

If the child has a urinary diversion and is wearing a prosthetic device, it is very important that he also be given specific times to use the bathroom. The urinary appliances also have a tendency to develop odors. This can be fairly well controlled by washing the appliance frequently, airing it on a routine basis, using deodorant or vinegar in the wash water, using deodorant tablets in the pouch, and keeping the child's skin clean and dry. The child should have at least two appliances so they can be alternated and aired adequately. There are several different varieties of appliances used. One utilizes a leg bag for collecting the urine, another has a pouch. The one with the leg bag is made of a soft rubber and is easy to keep clean. The advantage of this appliance is it creates less pressure on the stoma. Occasionally pressure from an appliance can cause the stoma to herniate. The disadvantage to this appliance is that the leg bag shows with girls and they are embarassed. The bag fits under the trousers of the boy so it is not as much of a problem (see Figs. 6–7).

The one with the pouch has the advantage of being easily concealed under clothing. But it is more difficult to keep odor-free if it is neglected (see figs. 8–9).

Both types of appliances are better connected to a urinary collection bottle at night. This facilitates better drainage. It also allows the child to move around freely without putting pressure on a bag of urine.

The bowel incontinence associated with myelomeningocele is more easily regulated. A program is established individually for each child. A convenient time for utilizing the toilet is essential. In large families this can be a problem. The child frequently needs extra time to complete evacuation. Suppositories are helpful in getting the pattern established. After a while, the child will usually evacuate without the suppository. The success of the bowel training may also be directly related to the dietary and fluid intake of the child. The mother and child should both be aware that any drastic change in the dietary intake may interfere

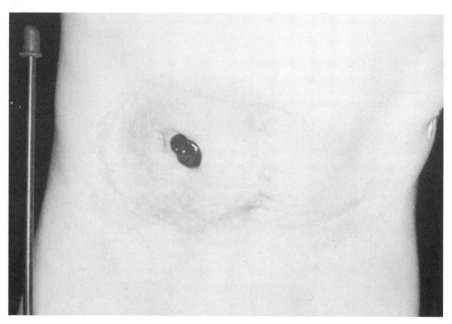

FIG. 6. A healed ileal stoma. The skin area around the stoma demands excellent care.

with evacuation and cause incontinence during the day. The bowel evacuation may be more successful if scheduled for evening. The morning hours may be too hectic in the household. Occasionally suppositories, an adequate diet, and good timing are not sufficient for evacuating the bowel. It may be necessary to resort to enemas. This is not a complicated procedure with the commercial enemas now available. The least amount of solution should be utilized to stimulate the movement. Again, the pattern of establishing a time, consistent from day to day, will cut down on the incontinence.

The bracing of the child will also contribute to the nursing responsibilities. The braces must fit properly if the child is to utilize them effectively. Also, the joints must move freely. Dust collects in the joints and must be removed. Oiling is also necessary. The child's skin should not have pressure marks from the braces. The leather parts should not be cracked. The leather can be preserved by the use of saddle soap. The braces must be checked frequently especially during growth spurts. The child's lower limbs do not grow as consistently as the rest of his trunk; however, he may gain weight and the braces may be too tight.

The child should be encouraged to use his braces. It is often easier to push him around in a wheelchair but this does not help him in his future adjustment to life. The emphasis should be on making the child as self-sufficient as possible.

FIG. 7. Ileal appliance with leg
bag for urine collection.

The nurse will also play an important role in counseling the parents and the child. The parents usually have many questions relating to growth, education, employment, finances, and so forth. Frequently the parents know the answers to many of their questions but they need an opportunity just to talk with someone. The children may need much more help in dealing with their questions. Their limited understanding prevents them from getting satisfaction from many of the answers given them. They find it very difficult to live in a world where their peers are so different from themselves. The child needs to learn to appreciate what he has and to focus less on his deficits. The child may fantasize that his body is perfect and this interferes with his understanding. If the child becomes too involved with fantasy he may need the help of a psychologist or psychiatrist.

FIG. 8. Mary is thirteen years old. She has a repaired myelomeningocele, arrested hydrocephalus, repaired bilateral dislocated hips, and ileo conduit. She is an outstanding student and gets around ably with the use of crutches and long leg braces.

DEFORMITIES OF LIMBS

A number of anomalies can be found in relation to the extremities. They may be obvious anomalies such as a missing limb or limbs or less noticeable such as a dislocated hip. The duration of care is frequently dependent upon the time lapse between discovery and therapy. For instance, a dislocated hip discovered in the nursery and treated immediately, will usually require only short-term therapy for correction. If the condition is not detected until the child is walking, the medical therapy will usually span a long period of time.

The child with a missing limb will require long-term care to guar-

FIG. 9. Here Mary illustrates the wearing of her urinary drainage appliance. The waist belt can be removed and washed or replaced. The bag is washed, dried and deodorant tablets inserted. Note she does not wear a leg bag and this appliance is completely covered by her dress.

antee that his prosthesis is functioning effectively. The skin areas also must be watched closely to prevent breakdown due to the added stress produced by the prosthesis.

Let us first consider the child with a missing or severely deformed upper extremity. The newborn clenches his fists. We do not know the exact reason for this but it would seem that the baby is comfortable in this position. The baby also sucks on his fists. The missing limb is important because of its absence. The baby may irritate the skin of the only limb. It may be useful to supply a pacifier to the baby to help compensate for the missing limb. As the baby grows he is ambidexterous. The baby with the missing hand is forced into a preference early unless a prosthesis is fitted to aid the child. The baby is able to use the prosthesis to assist with toys and later in learning to crawl and sit. The prosthesis helps to stabilize the body and provides the weight lost by the missing limb. The prosthesis becomes imperative when the child's neurological system begins to mature. He is capable of doing all types of two-handed activities and needs the prosthesis to complete his tasks. The early prosthesis is extremely simple. As the child grows he needs a prosthesis that can bend, grasp, lift, pull, and so forth. The early prosthesis demands much less care than the more complicated type. The infant and child prosthesis should be worn over a tee shirt to protect the child's skin from excoriation. The straps must be kept clean and in good repair. The child's prosthesis will also need attention to the rubber bands, the joints, and the cables. All parts must be in excellent condition in order to provide maximum function.

In addition to checking the prosthesis for functional ability, the nurse needs to encourage the parents and child to use the prosthesis consistently. The more uniformly the child uses the prosthesis, the more secure he will feel. The child who is permitted to go without the prosthesis for indefinite periods will develop one-handed skills and resist using the prosthesis. As he gets older, the one-handedness may incapacitate him.

At this point in time, the hook is far more functional than artificial hands. The child usually will want a hand to alternate with the hook for more formal occasions.

Lower-extremity prostheses are usually more readily accepted than upper extremity prosthesis. This is due to the almost impossible task of getting around on one leg. The length of the affected limb may influence this. One child with an almost perfectly formed leg refused to wear the prosthesis which provided him with a foot. The prosthesis slowed down his gait. He preferred to play sports without the prosthesis and consequently frequently injured the tissue at the end of the limb.

Injury to the tissue of the remaining limb is a critical problem. The prosthesis must be left off during the healing process. This necessitates an inconvenience to the child. It is wise to have a pair of crutches available in case this happens. Then the child will not have to miss school during this time. Care to the stump is best achieved by the use of a soap such as Dial. The area should be rinsed thoroughly and dried. In the hot weather powder may reduce itching. A stump sock made of virgin wool is placed next to the skin. This sock should also be washed daily. The sock should fit smoothly. The prosthesis fits over the sock. There is a tendency for stumps to shrink with time. The child should not attempt to remedy this by adding extra socks or stuffing cotton or the like in the prosthesis. The prosthetist should be consulted for all repairs or revisions to the prosthesis.

The school nurse should play a key role in introducing other children to the prosthesis. The child may be asked to demonstrate how he uses the prosthesis. The children need to be cautioned about pushing the affected child on the playground. They should understand that the affected child may need more time to master certain sports. They need to know that at times the child with a lower prosthesis will use crutches instead of his prosthesis. This introduction will help to erase the unknown element and help the children to appreciate the handicap.

The nurse should also talk with the teachers to help them understand the implications of the prosthesis. One important factor is that the child may tire more readily due to the added energy needed to use the prosthesis. The child may need a short rest period after gym, before beginning ordinary school activities. The teachers should try to treat the child as "normally" as possible but not to completely dismiss the possibility of fatigue. Gym should be encouraged, as well as swimming. An upper-extremity prosthesis may have to be removed during contact sports to protect the other children from accidental injury. Unless a special lightweight prosthesis is available for swimming, the regular prosthesis is removed and the child is taught to swim with one lower limb.

Much of the adjustment the child has in later life is dependent on his early experiences. Therefore, it is worth the extra effort in his early years to have the child adjust to his prosthesis. Even with much patience, it is not unusual for the adolescent to rebel against the prosthesis and the reasons for his anomaly. Every effort must be made to help the adolescent understand. If he has been given honest answers all along, it will be easier during his adolescent period. He may become quite hostile to the medical personnel providing his care or to his parents. Venting his feelings may be all that is necessary to make him feel better. He may need a period to talk over problems with others with similar anomalies. The adolescent may need help when he realizes that it is more difficult to achieve some of the developmental milestones, such as dating or getting a job. Too many failures may lessen his self-image. With the right professional counseling, the adolescent should be able to make an adequate adjustment.

In addition to the ways already spelled out, I think nurses can be helpful to children with prosthesis in the following ways:

1. The mother may need help in adjusting clothing to compensate for the prosthesis. Instead of disappointing the child because a garment does not fit, snaps or a zipper may be inserted in the side to accommodate the prosthesis. The use of Velcro strips on clothing can also be suggested.

2. When the child is hospitalized, the nurse should be sure the child wears the prosthesis whenever his condition warrants it. Failure to encourage the child to wear it may further his dislike for the prosthesis. He may get the idea that the nurses, too, think it is useless.

3. During hospitalizations make a place available for the child to wash his stump socks and to hang them up to dry. If the child is able to assume this chore he should be encouraged to do so. If not, the nurse should assume this for the child. The socks should not be sent to the laundry as the harsh detergent is not good for them.

4. The school nurse should check the gait of the child with a lower-extremity prosthesis. She may be the first one to detect an ill-fitting prosthesis or an irritation to the tissue. Children will frequently try to hide these facts so they do not have to go to the doctor.

The nurse's role in any of the handicapping conditions of childhood is dependent on the setting and the other professional personnel responsible for the child's care. The nurse must assume an active role in the care of children with prostheses. Her observations and guidance may greatly help the child and his parents.

The majority of cases of missing limbs are amenable to the use of prosthetic appliances. However, there are anomalies of the extremities which cannot be improved by prosthesis. Some children are born with severely deformed hands. For various reasons the hand may not be amputated to permit a prosthesis to be fitted properly. The nurse now has a more complicated role to play. She may be involved in devising appropriate utensils to teach the child to feed herself (see Fig. 10). Hopefully, an occupational therapist will be available to do much of the initial training. The nurse will then visit the home to see that the adaptations are being effectively utilized. Encouragement needs to be given to let the child feed herself. The nurse can help the mother protect the floor by using newspaper under the child's chair. The mother must realize that this may be a long and tedious process, but the end results will be worth the additional effort.

Other adaptations which may help the child to achieve successful self-feeding are the use of a deep dish with sides and a suction cup on the bottom of the dish. This will help the child by keeping the food on

FIG. 10. Utensils adapted for use with children with deficient hand function.

the plate and the plate on the table. The hand appliance then has a back edge to aid it in getting the food on the spoon. The suction cup on the bottom keeps the dish from moving out of the child's reach (see Fig. 10). The use of a "cobbler-type bib" will decrease the chances of the child soiling her clothes. When the child is ready to drink from a cup the training cup with the cover and spout will be useful. The wide cup without the handle will adjust to the deformity of the hand. The child will then grasp the cup on each side and raise it to her mouth. If the cup drops it will not spill much because the cover is on securely.

When the deformity does not lend itself to prosthesis application or an appliance, the child is taught to eat by the less socially acceptable way of holding the utensil in her toes. Fortunately, this is rare. I include the example just to show how much effort should be expanded to make the child self-sufficient.

There are several other types of congenital anomalies which have been omitted as they are more short-term in nature. The scope of this book is to focus on the ones that ordinarily require long-term care. According to Bramley, regardless of the nature of the disability, it cannot be overstressed that very few children will have severe emotional problems when the attitudes of the parents are essentially healthy ones. "We should remember that the child almost invariably mirrors the fears and the attitudes that his parents have about him and that, in general, the child will be a much happier individual when the parents regard him as a normal youngster, similar in his feelings to other children of comparable age and background (Bramley, 1963, p. 310).

I would also like to add that the child will be better adjusted if he can also trust and accept the medical personnel responsible for his care.

MINIMAL CEREBRAL DYSFUNCTION

This section will be concerned with the understandings and nursing care necessary in meeting the needs of a particular group of children with brain damage. The subject I wish to address myself to are those children whose brain injury presents itself as a difficulty with perception, conception, and/or a behavior problem—in other words, the children who are not primarily mentally retarded, or who do not have cerebral palsy, or a severe convulsive disorder, as a result of their brain damage. The children with learning disabilities as their major problem may, of course, also have these conditions as an additional minor problem.

There have been several names, over the years, given to these children. Doll (1932) and Strauss (1951) referred to them as brain-injured and distinguished them from generally mentally-retarded children. Basara (1966) refers to them as perceptually handicapped. I am certain more names can be found which have attempted to identify more accurately the syndrome which manifests itself in a number of overt ways.

Before I identify the signs, I should like to first point out that not every child will have all of these signs. He may have only two or three, or he may have many or all of them. In the book, *Helping the Brain Injured Child*, Siegel (1962) addresses himself to the following characteristics (not listed in order of importance):

      a) talkativeness
      b) awkwardness
      c) poor speech
      d) destructiveness
      e) animism
      f) distractibility
      g) hyperactivity
      h) impulsiveness
      i) perseveration
      j) irritability
      k) guilelessness
      l) aggressiveness
      m) social immaturity

Such an extensive list would indicate that almost any child could fit into the title of brain-injured. To further identify the children with whom I am concerned we can use as a working definition the idea that *when the brain is damaged, there is a complex field of forces disrupted, and this disruption makes it difficult for the child to interact, in the usual way, with his environment.* The extent to which this happens will be dependent on the extent and the locus of the damage. In a study by Schulman et al. (1965), it is stated that the only variable which approached unequivocal support as a correlate of brain damage, regardless of extent or location of damage, was distractibility. No evidence in their study supported the hypothesis that hyperactivity is a correlate of brain damage. They also found that autonomic lability may not be a direct correlate of damage, but rather that it may be related through its association with performative lability. I bring this out at this point as I believe that much of the literature in relation to these children has focused on symptoms which may not be the result of the brain injury itself, but rather may reflect environmental factors which might be controlled or manipulated to intervene before the child exhibits many of the behavioral signs listed by Siegel (1962).

In addition, we must consider that the response patterns of the brain-injured child will also be influenced by the psychological defenses utilized by the child. It becomes evident that we are dealing with a complicated reciprocal interaction between the biological defect and the psychological and environmental structures of each child. In order to understand the outcomes of these reciprocal interactions, one must evaluate thoroughly the biological, environmental, and psychological factors.

While many of the injuries are present at birth, there are others that are the result of an injury after birth. The child's progress prior to the injury should be evaluated to ascertain what progress he had made both psychologically and physically before the injury and what environmental support he received at the time of the injury. Generally, the earlier the injury occurred on the developmental scale, the greater is the potential for behavioral or psychological defects. The biological defect may affect three main areas: (1) normal maturation is interrupted, with the possibility of retention of primitive patterns, and/or a delay in acquiring new functions and abilities. Therefore, the child may exhibit behavior patterns of varying age levels. (2) The next area is in relation to perception and manifests itself as an interference with initiative and control of impulses. Another common result is (3) a "predisposition to anxiety."

For the remainder of this section, I shall refer to these children as children with minimal cerebral dysfunction. I have chosen this term as it clearly identifies to me that the child will have areas of normal functioning and areas of abnormal functioning depending on the part of the brain involved, and also that this damage may be minimal in nature—which permits a more optimistic outlook on the future for the child.

The nurse in the nursery has an increasing responsibility to identify early signs of brain injury. A good indicator of a problem is the baby's cry. The cry of the newborn normal infant is easily elicited by painful stimulation. The newborn with brain damage needs to be repeatedly stimulated to cry and the cry is weak, strained, and at times barely audible. A brain-injured child at one week of age may exhibit a cry with short abrupt bursts which have a shrieklike quality. These variations in cry should be quite evident to the nurse in the newborn nursery, who is in a good position to get early attention for this child.

As a child grows, his cry begins to have variations in pitch and rhythm with speechlike sounds intermingled. The brain-injured child's cry has a flat quality and lacks the speechlike sounds. Frequently the cry is gutteral in nature and seems to be forced rather than spontaneous. It is sometimes high-pitched and frequently shrieklike. These clues, evidenced by cry, should not go by without receiving adequate attention. The nurse's role is especially important in relation to charting the character of the cry and reporting this to the doctor. She may be instrumental in getting the doctor to listen to the cry. When the doctor examines the baby he may not hear the cry so an attempt to elicit a cry response may be all that is needed to get the child's attention. The delay in response and the amount of stimulation needed to sustain the response can be very striking.

The way the child feeds is another early cue to difficulty. The child with a brain injury is what is generally referred to as a "poor feeder." To be more concrete, the child does not suck well and must be stimulated frequently. He needs larger, softer nipples than normal babies of the same weight. He seems to lose parts of his feeding as he does not grasp the nipple and milk flows out the sides of his mouth. As the child gets older, he seems to drool a great deal of the time. When it is time for him to be tried on junior foods he is unable to chew meats.

The latter problems can be easily identified by the nurse when the baby is brought for well-baby supervision. In addition, she can check for other signs, such as the prolonged Moro reflex present in children with neurologic disturbances. The hands are a good indicator of disturbances in babies. Babies ordinarily prefer to clench their fists. The baby with fingers spread apart should alert the nurse to a possible problem. As the child matures physically, the developmental milestones are evaluated and deviations from the expected are evaluated to determine if they are biological or environmental in nature. Suggestions for altering environment to enhance developmental achievements is indicated. If the changed environment does not help, then biological conditions are probably the cause. Again, this is not a black or white thing, and a combination of the two is very common.

An example of changing the environment to enhance development might be observed in a child of seven months who is not sitting with support. You learn from the mother that she has never put the child in an upright position. The child spends the majority of the day in bed or lying in a play pen. The child is encouraged to be quiet so the mother can get things done. It is imperative that before the child is labeled retarded in developmental achievements he be given the opportunity to sit up with help and that he is stimulated by toys, voice, and other means to sit up for increasingly longer periods. In addition, the mother is encouraged to foster development and shown how to stimulate the child toward the next developmental goal if he achieves sitting before the next visit.

Earlier diagnosis puts new demands for treatment at an early age. The child with minimal cerebral dysfunction will need special classes. He will need consistent handling at home. The earlier the special classes are begun, the sooner the child may be able to transfer to regular classes.

Let us consider, for a moment, the handling of a hyperactive three-year-old. His daily pattern consists of running around the house, disrupting furniture, pushing the other children, destroying toys, and crying easily. His mother reacts with frequent outbursts of anger which tend to make the child more hyperactive. In advising the mother, the nurse should emphasize several points which may tend to lessen the frustrations. The child with minimal cerebral dysfunction finds it difficult to filter out stimuli. Therefore, he tries to react to them all at once. If he is watching TV and the wind blows the window, he tries to react to it and gets up and attempts to run to the window. His poor perception does not tell him the TV is in his way, and he runs right into it. His mother reacts by yelling a command, "Be careful," thus introducing another stimulus and further confusing his filtering mechanism. A therapeutic environment, for this child, would be one that controls stimulus.

The more "nude" the environment, the better. In fact, this child often does much better completely screened off with just one thing to concentrate on. Instead of TV he should be given simple block forms to work with or toys that are used to develop other senses which will help to make his visual sense more dependable.

It is very desirable to have fairly strict routines established as they tend to make the child feel more secure. He needs a definite sequence of events as he does not change easily from one activity to another. What could be considered a highly undesirable day for a normal three-year-old may be the best day for a three-year-old boy with minimal cerebral dysfunction.

In exploring the broken toys, it is frequently found that the child does not want to break the toy but he does not know how to use complicated ones. If the toy has wheels he may spin them until they fall off or if the toy has headlights he may become so entranced he pulls them out. Things that go around seem to fascinate him. Fewer and less complicated toys will tend to lessen the breakage problem.

In relation to pushing the other children, this may be caused by poor perception or it may be partially due to the poor body image the child has of himself. The child frequently feels the need to reach out and touch others and in our society touching others is not always considered appropriate.

The child also changes easily from one mood to another. He frequently cries and may almost seem to laugh and cry at the same time. He frequently gets scolded for his many unacceptable behaviors and crying seems to be his only way out. The nurse should try to help the mother see that the child who meets many failures during the day may feel very distraught. She must try to be sure to praise the child when he makes small gains, as the praise will help him to develop some self-worth. He needs praise desperately and his day will be much brighter if his failures are interspersed with some success.

In helping the mother to set limits and goals it is important to assess the child's assets rather than his deficits. His assets frequently get buried beneath his deficits and the child, as well as the parent, does not make sufficient use of them. Trying to find his strengths and building on them should be the goal of therapy. Frequently, the child is gifted verbally because he finds less confusion with this method of communication. He has learned by repeated failure that his performance only spells trouble. Therefore, education should include introducing things to help him with his verbal knowledge such as carving letters out of wood for him to trace as he says words, or showing him pictures to reinforce his words. Asking him to write the word "ball" may result in failure whereas spelling it verbally may result in success.

It is easy to predict that a three-year-old who exhibits these tendencies will not readily fit in a regular classroom situation when he gets older. Some authorities feel that medication may help to quiet the child and make it easier for him to pay attention. The reaction to the medication is not always favorable and frequently the child has an adverse effect producing exaggerated behavior. The parents and the child should know this is a possibility and they should realize that sometimes several medications will be tried before they find one that helps the child. They should also know that sometimes medication is not indicated.

Proper classroom placement is still not available for all these children, or even for a major portion of them. This means that many of them get into regular classes where they are a disrupting factor and their educational needs are not met. The teacher describes their behavior very nicely when she states they are in "constant motion," swinging their legs, tapping their pencils, destroying books, and seldom completing an assigned task. The teacher must be helped to give the child simple, direct instructions. If she punishes him by putting him in the corner facing the blackboard, he frequently does much better. She needs to know that it is not his reaction to the punishment that improved his output, but rather the decrease in stimulus. Also, the child with minimal cerebral dysfunction will need periods during which he can release his excess energy. After this release he is better able to return to work.

The school nurse should be aware that these children react poorly to minor stresses such as a toothache or a cold. Such a child may be unusually difficult to control and perhaps he would be better at home during these periods when additional stressful situations could be kept to a minimum. Other associated problems which may present themselves in school are the child's tendency to not step high enough and trip up stairs, or his seeming lack of knowledge that there is a step— so he falls down. He frequently misjudges and walks into the sides of doors. He may have difficulty getting his coat as he cannot reach high enough. If some of these things are kept in mind, intervention can be given which will aid the child and tend to cut down on his sudden outbursts when he meets the consequences of his actions.

In addition to the regular classroom work this child will benefit by "motor therapy." This is a conditioning process in which he learns to step down or step up. This can be done as a game making all types of obstacles for him to get over. At first these obstacles should be very simple, and then increased in complexity as he achieves and he masters a step.

Such children will frequently need help with reading as they see letters backwards and sentences seem to run together. The nurse can interpret to the parent and child his need for additional help. She may also help the parent to understand that it is not good to push the child to read at home because his reading skills are developed under very special conditions. Parents frequently find it difficult not to push the child as he looks so "normal" and they cannot understand why he does not progress like their other children.

The Hospitalized Child. When the child with minimal cerebral dysfunction is hospitalized, he often disrupts the entire unit. This is easy to understand when we take a minute to listen and watch the day and night happenings on the unit. His easy distractibility will make the hospital almost unbearable. Every attempt should be made to decrease stimuli. A private room, if available, can be very soothing. In contrast to the other children, treatment may be easier to do in his own room—where it is familiar, where he does not see myriads of equipment, and which is away from the mainstream of activity.

Even though we consider the hospital to be very "routine," it can frequently lack the consistency the child needs. A late breakfast may be intolerable to this child. A consulting physician may get greeted with hostility or the new nurse may get medications thrown at her. This child will frequently eat much better in his own room without all the usual things children like for eating time, such as music, dishes with pictures in the bottom, straws, and surprises. If the child wants to try eating in the group at another time, he should be given the opportunity. This does not guarantee that he will succeed but it does show him you know he is trying. If his behavior is completely disruptive to the entire group then this exposure should be discontinued. Types of disruptive behavior exhibited at meal time include taking everyone else's food, spilling the milk out of everyone's glasses, tearing up napkins, and throwing food on the floor.

NAP TIME.   Nap time may be a particularly trying time for the hyperkinetic child. Many parents have complained that these children are in constant motion all day and although they may appear exhausted, they never give in to a nap. Then they come to the hospital where a rest period is planned and they cannot tolerate the confinement. Putting them in bed may increase their irritability and may cause temper tantrums. When they are in bed they frequently rock, bang their hands, or shake the siderails. This activity can be best tolerated in a single room. The crib may need padding to protect the child from injury. It would be wise to have an understanding adult sit next to the child's bed during nap time.

HEIGHTS.   The child also has difficulty judging heights. When he is outside he falls down because he cannot judge curbs. In the hospital the nurse must be cautious in using bedside stools to assist the child when getting up. He will not be able to judge the distance and will fall the same as he does when he meets a curb outside.

This factor also is important when the child tries to negotiate stairs. He is extremely awkward and will need a nurse's hand as assistance.

HELPING THE CHILD UNDERSTAND HIMSELF.   The hospitalization provides the nurse with an opportunity to help the child to understand himself. Frequently he is frightened by his sudden outbursts; he is lonely and he feels isolated from the rest of the world. It takes a nurse who is not personally hurt by cutting remarks to work with this child. It also takes a nurse who can accept the idea that the child will have good and bad days and many more bad than good. She also needs to know that at times he will seem to regress and all her efforts seem to be in vain. She can introduce the school-age child to the book by Gardner (1966), which was specifically written to help the child learn to understand himself, and read sections with him. The book should be only a supplement to her counseling and not a replacement for it. The parents should also be introduced to the book. The parents should know which sections are currently being discussed with their child. The parents may appreciate knowing some of the child's responses to the book.

One of the most frequent reasons for hospitalizing this child is for diagnostic evaluation. This may be a very difficult period for the child as he is exposed to so many new things and people, frequently without proper preparation. The hospitalization may be extremely stressful for the parent, as they are anxiously awaiting a decision on just what is causing the hyperactive behavior. Many parents seem relieved when something is found to be organically wrong, as this then seems to somewhat justify the child's unacceptable behavior. A careful interpretation of findings is necessary so the parents know what the findings indicate. For instance, the parents may be told the EEG is normal and they think this means there is no brain injury. Other factors may be so much more relevant, such as the scatter performance on psychological testing and not the IQ number itself. Minor neurological deficits and history of behavior are also more significant than getting an abnormal EEG. There may be other parents who cannot accept the fact that their child is brain-injured and after a period of denial they may very well need a reinterpretation of what this means.

THE EEG.   An EEG (electroencephalogram) is a diagnostic tool frequently used in relation to neurological conditions. The procedure is used in conjunction with other diagnostic measurements and is not an independent tool for making a diagnosis. The EEG is a recording of the brain wave activity of the child. It is done to determine electrical abnormalities which may be present. It is an especially useful procedure for determining seizure activity.

Preparation of the child is paramount to decrease the anxiety which may accompany being taken to a strange room. The room is usually constructed to eliminate any distractions and therefore is usually very plain and isolated. The child should know about the room and the people that will be responsible for his care. There is usually a technician to do the EEG's.

The EEG can be done with the older child sitting in a chair. For younger children, it can be done lying down. Young children may need sedation in order to get an adequate reading because crying and excessive activity make a reading impossible to obtain. In older children maintenance medications such as phenobarbital and dilantin (anticonvulsants) are usually ordered to be withheld for 48 hr prior to the recording. This will provide a more accurate picture of the normal brain wave pattern for the particular child.

After the child is positioned, electrode compound is applied and electrodes are placed on the child's scalp. The child needs reassurance that these electrodes will not hurt him. The child may fear the unknown and also make self-explanations drawing on his limited body of knowledge. He may think he is being electrocuted and become unnecessarily alarmed. This is especially true of the child with minimal cerebral dysfunction. Each step must be explained very simply and the procedures done slowly. The nurse needs to help the technician understand the child's proneness to hyperactivity and overreactions to tests. If the child gets too upset, it may be necessary to postpone the procedure until another time.

After the child is adequately prepared, the technician asks the child to sit quietly while the recordings are taken. This may be impossible for the child with minimal cerebral dysfunction. Rest periods when he can move around should be liberally interspersed between quiet periods to help decrease the child's frustration.

After the recordings are completed, the nurse should remove all the electrode compound and be sure the child's hair is combed.

A Word to Parents.   Probably the best advice that can be given the parents is that they should try to see the child first and the brain injury second. While this may be difficult, it does provide for a better parent-child relationship. It also helps to provide the support the child needs as he is progressing through these difficult years. It is generally accepted knowledge that, with the right guidance and education, these children do improve by adolescence.

References

Alimentary Tract Obstructions of Infancy (Nursing Ed. Series, Pamphlet No. 4). Columbus, Ohio, Ross Laboratories, 1959.

Amador, L. V. Congenital anomalies. In Swenson, O. Pediatric Surgery 3rd ed. New York, Appleton-Century-Crofts, 1969, Chapter 74.

Basara, S. C. The behavioral patterns of the perceptually handicapped child. Nurs. Forum, Vol. V, No. 4, 1966, pp. 24–39.

Blakeslee, B., ed. The Limb-Deficient Child. Berkeley, University of California Press, 1963.

Bramley, G. L. The handicapped child—his attitudes and behavior. In Fishbein, M. ed. Birth Defects. Philadelphia, Lippincott, 1963.

Bruce, S. J. Reactions of nurses and mothers to stillbirth. Nurs. Outlook, 10:88, 1962.

Caplan, G. Mental Health and Consultation. U. S. Department of Health, Education, and Welfare, 1959.

Clemmens, R. L. Minimal Brain Damage in Children. In Rudick, E., ed. Pediatric Nursing. Dubuque, Iowa, Wm. C. Brown Co., 1966, pp. 82–90.

Ferrer, J. M., Jr. The esophagus. In Barnett, H. L., ed. Pediatrics, 14th ed. New York, Appleton-Century-Crofts, 1968, pp. 1519–1525.

Gardner, R. The Child's Book about Brain-Injury. Association for Brain-Injured Children, 1966.

Holt, J. L. A long-term study of a child treated for hypospadias. Philadelphia, Saunders, Vol. 4, No. 1, March 1969, pp. 27–37.

King, L. R. Hypospadias. In Swenson, O., ed. Pediatric Surgery, 3rd ed. New York, Appleton-Century-Crofts, 1969, Chapter 66.

Krupp, G. R., and Schwartzberg, B. The brain-injured child: a challenge to social workers. Social Casework, Feb. 1960 (Reprint).

Lehtinen, L. E. The brain-injured child: what can we do for him? Dallas Med. J. (special edition), March 1959, pp. 15–21.

Marlow, D. R. Textbook of Pediatric Nursing, 3rd ed. Philadelphia, Saunders, 1969, p. 107; pp. 173–175.

Martin, L., and others. Nursing care of infants with esophageal anomalies. Am. J. Nurs., 66:2463–2468, Nov. 1966.

Mathews, E. S., and Ransohoff, J. Hydrocephalus. In Barnett, H. L., ed. Pediatrics, 14th ed. New York: Appleton-Century-Crofts, 1968, pp. 847–853.

Solomon, G. Medication found beneficial in hyparactivity. Pediat. Herald., July–August. 1967, pp. 5–6.

Olshansky, S. Chronic sorrow: a response to having a mentally defective child. Social Casework, XLIII, No. 4., April 1962.

Owens, C. Parents reactions to defective babies. Amer. J. Nurs., 64:83–86, Nov. 1964.

Parad, H. J., and Caplan, G. A framework for studying families in crisis. In Parad, H. J., ed. Crisis Intervention. New York, Family Service Assoc. of America, 1965, p. 53–72.

Ross, A. O. The Exceptional Child in the Family. New York, Grune & Stratton, 1964.

Rothchild, B. F. Incubator isolation as a possible factor in the high incidence of emotional disturbances among prematurely born persons, Psych. Abstr., 42:52, 1968.

Schulman, J. L., Kasper, J. C., and Throne, F. M. Brain-Damage and Behavior. Springfield, Ill., Thomas, 1965.

Siegel, E. Helping The Brain-Injured Child. New York, Association for Brain-Injured Children, 1962.

Schulman, K. Meningomyelocele. In Barnett, H. L., ed. Pediatrics, 14th ed. New York, Appleton-Century-Crofts, 1968, pp. 857–860.

Smith, E. D. Spina Bifida and the Total Care of Myelomeningocele. Springfield, Ill., Thomas, 1965.

Solnit, A. J., and Stark, M. Mourning and the birth of a defective child. Psychoanal. Study of the Child, 16:523–537, 1961.

Steele, S. Children with amputations. Nurs. Forum, Vol. VII, No. 4, 1968, pp. 411–423.

———— The nurse's role in the rehabilitation of children with meningomyelocele. Nurs. Forum, Vol. VI, No. 1, 1967, pp. 104–117.

Stogdill, C. G. School achievement, learning difficulties and mental health, Canad. Mental Health (Supplement 48), Sept.–Oct. 1965, pp. 1–17.

Strauss, A. A., and Lehtinen, L. E. Psychopathology and Education of the Brain-Injured Child. New York, Grune & Stratton, 1947.

———— and Kephart, N. C. Psychopathology and Education of the Brain-Injured Child. New York, Grune & Stratton, 1955.

Strother, C. R. Discovering, Evaluation, Programming for the Neurologically Handicapped Child. National Society for Crippled Children and Adults, Inc., 1963.

Sugar, M., and Ames, M. D. The child with spina bifida cystica. Rehab. Literature, 26:362–366, Dec. 1965.

Swenson, O. ed. Pediatric Surgery, 3rd ed. New York, Appleton-Century-Crofts, 1969, Chapter 29.

von Schilling, K. C. The birth of a defective child. Nurs. Forum, Vol. VII, No. 4, 1968, pp. 424–439.

Zieman, H. F. The neurologically handicapped child. Amer. J. Nurs., 69:2621–2625, Dec. 1969.

10 CAROL REN KNEISL

Emotional Disorders of Childhood

The field of child psychiatry owes its emergence (1) to twentieth century psychoanalysts who began to focus on personality development and deviation and (2) to courts and correctional institutions who began to call attention to the need for prevention, treatment, and rehabilitation of juvenile delinquents. Out of these efforts the first child guidance and child treatment centers in the United States were established in New York, Boston, and Chicago.

Consequently, larger numbers of persons from many disciplines became involved in this field. The interdisciplinary range of child care workers is varied and includes nursing, psychiatry, pediatrics, psychology, social work, speech and hearing pathology, neurology, sociology, anthropology, and many other workers who engage in a wide spectrum of activities with disturbed or delinquent children. Earlier interests in the study of deviant or abnormal children turned to interest in the study of the well child or the normal child in the belief that one must understand normal development before one can understand developmental deviations.

Attempts to devise methods of bringing up children based upon understanding of growth and development have led to a number of absurd as well as common-sense or rational approaches. Historically, our beliefs about child care and parental responsibility vary along a continuum with the extremes of the continuum gaining the greatest attention from parents and professionals alike. For example, we have vacillated in our ideas about breast versus bottle feeding, parental permissiveness versus parental restraint, and demand feeding versus feeding on schedule for a number of decades. One of the most pragmatic helps available to parents concerned with child-rearing can be found in the beautiful prose below by Dorothy Law Nolte entitled "Children Learn What They Live." (Fig. 1.)

More recently, the emphasis is being placed upon the study of

CHILDREN LEARN WHAT THEY LIVE

If a child lives with criticism, He learns to condemn.

If a child lives with hostility, He learns to fight.

If a child lives with ridicule, He learns to be shy.

If a child lives with shame, He learns to feel guilty.

If a child lives with tolerance, He learns to be patient.

If a child lives with encouragement, He learns confidence.

If a child lives with praise, He learns to appreciate.

If a child lives with fairness, He learns justice.

If a child lives with security, He learns to have faith.

If a child lives with approval, He learns to like himself.

*If a child lives with acceptance and friendship,
He learns to find love in the world.*

Courtesy of Ross Laboratories.

animals, particularly primates. John Bowlby, who spurred interest in maternal and emotional deprivation as the result of his monograph published by the World Health Organization of the United Nations in 1951, has recently presented the thesis that the study of animal behavior, particularly that of primates, has extreme relevance to human psychology (Bowlby, 1969), an attitude which has previously been ignored, doubted, or denied. It has been proposed that consideration of growth and development is based upon certain inherent biological capacities through a long history of primate evolution combined with behaviors man shares with other primates and which is augmented through the use of a culture that is uniquely human (Morris, 1969). When considering the relationship of human behavior to primate behavior, one ought to keep in mind the fact that aspects of the uniqueness of human development are based upon infant behavior, which demonstrates not only intelligence but adaptability and flexibility as well, because the strategies invented by the infant when working within his limitations are plainly different from those of other primates (Bruner, 1968). And so the controversy continues in an attempt to refine and define those developmental characteristics and necessities which make for effective adaptation in living.

In 1961, the Joint Commission on Mental Illness and Health published the results and recommendations of their five-year study of mental health in America. While this report concerned itself mostly with adults and the establishment of community mental health centers, it did have some recommendations to make regarding children and their treatment in residential schools, clinics, and the community at large. The report noted the paucity of specialists in the area of children's mental health and recommended supplementation of state funds with federal funds in the training and education of professionals and lay people to augment the current number (Joint Commission on Mental Illness and Health, 1961). Impetus was given to these recommendations and to further study by the assassination of President Kennedy. President Kennedy's assassin, Lee Harvey Oswald, had been studied by the Bureau of Child Guidance in New York. Their recommendations, however, were never carried out. One outcome was an amendment to the Social Security law introduced in 1965 by Senator Abraham Ribicoff which provided funds for the establishment of a Joint Commission on Mental Health of Children. This project was a three-year study undertaken by a large number of professional organizations concerned with the mental health needs of children. The results were made public in May of 1969 (Joint Commission on Mental Health of Children, 1969). The Commission viewed as a national tragedy the lack of any unified or cohesive national commitment to children and youth. It called for drastic changes to bring about such a commitment and a "child-oriented society." Some of the changes recommended consisted of federal assistance for research, training, and treatment at every level of society to ensure effective implementation of programs designed to be of assistance to children. By May of 1970, one year after the publication of its report, the Commission regretfully announced in the communications media that not one community in the United States had yet provided adequate services. The seriousness of the problem can be deduced from the knowledge that at least 10 million young persons under the age of 25 have an emotional disorder.

This chapter will attempt to relate some portion of the problem to the student, although we humbly accept the knowledge that the magnitude and complexity of emotional disorders in children cannot possibly be dealt with within this volume.

Maladaptations and Neurotic Dysfunctions of Childhood

Neuroses or maladaptations of childhood were little recognized prior to the advent of psychoanalysis and the Freudian era although references were made in earlier centuries to the importance of child-rearing activities and the various thoughts, feelings and actions inherent in the parent-child relationship (Burlingham, 1951). However, the description of clinical cases concerning mental disturbance or disorder in children was treated as unique and highly unusual and curious, perhaps more appropriate for "Ripley's Believe It or Not" than for consideration by the professionals of the time.

One development which encouraged the use of the term "neurosis" when applied to children was Freud's analysis of the horse phobia of Little Hans at the turn of the century (Freud, 1936). In their study of hysteria, Breuer and Freud established the relationship between the experiences of living and neurosis, thereby drawing attention to the need to study childhood development (Breuer and Freud, 1936). The psychobiological approach advocated by Adolph Meyer, who utilized both analytic and descriptive psychiatry, also emphasized the importance of biographical study of the patient including childhood development (Lief, 1948).

Much of the knowledge concerning childhood neuroses comes from psychoanalytically trained therapists. Anna Freud's modification of the technique of psychoanalysis made it possible to study and treat children with neuroses (A. Freud, 1959). The play therapy techniques developed by Melanie Klein were analytically oriented and obviated the necessity for verbal confirmation required in the psychoanalytical treatment of the adult (Klein, 1932). Recently, professionals with varying orientations have been engaged in the direct study of children in child-study laboratories.

Some of the specifics which differentiate between the neurotic child and the adapted child are the following. The neurotic child fluctuates in behavior, and while he, at times, may respond appropriately in terms of age-expected behavior and reality, at other times he exists in a state of distress and has diminished capacity for testing reality. The neurotic child exists in a state of conscious and subjective mental distress, discomfort, or anxiety. His ability to call upon adjustment mechanisms or defense mechanisms to come to his rescue is diminished and, therefore, he is easily irritated and considerably excited by stimuli which others would perceive as relatively minor, nontoxic, or innocuous. Fortunately, complete disorganization of the personality or mental function does not take place even when the child's behavior appears disrupted to the onlooker. The symptoms the neurotic child exhibits indicate a self-orientation as, for example, is present in common signs such as daydreaming, masturbation, bed-wetting, fears, and neurotic compulsions and obsessions. One should not link such behaviors only to childhood neurosis, since both the quality and quantity of the behavior and/or symptomatology needs to be considered. What child has never been fearful? Or daydreamed? Although there are certain phenomena which can be unhesitatingly labeled neurotic (conversion hysteria is one), others need to be analyzed in terms of their frequency, severity, and duration.

It is difficult to assign any one single cause in the development of childhood neurosis. This difficulty has been well phrased by Cramer, who stated:

> Neurosis in childhood is caused by social experiences which are traumatic; that is, inappropriate in respect to the capacity of the mental apparatus of *that* child at *that* moment to contain and integrate them in a manner consistent with the maintenance of normal development. Since normal means something different depending on where one is, and especially depending on how old one is, adaptive devices of the child's mind find different responses in different environments and at different ages. Thus, differences in what constitutes a noxious stimulus may depend on various cultural influences (Cramer, 1959, p. 800).

Traumatic experiences, parental attitudes, and constitutional make-up are among the variety of factors generally present in the neuroses of childhood. Life experiences which may prove traumatizing to the child include loss of one or both parents when accompanied by unsuccessful mourning or inadequate substitutive figures, physical illness, injury, neglect, and traumatic acts of fate. Specific traumatic life experiences, parental attitudes, and constitutional make-up will be considered in view of the various neurotic and psychotic developmental deviations noted in this chapter. Before continuing, the reader would do well to review sources on personality development and adjustment mechanisms as background material necessary to an understanding of the emotional disorders of childhood. The author assumes that the reader possesses this necessary basic knowledge.

CRYING

When continuous, extensive, and unrelieved crying occurs in situations in which its presence seems unreasonable—that is, in the absence of physical pathology or physical discomfort—it serves as a signal denoting mental distress. Generally, parents learn to distinguish within the first few weeks of the infant's life between cries which signal hunger, pain, or bodily discomfort. They then require decreasing periods of time in which to diagnose and meet the unfulfilled need demanded by the infant. When crying persists beyond the point at which apparent needs have been met by the mothering one, the infant's experienced distress is likely to be mental rather than physiological. Further evidence that the infant's distress or anxiety is subtly communicated from the mother, and reflects her anxiety regarding mothering duties, may be seen in instances when someone other than the mother is able to reduce the infant's tension and anxious cry. The difference between these two individuals in handling the infant has to do with the quality of response.

Harry Stack Sullivan, a psychiatrist who devoted most of his time to the psychotherapy of schizophrenic adults, conceptualized an interpersonal theory of psychiatry based upon the belief that the quality of the early mother-child relationship was a crucial factor in determining the infant's later adjustment to the trials and vicissitudes of life (Sullivan, 1943). If the mother is insecure, unsure, anxious, she emphatically communicates this to the child, who responds with a like anxiety of his own. Out of such a pattern, a vicious cycle is born. The infant's increasing anxiety and discomfort add to the mother's anxiety, which in turn escalates the distress the infant feels. The cycle is broken when the mothering person feels secure, calm, and relatively nonanxious, thereby allowing the infant to experience similar pleasurable feelings. Crying infants do not become "spoiled" if they are picked up and held. During this stage of infancy children do not need, nor can they cope with, limit-setting and the delay of gratification. When their needs are met they will experience greater security, trust, and self-worth. Wise parents set limits, make demands, and impose restrictions when the child is able to handle delayed gratification.

FEEDING DISTURBANCES

Eating is one of the earliest meaningful experiences the child has and, concurrently, hunger is the most common cause of crying and discomfort in the newborn. The magnitude of the problem becomes evident when the review of the records of 110 preschoolers referred to the Child Development Center of New York City indicates that in 56 percent of the children, feeding problems were present, with the far greater majority present during the first year of life (Beller, 1962). Once physical disturbances such as allergy, pylorospasm, and inappropriate formula (which may account for feeding problems) are ruled out, emotional factors must be considered. Food refusal, colic, and vomiting are common disturbances of feeding. Less common disturbances are pica, obesity, and anorexia nervosa.

Jane W. Kessler indicates that when feeding problems occur, a mother may find herself repeating the same ineffective behavior of her own mother as she feels increasingly anxious, angry and guilty. Kessler makes the important point that:

> This is but one example of the important general principle that parents have special conflicts in handling problems which are a

repetition of their own. Whenever a parent has a blind spot, it is worth exploring for evidence of the same difficulty a generation earlier (Kessler, 1966, p. 105).

Food Refusal and Vomiting. With food refusal and vomiting, eating is associated with experiences of discomfort, as food often becomes the battleground in the mother-child relationship. What the infant is communicating is that he prefers the unpleasant state of hunger if his only other choice is to tolerate the interpersonal and intrapsychic discomfort which feeding brings.

Sometimes the problem is relatively simple. The mother simply needs to learn what to expect from the infant in terms of feeding and to readjust her own expectations of him. The mother who responds with rigidity in terms of the amount of food she believes should be eaten as well as the appropriate time in which to do so is likely to find herself faced with an unhappy infant who is forced to vomit because he has been overfed, or has waited too long, or cried too hard, and is unable to eat when the "magic hour" finally arrives. Resolution of some of these conflicts between mother and child can often times be reached through reeducation of the mother. Sometimes however, feeding problems may be indicative of the mother's deep-seated hostility toward the child. She may rationalize the need for a strict schedule, thereby forcing the infant to wait for the gratification of need, or may overfeed in an attempt to compensate for or to deny the resentment felt. In this case, an attempt is made to convert the gift of food into a gift of love. The person who refuses to play this game through the rejection of food which is the offered but dubious gift is the child. For example, a situation which has recently come to my attention is one in which a mother actually force-feeds the daughter when she refuses to eat. The child is placed on her back on the floor and is fed from a spoon while her mother sits astride her to keep her arms and legs flat. Needless to say, in this household mealtime has become battletime. Rational and logical explanations to the mother regarding her own behavior have no effect. It is likely, in such a situation, that an irrational and unconscious motive prompts this mother's actions. Her child is a candidate for more severe emotional disturbances in the future.

Colic. Sharp intestinal pain accompanied by loud crying which is unrelieved by holding or carrying the baby with flexion of the legs and abdominal distension is the generally accepted definition of infant colic.

Colic usually ceases by the third or fourth month of life. It may be classified as an eating disturbance because of some of the curious factors which surround it. For example, the infant seems to be most uncomfortable for three or more of the early evening hours, although he appears to be relatively comfortable during the remainder of the day. Most pediatricians and child psychiatrists believe that colic is likely to result from a combination of two circumstances: an immature digestive tract and disruption of the interpersonal relationships in the family.

Colic is distressing not only to the obviously uncomfortable infant but also to his parents, who become more and more frustrated when their well-meant intentions and attempts to alleviate the infant's discomfort are unsuccessful.

Babies who are colicky are often found to be more hyperactive than other infants. They are often called tense, vigorous, lusty, and easily stimulated and startled. This may be an indication that the role of inborn constitutional differences may be important in producing colic.

The correlation between infant colic and its appearance in the evening hours may be the arrival home of the father who has been absent during the day while at his job. It is likely that the father's appearance alters the mother-child relationship. For example, the immature man may resent the time his wife spends with the child, or his return and the need to prepare dinner for the family realistically takes the mother away from the child for a longer period of time, or perhaps the mother does not look forward to her husband's return home in the evening. Any one of these factors is bound to disrupt the infant-mother relationship, particularly if anxiety is an accompaniment.

Because of the distressing nature of infantile colic, parents inevitably embark upon the search for a solution which often takes them to the pediatrician's office in search of alterations in the formula. Occasionally, formula alterations can be helpful when an immature digestive tract is present. Unfortunately, formula alteration is not always helpful and some parents may request the pediatrician to suggest formula changes every few days or may even embark upon the search for a pediatrician who will be able to offer some sort of "cure."

As such behavior continues, the relationship between the child and his parents becomes more frustrating and unrewarding and fraught with anxiety. At such times, both parents and baby deserve a respite from each other, a vacation, if you will, to interrupt the escalation of dissatisfaction. The empathic nature of anxiety becomes more evident when colic cannot be attributed to physiological problems or constitutional defects.

Attempting to soothe the infant may be temporarily helpful and at least offer some relief to both parents and child. At the same time, they could be encouraged to become aware of the pattern of colic and attempt to correlate it with their activities and the environment in the home. They perhaps may be able to determine events that increase their own anxiety communicated to the infant, and thereby alter their behavior or the environment.

Pica. Pica, the ingestion of substances generally considered inappropriate, such as clay, plaster, charcoal, and wax among others, is an expected state of affairs until approximately one year of age. During this first year of life every child who explores and tests the world around him is likely to have eaten a variety of unusual and generally unappetizing substances. The child who purposefully seeks out certain objects to eat, such as sand or paper or whatever, and remains persistent in his efforts evidences a feeding disturbance. Environmental and cultural conditions seem to play an important role in the development of pica.

Numerous research studies have been carried out in attempts to determine the influence which such factors as socioeconomic status, race, intelligence, and nutrition have in cases of pica. The results of the investigations are oftentimes contradictory. For example, some studies have indicated that children with pica are often severely retarded and almost always of subnormal intelligence while other investigations conclude that pica has no relationship to level of intelligence. The influence of nutrition is also unclear. While some children who eat plaster have been found to have a calcium deficiency, others have not. Dietary lacks have not consistently correlated with the presence of pica. In her study of pica, Cooper indicates a higher incidence of pica among Negroes and in lower socioeconomic groups (Cooper, 1957). Among these groups, pica may be considered a somewhat natural state of affairs since of the more than 700 mothers interviewed, 171 reported it upon questioning while only one mother spontaneously offered this information. Cooper's results have been corroborated by others (Gutelius, et al., 1962). Physical environment may be an important factor since the active child who does not have an interesting and constructive way in which to release his energy may well turn to chewing furniture, clothes, or windowsills. Consistency is absent here since children who are stimulated and even overstimulated have developed this particular feeding disturbance. This may indicate that relationships between the child and the significant persons in his environment need to be investigated further in an attempt to determine etiological factors.

Although pica generally disappears by the time a child is about six years old, there are numerous instances of pica in school-age children and adults, particularly in pregnant women.

Anorexia Nervosa. Anorexia nervosa, which occurs most often in girls, is a condition in which food is perceived as revolting and inedible. The anorexic patient refuses food, or regurgitates food which has been taken, resulting in excessive weight loss and malnutrition which can proceed to the level of starvation.

The anorexic patient seems to be caught up in a power struggle with those persons who are attempting to cajole, persuade, threaten, or punish her into eating. According to a variety of points of view, anorexia nervosa may be an unconscious method by which the fear of sexuality, or anal aggressiveness toward the self or others may be expressed. When it is part of a psychotic disturbance such as schizophrenia it may relate to withdrawal from the unsafe, external world to a safer, internal one.

Certain commonalities have been identified as present in anorexic children and adolescents. One factor is that food has a special importance and meaning to the child's parents who often eat or drink to excess. In addition, food and eating is not newly important to the patient herself since the developmental history frequently indicates earlier power struggles with parents over food in various forms. The youngster has often been overweight before this symptom developed and engaged in bouts of compulsive eating. Third, there seems to be evidence of unwillingness to grow up, mature physically and become heterosexually oriented (Kessler, 1966).

These commonalities were evident with Margie, a 14-year-old girl who was hospitalized when she was near starvation. Margie refused all food and when forcefed by one or both parents would regurgitate. She was badly emaciated and so weak that she was unable to walk.

Margie's mother drank heavily on a rather sporadic basis, and when she did, she was in no condition to prepare lunch or dinner. It was often up to the patient herself to assume responsibility for preparing food for herself and a younger brother and sister. The mother's drinking bouts coincided with the father's absences from the home for business reasons. Margie's mother questioned his absences and suspected that her husband was interested in other women.

Before the onset of these symptoms, Margie's mother described her as "fat, sloppy, and unattractive." She often berated her daughter for her appearance and compared her unfavorably to other children who lived in the neighborhood. Margie often heard her mother say that she would "give anything to have a daughter I could be proud of." Suddenly after one of the mother's alcoholic periods, Margie refused to fix lunch or dinner for herself or the other children, and refused food prepared by others.

The day she was admitted to the hospital, Margie wore a pullover sweater. It was only since her excessive weight loss, her mother said, that Margie would consent to wear sweaters. She previously refused to wear them and often commented that "my bust shows up too much." Margie expressed joy over the fact that she had not had a menstrual period for months.

Initially, Margie was given intravenous feedings since the malnutrition was at a critical level at which irreversible damage could take place. Although one does not want to be caught up with the anorexic patient in the power struggle over food, intravenous feedings may be necessary to save the patient's life. In addition to medical management, psychotherapy was instituted with Margie and her parents as well. While Margie was being treated by a child psychiatrist, her parents' psychotherapy took place in a marital couple's group led by a psychiatric nurse clinician. Eventually Margie consented to chewing fruit-flavored gum and proceeded from there to eat one soft boiled egg daily. As both Margie and her parents began to work through individual and mutual conflicts, Margie's symptoms abated and she began to gain weight. The last time that staff members saw Margie they found her to be "a little thin but cute." She informed them that her mother had agreed to her request to remain late after school one day a week to take ballroom dancing lessons.

The prognosis is not so favorable when anorexia nervosa is only one of many symptoms present in a psychotic youngster.

SLEEPING DISTURBANCES

Disturbances of sleep seem to have to do with the fear of being left alone. The child, who is totally dependent upon his parents for his survival, needs to experience feeling secure and wanted and knowing that his needs will be met and his discomfort eased. Such security comes about through experiencing gratification, time and time again, in the meeting of needs. The child who is not sure whether his needs will be met will exist in a state of uncertainty and apprehension and will experience difficulty in learning to trust. Such a child will be fearful of being alone and in the dark, for it brings with it a state of uncertainty since the child's expectations of what will, or will not, happen to him are not clear.

Many times disturbances of sleeping, as well as the other neurotic disturbances previously mentioned, are encouraged by parental beliefs that meeting children's needs will "spoil" them, and so they purposefully delay the child's gratification. What the child will learn from such experiences, however, is that people cannot be trusted and that he cannot depend upon others. He will constantly feel threatened for his own safety and well-being, since the persons his physiological and emotional survival depends upon most have proven themselves to be untrustworthy.

Young children with problems of sleep are often fearful of their own aggressive impulses and loss of control associated with sleeping. These fears can generally be linked with the child's developmental stage and the current difficulties and stresses he faces. Nightmares reach a peak between the ages of four and six and are infrequently reported by younger children. When sleep disturbances are severe and chronic in nature they can be deemed pathological and indicate that the level of anxiety experienced by the child cannot be reduced by the mechanisms known to him. In such instances, psychotherapeutic treatment is useful and generally effective within a short period of time.

THUMB-SUCKING

Thumb-sucking is an important method of self-gratification enjoyed by the infant. Generally, after the first year of life, thumb-sucking decreases and loses its fascination for the child. When it remains a persistent behavior and chief source of gratification it can be considered a sign of mental conflict. Attitudes toward thumb-sucking can be equated with the swinging pendulum. At the present time in our society a rather permissive attitude toward thumb-sucking is uppermost. Relatively few parents continue with earlier forceful repressive measures in attempts to suppress or prevent thumb-sucking in their children. Parental indulgence or permissiveness have not negated the need for thumb-sucking and in this sense it is as much a failure as bandaging the child's hands or coating them with an unpleasant-tasting liquid. The reason rests in the fact that thumb-sucking, just as any other symptom, while partially or temporarily relieving the anxiety associated with intrapsychic or interpersonal conflict, does not cure or resolve the child's troubles.

Thumb-sucking may be considered more serious when factors of age, quantity, and association with other symptoms occur. The older child who sucks his thumb persistently and frequently while indulging in other symptoms indicative of immaturity or neurosis is certainly in greater emotional difficulty than the child who regresses to thumb-sucking upon the advent of a critical event or physical trauma. Temporary regression usually reverses itself when the critical event or physical trauma assumes a less threatening nature. In the case of the immature or neurotic child whose thumb-sucking occurs in conjunction with a multiplicity of symptoms, psychotherapy and parental education may be required.

PHOBIAS

Like sleep disturbances, phobias in childhood are common and are regarded as developmentally normal when they occur at an early age, at which they are transient in nature. However, phobias of children at the age of five and older can be disabling to the child when they are severe in nature. Severity is indicated when the child is preoccupied with the situation, event, person, or thing he fears so that he seems to be existing in a constant state of dreaded anticipatory anxiety.

Although numerous theorists attempt to explain the cause or causes of phobias, most include the onset of a frightening experience which arouses anxiety and guilt leading to repression. A phobia gives the child something tangible to fear and, as frightening as it may be, is not so intolerable as the uncanny dread experienced during anxiety, an inner event.

The most frequent childhood phobias are of animals, transportation, and schools. Although horse phobias such as that of Little Hans, reported by Freud, are rare, dogs and insects seem to be leading contenders. The phobic object gives a clue to the unacceptable thought, wish, or impulse being repressed by the child. For example, insects are often feared because of their association with dirt, horses are feared because they are equated symbolically with the father, and the fear of snakes indicates the projection of sexual feelings.

Phobias involving transportation interfere more significantly with the child's life and that of his parents. It is for this reason that treatment is more often sought and needed than in the case of an animal phobia.

School Phobia. School phobias are those which present the greatest concern and problem for the child, his parents, and his teachers.

Since legalities are involved a child's frequent and prolonged absence from school cannot be ignored. For this reason, school phobias are those most often treated and talked over in circles of parents, educators, school psychologists, and others.

Although school phobias may occur at any age, they are generally associated with the lower elementary grades and with transient somatic symptoms such as vomiting, diarrhea, or headache which diminish once the child is assured that he does not have to go to school. The interesting phenomenon that children with clear-cut learning difficulties, or those in real danger of failing, do not develop school phobias has been noted (Kessler, 1966).

School phobia is another instance of the empathic communication of anxiety between mother and child, specifically, a fear of separation. This mutual dependence forces the child into a rather strange role— that of meeting another's needs while striving to have his own met. The child's unacceptable thoughts of aggression and hostility are believed by some to account for his regression to an earlier stage of dependency.

The treatment of school-phobic children must also include the family and the school in a collaborative process. It may include a variety of methodologies in the psychotherapeutic process ranging from psychoanalysis to play therapy to classical and operant conditioning.

PROBLEMS IN SPEECH AND LANGUAGE DEVELOPMENT

Difficulties in speech and language development are not at all uncommon among children referred to child guidance clinics. Many of the problems of enunciation and articulation are treated solely by professional speech pathologists. Such difficulties as stammering, or stuttering, and the delayed speech often present because of organic causes or functional psychoses are those which are most often brought to the attention of mental health professionals in the area of child psychiatry.

Stuttering. Stammering, or stuttering, indicates a disturbance in the flow of speech due to muscular contractions or spasms and is most often observed in male children. The onset generally occurs between the ages of two and four.

The most problematic feature of stuttering is the social alienation which frequently results as the stutterer bizarrely attempts to control his speech through facial grimaces, slapping himself, using unusual body gestures, and substituting other words or phrases for those originally intended.

Many researchers have focused upon the identification of personality characteristics of the stutterer and to date have not been able to pinpoint a special personality type. There does seem to be general agreement, however, that the interruption of the flow of speech displays conflict and indicates withholding rather than giving. Theories as to the nature, origin, and identification of this conflict are varied and run the gamut. Basically, physiological views are those which consider the cause of verbal difficulty as related to a constitutional predisposition ranging from that of identifying stuttering as a miniature epileptic seizure to associating it with metabolic disturbance. Most theorists now allow room for a psychogenic variant which either stands alone or is associated with a somatic one. The widely accepted theory of mixed cerebral dominance propounded in the 1920s and 1930s has fallen into disfavor. This theory held that an existing physiological rivalry between the two cortical hemispheres, if one was not sufficiently dominant, accounted for a poorly synchronized speech musculature which resulted in stuttering (Travis, 1931). However, more recent studies have indicated that children who stutter are not particularly ambidextrous, or left-handed, or have had their handedness changed by parents or teachers (Bloodstein, 1959).

Psychological views of stuttering often focus on the intrafamilial relationship. Stuttering has been attributed to disturbances in the mother-child relationship (Wyatt and Herzan, 1962), an approach-avoidance conflict (Sheehan, 1962), a conflict of gratification of instinct according to the psychoanalytic view (Fenichel, 1945), and undue parental criticism which fixates the symptom by calling attention to it (Johnson, 1955).

Children who stutter and are anxious about it often need the direct help which psychotherapeutic treatment offers. Behavior shaping based on learning theory has been found to be effective also, as has speech therapy with a properly educated speech therapist. Parental education is important for the attitude of the parents can serve to either increase or decrease the child's anxiety and his stuttering. A well-written pamphlet which ought to be recommended to the parents of children who are beginning to stutter was authored by a speech pathologist, Dean C. Engel, and a clinical psychologist, Isadore Helfand. Entitled "Stuttering is a Family Affair," it is available through the Cleveland Hearing and Speech Center, Cleveland, Ohio 44106.

PROBLEMS IN TOILET TRAINING

Problems in toilet training often reflect the interpersonal battle between parents and child and in this way are similar to feeding disturbances. The toilet, anus, and genitals are often sources of taboo and constraints imposed by parents in their attempt to acculturate their young in a way that will make them hygienically clean and acceptable members of human society at large. Because of the importance placed upon the bodily functions of micturition and defecation a child's refusal to play by the rules of the game can wreak intrafamilial havoc.

Eneuresis. Eneuresis, or wetting, when occurring occasionally and at night in children younger than eight is considered usual and of little consequence. As with stuttering, there has been no consistent identification of a consistent personality type or behavior associated with eneuresis, although it is seldom found as the only sign or symptom of emotional disturbance or emotional immaturity in a child. In fact, these children are often found to be thumb-sucking, masturbating, nose-picking, nail-biting, and so forth, for longer periods in their lives than the majority of children. Leo Kanner, who makes the point that symptoms of emotional disturbances and emotional immaturity were generally present in eneuretic children categorizes them as follows (Kanner, 1957, p. 448):

Aggressive, fighting, mischievous, cruel	8%
Whining, complaining, moody, irritable	32%
Restless, overactive, fidgety, excitable	21%
Disobedient, impudent, spiteful, stubborn	14%
Timid, shy, bashful, seclusive, unusually quiet	8%
Listless, indifferent, apathetic	5%
Overconscientious, serious-minded	3%

Kessler has regrouped Kanner's categories to focus on the way the child handles aggressive impulses. She notes that the first four categories, or 75 percent, include aggressive children, while the second four, or 25 percent, include children who have turned the aggression inward against themselves. (Kessler, 1966, p. 120) She has also identified what she believes to be common dynamic patterns in children with eneuresis: regression as a response to separation from the significant person originally responsible for toilet training, confusion and/or ambivalence over sexual identity, and "revenge eneuresis" as a way of expressing felt anger toward the parents. (Kessler, 1966, p. 122).

Attempts to explain eneuresis as a purely physiological event have met with little success. Eneuretic children do not have electroencephalographic patterns which differ from those of noneneuretic children, they do not have smaller bladders, nor do they wet their beds because they sleep more soundly. Children have been eneuretic on occasion for a variety of physiological reasons and certainly bladder infection and its accompanying symptoms may encourage nighttime bed-wetting. However, these instances are the unusual rather than the usual. Unfortunately, when parents subject their children to a variety of diagnostic urological procedures which focus upon the genitals, it often adds to their fearful fantasies regarding differentness and genital mutilation.

Helpful measures for the eneuretic child include environmental changes which realistically encourage the child to assist himself. They may include a night-light for the child who fears walking to the bathroom at night, removing diapers and/or rubber pants which set up the expectation that the child will wet and is unable to control his bladder, and firm but kindly encouragement from the parents.

The approach may be very different, however, when eneuresis occurs not infrequently but has become an established pattern. Conditioned response therapy is frequently employed, which focuses upon the removal of symptoms through the process of retraining. Commercial products are often sold which produce an unpleasant sensation for the child, which are triggered by moisture when urine comes in contact with the apparatus. Children who do not respond to any of the treatments previously outlined are candidates for psychotherapy.

Encopresis. Encopresis is the term used to indicate soiling with feces. Although it may occur through anatomical defect, impairment of the nervous system, or in the mentally retarded or child who is not toilet-trained, it is considered a severe neurotic symptom when it occurs in physiologically normal children who have passed the stage of toilet-training. As with many of the feeding disturbances, disturbances of toilet-training take place on an emotionally invested battleground. The struggle of child against parent and vice versa may subvert and minimize all other aspects of the parent-child relationship while the war over power and control takes place. It often brings to the fore the latent and not-so-well-hidden hostility of both parents and children as each attempts autocratically to rule the other. For example, not too long ago an acquaintance asked what she ought to do about her five-year-old, Tessa, who continued to soil herself and withhold feces even if on the potty seat for hours on end. When I asked the mother what she had done so far she responded with: "Everything I can think of. I've spanked her, I've shouted at her, I've embarrassed her in front of her playmates, I've sent her to bed without supper. I've even rubbed her face in her soiled diaper and refused to change it all day, but even that doesn't help. I've tried everything!" It seems to me from what she continued to say that this mother had not tried affection, increased attention, or attempted to diagnose the basis for Tessa's behavior and her responses to it. Instead of making these points evident to Tessa's mother, I asked her if she had any ideas about what she might do next. When she said that she was planning on phoning a child psychiatrist for an appointment, I encouraged her in her wise decision and attempted to prepare her for the visit. To have chastised this mother for her behavior toward Tessa would only have increased her guilt and anger.

When combined with withholding and eneuresis, soiling takes on a more pathologic form and calls for psychotherapeutic treatment. In such instances it may signal nascent antisocial disturbances or psychoses. However, when soiling occurs because of training failure or is regressive in nature, as upon the birth of a baby brother or sister, it often resolves itself when the significant persons in the environment recognize the child's temporary, albeit increased, needs for love and attention.

RITUALISTIC AND STEREOTYPICAL BEHAVIOR
AND THINKING (COMPULSIONS
AND OBSESSIONS)

Ritualistic and stereotypical behavior and thinking, or compulsions and obsessions, exist together—although one may be a predominant mode of expression over the other. Obsessions take the form of recurrent unpleasant or anxiety-producing thoughts, while compulsions are ritualistic acts designed to reduce the anxiety to a level that can be tolerated, at least temporarily.

Obsessional compulsive symptoms may be present during normal growth and development. For example, it is not at all unusual for children about the age of two or three to be greatly worried about preventing messiness or dirtiness or to insist upon changing clothes as soon as they become soiled. The child is simply overresponding to his newly learned rules and regulations and superego restrictions resulting from toilet training. School-age children in their efforts to attain and maintain perfection in self-control will often engage in ritualistic behavior such as that identified by Benjamin Spock:

> The commonest is stepping over cracks in the sidewalk. There's no sense to it, you just have a superstitious feeling that you ought to. It's what a psychiatrist calls a compulsion. Other examples are touching every third picket in a fence, making numbers come out even in some way, saying certain words before going through a door. If you think you made a mistake, you must go way back to where you were absolutely sure you were right, and start over again.
>
> The hidden meaning of a compulsion pops out in the thoughtless childhood saying, "Step on a crack, break your grandmother's back." Everyone has hostile feelings at times toward the people who are close to him, but his conscience would be shocked at the idea of really harming them and warns him to keep such thoughts out of his mind. And if a person's conscience becomes excessively stern, it keeps nagging him about such bad thoughts even after he has succeeded in hiding them away in his subconscious mind. He still feels guilty, though he doesn't know what for. It eases his conscience to be extra careful and proper about such a senseless thing as how to navigate a crack in the sidewalk (Spock, 1963, p. 390).

However, when obsessions and compulsions are allied with phobias, tics, and hysteria, the child finds himself severely limited and handicapped in relation to other people, his environment, and even himself. In these instances it has been found that many children with this combination of symptoms have been mistakenly diagnosed as psychotic (Despert, 1955). Because of the extremely limiting nature of obsessive compulsive neurosis with its resultant restrictions upon the growing child who should be exposed to newer and different learning experiences, individual therapy is the recommended method of treatment in an attempt to assist the child in relaxation of his superego controls.

HYSTERIA

Hysterical symptoms occur when the attempt to repress forbidden wishes, desires, or impulses fails and the previously repressed thoughts begin to come to the surface and are more available to consciousness. They take various forms such as sudden uncontrolled outbursts that border on panic, conversions such as hysterical blindness, dissociative reactions such as amnesia and sleep walking or multiple personality made famous by the case of "the three faces of Eve," tics, and even hallucination. Fewer cases of hysteria in childhood are seen today. Some ascribe it to the fact that the repressive child-rearing practices of the Victorian era have given way to overindulgent and permissive practices more likely to encourage hedonism, pleasure-seeking, and character disorder rather than hysteria (Wallder, 1960). It has also been suggested that hysterical reactions are responses to extreme inconsistency between word and action particularly when parents link their children's sexual feelings with evil and punishment while at the same time encouraging them through their own seductive behavior (Proctor, 1958).

Because hysterical persons are so suggestible and easily influenced, a symptomatic cure can generally be quickly obtained in psychotherapeutic work. Maintenance of the "cure" may depend upon a continued relationship with a therapist to prevent either a relapse or the appearance of a different hysterical symptom. To resolve the tendency to acquire new symptoms may require intensive psychoanalytic treatment.

Psychotic Dysfunctions of Childhood

It is always much more difficult to talk about the psychotic dysfunctions of childhood because of the constant controversy over etiology, treatment, diagnosis, and nomenclature that rages in professional circles. While some of the emotional disturbances discussed in this section may be considered more severe than neurosis in both quality and quantity, others may not be considered along the same continuum and may be viewed as entirely separate.

Despite the fact that psychosis is relatively rare in childhood, approximately 2000 volumes concerning these severe disturbances have been written within the past 30 years while, in comparison, the literature is relatively scant regarding the less severe and more frequent maladaptations discussed earlier. Perhaps the reason may be found in the fascination which childhood psychoses hold for the researcher, the clinician, and the theoretician, and the startling uniqueness often presented in the case studies of such children and their families.

Psychotic dysfunctions in childhood differ significantly from those which make their appearance later in life. In adulthood, the most common form of psychosis is schizophrenia, followed in frequency by the affective psychoses and organic psychoses. Although classical schizophrenia may appear during adolescence, the childhood psychoses discussed here are those with onsets by the time the child is five years old. Symptoms often begin to be observable within the first year of life when the child responds to and communicates with others in a strange and often bizarre way. The signs which Kessler has identified in behavioral terms are the following:

... the most important single sign is a severely disturbed relationship with people. This may take the form of a lack of interest in, or awareness of people (i.e., autism) or it may take the form of an inability to separate from another person (i.e., symbiosis). From this distorted relationship with people arise difficulties in communication . . . inability to imitate or to engage in normal play, extraordinary preoccupations with inanimate objects, and clinging to a mechanical, routinized, compulsively repetitious mode of living. Neurotic children, of course, also have disturbed relationships with people, but not to the same extent and without side-effects which encroach upon every aspect of their functioning (Kessler, 1966, pp. 263–264).

Children who fit these categories will be considered in the sections dealing with hospitalism and anaclitic depression, autism, childhood schizophrenia, and symbiosis. A separate section on behavior disorders and delinquent behavior follows. The author wishes to avoid a long discussion of nomenclature and semantics which she believes serves only to cloud the issue rather than to illuminate the student's understanding of the severe and psychotic dysfunctions of childhood.

HOSPITALISM AND ANACLITIC DEPRESSION

Effects of emotional and social deprivation have historically aroused the curiosity of others. The literature and nonfiction of old include tales of the study of children found roaming the countryside or living in forests supposedly being reared by wild animals. In colonial America and in Victorian times, children who were reared in attics, closets, or secluded rooms because they were "possessed," retarded, or illegitimate have also been studied. The interest in the study of such deprived children continues today since a reawakening of interest in the 1940s when a number of child psychiatric workers began studying the effects of maternal separation on children being raised in institutions such as hospitals and particularly orphanages. In 1940, L. G. Lowrey, an American psychiatrist, reported upon his observations of children who had spent the first three years of their lives in orphanages (Lowrey, 1940). He described a clinical syndrome consisting of self-centeredness and an inability to give and receive affection coupled with aggressive behavior and speech impairments. Interestingly, he did not find this behavior pattern occurring in children who entered the orphanage after the age of two or three. His observations were supported by Margaret Ribble (1941), who emphasized the personality disorganization and its relative irreversability which occurred through deficient mothering, and by W. Goldfarb (1946), whose study of children reared in an orphanage indicated that those deprived of family life in early childhood were less intelligent, had poorer memories, and showed marked impairment in language development and school adjustment when compared with children who had been fostered out as soon as they arrived at the orphanage. Another early investigator who reported the results of his studies of emotionally deprived children was René Spitz. The results of his studies were the identification of two clinical syndromes in infancy which he called hospitalism and anaclitic depression.

He described hospitalism as a condition in which the infant is physiologically and socially deteriorated as the result of long confinement in an institution. In his first and now classic study, Spitz studied 164 children in two institutions—a foundling home where infants were cared for by staff members and a nursery in a penal institution where infants were cared for by their mothers, who were incarcerated there (Spitz, 1945). Spitz demonstrated that infants cared for during their first year of life by the mother, even in such an unfavorable setting, surpassed the infants cared for in the foundling home in a number of ways. For example, they were more agile, active, vocal, and physically healthier, while the infants in the foundling home were more prone to illness, sustained a great mortality rate and lagged behind developmentally in a number of ways. It should be noted that in the foundling home, for "ease of care," the children were isolated from one another and adults by covered crib sides and received almost no stimulation except at feeding time. Since they received food, medical care, and housing to the same extent as did the children in the penal institution nursery, Spitz concluded that their developmental lag and general deterioration was the result of a lack of mothering. His follow-up study two years later supported his original conclusions (Spitz, 1946). He found that the children in the foundling home continued to deteriorate in a number of ways. Not only was the earlier deterioration present but they also failed to adapt to toilet-training, were underweight and undersized.

Anaclitic depression, on the other hand, is a specific reaction of the infant to separation from the mother occurring once an established interpersonal relationship, particularly a good one, between mother and infant is disrupted or discontinued. Such infants develop a severe mourning response to the loss of the mother which progresses to depression, withdrawal, physical debilitation and severe disturbance in relationships with others. Spitz described this syndrome in 1946 when he found 19 severe and 26 mild cases of anaclitic depression among 123 infants in an institution (Spitz, 1946a). He also found that the syndrome developed only in infants whose mothers assumed the full care for them until between six and eight months of age when they were removed from the child for a period of at least two to three months. These infants wear a constant sad expression on their faces, become rigid, insomniac, withdrawn, apathetic and eventually apprehensive and fearful of human contact to the point at which the infant screams at the approach of another human being. When the mothers are restored the infants seem to recover and become happy again. When the mothers are not restored the deterioration and depression continues through apathy, to a catatoniclike state, and often to death within the year. Research still is incomplete, however, for not all infants deprived of mothering develop anaclitic depression. In addition, separation from the mother before the age of six months does not result in this syndrome. This seems to indicate measures which might be taken to prevent and reduce cases of hospitalism and anaclitic depression among infants. For example, other studies have indicated that the critical period seems to be between six and eighteen months of age and that therefore, it is possible for institutional staffs geared to the recognition of the emotional needs of children to provide adequate substitute mothering and intellectual stimulation at this particularly critical time (Rheingold, 1956; Rheingold and Bayley, 1959; David and Appell, 1961).

Another researcher whose work substantiates the detrimental effects of maternal deprivation is John Bowlby. An early study of Bowlby in 1946, which concerned itself with juvenile thieves, demonstrated that out of the total 44 youngsters studied, 17 had undergone early or prolonged separation from the mother or mother figure during the first five years of their lives; this was a much higher percentage than that of a control group of children being treated at the same clinic (Bowlby, 1946). In addition, these children had been described with many of the same adjectives used in the description of children with behavior problems, delinquent behavior, or sociopathic and antisocial tendencies. Bowlby spurred further interest in research in maternal and emotional deprivation as the result of his monograph published in 1951 and his more current work dealing with the infant's dependence on its mother (Bowlby, 1957, 1969). Since Bowlby's early work, large numbers of researchers, theoreticians, and clinicians have been interested in the effects of separation as a basis for child-rearing and social welfare practices. The result has been that until recently, the opinion has been that any mother is better than no mother at all with a resulting tendency away from group care of children. More recent work in the Israeli kibbutzim and in group care homes in other countries may be indicating that the advantages of group care when mothering is absent, negligible, or hostile have been unfortunately discounted in the past (Wolins, 1969; Bettelheim, 1969). Other eminent authorities have begun to sternly criticize the group care offered in settings such as kibbutzim, which they believe hamper the initiative and creativity essential for future leaders.

Although the unfortunate results of hospitalism and anaclitic depression are generally understood to be the result of emotional and maternal deprivation, the questions which remain to be answered revolve around the best means to prevention and effective treatment modalities. At this time, the pro's and con's remain unresolved.

AUTISM AND CHILDHOOD SCHIZOPHRENIA

The clinical entity of autism was first described in 1943 by Leo Kanner, who used the term early infantile autism to describe children whose behaviors seemed to constitute a unique syndrome which he believed to be a form of childhood psychosis (Kanner, 1943). Prior to Kanner's definition and indentification of the syndrome of autism (from the Greek word for self) most doctors believed that these children were mentally retarded and most often recommended that they be placed in an institution for the mentally retarded to receive the custodial care given at that time. Kanner believed that the condition was innate and probably incurable, while noting that parents of autistic children were highly intellectual but tended to be emotionally cold. In fact, Kanner labeled them "refrigerator parents." This belief and similar beliefs are held by most experts in child psychiatry regardless of their theoretical orientation or their ideas regarding treatment. Other believe that such attitudes have only served to saddle parents of autistic children with useless and harmful guilt; these workers note that some of the symptoms of autism or differentness become noticeable in infancy even before strong parental influence upon the child's behavior is regarded as likely. Indeed, approximately five years ago an organization called the National Society for Autistic Children was founded by a group of parents of autistic children in order to give one another moral support, to educate themselves and the public at large, and to stimulate research to arrive at causes of autism—particularly biological ones. Many hope that autism will turn out to be similar to cretinism and PKU (phenylketonuria). The belief in Great Britain is that some heretofore undiscovered biochemical abnormality of the brain based upon hereditary factors lies at the root of autism (Wolff, 1969). Increasing numbers of child care experts seem willing and eager to avoid the blame label and the etiological roots of autism in an attempt to concentrate on helping the autistic child and his family.

Many autistic children are not identified or receive treatment before the age of two, and usually three or four, when the signs of autism are readily recognizable even to the casual observer. Some advice given to family doctors on recognizing the autistic child is helpful and merits repetition here.

How to Spot the Autistic Child

* The child does not speak properly for his age, or at all.
* He has no awareness of his identity.
* He is pathologically preoccupied with a particular object.
* He resists change around him, struggling to maintain or restore the familiar.
* He is excessively anxious without any apparent reason.
* His emotional relationships are grossly impaired.
* He may twirl, rock, walk on tiptoe, or remain rigid for sustained periods.
* He appears to be seriously retarded but has flashes of normal or exceptional intellectual function.[1]

[1] From "Breaking Through to the Autistic Child," *Medical World News,* October 28, 1966, p. 92.

However, parents quite often report instances of strange and bizarre behavior in their children before they reach this stage and while they are babies in cribs. As infants they may be described as never cuddly or smiling, seemingly uncaring about whether mother or father is in the room, never physically reaching out to be lifted, hugged, or touched, being contented in being left alone without apparent distress over separation, and failing to imitate gestures such as waving bye-bye, or participating in early games such as peek-a-boo and pattycake.

In addition it seems evident that autistic children are much more object-oriented than they are people oriented. For example, they may be fascinated for months on end, to the exclusion of all else, with toys or objects which spin, reflect light, or can be rolled, manipulated or twirled in some way. However, they seldom relate to gestures or verbal cues from persons to the extent that many are suspected of being deaf and are often known to hearing and speech clinics. When thwarted in their desires, autistic children may resort to primitive atavistic behavior such as screaming and tantrums which, with their frightening consequences of hurting the self or others, may result in parental responses that have as their goal ending or supressing the primitive behavior. Some parents have reported being autocratically controlled by their autistic child to the point at which they might have to stand guard over the child or his environment in order to protect him. In this way, many autistic children are despots in their demands, and essentially have unyielding control over the lives of others in their environment.

It is not unusual to hear experts say that autism is a rare illness. In fact, such a statement may be found in almost any textbook concerned with child psychiatry. Such statements seem inconsistent with the findings of a recent survey which indicate that between four and five out of every 10,000 children is autistic (Lotter, 1966). It is alarming to note that the frequency of autism is greater than that of blindness and almost as great as that for deafness in children (Lotter, 1965). Labeling autism as rare seems to minimize its seriousness and frequency. No one yet seems to be able to explain the additional fact that four out of five autistic children are boys.

Whether such a condition as childhood schizophrenia exists or not is a moot question. While some authorities classify autism and symbiosis as varying forms of the overall rubric of childhood psychosis, others consider childhood schizophrenia as a separate category and often reserve it for children who seem to develop symptoms after the age of five years or in children whose disordered behavior appears after an initial period of normal development. Many liken the illness to a juvenile form of adult schizophrenia. In speaking of childhood schizophrenia most authors quote Lauretta Bender who classified numerous organic as well as emotional disorders under this general heading. Her methods of diagnosis and statements of observed signs are couched in physiological terms in accordance with her belief as to cause (Bender, 1947). She includes withdrawn and autistic behavior as only one of many signs of childhood schizophrenia. Others, such as Mahler et al. (1959) do not acknowledge childhood schizophrenia as a separate category. Although they include both autism and symbiosis, their third category of more benign childhood psychoses is composed of a syndrome in which children may alternate between autism, symbiosis, and the neurotic states discussed earlier.

SYMBIOSIS

Another subcategory of the overall rubric of childhood psychosis is symbiosis, which was not so defined until Margaret Mahler's now classic publication of 1952. The symbiotic child, rather than being content to be alone and in fact desiring a paucity of interpersonal relationships as does the autistic child, experiences extreme difficulty in separation from his relationship with the mother. The closeness of his association with his mother and the extent of the dependency is demonstrated by the fact that even brief and temporary separations such as mother's walking into another room may produce panic.

Symbiotic children are seldom conspicuously disturbed as infants. Symptoms manifest themselves between the ages of two and five with a peak at four years of age. The behavior of the child appears to be an attempt to reestablish the mother-infant-as-one phase before the developing ego assists the child in separating himself from others and coming to understand the "me." In the course of normal development infants naturally undergo a state of symbiosis. In fact, the unprotected infant must indeed rely upon his parents for his life. When he becomes a toddler at about 12 to 15 months of age, his growing sense of ego identity assists him in his gradual separation from mother as he begins to gain some independence. He can tolerate going away from mother because he knows she will come back. This has been termed the beginning of the separation-individuation phase of personality development which has been described as a kind of second birth (Mahler and Gosliner, 1955).

It can be noted that the environment of the symbiotic child cannot generally be said to encourage gradual separation from the mother, emergence of the ego, and establishment of interpersonal relationships with others. Although the possibility exists that constitutional predisposition may be a factor in determining symbiosis, there is little evidence at this time which would support such a belief. Mothers of symbiotic children have often been identified as overprotective, however. It remains to be determined whether the mother is simply rsponding to the needs of a dependent symbiotic child, or if the response of the mother encouraged symbiosis. Overprotection includes excessive contact between parent and child, prolongation of the stage of infancy, and the prevention or suppression of independent or autonomous behaivor. Dynamically, maternal overprotection is closely related to maternal rejection. A number of researchers have found that mothers who were rejecting before the birth of the baby underwent a reaction-formation against their unconscious hostility and responded by being oversolicitous, compulsive, and smothering in the care of their infants. In fact, such maternal overprotection has also been linked to pervasive learning disorders in children (Buxbaum, 1964).

Symbiotic children have often been described by their mothers as extremely sensitive infants who were frequent criers. The symptoms of psychosis become more readily identifiable as critical developmental periods which have to do with increasing independency. To the symbiotic child, these periods are not viewed as milestones to be surpassed with delight, but rather are viewed as cruel and unwanted crises. Bergman and Escalona (1949) have described an unevenness of growth and extreme vulnerability to frustration as some of the unusual sensitivities demonstrated by the symbiotic child. For example, parents often report unusual reactions to small failures to the point that a symbiotic child may give up locomotion and all attempts at locomotion for months because of a fall or bump in the learning process. Perhaps part of this response may be explained by the fact that locomotion might serve to take the child away from mother as well as to her.

Some authorities now believe that the symbiotic child who finds his state of continual panic at the thought of separation unbearable regresses to the use of autistic behavior in an attempt to arrive at a solution through a form of secondary retreat (Mahler et al., 1959).

Asocial, Antisocial, and Delinquent Behavior

The term juvenile delinquency is generally not applied to children below the age of adolescence. While younger children are often labeled as asocial, antisocial, or having behavior problems or conduct disturbances, similar dynamics are in operation as in the older child or adolescent.

Delinquent behavior has been a social problem throughout recorded history. Writings on papyrus and cave walls tell of community and individual concern with the problem behavior of youth. It was not until the eighteenth century, however, that children were treated differently than were criminal adults. At the present time, most persons view asocial, antisocial, and delinquent behavior as that opposed to or detrimental to the beliefs, attitudes, and laws held by society at large and our culture in particular.

This section will consider the individual delinquent—the youth whose behavior is intrapsychically or interpersonally determined—and the gang delinquent, the youth whose behavior is sociologically or culturally determined. Kessler's classification referred to the cause of juvenile delinquency as disorder in the superego regarding the following:

1. The absence of a superego because of early neglect, deprivation and failure to establish meaningful relationships at the earliest level (also called the "psychopath" and the "unsocialized aggressive").
2. Identification with socially inadequate models, incorporation of antisocial values, inability to achieve satisfaction in socially acceptable ways because of either deficiencies in ego functions or lack of opportunity, or both (the "normal delinquent"; the "socially delinquent").
3. Lacunae in superego resulting from the conscious sanctioning by the parents of behavior which they pronounce to be wrong.
4. Weakness of the superego in coping with instinctual desires (e.g., as in the narcissistic, hysterical person who "does it now, regrets it later").
5. Abeyance of the superego because the delinquent behavior is an unconscious means of expressing aggression toward the parents or of acting out a special unconscious fantasy, or is a way of obtaining punishment for an unconscious sense of guilt ("neurotic delinquency") (Kessler, 1966, p. 303).

Attempts have frequently been made to align delinquency with any one of various causes, predispositions, or tendencies. For example, in the early part of the twentieth century much attention was paid to the morphological and anatomical differences which were thought to characterize persons with various mental disorders and delinquency as well. It was thought that the cranial structure of the criminal might be different as well as the general musculature, which was termed mesomorphic. Age and onset of puberty have been linked with criminal and antisocial behavior, the belief being that decreasing age of puberty may be a factor contributing indirectly to the increase in juvenile delinquency, particularly among girls. Recently, the idea that a person's genetic make-up may be responsible for his committing acts of violence has found favor with the identification of the XYY chromosomal constitution. Rather than the usual XY chromosome composition in the reproductive cells, this person has an extra Y chromosome which is thought to elevate aggressiveness potential. Since 1965, studies of men in penal institutions have tended to support this belief. Within the past few months, researchers have begun to criticize the validity of some of these studies and propose that chromosomal differentness as a solitary factor is insufficient grounds for the suspicion of violent or aggressive behavior. It is difficult to think about problems of research methodology when examination of persons who have committed violent acts indicates the presence of the XYY chromosome as in the case of Richard Speck, the convicted murderer of eight nurses in Chicago in 1966.

THE GANG DELINQUENT

Sociologists and cultural anthropologists are highly concerned with gang delinquency which, although viewed as deviant behavior, may only be an expression of the accepted pattern of behavior of a subcultural group. In such a circumstance, while the child is considered delinquent by the larger society, he is considered "normal" by the smaller society which comprises the environment in which he exists (Miller, 1958).

Since gang delinquency is primarily a working-class phenomenon, it has been connected with lower socioeconomic class neighborhoods, which are more prone to a lack of social unity and organization (Cohen, 1955). In addition, some believe it to be a reaction-formation regarding the unattainable middle-class standard (Cloward and Ohlin, 1960). It is a way for the gang to outwardly turn against those values and standards which it covets. This suggests that the discrepancy between what lower-class youths want and what is available to them accounts for difficulty in societal adjustment.

In terms of treatment, it is important to determine whether a child's delinquent or antisocial behavior fits within this category since the treatment approach varies from that of the individual delinquent and his parents. Problems of gang delinquency are problems for the community at large and all of the resources of that community must be mobilized for a broad-base community attack if it is to be effective.

THE INDIVIDUAL DELINQUENT

The individual delinquent who fits into Kessler's first, third, fourth, and fifth categories is one whose intrapsychic conflicts, whether they be neurotic or psychotic, or whose interpersonal conflicts regarding significant persons indicate a psychopathological or emotionally disturbed bent either within the child himself or within the framework of his family. A review of these categories indicates the involvement apparent in the parent-child interaction.

Individual delinquency has often been ascribed to maternal deprivation and rejection in the early years, as well as paternal rejection in the later years. Many now believe that, after dozens of years of emphasis on the importance of the mother in the development of the child, the pendulum is finally beginning to swing where it belongs—with a focus on *both* parents.

Treatment of the individual delinquent has a greater focus upon psychotherapy in attempts to resolve the conflicts present in both the child and other family members. Approaches range from family therapy to group therapy to individual therapy either on an outpatient basis in a child guidance or family therapy setting to residential treatment in facilities where staff can work toward reeducation efforts with the youngster.

Whichever the method of approach for either of these two types, most experts today agree that incarceration within penal institutions comprises punishment and not treatment or rehabilitation and that in the very institutions ostensibly designed to protect society and the child, the child learns to improve his criminal "skills" and emerges a hardened and wiser criminal and societal problem.

Treatment Approaches

A wide variety of disciplines is engaged in work with emotionally disturbed children and youth in multiple settings. In many areas of the country the traditional child mental health workers are considered to be psychiatrists, psychologists, and social workers. Child psychiatric nursing as a specialty is a relative newcomer to the field, particularly since the care of emotionally disturbed youngsters is moving out of the psychiatric hospital setting. There may be reluctance at times to utilize child psychiatric nurses in facilities other than in-patient services. Some of the reluctance may be attributed to professional jealousy and insecurity among mental health workers. Most of the reluctance, however, can be attributed to two factors—the lack of child psychiatric nurses prepared at comparable educational levels (master's and doctoral degree holders) who can communicate with other professionals by sharing the same universe of discourse as well as willingness on the part of nurses to retain the comfortableness of the safe hospital setting in the assumption of managerial rather than clinical skills. The role of the child psychiatric nurse clinician will be discussed in a section following this one.

Having read the earlier data in this chapter, the student should be well aware that psychiatric treatment, if it is to be effective, cannot always focus only on the individual identified as the patient. Indeed, treatment of whole communities for their social ills may be necessary. Programs of treatment and education are particularly important for the parents and siblings of the emotionally disturbed child. The need for a focus on parents in terms of the parent-child interactions previously described should be particularly apparent. Knowledge of growth and development makes apparent the needs of the siblings of the emotionally disturbed child. Better still, one hopes for a future in which preventive psychiatry will reduce the incidence, duration, and prevalence of mental disorder as well as the resulting impairment.

THE PSYCHOTHERAPIES

Psychotherapeutic treatment may take place in a variety of ways in a variety of settings. Treatment of the child may be dependent on an individual relationship with a therapist or a relationship with a therapist and a group of other children.

Child analysis or psychoanalytically oriented psychotherapy is based upon the achievement of insight for the child as well as change in the life-style and psychic structure of the child (Anna Freud, 1946). Although psychoanalytic techniques vary with the age and abilities of the individual child they are geared toward an intensive relationship requiring sessions with the child analyst as much as five times weekly. Child analysis is predicated on the ability of the child to relate verbally with the analyst. Although the medium of play may be introduced within the psychoanalytic relationship, its use and effectiveness in analysis is determined by verbal consideration of the conflicts expressed by the child (Klein, 1955). These points indicate that psychoanalysis is certainly not the treatment of choice for children when certain pragmatic considerations are taken into account. For example, the autistic child who does not relate at the required verbal level would not be an appropriate candidate, nor is the prohibitive cost of three to five weekly sessions with an analyst within the financial means of the great majority of parents.

Group psychotherapy with children offers multiple stimuli. Rather than an intensive relationship with one therapist it offers a variety of relationships with others. In a group, children learn from one another; therefore, a mix between children who are aggressive with those who are passive and/or withdrawn offers opportunities to all to incorporate the positive aspects of the other and to receive pressure to change regarding their own negative behaviors (Slavson, 1952).

Family therapy is group psychotherapy with the members of the family, based upon the belief that the origins and stimuli toward emotional disturbance may lie within the family group. Whether this is determined to be so or not, there is no doubt that emotional illness in one member of the family affects the others and, in Ackerman's (1958) view, is an expression of family pathology. In many situations, a combination of techniques may be used. A number of workers may engage themselves therapeutically with various members of the family in an individual relationship which is enhanced through the use of family therapy as an additional treatment tool.

Another approach utilizes the learning principles originally identified by experimental psychologists and based upon the premise that neurotic and even psychotic behavior is learned and therefore can be unlearned (Eysenck, 1960; Ferster, 1961). Psychotherapy in this way emphasizes societal norms or behaviors which are considered socially acceptable. Generally it requires a consistent environment in which all staff carry out measures designed to extinguish unwanted behavior. For this reason, behavioral techniques are usually employed in residential treatment centers.

Play therapy may also be used as a treatment technique employed by itself or in combination with other forms of treatment. The particular theoretical approach of the therapist will determine the manner in which play therapy is instituted and utilized, and will vary according to the situation. Play as a nondirective therapeutic means which focuses on the relationship between child and therapist as the crucial factor in the outcome of the therapy is discussed by Virginia Axline (1969), who emphasizes the naturalness and spontaneity of the technique, whereas Kleinian analysts may use it for symbolic interpretation of unconscious conflicts (Klein, 1932).

THE SOMATOTHERAPIES

The somatotherapies or physical treatments for mental illness are all but discontinued in the treatment of emotionally disordered children except for the occasional use of medication which may be helpful in some cases to a lesser extent than in the adult. One strange paradox of drug treatment for children involves the child whose hyperactivity poses a learning problem for him in school. Such children have their hyperactivity diminished through treatment with a central nervous system stimulant which has entirely the opposite effect in adults.

In the late 1940s and the early 1950s electroshock therapy was employed in the treatment of emotionally disturbed children, as was psychosurgery such as lobotomy. Fortunately, these methods employed in the treatment of disturbed children in the psychiatric hospitals of the time have been discontinued.

THE SOCIOTHERAPIES

Sociotherapeutic or milieu therapy approaches may be employed in residential treatment facilities when it seems wisest to treat the child away from the home setting. The trend seems to be toward a greater application of therapeutic environment in the treatment of the child although there still are in existence a number of facilities which serve simply as places to live rather than as treatment facilities.

This form of treatment requires that everyone in the milieu contributes to the therapeutic effort so that in an institutional or residential setting efforts must be made to help maids, janitors, cottage parents, and secretaries become, if not milieu therapists, then at least therapeutic manipulators of the milieu. Kessler's excellent chapter "Treatment Away from Home" is a recommended reading for those interested in the influence of milieu (Kessler, 1966).

The Child Psychiatric Nurse Clinician

The pattern of specialization in clinical nursing is one of the most important and salient trends in professional nursing today. Although the term specialization was used as early as the mid-1930s, it signified the nurse who provided the bedside or administrative and management care for patients whose illnesses fell within the classification accorded certain diseases, conditions or ages. More often than not, a nurse was considered to be a "specialist" in an area of patient care by simple virtue of the fact that the agency or institution which employed her was restricted to the care of tubercular, psychiatric, obstetric, medical, or pediatric patients. The longer the nurse cared solely for the tubercular patient, for example, the more of a "specialist" she became as experience became equated with specialization.

Today, the pattern is changing. The committed professional nurse who is a master practitioner actively engaged in the provision of excellence in patient care has been dubbed the "nurse clinician" by Frances Reiter (1966). It is Miss Reiter's definition which is referred to here to avoid confusion with other terms which may be favored by others.

Clinical expertise in psychiatric nursing focuses upon the subrole of counselor or psychotherapist. The nursing subroles of mother-surrogate, technician, manager, socializing agent, health teacher, and counselor or psychotherapist were identified by Hildegard Peplau, one of the foremost psychiatric nurses in the United States. She identified the counselor-psychotherapist subrole as the emphasized one for the psychiatric nurse clinician. The remaining traditional subroles assume lesser importance for the nurse clinician and remain chiefly within the province of other nurses who assume management and administrative duties or perform patient care under the guidance and supervision of the clinical expert.

In order to effectively carry out the expected functions inherent in rendering expert clinical patient care in the psychotherapeutic role, the nurse clinician must have depth in theoretical knowledge and the skills of psychotherapeutic nursing. She must be able to observe, assess, interpret, intervene, and evaluate in order to render expert direct and indirect psychiatric nursing care and to function as a change agent. The functions have been specifically noted and defined for child psychiatric nurses by Agnes B. Middleton:

> Child psychiatric nursing may be defined as direct care to the emotionally disturbed child, usually within the matrix of his primary group—the family. The child psychiatric nurse is therapeutically involved in the exploration and resolution of the crises of childhood. The nurse directs her therapeutic influence on children, their families, and the settings within which interactions take place. She becomes involved with children who may have a variety of labels—"emotionally disturbed," "mentally ill," "behavior problem," "delinquent," "learning problem," or even "mentally retarded." Another way of describing child psychiatric nursing is that the nurse becomes involved with children who themselves may feel distressed or unhappy or who by their behavior cause distress to others. The involvement may occur in a variety of settings—the home, school, outpatient clinic, the pediatric ward of a hospital, or a residential unit in

a treatment center or hospital for emotionally disturbed or mentally retarded children (Middleton, 1967).

The child psychiatric nurse clinician accomplishes these goals through using a variety of methods which have as their core the nurse-child relationship. She may utilize the one-to-one relationship, play therapy, sociotherapy or manipulation of the milieu, behavior shaping based upon learning theory, and group therapeutic skills, among others. Of additional importance is the necessity to collaborate with other disciplines who also contribute their skills as members of therapeutic teams.

As such requirements and techniques are spelled out, it becomes evident that experience no longer qualifies the nurse as a clinical expert in the area of child psychiatry. One is not fated to assume such a role from birth, although some individuals by virtue of their experiences in living assume the role with greater ease than do others with like academic and professional experiences. Some of the experiences in living which are especially significant for the child psychiatric nurse are those concerning punishment, limit-setting, authority, sex, and competiveness. Therefore, in addition to depth in theoretical knowledge and the skills of psychotherapeutic nursing she must engage in preceptory or clinical supervisory relationships with a more experienced and knowledgeable nurse clinician, to assist in the identification of conflicts and the resolution of anxiety.

The combination of these three essentials can be found in graduate programs in psychiatric nursing which lead to a master's degree. Table 1 lists Master's programs accredited by the National League for

TABLE 1

NLN ACCREDITED MASTER'S PROGRAMS IN CHILD PSYCHIATRIC NURSING

NAME AND ADDRESS OF UNIVERSITY	CURRICULUM OFFERINGS	APPROXIMATE LENGTH
Boston University	Juvenile Delinquency	2 semesters
635 Commonwealth Avenue	Child Psychiatry	4 semesters
Boston, Massachusetts 02215		
New York University	Child Psychiatry	4 semesters
Washington Square	Parent-Child	3-4 semesters
New York, New York 10003		
University of California	Post-Master's in	
San Francisco Medical Center	Child Psychiatry*	6 quarters
San Francisco, California 94122		
University of Cincinnati	Child Psychiatry	6 quarters
Cincinnati, Ohio 45221		
University of Maryland	Child Psychiatry	4 semesters
624 W. Lombard Street		
Baltimore, Maryland 21201		
Wayne State University	Child Psychiatry	6 quarters
Detroit, Michigan 48202		

* Upon completion of 3 quarters master's program in adult psychiatric nursing.

Nursing. The student interested in such a program should remember that programs may change, and new programs may be added. Specific information regarding the academic programs should be sought from individual colleges or universities. Programs which have as their major emphasis the preparation of teachers or administrators, rather than child psychiatric nurse clinicians, have not been included in this listing.

References

Ackerman, N. W. The Psychodynamics of Family Life. New York, Basic Books, 1958.

Aichhorn, A. Wayward Youth. New York, Viking Press, 1935.

Axline, V. Play Therapy, rev. ed. New York, Ballantine Books, 1969.

Beller, E. K. The Clinical Process. New York, Free Press of Glencoe, 1962.

Bender, L. Childhood schizophrenia. Amer. J. Orthopsychiat., 17:40, 1947.

Bergman, P., and Escalona, S. Unusual sensitivities in very young children. In Psychoanalytic Study of the Child. New York, International Universities Press, Vol. 314, 1949.

Bettelheim, B. The Children of the Dream. New York, Macmillan, 1969.

Bloodstein, O. A Handbook on Stuttering for Professional Workers. Chicago, National Society for Crippled Children and Adults, 1959.

Bowly, J. Maternal Care and Mental Health, 2nd ed. Geneva, World Health Organization, 1951.

Bowlby, J. Attachment (Volume I of Attachment and Loss). New York, Basic Books, 1969.

Bowlby, J. Forty-four Juvenile Thieves: Their Characters and Home Life. London, Bailliere, Tindall & Co., 1946.

Breaking through to the autistic child. Med. World News, October 28, 1966, p. 86.

Breuer, J., and Freud, S. Studies in Hysteria. New York, Nervous and Mental Disease Pub. Co., 1936.

Bruner, J. Processes of Growth in Infancy. Clark University Press, Barre Publishers, 1968.

Burlingham, D. T. Precursors of some psychoanalytic ideas about children in the sixteenth and seventeenth centuries. In The Psychoanalytic Study of the Child. New York, International Universities Press, 1951, Vol. 6.

Buxbaum, E. The parents' role in the etiology of learning disabilities. In Psychoanalytic Study of the Child. New York, International Universities Press, Vol. 19, 1964.

Caplan, G. Prevention of Mental Disorders in Children. New York, Basic Books, 1961.

Caplan, G. Emotional Problems of Early Childhood.

Cloward, R., and Ohlin, L. E. Delinquency and Opportunity: A Theory of Delinquent Gangs. New York, Free Press of Glencoe, 1960.

Cohen, A. K. Delinquent Boys: The Culture of the Gang. New York, Free Press of Glencoe, 1955.

Cooper, M. Pica. Springfield, Ill. Thomas, 1957.

Cramer, J. B. Common neuroses of childhood. In Arieti, S., ed. American Handbook of Psychiatry. New York, Basic Books, 1959, Vol. 1, pp. 797–815.

David, M., and Appell, G. A study of nursing care and nurse-infant interaction. In Foss, B. M. Determinants of Human Behavior. London, Methuen & Co., Ltd., 1961.

Despert, L. Differential diagnosis between obsessive compulsive neuresis and schizophrenia in children. In Hoch and Zubin, eds. Psychopathology of Childhood. New York, Grune & Stratton, 1955.

Eisenberg, L. School phobia: a study of communication of anxiety. Amer. J. Psychiat., 114:712, 1958.

Eysenck, H. J. Behavior Therapy and the Neuroses. London, Pergamon Press, 1960.

Fenichel, O. The Psychoanalytic Theory of Neurosis. New York, W. W. Norton, 1945.

Ferster, C. B. Positive reinforcement and behavioral deficits of autistic children. Child Devel., 32:437, 1961.

Freud, A. The Psychoanalytical Treatment of Children. London, Imago Publishing Co., 1946.

Freud, S. Analysis of phobia in a five-year-old boy. In Collected Papers. New York, Nervous and Mental Disease Pub. Co., 1936.

Goldfarb, W. Effects of psychological deprivation in infancy and subsequent stimulation. Amer. J. Psychiat., 102:18, 1946.

Gutelius, M., et al. Nutritional studies of children with pica: Part I, Controlled study evaluating nutritional status: Part II, Treatment of pica with iron given intramuscularly, 1018; Pediat., 29:1012, 1962.

Johnson, W. Stuttering in Children and Adults. Minneapolis, University of Minnesota Press, 1955.

Joint Commission on Mental Illness and Health. Action for Mental Health. New York, Basic Books, 1961.

Joint Commission of Mental Health of Children. Crisis in Child Mental Health: Challenge for the 1970's. New York, Harper and Row, 1969.

Kanner, L. Autistic disturbance in affective contact. Nerv. Child, 2:217, 1942–1943.

Kanner, L. Child Psychiatry, 3rd ed. Springfield, Ill., Thomas, 1957.

Klein, M. The psychoanalytic play technique. Amer. J. Orthopsychiat., 25:223, 1955.

————The Psycho-Analysis of Children. London, Hogarth Press, 1932.

Lapouse, R. Who is sick? Amer. J. Orthopsychiat., 35:138, 1965.

Lotter, V. Epidemiology of autistic conditions in young children: I: prevalence. Soc. Psychiat., 1:124, 1966.

Lowrey, L. G. Personality disorganization and early institutional care. Amer. J. Orthopsychiat., 10:576, 1940.

Mahler, M. S. On child psychosis and schizophrenia: autistic and symbiotic infantile psychosis. In Psychoanalytic Study of the Child. New York, International Universities Press, Vol. 7, 1952.

Mahler, M. S., and Gosliner, J. B. On symbiotic child psychosis. In Psychoanalytic Study of the Child. New York, International Universities Press, Vol. 10, 1955.

Mahler, M. S., Furer, M., and Settlage, C. F. Severe emotional disturbances in childhood: psychosis. In Arieti, S., ed. American Handbook of Psychiatry, New York, Basic Books, Vol. 1, 1959.

Meyer, A. The Common Sense Psychiatry of Dr. Adolph Meyer, Lief, A., Trans. New York, McGraw-Hill, 1948.

Middleton, A. B. Introduction to child psychiatric nursing: the role of the clinical specialist. In Kalkman, M. E., ed. Psychiatric Nursing, 3rd ed. New York, McGraw-Hill, 1967.

Miller, W. B. Lower-class culture as a generating milieu of gang delinquency. J. Soc. Issues, 14:5, 1958.

Morris, D. The Naked Ape, Dell, 1969.

Proctor, J. T. Hysteria in Childhood. Am. J. Orthopsychiat., 28: 394, 1958.

Reiter, F. The nurse-clinician. Amer. J. Nurs., 66:274, 1966.

Rheingold, H. L. The modification of social responsiveness in institutional babies. Mono. Soc. Res. Child. Devel., 21:1956.

———— and Bayley, N. The later effects of an experimental modification of mothering. Child. Devel., 30:363, 1959.

Ribble, M. Disorganizing factors in infant personality. Amer. J. Psychiat., 98:459, 1941.

Rutter, M. Classification and Categorization in child psychiatry. J. Child. Psychiat., 6:71, 1965.

Sheehan, J. G. Projective studies of stuttering. In Trapp, P., and Himelstein, P., eds. Readings on the Exceptional Child. New York, Appleton-Century-Crofts, 1962.

Slavson, S. R. Child Psychotherapy. New York, Columbia University Press, 1952.

Spitz, R. A. Hospitalization. In Psychoanalytic Study of the Child. New York, International Universities Press, 1945, Vol. 1.

———— Anaclitic depression. In The Psychoanalytic Study of the Child. New York, International Universities Press, 1946a, Vol. 2, 313.

———— Hospitalization: a follow-up report. In The Psychoanalytic Study of the Child, New York, International Universities Press, 1946b, Vol. 2, 255.

Spock, B. Baby and Child Care. New York, Pocket Books, Inc., 1963.

Sullivan, H. S. The Interpersonal Theory of Psychiatry. New York, W. W. Norton, 1943.

Travis, L. E. Speech Pathology. New York, D. Appleton and Company, 1931.

Trieschman, A. E. Temper, temper, temper, temper, temper. The New York Times Magazine, April 12, 1970, p. 99.

Wallder, R. Basic Theory of Psychoanalysis. New York, International Universities Press, 1960.

Wolff, S. Children Under Stress. London, Penguin Press, 1969.

Wolins, M. Group care: friend or foe? Social Work, 14:35, 1969.

Wyatt, G. L., and Herzan, H. M. Therapy with stuttering children and their mothers. Amer. J. Orthopsychiat., 32:645, 1962.

11 SHIRLEY STEELE

Nursing Care of the Child with Burns Requiring Long-Term Care

Burns are responsible for a significant number of deaths in children under five years of age. According to Donnellan (1969), in the United States alone, 2200 to 4000 children died each of the past 10 years from this painful injury. The toddler or preschooler, with his innate curiosity, explores everything. His curiosity can easily result in spilling hot liquids or igniting his clothing. It takes an especially conscientious mother to remember always to turn the handle of pots inward when cooking, or to keep chairs away from the stove, or to put hot liquids away from the edge of the table. Despite the most careful attention to these precautions, children can still manage to burn themselves. They move chairs near the stove and climb up to explore the pots or they pull the overhanging tablecloth and the hot liquid slips over the side of the table.

In addition, there are the inconsistencies in the environment which confuse children. If they are allowed to touch the burners of the stove when they are turned off, then they are likely to try the same thing when the burner is on. If they are allowed to lean against radiators or space heaters when they are off, they are likely to do the same when these devices are turned on. Teaching has to be consistent for the young child who does not yet know the concepts of hot and cold or off and on.

Another contributing factor to this high incidence of burns is the many and varied materials now used in producing clothing. Many of them are highly flammable and when they begin to burn they burn quickly; the child usually runs, which fans the fire. School-age children often burn themselves by playing with matches or fire.

The severity of the burn is usually determined by the duration of the exposure and the intensity of the heat. Other contributing factors are the way the heat was applied, the size of the child and the body surface involved, the age of the child and the protective aspects of his skin and vascular system, and the type of burn received.

Therefore, some of the initial questions that need to be asked when a child is admitted to the hospital include the following:

1. When did the burn occur?
2. What was the causative agent?
3. Approximately how long was the child exposed to the agent?
4. If the burn occurred in a closed area, were fumes and heat inhaled?
5. What was the child's last recorded weight?
6. Was the child in good physical health prior to the injury?

These questions will help to establish what the child's physical appearance and health status were prior to injury. This information is valuable in helping to establish the child's chances of recovery.

Other questions which need answering to permit adequate therapy are the following:

1. What first-aid treatment, if any, was given at the time of the injury?
2. Was any medication given (such as a tetanus shot or pain medication)?
3. Does the child have any allergies?
4. Has he had much pain from the burn?
5. Is he having pain now?
6. Does the child have any illness or medical condition (such as a cold or diabetes)?

This list of questions will help establish priorities for treatment. If the child has not had a tetanus injection, it will be included soon. If he has a concurrent illness, that will also be considered in the care plan.

Classification of Burns

Burns are commonly classified as *first, second,* or *third degree* according to the severity of the injury. *First degree* causes vasodilatation and damage to the epidermis and heals rapidly. *Second degree* burns, or partial-thickness burns, cause damage to the capillaries and involve the epidermis and upper portions of the dermis; there may be blebs containing fluid. *Third degree burns*, or full-thickness burns, destroy the epidermis and dermis layers, have thrombosed capillaries, and result in formation of eschar (dead tissue).

Calculating the extent of the burn can be a difficult process. It is possible to overestimate the severity of the burn and it is also possible to have second degree burns advance to third degree by bacterial infiltration.

The care during the acute stages demands very skilled personnel as the child's recovery depends on proper replacement of fluids and electrolytes, prevention of infection, prevention of further damage to the tissue, and early recognition and treatment of complications.

The long-term care of children with burns may be directly or indirectly related to things which happen to the child during the acute stage. Some of the long-term problems result because of omissions in care during the acute stages.

Implications of Diet

During the acute stages, the body is faced with meeting the changes produced by exchanges of electrolytes, hormonal changes, fluid changes, and destruction of tissue. During this period it is imperative to replace fluids and provide adequate nutritional requirements to cope with the insult. Initially the fluid and electrolyte replacements may be adequately handled by the intravenous route of administration. This leaves the child free of the responsibility of accepting the medical routine. As replacement is established and the child begins to respond, he is given the responsibility for accepting the diet and fluids to restore him to optimal health. The effects of hormonal changes, as well as that of destroyed tissue and pain, may make this request seem unreasonable to the child. In addition, he is faced with decreased activity due to bedrest, and frequently isolation. He is not hungry enough or interested enough to want the food that is offered. His anorexia becomes a real challenge to the nursing personnel. Their interest in getting the child well increases their persistence to get the child to eat. The condition created by lack of interest on the child's part in eating and increased interest on the nurses' part in getting the child to eat can be detrimental to the long-term care of the child. He begins to dislike the nurse that insists on his eating and to distrust the people giving him care. He misinterprets their interest as antagonistic to his well-being. Even after his appetite begins to return, he may dislike food as it evokes such unhappy remembrances for him.

The problems of providing adequate dietary intake may be lessened by including the parents' participation. The parent is able to provide helpful hints about the child's likes and dislikes in relation to food. They are also helpful in providing supplemental foods. The parents are frequently amenable to preparing foods at home and bringing them in to the hospital. While we do not want to impose unnecessarily on the parents, their contributions cannot be underestimated. They can also provide nutritional requirements during periods when the hospital dietary facilities may not be operating. The child does not understand that he is supposed to get hungry at only the times that meals are scheduled. He may wake up during the night and request a hamburger. By working with the parents and the dietary staff, this request need not be impossible to meet.

Another implication to long-term care is the type of diet offered during the acute stage. It is usually high in protein, carbohydrates, calories, and some vitamins. To provide these requirements, nurses frequently resort to milk shakes and other high caloric liquids. The child may learn to like this very rich diet, and as his convalescence continues he may become obese. He may also develop eating habits which are much too expensive and selective for the family to provide.

Implications of Isolation

Another area which needs exploring is the use of isolation for children with burns. Isolation has been readily accepted practice as it "cuts down on infection." It is now evident that isolation also cuts down on the child's interest in living. He is cut off from his parents by masks, gowns, and frequently by touch. He is also cared for by personnel who are silhouetted by gowned bodies, exposing only their eyes for him to receive nonverbal communication clues. He is frequently in an area where there are other acutely ill children who need similar demanding care. He may be in a sideroom and frequently has a cradle over his bed. He may even be on a Foster frame or Circulo-matic bed. He frequently has side rails up and often does not have a pillow. This bed is a far cry from the one he is used to at home. It isn't familiar, or for that matter, it may not even be comfortable for him.

Let us examine this isolation room. Despite his previous family conditions, the child is placed in a single room in a bed by himself. These two factors, a single room and a single bed, may be unknown to him—especially if he comes from a large or poor family. The stimuli in this room are medical in nature, and may very well be more depressing than stimulating.

He may be interested, at first, in the intravenous bottle or the equipment for checking specific gravity, or in listening to his heart beat with a stethoscope. These stimuli quickly change to boring ritualism, and the child becomes disinterested. The room may be air-conditioned and this provides an auditory stimulus for a short period. This noise quickly becomes agitating and tends to lead to disorientation over a period of time. The disorientation is further enhanced by the lack of clocks, calendars, and other daily reminders to the child of time and place. Reminders such as the school bell's ringing at 9:00 A.M., the factory whistle's blowing at noon, the mailman's coming in the morning, and the breadman's coming in the afternoon are all removed and the child's immature sense of time is destroyed completely.

The isolation may indicate to the child that what he has is "bad." This connotation sets the stage for the child's feeling towards his burns and his revised body image. The child who is burned frequently feels the burns are punishment for his "wrong-doings," and the isolation serves to accentuate this feeling. The child who received his burns as a result of playing with matches or fire is especially prone to this re-action. He has probably been cautioned many times not to play with fire and he disobeyed his mother's wise counsel. Now he is receiving the punishment given to children who disobey their parents.

The isolation further adds to the separation of child and parent and nurse and parent. It puts a barrier on communicating in a usual manner. A frequent use of touch is utilized in normal adult-child rela-tionships. The child learns early to cuddle and caress. He receives a great deal of gratification from this touch no matter how frequently or infrequently it is utilized in his early childhood. As he grows older, he relies less and less on this touch, but he frequently resorts to it in time of illness. The isolation, whether complete or partial, hampers the grati-fication the child receives from touch. Complete isolation is the term I use to describe when parents are forbidden in the room and partial isolation is the term used when sterile gloves interfere with granting of the normal touch sensation.

TOUCH DEPRIVATION

The effect of this isolation is that the child is deprived of the normal comforting sensation of touch. The touch he receives is usually only painful, as it is provided when turning the child. Turning can be a very painful experience for the child who is burned. Because the child learned to associate touch with pain he soon learns to prefer not to be touched.

During the long-term care it is necessary to help the child feel good about his body and to begin to get some gratification from touch. De-pending on the severity of the trauma, the nurse can begin to reintro-duce the child to kinesthetic sensations. She can utilize soothing lotion and gently rub it on the scar area. The soothing, relaxing motion with the warmth and tenderness of her fingertips can bring real joy to the child. At first, his tolerance may be extremely low, but it will increase with time. From this beginning she can then proceed to have the child apply the lotion himself, or to have his mother apply it and then the child. If the child is an adolescent, some of the cosmetic lotions can be utilized that mask some of the scar and have the same color tone as his skin.

The younger child may need to start by applying the lotion to the nurse. This gives him an excuse to get close and still does not threaten his will to be alone. The younger child might also enjoy applying lotion to a doll.

A convenient method in reuniting the child with touch is estab-lished when the child is started on tub baths. In the tub it is perfectly acceptable to touch the child. As the child is being taken out of the bathtub, the nurse should lean over and make her neck readily accessi-ble for the child to reach for support. The child reaches up and to his surprise finds the sensation satisfying.

AUDITORY DEPRIVATION

The auditory effects of isolation are usually reversed as soon as isolation is discontinued. They can, however, be prevented by providing music, radio, and normal voices during the isolation period. It is possible for young children to forget their parents' normal voices when separated from them for long periods. This is important to keep in mind, as the parents' voices may sound very different and foreign through a mask. If it is not permissible for the parents to enter the child's isolation room, an intercom can be successfully utilized between the parent and child. Many children play with intercoms as toys, and they are well-known items to today's child. Intercoms can be bought very inexpensively if the hospital is not equipped with them. The value of getting a set especially for the child is that the parent can stand by a window so the child can see him as well as hear him. In some of the more progressive hospitals closed-circuit television is also utilized and the child can see and hear the parent who is located in another area such as the lobby. This is also a means to have the other siblings communicate with the hospitalized child. The disadvantage is that the child is not able to answer back directly. This can be improved by having the child dictate his questions and answers to the nurse and have them delivered to the siblings. The burned child may be very interested in asking his other siblings about his dog that was close by at the time of the accident. He may fear the dog is also burned. Or he may wonder about his friends or his toys during his absence. These are child-type questions and he wants an answer from another child who understands his concerns. This may be an example of the communication gap between adults and children, and the great satisfaction derived from communicating with children his own age.

Isolation may even occur when the child is simply subjected to long periods of hospitalization. He need not be in an "isolation technique" to be isolated. The isolation may be due to a decrease in normal developmental experiences. For instance, the child who is burned may be hospitalized during a very important spring. Spring to a toddler or preschooler is essential to introducing him to the rebirth of flowers, grass, and trees. The one-year-old child does not have the capacity to appreciate the buds. The toddler or preschooler does, and it is important to expose him to them at the time that he is developmentally ready for this experience. The nurse must provide substitute ways of providing the child with such an experience. Books with simple stories about spring are useful as a starting point. The stories can be read and then the books left with the child for his own exploration. A garden can be started in his room. He can plant seeds to watch the beginnings and various stages of growth. House plants which flower can be added for variety. In addition, the child should be placed near a window so he can see changes outside. Binoculars may be needed to bring things into closer focus. The family can be encouraged to take photographs of their yard and home during the season to keep the child up to date on his familiar environment. A bulletin board can be utilized to put up pictures which help to orient the child to time. Very appropriate pictures for display are those drawn by his peers or siblings. The bulletin board should be easily movable so the child can change it if he is old enough to participate in the activity. If he is too young the parents or health personnel must assume responsibility for up-dating it frequently. Other helpful items are peg-boards, blackboards, magic slates, and drawing boards. All of these can be utilized to help cut down on the child's isolation and to nurture developmental progress.

CHILDREN'S VIEWS OF ISOLATION

In a study by Pidgeon (1967), children were interviewed regarding their understanding of isolation. Pidgeon found that 71 percent of the 3.6- to 6.11-year-olds gave incorrect responses to her questions regarding the cause and effect and rationale for isolation. This high percentage indicates the real need for nurses to work with children to help them understand *why* they are isolated. The older age groups had a better understanding but still demonstrated the need for factual information regarding isolation. The younger age groups illustrated the idea that the cause of isolation was related to psychological or moral issues. The school-age children were able to draw upon more experience and could identify physical aspects as the causative agents. In the adolescent age groups, 92 percent of the youngsters interviewed gave correct responses regarding their isolation. The findings suggest that a great deal needs to be done to help preschoolers understand isolation, while the school-age child and adolescent seem to need lesser professional help to supplement their other resources. The real challenge with children who are burned is to help them cope with the guilt which may exist. It is necessary for the child to be able to do more than just verbalize his knowledge. He must also be helped to deal with the information in a realistic way. For example, John, a 10-year-old, was admitted with 35 percent of his body burned. He was placed on strict isolation in a side-room. When asked if he understood the reasons for the isolation he gave this response: "I am being treated on open technique. I am isolated to cut down the possibility of infection."

Initially, that response sounds like John thoroughly understands his isolation. However, after John feels more comfortable communicating with the nurse, he adds this statement: "I know why the doctors says I'm isolated, but do all kids get put in these rooms when they play with matches?"

This additional statement opens the way for the nurse to explain that isolation is not punishment, that playing with matches is not the reason for isolation, nor is isolation used unless it is absolutely essential for the best possible care of the child. It is also helpful to explain that, as a nurse, you do not like to isolate children and you are willing to help children in any way possible to tolerate isolation. A question such as, "Is there anything I can do or get you which would make you feel comfortable while isolated?" Or, capitalizing on the child's imagination: "If you could wish for anything to have right now, what would it be?"

It is not always possible to provide the child with his wish but at least you can begin to find out how he feels and what he would like. You may even find by making some trade-offs that you can provide something which closely approximates his wishes without interfering with the isolation technique.

PARENTS AND ISOLATION

The effects that isolation can have on the parents can be as detrimental as the effects on the child. The parent is placed in an awkward position by virtue of the child's being burned in the first place. Burns are referred to as preventable accidents in childhood. But the prevention is not as easy as prevention provided by periodic immunizations. It is prevention which requires almost constant supervision of the child. Burns may occur despite the most conscientious guidance, or, conversely, they may occur as the result of a battering parent. The wide range of causation behooves us to work diligently with the parents, from the onset.

Bright (1967) identifies a tool which she used to record, assess, and plan care for the parent. I feel such a tool can be useful when isolation interferes with a close mother-child relationship. This is especially significant for children with burns as there is a high incidence of disturbed mother-child relationships in this pediatric population. What can the tool do? It can begin to identify the way the parent reacts and responds when isolation is a major obstacle to effective communication. It can also help to identify areas of concern which cause anxiety in the parent and further adds to the communication gap.

Recordings such as the following may help to identify ways the nurse can begin to help the parent and child to understand one another.

One mother stated: "Jerry always does the darndest things! He's my trouble maker. He got what he deserves!"

This statement, along with the following description of the mother, are recorded on the tool for use by the professional team.

Mrs. M. spoke with real feeling. She emphasized the words *he*, *troublemaker*, and *deserves*. She maintained eye contact during the conversation and her facial expression was stern and determined.

From first glance, this information reveals a mother and child who may be temporarily *helped* by the isolation technique. It would not be beneficial to Jerry to hear his mother talk this way. The isolation also provided an opportunity for the mother to release these negative feelings to a helping person.

There is, however, much more to be done for this family. Parod and Caplan (1960) bring out the important fact that when one is dealing with families in crisis, it is possible to help them resolve the acute stress situation and at the same time to help them also bring satisfactory solutions to unresolved problems. They found that people can "rise to the occasion" and seem to find new strength to deal with the current crisis, and in the long run resolve other situations which have interfered with healthy family relationships.

The situation quoted would seem to need this type of intervention. How can we help the mother to see her responsibility to her child during this acute crisis and perhaps at the same time improve her feelings toward him when he is well? How can we minimize the effects of isolation to help meet our overall objectives? First, we must help the mother understand that her presence is essential despite her present feelings. A statement such as, "I know how frustrated you must feel, but please try to believe that Jerry needs you." Or, "Isolation is only to prevent infection, we do not use it to separate the child and parent. We thoroughly believe that parents are the *best* therapy for their children."

Isolation is a barrier which interferes with the expression of motherly instincts when they are at their height. For instance, Mrs. M's first reaction might be to rush to Jerry and hug him and ask his forgiveness in an effort to release her guilt. Because he is isolated, she is deprived of this experience and must try to relieve her guilt without the help of her son. Despite a strained mother-child relationship prior to the insult, she might have benefited from this experience. Jerry might also have benefited by witnessing his mother being genuinely interested in his welfare and asking for his understanding. Each might have begun to see the other in a different light, but isolation blocked out this opportunity.

We can minimize the effects of isolation by helping the mother to verbally express her feelings to Jerry.

The nurse might say, "Don't be afraid to tell Jerry how you feel. Let him know you are sorry he must withstand the pain."

When working with Jerry you can help further by sharing with him his mother's desire to help despite the limitations created by the isolation. For example, "Your Mom would love to be able to come in the room. As yet, the doctors still feel it is best not to let her come in. Is there anything you want me to tell her?"

The success of intervention will greatly depend on the ability of the nurse to provide opportunities for the parent and child to interact in a meaningful way, despite the isolation, and to draw upon their hidden capacities to resolve conflicts which interfere with coping with acute stress.

Implications of Whirlpool

The use of whirlpool during the acute stages is commonly accepted practice. The whirlpool helps to cut down on infection and reduces the odor from decaying tissue. This very useful procedure has lessened the use of soaks to the burned area. It can be an extremely soothing procedure. The way it is introduced to the child is most important and especially so if the child has been burned by liquid. The whirlpool may ignite uncomfortable memories for the child. If the original introduction to the procedure is handled correctly, the long-term use of the therapy is easy. Children innately enjoy water play and the whirlpool can be utilized this way. The use of squirt guns, boats, sponges, etc., help to make the therapy a treat instead of a treatment.

The trips to whirlpool should not be used as a bribe for good behavior. They should not be withheld for "uncooperative" behavior. This method of control interferes with the long-range satisfactory use of whirlpool in the child's care. Withholding whirlpool therapy may meet a short-term goal of care, but it readily interferes with the long-term care of the child. In long-term goals, we want the child to appreciate and enjoy the whirlpool as a method of enhancing his grafting and promoting a return to health. As a part of the long-term therapy, we want it to have only positive connotations to the child.

Contractures

Contractures are a frequent result of burns. Some are the result of scar tissue while others are caused by lack of adequate protection during the acute stage. Positioning of the child with burns is of prime importance. The child has the tendency to put his body in the position which is the least painful. The position may cause a contracture or contractures and necessitate additional surgery. The key to good results is to place the body in good alignment, use a footboard, place pillows and sandbags as needed, use splints if necessary, and change positions frequently. These rules carry through during the skin-grafting stages, also. It is equally important to control contractures during all periods of hospitalization. Frequently even during discharged periods, areas are splinted to keep them in good alignment. Even the smallest finger must be protected. A small splint made from a baby tongue blade can be used for this purpose. Splinting is especially useful if the child is unable to control and exercise the part involved. An arm that has been burned can be splinted with a padded arm board. Care must be taken to check for proper circulation.

The armboard is removed for whirlpool and exercises and then reapplied. Passive exercises are given to parts that are not immobilized by skin grafting. These exercises should be given during all hospitalization periods and taught to the mother for home use, if indicated. The exercises can be achieved through the use of toys that necessitate movement of the involved part. If it is a hand involved, throwing and catching a ball is useful, or playing pool in the case of an older child. If it is finer coordination, turning the pages of a book will suffice. Stretching of the neck muscles can be achieved by placing the child's bed so he must turn to see TV or to see who is entering the room. The conscientious care taken to prevent contractures may save the child periods of being in traction or even surgical correction to release contractures.

Pressure Sores

Fortunately, in the care of children we have fewer situations in which pressure sores are a problem. However, children who are immobilized due to the burns or grafting are good candidates for developing them. The positioning and turning done to prevent contractures will also aid in the prevention of pressure sores. If the child is immobilized for very long periods, an alternating-pressure mattress may be a helpful addition. Pressure sores are easily started on already destroyed tissues, such as burns, so close attention should be paid to the burned areas.

The treatment for pressure sores must be selected carefully. Routine care, offered in some hospitals, should not be instituted without checking with the physician. The application of a heat treatment with use of a light bulb can further aggravate the burn. The application of ointments can interfere with the therapy being given. The best treatment may very well be to keep the area clean and exposed to the air with additional consideration given to not putting pressure on the already involved area.

The child frequently likes to wear jewelry or clothing which may cause constrictions and result in pressure sores. Removal of all constricting bands will aid in circulation and help in prevention of pressure sores. If the constricting band is a "good luck charm" the child can choose another area in his room where it can be kept. He may want it taped to the foot of his bed, or hanging on a mobile. I have found that children will cooperate in removing such articles if they have been consulted in the decision rather than forced into it. Making a game of where the article can be placed is good fun. A little child may even enjoy the magic of having the charm change places and guessing where it is, providing the charm is not kept out of sight too long. This same charm may reappear on every admission and the child will expect the same attention to be given to it.

Dependence on Adjunct Therapy

One of the concerns of long-term care with children who are burned is the dependence they may develop on measures taken to lessen their pain or help them progress. One of these measures is the use of narcotics. The older child quickly learns that the stick of the needle is worth the relief he gets from the medication. As the time passes, either on the first admission or on following admissions, it becomes necessary to evaluate the child's real need for the narcotic. This can be a real challenge. Each child's pain threshold is different and no one wants to expose the child to severe pain when it can be alleviated. The greatest adjunct to relief of pain is the alleviation of fear. The child who is afraid frequently requests pain medication so he can go to sleep and forget everything. I contend that providing means to lessen the fear will lessen the amount of medication needed, especially during convalescent periods. (Injections are considered again under the section on handling stress.)

To lessen fear, we must look at some of the things children fear and how they can be handled. Many children fear darkness. The use of a light in the room can take partial care of this. Close approximation to the nurses' station will allow him to see people when he wakes up. Some children fear being left alone. The use of volunteers or other roommates can lessen this fear. Some children fear unfamiliar noises. This is harder to control in a hospital. However, if each time a noise is made, no matter how familiar it is to the nurse, it is explained to the child, it will eventually become familiar and less of a threat. Some children fear unfamiliar voices. This is especially so when positioning keeps the child from seeing the person. The common courtesy of adults' identifying themselves by name and function, when entering the room, can lessen this fear. Some children develop fears because the hospital does not conform to his home routine. If the child is used to sleeping with his door open, or with a radio playing, or with a favorite toy, the change in routine may cause him concern. Any return to normal conditions for the child will help to make him more comfortable.

One way to determine whether a child really needs a narcotic is to watch closely the times and conditions when the request is made. The child may request narcotics when he wishes to withdraw from a situation, such as when exercises are scheduled. He may request it when his parents visit. This request may be made because he wants them to know how painful the burns or surgical procedures really are. He may request them to make the parents feel guilty for his confinement. He may request them so he is conveniently asleep when the parents visit or when meals are served.

These types of clues can help you determine the use or misuse of the narcotic at a particular time. While it is certainly important to have the child as free of pain as possible it is not fair to have the child become dependent on narcotics. Careful evaluation of the foregoing factors will help you make a more realistic evaluation of the child's need for the narcotic to alleviate physical pain. The emotional pain he has is more adequately treated by other methods.

It is also necessary to search for clues which might indicate that the child is having pain but will not request medication because he does not want another needle. The child must be told that after the "stick" he will soon feel relief of his pain. He should also know that at this time only a "needle stick" can be used to give the medication. He should know that you do not enjoy hurting him but you know that children do feel better after they get the medicine.

The parents will also need to know that narcotics are not used without jurisdiction. With the current emphasis on narcotic addiction by youth, they may have real concern about introducing the child to drugs.

The parents should also know that occasionally a child may request narcotics when they cannot be given. They need to be assured that our aim is to make the child as comfortable as possible but also to assure safe delivery of medications.

Another adjunct to burn therapy, but one that is decreasingly necessary, is the use of tracheostomy, when the area around the face and neck are involved or when caustic inhalants are involved. The child can become very dependent on the tracheostomy. The longer it is utilized the more difficult it usually becomes to close it off and remove it. Partial "corking" can be attempted while the child is sleeping. During sleep it is easier to evaluate the child's need for continuance of the therapy. If the partial "corking" is successful, the next night complete corking is tried. When it is quite clear that the child can breathe with the tube corked, he can be introduced to the idea. This does not mean that the child will still not become anxious and develop respiratory difficulty, however. Very close supervision is still warranted and removal should be done when the child is calm. Occasionally repeated attempts at corking fail and removal is done under close supervision. The child should not be left alone during this time and sterile equipment must be close by in readiness for reinsertion.

It is sometimes necessary for the child to be discharged with the tracheostomy. The nurse is responsible for teaching the parents the proper care and danger signals. A referral to the local community health nurse is also indicated. The child should not be discharged until the equipment is in the home and the community health nurse has checked it for proper size and functioning. The community health nurse is able to check for outlets for the suction machine, evaluate home facilities for cleaning equipment, talk with the mother about her concerns, be sure that emergency telephone numbers are available near the telephone, and elicit the parents' understanding and willingness to assume the responsibility for the child's care.

Psychological Problems

The area of emotional or psychological responses is a very large one. I have chosen to present case material to illustrate this area.

CASE STUDY PRESENTATIONS

My first meeting with Marty was momentary because it took immense concentration and stamina to bear the sight of him. Wearing a diaper and striped shirt, he lay in a bed on his back with his head held up, his legs and knees flexed and his right hand swathed in cumbersome bandages. He rocked back and forth, he wailed and moaned. Light brown hair on his head was sparsely interspersed with patches of scarred scalp tissue. As I dared to approach him he turned his head and looked at me. Mucus bubbled and streamed from his nose. Tears poured down his face although his sobbing abated as I drew closer. Reddened scar tissue encompassed his face, his features were twisted and taut, the musculature about his mouth was particularly puckered and tight. Could he open his mouth sufficiently to eat or to speak I wondered? His left ear was bent over upon itself, his right ear was whole but disfigured, then tissue tags adhered to both upper and lower eyelids near the inter-canthus of his eyes, there were eyelashes but only a resemblance of an eyebrow over his right eye (Slamar, 1967, p. 212).

This is but one descriptive picture of a child with burns. While it is not a pretty picture I feel it helps to set the framework for planning nursing care for children who are severely burned.

I was asked to be the keynote speaker at a two-day institute on children with burns and was presented with the following picture of a burned child. Randy was a four-year-old child from a lower-socioeconomic family in a black community, in a major city in the United States. His family was completely eradicated by a fire with Randy the sole survivor. Randy was severely burned in this fire and had been hospitalized for a long period of time in a county hospital. He was to be part of an interracial family on his return to the community. The mother's sister was to be his legal guardian. In his own family Randy was the youngest boy of five children. In his new family Randy would be the youngest child with two older sisters. The new family was more highly educated than his own family, and they came from a middle-class neighborhood in an integrated community. Before planning any nursing action, it is imperative to look at some of the sociological and psychological implications for this child. If we are to look at ordinal position and if indeed it is so that the three most vulnerable children in any family are the oldest girls, the youngest boy or the only child, then I think we can visualize that Randy in either of the two families was a vulnerable child—the "plus" factor being, of course, that he was in the same ordinal position in both families. Perhaps an additional factor was that there were other boys in his own family and in his new family he would be the only boy. It is also important to know that there was a wide range in ages in his new family. The aunt who was to be his legal guardian realized fully that she was going to have a great responsibility in assuming care of Randy. She changed to a part-time basis in her well-paying job to spend more time at home with him. Randy's own mother was a full-time homemaker. If we assume that man is a dependent animal, that he prefers to exist in groups, that his conformity is based on dependency, and that we cannot separate him from his environment, then I think we can say without any hesitation that even though the family to which Randy would return was different from his own, it was a plus factor that he would be part of another family. It is also well known that when the number of people in a family increases, the number of interpersonal relationships increases drastically. The addition of Randy into this family would make changes in the family constellation for the new family as well as for Randy. While Randy would be decreasing the numbers of relationships that he had within the family, the members of the new family would be increasing their numbers of interpersonal relationships.

FACTORS INFLUENCING THE WAYS A CHILD HANDLES STRESS

For this discussion, stress will be considered as being any situation or condition which is inherent in the environment and which poses a threat to the child's emotional state and causes him to make certain adjustments in order to cope with the situation. This stress may be of a minor nature or of major magnitude. The degree of severity is not necessarily portionate to the response it causes.

Stress affects the psychological as well as the physiological functioning of the child. For instance, the child may be able to conceal his psychological response to an incident but his physiological response of a blushed face is readily evident. Or conversely, the child may scream loudly in response to stress but his bounding pulse may not be evident to the nurse.

Students are usually painfully aware of their own stress in the clinical situation and therefore may be more atuned to the child's stress. I think this is especially so in relation to painful procedures which the student must do to the child. This awareness can help the student appreciate the need for paying special attention to the child after the procedure has been completed. However, the student is sometimes so relieved to have her own stress alleviated that she forgets the aftercare of the child. This situation is prone to occur when giving the child with burns an injection (actually it applies when giving an injection to any child). The student frequently dislikes giving injections to children and she realizes that children fear receiving them. After the student mobilizes herself to go to the child's bedside, she is aware that her presence increases the anxiety of the child (Torrence, 1968). This knowledge may also increase the stress of the student. After the child is prepared for the injection and receives the injection his psychological and physiological states begin the return to his prestress level. The student is similarly going through the same cycle. The fact that the student also receives relief can help her to gain confidence in her own ability to give injections to children. However, the same situation does not necessarily give the child any confidence and it may actually increase his anxiety regarding injections and serve to heighten his fears in the future. The next time the student attempts to give the same child an injection he may have an increased reaction to stress, which causes the student to lose some of her confidence. This reciprocal interaction tends to influence both the student and the child in relation to their stress responses.

What can be done to help lessen the child's stress with respect to injections? To answer this question it is necessary to consider many and quite complicated contributing factors. First, it is generally accepted from clinical evidence that all children dislike to receive injections. If you ask them what they dislike most about nurses, doctors, or hospitals they almost all reply "shots." The degree to which the child experiences stress from injections is not consistent, however. Even infants seem to recall receiving injections because they begin to cry when returning to the doctor's office or well-baby clinic where they previously received an injection. Their dissatisfaction with injections does not seem to be lessened by any type of preparation. It likewise seems clear that toddlers' and preschoolers' stress is not diminished by preparation for the injection. However, the school-age child and adolescent seem to benefit from preparation which includes simple explanations of what the injection means to their bodily function.

According to Torrence (1968), the physiological response of heart beat increased when the nurse entered the child's unit with the injection. The study was limited to children 3.2 years to 7.2 years and specifically addresses itself to responses of these particular age periods. The information is valuable as it clearly identifies that stress is heightened as the threat becomes more intense. Although the study involves limited ages, clinical evidence supports that children of other ages may respond similarly when the threat of injection becomes inevitable. School-age children show signs such as clenching of lips, clenching of fists, facial grimacing, raising of shoulders, inhaling of breath with resultant rigid abdomen, tightly closed eyes, downturning of toes, tightly crossed arms, cracking of fingers, or hiding under the sheets. If these children were studied under similar conditions, they probably would have an increased heart rate, also.

In light of this information, it would seem logical that injections should be given without unnecessary delay in order to decrease stress. A simple and quick explanation should be given followed by the injection. This method would be superior to entering the unit with the syringe and then delaying the process by attempting to decrease the child's anxiety by playing with his toys or attempting to engage him in a conversation.

Another factor which needs to be considered is the way the child perceives the size of the syringe and needle. If you ask the child to indicate how big the syringe is, he will usually give a size far too large to store in most drawers. His description of the syringe and needle may closely resemble the threat he feels from the injections. This fact is good to keep in mind, as nurses are sometimes tempted to show the child the small amount of solution in the syringe to try to convince him it will not hurt too much. The child sees the syringe and needle and the amount is not so significant to him as it is to the nurse.

After the injection is completed, the child can be helped to resolve the stress by being comforted by the nurse, by being allowed to act out his hostility, and by being protected from other stress situations before he has resumed his composure.

Injections might be better tolerated if they could be given at optimal time periods rather than on a regularly scheduled basis, as commonly ordered. For instance, the child with burns may be ordered to receive penicillin 300,000 units every 8 hrs. The injection may be due when the child has just completed another painful experience and the child is poorly equipped to handle this additional stress. He reacts strenuously to this new stress and it is possible that this reaction is lessening his capacity for recovery. At a later time, the injection might possibly be less of a threat as the child has had time to recover and he feels less threatened by the same injection. If the injection is ordered only on a daily basis it is easier to vary the time of administration and to judge the most optimum time for delivery.

The fact that any experience with a needle is considered as a "shot" by the child further adds to the confusion. The child who had a large amount of blood drawn after several painful attempts to find a vein, may remember this experience and expect it each time he gets an injection. His level of anxiety may go up in relation to that experience and expect it each time he gets an injection. His level of anxiety may go up in relation to that experience for a long time before he learns to adjust to what seems to be a lesser threat, that of a single injection. It is important to note, however, that the single injection may actually be as threatening as the more painful procedure and the child's anxiety may not be lessened.

There are other factors which could be added, but this list tends to illustrate the complexity of the situation and helps to identify the ways a nurse can be instrumental in helping the child cope with one of the many situations that he will face.

The way the child handles stress and the anxiety and tensions produced by stress are related to a number of factors. In planning nursing care it will be imperative to give attention to these influences. I will list a few: (1) the age of the child and the status of his personality development prior to stress; (2) his past ways of dealing with new and difficult situations; (3) the immediate emotional surroundings of his illness; (4) the nature of his illness and its acuteness, as well as the severity, duration, and type of symptoms; (5) the degree of discomfort involved in the diagnostic procedures; (6) the meaning of illness to the child and his preexisting feelings regarding health and disease; (7) his specific fears and fantasies; (8) the attitude of his family toward illness; (9) the child's relationships with physicians, nurses, and other hospital personnel, and their attitudes and feelings about children;

(10) the nature of the hospital setting, and its policies and practices; and (11) the preparation of the child for the experience.

NOW TO RETURN TO RANDY

When we look over this list of items it becomes evident that Randy was certainly extremely vulnerable. He was at an age when it was especially important to him to have his parents and especially his mother. He also had very little in the way of past experiences to prepare him for such an acute situation. He was never previously hospitalized. His experiences with health personnel were limited to inconsistent visits to a well-baby clinic and an occasional visit to an outpatient department for minor acute illnesses. Randy was familiar with a community health nurse who visited the family, but he did not receive any direct services.

It was rather difficult to elicit any information on how Randy handled past stress situations. His aunt described him as a "good boy."

Because of the nature of his illness, Randy would be exposed to many painful procedures. The illness would have all stages, with an acute phase right through a long convalescent period with periodically recurring acute phases due to skin grafting. There would be a great deal of discomfort from his illness. Randy's age range would make him particularly dependent on fantasies, and unfortunately many of these fantasies would be based on a great deal of reality because of the fire and the resultant destruction of all of the other members of his family and his home. In developing a plan of care for Randy or any other burned child, it is important to know the current stage of the burn. This is important as the care is very different during the acute stage from what it is during the convalescent stage. It is my personal opinion that during the acute stage of illness the child gets a great deal of support from the many people who cluster around him and are doing things for him. Most of the children fear death, and intense activity provides them with some satisfaction that people are trying to save their lives.

I have already indicated that Randy was hospitalized for a long period of time. My introduction to him came during his convalescent stage of illness. In designing a plan of care for Randy, or in offering suggestions as a consultant, I like first to look at the child's assets and later look at his deficits. I believe this is especially important because one can become overwhelmed and easily discouraged by the number of deficits in a situation. In examining the assets of this child I was fortunate enough to meet the child's aunt and to explore informally with her some of her feelings about Randy. When I first met her, I thought she was wearing a very attractive wig. I commented on the hair-do and she told me that it was a wig. I felt that this could be very important for Randy, as all of his hair was burned and his head was covered with scar tissue. I felt this was an asset as Randy was already familiar with people wearing wigs. I have seen, particularly in children who have lost their hair due to chemotherapy, that while the wig does improve their appearance it seems that the parents put a great deal of emphasis on the child's wearing the wig so that the child rebels and refuses to wear it. This was a more normal situation—that is, adults in the family thought it made an improvement in their appearance and wore them willingly. His aunt also told me that she had several different colored and styled wigs, and her enthusiasm for them was certainly going to be another very positive factor. I pointed out to her the importance of Randy's seeing her, not only with the wig, but also putting on the wig. He could then develop a pattern of wearing the wig without any push on her part. I was able to discuss with her that there would be times when he perhaps would not want to wear it and should be allowed to go without it if he so desired.

Another asset was that Randy knew his new family quite well. His familiarity with them diminished the ill effects despite the fact that in comparing the two families they seemed very different. Randy had stayed for weekends with this family and certainly knew some of the differences. If he didn't recognize them, at least he seemed to fit in the family and enjoy his visits. The financial burden that Randy might have on this new family was certainly of concern to the aunt. She was being helped through the social service worker of the hospital to meet the financial obligations. An attempt was being made not to disrupt the economic standing of the family.

The fact that a two-day conference was being planned around the needs of one four-year-old child indicated to me that there was something similar to a crisis situation existing. The crisis situation did not seem unique. A review of the literature concerning burned children shows that nurses need release from the constant care of these children and that the care is more difficult at some stages than others. The period of time for which this conference was planned was when the child was discharged from the hospital into the community. He would be readmitted to a different hospital for his skin grafting. There were a large number and variety of nurses involved in his care at various periods of time. In evaluating the situation the hospital nurses had on many occasions been very frustrated in dealing with Randy and had derived a great deal of support from a child psychiatrist who had given consultation to the clinical unit. They had also received a great deal of guidance and support from a clinical nurse specialist in the area. It seems evident to me, however, that the support they received supplied only a patch to an almost explosive situation. Little was yet to be accomplished in trying to creatively develop some new nursing approaches to meet Randy's needs.

The hospital that supplied Randy's medical supervision during his acute phase had become a very integral part of his life. He became extremely comfortable within this situation. It provided a shield for him from the community to which he would have to return with his very severe scars. For this reason, he liked his long hospitalization. He had also learned that during his convalescent period the diagnostic procedures were not as painful as they were during his acute phase, and he felt reasonably safe in the environment. He also developed some close relationships with some of the nursing personnel that he did not want to see destroyed in the same way that his relationships with his family had been severed. To make his transition to home easier, the hospital had sent a community health nursing referral. The nurse was new to Randy and the family situation and felt rather inadequate in her role because she could not identify any overt needs for Randy at this point in time.

During the conference we identified certain things that we felt would be essential for her to do, especially considering that Randy would be readmitted on numerous occasions to the hospital for skin grafting and reconstructive surgery. She would then be utilized as one person who could prepare or help to prepare Randy for hospitalization. She could also visit him in the hospital when he was hospitalized. This we felt would be especially important because Randy was going to a different hospital which had extremely limited visiting hours for children. When we had the conference, it was almost impossible for Randy's aunt to visit him even during these restricted hours. I might add that the participants in the conference did write letters to the hospital requesting a change in policy for visiting of children. The community health nurse was also able to make herself available to the aunt to discuss emotional reactions of Randy in his new family setting. We felt as a group that it would be very important to continue community health nursing services throughout Randy's long period of rehabilitation.

In working with children who have been burned, one should keep in mind—as we have mentioned earlier—that the child frequently feels great guilt for the burn and that he is very quick to blame trusted people for letting him get burned. In the case of a four-year-old, the blame is frequently placed on the parent. It is also important to keep in mind that the newly learned skills of the child may be stopped at the time of the burn and that the child needs a period of time to readjust and to begin to relearn skills during his convalescent state. In planning Randy's care during the convalescent stage, it was important to provide a means for the child to act out his fears and anxiety through play. It was planned to do this during his repeated hospitalization. The child needs to be allowed to explore the same equipment that has been used with him, and his play involving this exploration may be directed at a doll or other appropriate toy. If the child is not able to play out his fears, he must be encouraged to do so at least verbally. This is frequently a much more difficult response to elicit from the child. Because he is used to using play as a communication tool, the results are usually better when play is utilized. Randy's nursing care plan included the following.

1. Frequent community health nursing visits to Randy's aunt to elicit responses to Randy's integration into his new family.
2. Periodic monitoring of financial situation to be sure it does not get to be a burden on Randy's "new" family.
3. Help from community health nurse in preparing Randy for hospitalizations.
4. Community health nursing visits to Randy when he is hospitalized.
5. Meeting with nursing staff in "new" hospital setting to explain special needs of Randy.
6. Send nursing report of Randy's past hospitalizations to "new" hospital.
7. Encourage new developmental tasks despite serious physical handicaps.
8. Help Randy develop resources for handling his changes in body image (e.g., wig).
9. Continue to focus first on Randy's assets in planning intervention and later on his deficits.
10. Encourage integration into his new community to lessen "cultural" shock when starting school.
11. Provide aunt with telephone numbers to call for information and guidance both when Randy is at home and when hospitalized.
12. Encourage means of communicating with Randy when he is hospitalized (e.g., revision of visiting hours, sending pictures of family, postcards, tapes of family interaction).
13. Continual adjustment of plan to allow for changes in age and changes due to grafting procedures.

Another Case Discussion

BOBBY

This patient required day-to-day brainstorming in order to meet his needs. Bobby was eight years old at the time he was transferred to our clinical area. His immediate care had been given in a small local hospital with a very small pediatric census. When Bobby was transferred, he was having nightmares and would scream out during the night or whenever he fell asleep. He had many fears of being left alone and these fears were interfering with his recovery tremendously. It was believed on the initial evaluation that Bobby would benefit a great deal by special nursing services. He had the good fortune to have a male nurse on the night tour of duty and Bobby gained a great deal from this relationship. After the really acute stage, when his condition varied almost minute-to-minute, the private duty nurses were released and Bobby was on floor care. At the time this decision was made, it was felt that Bobby's condition was such that he would not suffer from withdrawal of the nurses and that he might progress faster in a less dependent role. This was not the case and Bobby's condition worsened as he again felt very threatened by being alone. With this in mind, a night nurse was assigned with Bobby and he was on floor care during the day and evening shifts. Bobby was particularly fearful of moving his limbs as the exercise program planned for him was quite painful. One of the things that helped Bobby tremendously was the nurse's convincing the physician that Bobby should be out of bed, riding a tricycle. This would stretch his contractors much more successfully than the exercise program. It was very rewarding to see this child, despite the pain and discomfort, "light up" and become very enthusiastic about his therapeutic plan of care when it was something that was so common and familiar to him as a tricycle. Bobby was also told that at the times he was scheduled for skin grafting, he would have to be separated from his tricycle. Although this was particularly difficult for him to do, he did accept it as reality.

Bobby showed one of the typical reactions of a child who has been severely burned, that of a great deal of antagonism, especially for the nurses who provide his care. These nurses do many painful procedures to the child. The child interprets these painful procedures as punishment—another punishment, in addition to the one he has already received—for what he thinks are his wrongdoings.

In reviewing the literature of burned children, especially children who have played with matches, as Bobby had, we see that frequently these children had some disturbed emotional development prior to their injury. This was the case with Bobby. Bobby and his mother were having a real conflict with one another and on repeated occasions she told him not to play with matches. On this particular day he was playing with them and set his clothing on fire. His mother's immediate response to the injury was, "Didn't I tell you so?" This theme was carried through on the infrequent visits she made to Bobby. It was possible for his mother to protect herself from having to see him during his acute stages by just staying home. Because of her many responsibilities to her other children and because of the transportation problems, she was able to justify to herself her long periods between visiting. However, we were not able to justfy them to Bobby. At times he would verbalize that he didn't want to see her anyway and this probably was very true. However, it was sometimes very evident that he wanted very much to see her despite their poor relationship.

I was an instructor in the clinical setting where Bobby was hospitalized. My office was in the clinical area. Bobby would frequently come to my office, as this was an extremely safe place for him to be. However, I did feel that I could not make it consistently comfortable. Bobby needed someone that he could talk with, and after a period of time he would come in and play with the toys that were on my desk. He began to talk through the toys to me about his feelings, about his fears, and about his reluctance to go home.

Bobby had already experienced the uncomfortable feeling of people staring at his disfigured body. He could deduce that he would get a great deal of the same when he was returned home. He frequently would mention that he never wanted to return to school, that he hated other children, and that he would just like to stay in the hospital forever. One of my responses to such a statement was, "You do not like it when people stare at you, do you Bobby? I can understand why you would not like it." At first such a response would just bring a flood of tears from Bobby, but as he developed trust in me, he was able to say with a great deal of feeling and hostility, "No, I hate them when they laugh at me or stare at me." Over a period of time we were able to discuss how some of the surgery which he considered extremely painful could improve his appearance. While he did not like to go for skin grafting and reconstructive surgery because of his extreme discomfort to him, its end result was frequently an improvement in his outward appearance. We also discussed some of the clothing that he could wear to cover some of his more severe scars. We discussed, too, some of the things that could make him a very fine companion to other children despite his scars. Although I'm sure Bobby had many concerns to which there were no easy answers, and concerns to which he would not accept answers, the very fact that somebody was there to discuss some of his feelings seemed to relax him. I believe this is a role that nurses should offer to all burned children. I also believe the fact that I was somewhat of an outsider helped our relationship and perhaps this type of person can do the listening to the child better than the person who has to do the painful procedures and assume daily responsibilities for his care. As stated earlier, much antagonism is exhibited by burned children toward the people who deliver their care, and it would not be humanly possible for the professionals not to feel some negativism in response. It has been pointed out that nurses need relief from the care of severely burned children and I believe that, by supplying an outsider to the situation, nurses can get some of this relief. In addition, the more obvious ways of providing a particular nurse relief, such as not assigning her to this child for a period of time or rotation of staff from one area or shift to another, can be beneficial. It would seem very important for a child with burns to have a consistent person in his environment; and this consistent person should be one who has a great deal of maturity and insight. Even though she does not provide direct nursing care to the child, she should be available to visit with him each day. This person should plan to attend the team conferences relating to the care of the child. She should be able to offer, without a great deal of personal involvement, some of the things that the child is thinking. She can contribute only those reactions to the people giving him his care that will influence changes in his care plan.

There are a few other aspects in relation to Bobby that I would like to include. One was the way in which he was reunited with his family. We started by writing postcards to his family, and the other children in the family returned postcards to him. Then we advanced to the more personal contact of calling his home and allowing him to talk to his family. The nurse was working with his mother to encourage her to call in to Bobby. These phone calls were arranged at times when the phone would not be particularly busy and it would not inconvenience the staff to get Bobby to the phone. The mother also was encouraged to try and plan to visit more frequently. While there were not treatments that were going to be her responsibility when she was home, she needed to become more familiarized with the very changed body of her child. I cannot say that there was much of a change in attitude between the mother and child before the discharge. It was hoped at least to have nurtured a little understanding before reuniting them. A report was also sent to the private pediatrician and a copy made available in case he wanted to send it to the local hospital where he had cared for Bobby. There was a possibility Bobby would be readmitted to the local hospital for more skin grafts, in the future. This report had an extensive section by the nursing personnel spelling out many of the fears that Bobby had when hospitalized and also some of his feelings regarding discharge. It was hoped that if Bobby was readmitted, emphasis would be put on some of the factors that helped to make him feel more secure in the hospital setting.

COMMENTS

I should like to conclude with just a few isolated things that I have gathered working with a great number of children with burns. One is the idea that we must report very objectively about the child to people who do not know him. For instance, I had a group of beginning nursing students in a clinical area and we received the report that Johnny was a darling little two-and-a-half-year-old who was the delight of the entire ward. From this description the student assigned to care for him gained the impression of a very cute little boy and accordingly felt fairly secure about meeting him. When the student went to see the child, she was extremely repulsed. She came out with her face all scrunched up, and her almost breathless approach to me was, "O, Miss Steele, what did happen to that child?" I went in to see the child myself and the child I saw was not the one reported to me either. This was a child whose entire face was scar material. He had no eyebrows, no eyelashes, no hair, his little arms were extremely deformed, and he was extremely pale. In one short glance, one could not see behind this exterior to the very charming child who was described in the report. I do not think that it is fair to have the student given this false impression and I feel that we do this a great deal in nursing. The people that are in the situation become extremely attached to some of these children and do indeed feel very warmly about them. I am sure it is not because of their exterior appearance, but rather because of what they have learned to appreciate of the child's assets.

Another thing that I have found consistently in relation to children with burn scars is that they misinterpret many of the things that we do to them, and one of the things that they frequently seem to misinterpret is the grafting procedures. I have had many children say to me, "You are skinning me alive" or "Everytime you put me to sleep you take away my good skin." Postoperatively, I have seen more of them overprotect the donor sites than the recipient site and I think this is because of their misinterpretation. I think perhaps we should take a new approach to what we do to children and perhaps admit to them that some of the things we are doing are not for them but are done for us, such as, "I need to know what your blood pressure is and so I am doing this for my information." Or, I need to know your blood pressure to be able to monitor your care." I think if we put more of the painful procedures on this basis, then the child would be more willing to accept some of the things that we do *to* him and not *for* him. Then, the things that we do specifically for him, such as provide him with play activities, would be more meaningful. He could see the direct relationship between what he likes and what he gets and what he dislikes and what he has to accept anyway.

Another area which I feel causes great concern to the child is the need for isolation, and I believe it is fortunate for us that the trend to isolate the child with burns is decreasing in importance. Extreme isolation has many ill effects as we well know. It is especially traumatizing to a child who already has so many fears and especially the fear of death. When we leave them isolated for long periods they have much more time to think about death. Those of us who have witnessed a child die, and the postmortum examination finds that physiologically there was no reason for him to die, have certainly a reason to believe that the psychological aspects of the burned child carry a great deal of import on his overall condition. Conversely, there are children, very severely burned, who seem to live despite unbelievable odds. Their will to live is fostered by coaxing and support from caring adults.

Another area of concern is the one in which parents may be "overprotective." This term is rather broad and it has different connotations to different people. I shall use the term to denote a relationship which interferes with the child's ability to return to normal independence. Thus, a parent who does not allow the child to participate, at all, in his personal care is being overprotective. The nurse working with the child also needs to be working with the parent. She needs to set limits for the parent as well as the child. For example, "Mrs. G., John needs to use his hands to prevent contractures. He is capable of washing his own face." And, "John, your fingers need exercise. It may hurt a little to use them. Here, try washing your face with this washcloth!"

The nurse and Mrs. G. offer support to John during the procedure. If John is capable of doing more of his bath he is encouraged to do so. If he is not, Mrs. G. may finish the bath if she wishes to participate in this way.

After the bath is completed recognition is given to John for his efforts. Praise is given only if justified. A word of encouragement for future participation is also given.

Then the nurse talks privately with Mrs. G. She gives her an opportunity first to express how she felt about the experience. Then the nurse explains to Mrs. G. that it is very important to John to help him to be self-sufficient. A statement such as, "It is painful for you to watch John try, isn't it?" or "Does it hurt you to watch John try so hard?" is appropriate. It is also important to help Mrs. G. understand that with your nursing knowledge you will have to make decisions in the best interest of John. You explain that periodically you will discuss with her areas which will need revision in accordance with John' progress.

You attempt to establish an open line of communication so you can readily intervene if the child is being overprotected. This seems like a simple example and one which can readily be handled. The seriousness of it lies, however, in the results which may ensue. Early intervention may be the difference between functioning or nonfunctioning fingers. Another factor to be considered in whether to ignore early signs of overprotection is that frequently the problem grows in magnitude as the hospitalization continues. It is frequently easier to cope with the smaller problems than the larger ones which can follow. For instance, the mother may then wish to keep her child isolated from other children. If we have allowed her to overprotect him when it related to personal hygiene then why shouldn't she continue to overprotect him? If we have not guided her and shared our intellectual knowledge regarding the seriousness of overprotection in the past, then it is difficult to start interceding at this point. Periodic intervention helps to maintain an open channel of communication with the parent. If she is used to exchanging ideas with the nurse when things are going well, then she is less likely to be defensive or uncooperative when change is necessary. The well-being of the child is always of utmost importance. If our requests are centered on a more therapeutic environment for the child with emphasis on rehabilitating him to his maximum potential, parents will rarely disagree with the plan of action. The plan is further strengthened if the parent and child are included in its construction.

Case Presentation and Study Questions

Amy is a six-year-old with 45 percent of her body covered with burn scars. Her burns were the result of getting too close to the stove in a flimsy nightgown.

Amy comes from a family of two children. She has a sister two years older than herself. Mr. and Mrs. M. appear to be a happily married couple and show deep interest and concern for their family.

Amy has been hospitalized on four previous occasions. She has a tracheostomy in place since the initial insult three years ago.

At the time you meet Amy she is in a rooming-in situation with her mother. She is admitted for release of contractures of both arms. Amy has had the surgery and is receiving postoperative physical therapy. When Amy is not at physical therapy her arms are restrained up over her head. She is allowed out of bed, walking 15 min per day.

Consider the following questions in providing nursing care for Amy:

1. What are nursing considerations when a child is restrained in the described manner? How would you introduce the mother and child to the plan of restraints?
2. What types of intervention should be planned for the child's 15 min of ambulation? When should the plan be established? Who should be included in making the plan?
3. Who should assume the responsibility for the tracheostomy care? What factors will determine this decision? How should the child and family be prepared for removal of the tracheostomy of long-standing?
4. How can both Mrs. M. and Amy keep in touch with the other child and Mr. M.?
5. What types of activity are realistic for Amy after discharge?

References

Blake, F. G., Wright, R. H., and Waechter, E. H. Nursing of Children, 8th ed., Philadelphia, Lippincott, 1970, pp. 321–326.

Bright, F. Parental anxiety—a barrier to communication. A.N.A. Regional Clinical Conference, 1966. New York. Appleton-Century-Crofts, 1967, pp. 13–19.

Constable, J. D. Pre-injury emotional instability held clue to difficulties with many burned children. Pediat. Herald., Sept.–Oct. 1968, pp. 1–2.

Donnellan, W. L. Burns. In Swenson, O., ed. Pediatric Surgery, 3rd ed. New York, Appleton-Century-Crofts, 1969.

Ducharme, J. C. Burns and pediatrics. Canad. Nurse, 57:851–853, Sept. 1961.

Einhorn, A. H., and Jacobziner, H. Accidents in childhood. In Barnett, H. L., ed. Pediatrics, 14th ed. New York, Appleton-Century-Crofts, 1968.

Gould, M. A child with burns. Amer. J. Nurs., 61:101–102, Dec. 1961.

Little, D. E., and Carvevali, D. L. Nursing Care Planning. Philadelphia, Lippincott, 1969.

Long, R. T., and Cope, O. Emotional problems of burned children. New Eng. J. Med., 264:1121–1127, June 1961.

Parad, H. J., and Caplan, J. A framework for studying families in crisis. Social Work J., 25:3–15, 1960.

Pidgeon, V. A. Children's concepts of the rationale of isolation technic. A.N.A. Regional Clinical Conferences, 1966. New York, Appleton-Century-Crofts, 1967, pp. 21–27.

Quinlan, E. Dietary treatment of burns. Canad. Nurse, 61:375, May 1965.

Rubin, M. Balm for burned children. Amer. J. Nurs., 66:297–302, Feb. 1966.

Slamar, C. Behavioral interaction between a three-year-old child with burns scars and his nurse. A.N.A. Regional Clinical Conferences, 1967. New York, Appleton-Century-Crofts, 1968, pp. 211–217.

Torrence, J. T. Children's reactions to intramuscular injections: a comparative study of needle and jet injections. Ohio, Frances Payne Bolton School of Nursing, Case Western Reserve University, 1968.

Woodward, J. Emotional disturbances of burned children. Brit. Med. J., No. 5128:1009. 1959.

———— and Jackson, D. Emotional reactions in burned children and their mothers. Brit. J. Plastic Surg., 13:316, 1961.

12 SHIRLEY STEELE

Nursing Care of the Child with Juvenile Diabetes

The importance of diabetes as a long-term illness of childhood cannot be underestimated. The disease has its onset in various age groups and includes the newborn period as well as adolescence. Advances in treatment have expanded the life expectancy. Diabetes is a hereditary disease transmitted by a recessive gene. The hereditary factor is responsible for some unique factors which contribute to the nursing care of the child and the family. These factors will be described in greater detail later in the chapter.

A brief explanation of the clinical entity is essential to understanding the disease because nursing care in all of the age groups will be influenced by the pathology and the physiological response of the body.

Pathology

Diabetes reflects a disturbance in carbohydrate metabolism. It is caused by a deficiency in insulin with a resulting hyperglycemia and glycosuria. The complicated process also results in an abnormal metabolism of proteins and fat. The pathological process is aggravated by the loss of water and electrolytes by diuresis. These losses take place from both the extracellular and intracellular compartments. Hemoconcentration and dehydration occur as a result. Renal dysfunction occurs as a result of the dehydration and hemoconcentration.

This situation is further complicated by tissue breakdown. The body is unable to utilize glucose, so protein and fat are utilized in an attempt to compensate. The increase in fat breakdown in the liver results in an overproduction of ketones. These ketones are released

475

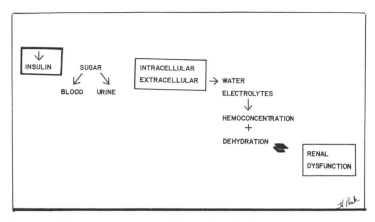

into the circulatory system and overload the excretory system. The accumulation of ketone bodies is of particular importance when the diabetes is out of control.

The above explanation is, of course, a simplification. For a detailed explanation the student should consult a medical text.

The etiological process is usually abrupt in juvenile diabetes. In the obese adolescent the onset more generally resembles the adult response to the illness. Another variation of onset in children is one described as a latent phase of the disease (Weil, 1968). Weil describes children with hyperglycemia and glucosuria resulting from surgery, acute stress situations, or illness as being in a state of latent diabetes. He states that these children frequently become overtly diabetic in later years. The child is usually underweight as opposed to the adult patient who is generally overweight at the onset. The symptoms which are common in juvenile diabetes include loss of weight, increased thirst and appetite, and polyuria. The child may be seen in coma or stupor due to an acute infection. The symptoms which may precede the coma are flushing, drowsiness, dry skin or skin lesions, abdominal pain, nausea and vomiting, or generalized body pain (Nelson, 1960).

The initial disbelief of the parents and the child is very understandable when a disease has such a rapid onset. The child may have a mild skin or throat infection and become acutely ill. He is admitted to the hospital and blood tests reveal juvenile diabetes. The child is treated vigorously and has a remarkable response to therapy. The parents are usually very relieved to see the dramatic improvement in their child. Their elation is short-lived as they begin to realize the implications of the disease to their child and the family.

It is usually easier for the parents to understand the possibility of their child having diabetes if close relatives in the family have the disease. Even though it is easier for them to understand, this may not be a "plus factor" as they may have some misconceptions and fears because of their previous experiences with the disease. However, it is especially difficult for parents to understand how their child can be the "first" to have the disease. There are a substantial number of these "childhood firsts" as documented by the fact that "over a 20-year period of history-taking only 57% of the children with diabetes had a positive family history" (*Juvenile Diabetes*).

The incidence of juvenile diabetes in the United States is estimated at between 150,000 and 300,000. The disorder affects both sexes with equal frequency as opposed to the adult type which is more than twice as common in females. The age of onset varies slightly with the sex of the child. The girls' peak incidence is 11 years while in boys it is 13 years (*Juvenile Diabetes*).

The increase in juvenile diabetes is a result of better medical supervision of pregnant diabetic women and close supervision of their newborn infants. "The newborn child of the diabetic mother is frequently larger and overweight. The face is swollen, often moon-like, as in Cushing's syndrome. The abdomen is tense, shiny and protruberant" (Anderson, 1964, p. 6). The baby is placed in a neonatal suspect nursery or in the premature unit so that he can be observed closely. However, there is still an increase in neonatal mortality of infants of diabetic mothers despite close supervision. The most accepted theory to explain this is that the baby dies of hypoglycemia. This theory is disputed by some and consideration is also being given to the respiratory and metabolic acidosis found in many of the infants (Gellis, 1960).

In addition to an understanding of the disease process itself the student needs to appreciate the prognosis and complications of juvenile diabetes.

It is well to keep in mind that this disease is somewhat more difficult to control than the adult variety of the disease—hence the frequently used expression that the child is a "brittle" diabetic. Children are prone to periods of hypoglycemia and acidosis at any time. They are also prone to infections, neuropathies, and vascular changes. The degrees of control does not necessarily influence the onset and severity of these changes.

The student needs to keep in mind that the child is faced with a long-term condition that he is unable to forget for even one day. The administration of insulin at least daily and the frequent testing of urine are constant reminders of his disease process. In addition, he must pay more attention to his activity than the ordinary child. This is important as his insulin requirements will vary with his activity. The child's nutritional requirements must also be monitored more closely than the ordinary child. (Diet will be discussed in greater detail later in the chapter.) Great emphasis is also placed on good skin care. This may be particularly frustrating to the school-age child, who is very lax about his personal hygiene. If he slips, an infection may quickly develop. This is most unfortunate as the healing process is also delayed.

Parents' Reaction

According to Hughes (1967), parental acceptance, adjustment, and cooperation are hindered by several factors: (1) long-term nature of the disease; (2) dangerous immediate complications, arousing fear; (3) well-known later complications, causing chronic anxiety; (4) worries about future vocation; (5) thoughts of marriage and transmission of disease; and (6) monotonous problems of proper management.

While the list of six items may seem short, the magnitude and scope of the problems can present unlimited problems in gaining parent cooperation. It is easy to see why at certain periods in time, the parents will be able to accept the disease more readily than others. For instance, when the child is of school age and has been controlled on a constant amount of insulin for a period of time, the parents may be comparatively relaxed. When the child reaches the preadolescent growth spurt and the insulin requirements are radically changed, the child is frequently absent from school because he feels sick. The mother becomes very anxious because the child is not well; she becomes impatient with the doctor because he cannot get the insulin adjusted; she worries about the child's falling behind in school work. The constant worry generated by the uncertainty makes the disease seem terrible. Her once relaxed attitude has been disrupted by this new need to focus on the disease. Her ordinary routine is disrupted and this can cause anyone to be impatient with the causative agent. Her anxiety influences other members of the family and particularly her husband.

The parents' reactions are of utmost importance because they have such a strong influence on the way the child accepts or copes with the disease. The child's emotional adjustment prior to the illness is another important element in the child's adjustment. If the child has a firm foundation to build on he is in a better position to make the needed adjustments. The basic emotional needs of the child are unchanged by illness. He still has a strong desire for parental love and acceptance. If the parents are too overwhelmed by the situation, they may be immobilized and unable to provide these basic needs.

Planning Care

The student can avail herself of many aides in preparing to give care. Numerous pamphlets and guides are available for use in teaching.

An example of this is the comic book supplied by Lily Drug Company entitled *Keith and Ellen Win a New Look On Life*. This is geared to the juvenile diabetic and offers a relaxed way for the child to learn about the disease. In addition, there are pamphlets prepared for the adult diabetic which can be adapted to meet some of the needs of the juvenile diabetic. A list is included at the end of the chapter.

The student would also benefit by reading an excellent lay publication on juvenile diabetes. It is a chapter entitled "The Chirping of a Sparrow" in *Thursday's Child Has Far To Go*. The chapter will help the student understand how a particular child and her family react when they are faced with the problem. It is written from a lay person's standpoint and probably more clearly identifies some of the feelings experienced than the majority of the professional literature does.

Nursing care for the newly diagnosed diabetic is somewhat more detailed than for the child with a history of diabetes. The student will need to develop a plan of care utilizing what the child knows already, as repetition is particularly boring.

The new diabetic is usually taught a few simple facts about his disease, determined by the age of the child. A toddler may only be told that he has to get needles to help him stay well. It is very difficult for a toddler to understand this concept and he may think it is better to be sick than to get stuck every day. The preschooler can understand a little more but he is not any happier to get needles than the toddler. It may be helpful for him to talk to a school-age child with the disease and observe the other child also taking injections. The school-age child is usually the most cooperative in learning and assuming responsibility for his disease. However, he, too, will have periods when it becomes a drag and he will need assistance. During adolescence the child's natural tendency is to rebel and the disease receives its share. The actual degree to which the adolescent does rebel, however, does not seem well documented in the literature. Utilizing factors of normal growth and development we have assumed that the child will rebel— but, again, it is probably more related to each child's individual emotional make-up than to the adolescent group as a whole.

After the child has been told about his disease in a manner commensurate with his age, a next step is to have the child learn to test his urine. The school-age child or adolescent is ready for this task. He becomes quickly aware that urine specimens play a large role in his disease process. From the moment he is hospitalized people start asking him for specimens. Therefore, he should have some natural curiosity about what is being done with the specimen. The student should prepare a place in the utility room and set up a teaching session. It need not be the time for a urine to be tested (see Fig. 1). This will allow more time for teaching and discussion. The child should be taught to test his own urine and record the results. He should also be shown how to clean and replace the equipment. The parents should also learn this procedure as it will be their responsibility if for any reason the child is unable to assume the role. The toddler is too young

FIG. 1. A separate area should be set aside in the utility room for the child to test his urine. All equipment should be readily available.

to understand this procedure. The preschooler may be interested in seeing it done, but he is too young to do it himself. The parents of these younger children must assume total responsibility for the child's urine testing (see Table 1).

TABLE 1

SUGGESTED PROCEDURE FOR TEACHING URINE TESTING

1. Select time mutually acceptable to child and nurse
2. Select place free from distractions
3. Have equipment ready
   - (a) test tubes
   - (b) medicine dropper
   - (c) water supply
   - (d) Clinitest and Acetest tables
   - (e) appropriate color charts
   - (f) place to record results
4. Have place to store supplies after use

At first, the child gets real satisfaction from achieving this task as it is new to him. It must be remembered, however, that the repetitive nature of the task may convert it to a chore and the child may lose interest. The strict routine of testing frequently should be replaced as soon as possible. In fact, there may be some value to the nurse's testing the urine while the child is hospitalized. This is, of course, debatable as some authorities believe the child should accept this chore as any other of his daily tasks. It must be remembered that even the brushing of teeth and washing are not done willingly by the child and one could question whether the child does indeed accept them as daily requirements.

Whether the child or nurse assumes the responsibility for the urine testing is not so important as what is done with the results. Talking with the child about the results will help him to correlate how he feels when a urine is +4 as opposed to negative. He will begin to see the relationship between what he eats and the amount of activity in which he engages and the urine test results.

We here assume that the child is hospitalized during the initial stage. However, some physicians prefer to regulate the child at home. This allows for more accurate assessment of the child's activity as related to his insulin needs. The community health nurse will probably be the one to teach the child and parents the urine testing, or it may be done by the doctor's office nurse.

If the child is hospitalized, there is usually sufficient time to space the teaching. It is not necessary to immediately begin to teach the child to give his own insulin. Timing is important in obtaining the child's cooperation. If he is feeling depressed from learning about his disease, he does not have enough energy left over to assume new tasks. After he has had time psychologically to internalize the disease, he is in a better position to proceed with teaching.

Again, there is not total agreement by medical personnel whether the school-age child should be expected to administer his own insulin. Utilizing the developmental factor that the child of this age has good eye-to-hand coordination, it is assumed that he is capable of the task. The decision would better be made on an individual basis, taking into consideration the way the child and parents feel about the procedure.

Assuming that the child is to take the responsibility for the task, a lesson plan should be prepared for teaching the procedure. The time allocated to teaching nursing students to give injections should be used to determine the time. Frequently, the nurse expects the child to learn this task in far less time than it took her to do it. The equipment utilized should be equivalent to the equipment that will be used at home. If disposable syringes will be used then it is realistic to use them in the hospital. If a glass syringe is to be used and boiled each time, then this should be utilized for teaching.

The principle of sterility may be an entirely new concept to the child. He may need considerable help in understanding it. Proper handling of a syringe is built on knowledge of what is or is not sterile. He can be taught to sterilize his syringe in the coffee basket of a coffee pot bought specifically for this purpose (see Fig. 2). This method of sterilization cuts down on the possibility of the child's burning his fingers in boiling water. It also lessens the possibility of the water boiling over or boiling dry. The safety factors are of utmost importance with the school-age child, who probably has had limited experience working with a stove.

The community health nurse should also be utilized to be sure that the home situation can accommodate the procedure. Frequently, parents are too embarrassed to say that they do not have the necessary equipment at home. Or they may not realize what it is we are requesting. The parents need to know exactly what they will be given by the hospital and what is their responsibility to have purchased, prior to the discharge. If the child has not been hospitalized the home is probably better equipped as they have had to assume the full responsibility from the beginning (see Table 2).

After the initial session, the child will need time to practice handling the equipment. He will need encouragement to transfer what he has learned using the orange to his own person (see Fig. 3).

A chart of the sites utilized for injection should be made available. The child is taught the necessity of rotating sites and he establishes a pattern for himself.

FIG. 2. An ordinary coffee pot can be used to sterilize the needle and syringe.

Table 2

Suggested Procedure for Teaching Insulin Injection

1. Prepare simple chart of role of insulin in body
2. Select time acceptable to nurse and child
3. Select place free from distractions
4. Assemble equipment
   - (a) syringe
   - (b) needle
   - (c) alcohol and cotton ball
   - (d) sterilization equipment (coffee pot)
   - (e) appropriate insulin
   - (f) orange
5. Explain each of the objects to the child
6. Demonstrate sterilization of syringe
   - (a) separate syringe and needle
   - (b) place in coffee basket
   - (c) put water in coffee pot
   - (d) place coffee basket with syringe in coffee pot
   - (e) place cover on pot
   - (f) place pot on burner of stove
   - (g) boil for 10 min
   - (h) let cool
   - (i) remove plunger of syringe by lifting near end
   - (j) remove barrel of syringe and place plunger inside
   - (k) remove needle by hub and attach to syringe
   - (l) draw up correct amount of insulin
7. Place syringe in appropriate spot to maintain sterility
8. Cleanse area with cotton ball saturated with alcohol
9. Inject insulin into orange
10. Pull back on plunger
11. Remove needle and cleanse area with alcohol sponge
12. Rinse syringe and return to appropriate storage place
13. Discard cotton ball
14. Free discussion

FIG. 3. Child learns to give her own insulin. The sites are rotated on a planned sequence.

As soon as his insulin requirements are established, the child is given an explanation of the type or types he will receive and their expected action. He needs to know that regular insulin is quick acting and results begin in ½ hr. Its peak action is in 3 hr and its activity is over in 6 to 12 hr. Regular insulin is usually given in combination with a long-acting insulin such as Ultra-Lente or protamine zinc insulin (PZI). These long-lasting insulins have an effect 4 to 8 hr after injection. Two other frequently used intermediate-acting insulins are NPH and Lente. The child will be less confused if he is only introduced to the particular types he will be receiving. Just mentioning that there are other types available will be enough. He needs to know whether he can combine the long- and short-acting forms he will receive. Most of them can be combined, but PZI should not be combined with the short-acting type ordered.

Another area of importance in teaching about insulin is the area of U40 and U80 insulins. The child and parents must remember that U40 insulin is used with a syringe calibrated with U40 markings and that U80 insulin must be used with U80 markings. An inaccurate dose will result from mixing the wrong insulin with the wrong scale. The bottles are clearly marked and the differences in labels should be shown to the child and his parents.

In helping the parents to determine whether to use disposable syringes, the cost factor is of utmost importance. Occasionally the

FIG. 4. A home visit by the community health nurse readies the father for the return of his son, with newly diagnosed diabetes.

parents feel the cost is minimal compared to the convenience obtained. Some parents decide to use the glass syringe but get a couple of disposable ones to have on hand for travel or in case the glass syringe is broken. Regardless of which type is chosen, more than one syringe should be bought so there is always one available (see Fig. 4).

Diet: Free or Restricted?

The next area which plays an important part in the life of a diabetic is his diet. The dietician should be contacted to be a team member. There are basically two types of diets prescribed. The one receiving the most attention at the present time is the so-called "free diet." The other type is the restricted diabetic diet most well-known to adult diabetics. Regardless of which is chosen, the main emphasis is on supplying adequate nutrients to promote normal growth. The emphasis on supporting growth is the clue to why the diet must be frequently changed if the child is placed on a restricted diet. The "free diet" probably is more satisfactory to children as they are able to eat until they are satisfied. It should be established immediately which dietary plan is to be followed so the child does not have to be disappointed by a change in plan.

The "free diet" varies the least from the ordinary diet of the family. Therefore, dietary discussion will center around a good nutritional diet with avoidance of foods with too much carbohydrate content. Discussion of the ordinary dietary intake is necessary as many children have very poor dietary habits. A breakfast of potato chips and doughnuts will not do. However, some of the culturally determined breakfasts may be as adequate as the basic four requirements of the textbook diet.

The restricted diet will take more time to understand. The exchange lists are utilized in meal planning. The parents and child will need to study the exchange lists and check them against the diet served in the hospital. It is very important to elicit the child's likes and dislikes and include them in planning. This will cut down on the amount of replacements needed to supplement the food the child refuses to eat. From time to time the child's likes and dislikes change. He may also find that some of his favorite foods are not as palatable in the hospital. Reevaluation is an essential part of the diet plan.

It is generally believed that the less emphasis placed on the diet and its restrictions the better. The child should not feel that he has to steal food to have his appetite satisfied. Neither should he have to be laughed at or teased by his peers for being on a specific diet.

The school nurse and teachers need to know the child has diabetes. They should know that the child may need supplements during school hours. The child should carry hard candy with him for periods when he feels weak. Also, if a snack is necessary during school time, it can be planned so the child does not appear to be getting special privileges.

An important consideration when one is planning the child's dietary intake is the amount of activity the child will be having. In keeping with the emphasis on a "normal life", adjustments will have to be made for increases in activity. On a day when the child has gym, he will need a decrease in insulin because of the increase in activity. His lunch may be changed slightly to include additional protein. This protein is valuable as it maintains the blood sugar level more adequately than do carbohydrates. A candy bar would give quick energy but it is rapidly metabolized and the blood sugar would drop quicker.

An appropriate way to teach the child about this requirement is to plan strenuous activities for him and have him compare how he feels and also to keep a record of his urine testing and the amount of insulin he received. He will soon be able to see the relationship between his activity and insulin requirements.

Teaching About the Disease

Thus far the teaching has been based on the tasks necessary to have the disease kept under control. This is only the beginning in helping the child and his parents understand the disease. A simple explanation of the "3Ps," such as the one that follows, is essential:

(1) Polyuria—increased amount of urine due to the sugar accumulation in the blood and ultimate excretion by the kidneys.

(2) Polydipsia—increased thirst caused by the excretion of large amounts of fluid with the sugar.

(3) Polyphagia—increased appetite due to the body's inability to utilize starch and sugars adequately.

The student should consult a textbook on fluid and electrolyte balance for a more detailed explanation of the effects caused by the "3Ps".

The parents and child also need to know the signs and symptoms of impending danger, such as light-headedness, sweating, restlessness, or rapidly beating heart, which are the result of too much insulin. Sugar should be taken immediately. The child may have to actually experience some of these conditions before he really understands the states we are describing. The child also should be able to get to the "sugar" without too much disruption of his ordinary schedule. This will decrease the chances of the child's using imaginary excuses to get special attention. An illustration would be as follows. The school-age child is frequently pressured by ordinary school routines. He is not allowed to escape from this pressure but rather he is forced to work under it and to cope with the situation. The child with diabetes could easily decide he is having an insulin reaction and leave the room to get his sugar supply. It is better to have the sugar in his desk or pocket and have him get it without leaving the room. Then the child is not tempted to try to use his disease as an escape hatch when the going gets rough.

SKIN CARE AND FOOT CARE

The exact importance of cleanliness has never really been proven. However, there is reason to believe that it is important for the child with diabetes to have clean skin. This is especially important as any child is prone to receive many cuts and scrapes which easily become infected if they are not kept meticulously clean. The healing process in diabetes is longer, and prevention is the best adjunct to care.

Foot care also is very important. Few people actually cut their toenails correctly. The child should be shown how to cut his toenails straight across and not rounded as is frequently the practice. Correct footwear is also imperative. If the child's shoes are too tight, his feet easily become prone to ingrown toenails and secondary infections. Well-fitting shoes will also cut down the number of callouses the child develops. If he does develop foot problems, he should get early medical attention before the condition has a chance to advance. Bathing of the feet with proper drying and an application of talcum powder is encouraged. The area between the toes should be given special attention. If the skin is dry it may be necessary to apply a soothing lotion. After daily bathing, a clean pair of well-fitting socks should be worn. Because the blood supply to the feet is frequently diminished in diabetics, the child may feel more comfortable in a heavier sock than his peers wear. He may also need a slipper sock or loose woolen socks to wear to bed.

HEREDITARY ASPECTS

Studies of the genetic nature of the disease suggest that the occurrence of overt diabetes in certain circumstances may be multifactoral, with different modes of inheritance (Weil, 1968). This statement clearly illustrates why it is so difficult to answer parents' questions in relation to "how their child got the disease." The student can only make statements which are general knowledge—such as the gene for diabetes is extremely common in our population. She should then refer the parents to their physician for a more thorough explanation.

The parents frequently feel a degree of guilt for the child having the disease. If they have questions regarding whether to have more children, they should be encouraged to speak to their physician or seek genetic counseling.

ADDITIONAL PREPARATION FOR LIFE

The child with diabetes needs a consistent plan for living comfortably with his disease. The plan should include the normal things which children enjoy doing. The child should be encouraged to go to summer camp. If he is not accepted at a regular camp, there are specific camps for diabetic children. The child may benefit from having contact with an older diabetic. He should be encouraged to call this acquaintance when he needs answers to specific questions about coping with his disease. It is best to have as the older diabetic a person who had his disease during childhood so he knows what the diabetic child is going through. It is also important for the child to feel free to contact the people in charge of his medical supervision. The child is the best judge of how he feels and he can explain it best to the professional personnel. A simple phone call may be all that is needed and the child may be able to avoid missing school an entire day to go to the doctor's office or clinic.

The child should also be given the opportunity to wear an identification bracelet or necklace describing his physical condition. He should also be offered a card to be placed in his wallet. These ideas are not always received kindly by the child. He does not like to be different and he frequently interprets these measures as overt examples of how he is different. They should be introduced by a person who is willing to spend time talking over the reasons for having such identification. The child can then make his own decision as to whether he feels they are essential.

THE NEED FOR INSULIN

Another question which is frequently asked by child and parent is why the child cannot be treated with "pills instead of injection," or, when the child gets older, will he be able to switch to the pill instead of insulin? The explanation is fairly simple but the child and parents may need to ask frequently as they do not want to accept what they hear. The juvenile diabetic is unable to be regulated orally because these agents' action is to produce insulin. The juvenile diabetic has no capacity to produce insulin so that stimulation by the outside agent is useless. The more intelligent child or parent may need additional information. They may need to know that the islands of Langerhans are nonfunctioning and, therefore, it is impossible to stimulate production of insulin. This is not the case in the adult type of diabetes, and, therefore, the oral agents can be utilized effectively. The parent may know of another child who has received oral agents. This can be explained on the basis of the early management of diabetes, when temporarily insulin production is possible. However, if the parent checks further she will probably learn that the agent has decreasing effectiveness as the disease progresses and it is probably being used in combination with injectable insulin.

The parents and child should also be aware that as the child grows he will probably need larger doses of insulin. This factor will help them to understand that growth needs alone will necessitate close medical supervision. When the additional units are prescribed it may help to cut down on their anxiety regarding the condition's becoming "worse."

There is an early response to insulin which was not included in the section on teaching about insulin. It does not happen in all cases of diabetes but it still merits mention here. The new diabetic may have some function of the pancreas. When the regimen of insulin injection is begun, the pancreas may recover the ability temporarily to secrete insulin. This ability makes it essential to monitor the child closely to prevent insulin shock. If the child is being regulated in the hospital, this reaction will be easily detected and allowances made for it. If the child is being regulated at home, the parents should be aware that this can happen and that its most common occurrence is around the second week of therapy. However, the response may not take place for six weeks after onset. The child's insulin will be adjusted accordingly and then the child's condition will usually remain stable for periods varying between two months and two years (Weil, 1968). The large variation in figures will help the parent to understand how individualized the plan of care must be for each child. The period of improvement should not be overemphasized as the parents may believe that their child is recovering from the disease. The emphasis should be on the long-range reactions, with this period as a small part of the overall course of the disease.

As we learn more about the transplants of organs, the outlook for juvenile diabetes may improve. However, at this point in time, it is safest to tell parents and children that they will have to take insulin daily in order to maintain and regulate their health.

INFECTIOUS PROCESSES

Although we do not want to make the parents overly anxious regarding the disease, we must make them fully aware of the dangers of infection. As was stated earlier in relation to the onset of the disease, the child is prone to develop acidosis as a result of a relatively minor infection. This factor also holds true after the initial period. Children frequently develop infections which they do not call to the attention of their parents. Anything which does not incapacitate them is frequently ignored. A throat infection, in its early stages, is not evident to the parent. Unless the child makes it known, the parent considers the child well. In combating the infectious process, the body may develop a slight temperature elevation. This, too, can go unnoticed by the parent. This elevation influences the body's metabolism. When the metabolic rate is changed, the insulin requirements are also affected. The child needs additional insulin, if he is satisfactorily to combat the infection. The child's cooperation in reporting early signs of sickness is imperative. The parent then must seek medical advice regarding an alteration in insulin requirements, dietary changes, or changes in activity. The parents should be cautioned against altering insulin dosage on their own.

In addition to early recognition of infection, parents should be cautioned about having the child unduly exposed to other children with infectious diseases. They should also be encouraged to have the child's immunizations kept up-to-date. Periodic review of the child's immunization is important as information in relation to current immunization protection emerges. It is also necessary as new immunizations are developed to have the child receive the benefit from them. The child will offer some resistance to receiving additional injections but his objections should be overruled because of the benefits derived.

If the child is exposed to another child with a severe infectious process it is also important to talk this over with the child's physician to see if prophylactic therapy is indicated.

During an infectious process urine testing is especially important. Urine testing may be relegated to a lesser position by the child when he is doing well. But during times of infection the urine must be monitored very closely. In addition to testing for sugar, acetone is also checked. The degree in normal variations is what is significant. Physicians differ as to what is the best maintenance for the child. If the physician prefers the child to have +1 sugar in his urine, then the deviation from +1 is what is significant. If the child has been maintained on negative urines then the deviations of +2 will be more significant to this child. All children are maintained without acetone secretion, so any acetone will be significant. A doctor should be called if acetone is present. One of the best suggestions to the parents regarding infection is, "When in doubt, call."

EYE CARE

Another important consideration in treating the child with diabetes is the care of his eyes. It is well known that in older diabetics there is a proneness to blindness. There is reason to believe that in juvenile diabetics there is a greater than normal possibility that they will have changes in vision. However, the onset of changes in vision is not well documented; neither is the relationship between the severity of the disease and the severity of the changes in the eye. The changes in vision may be of a temporary or permanent nature. The important aspect for the nurse is to remember that vision changes can be in direct relationship to fluctuations in the blood sugar; therefore, a child who is out of control may have blurring of vision which is only temporary in nature. The parent and child should both be aware of the necessity of having frequent eye examinations.

OTHER COMPLICATIONS OF DIABETES

The juvenile diabetic is prone to other changes in addition to those affecting his vision. The degree to which the parents will be introduced to these possibilities is extremely individualized. With the new diabetic the possibilities may not be brought up at all; however, as the child grows, it is important for the parent to be introduced to some of these additional possible complications. The introduction will be done according to what a physician thinks the parents should know at any one given time. For instance, it is well known that the juvenile diabetic may develop arteriosclerosis. This concept may sound very simple to people in the medical profession but it is extremely foreign to the lay person. A very simplified explanation must be given, and one that the parent can utilize effectively. According to Engel, "patients certainly, regardless of their level of education and sophistication, prefer to blame their illness on something they caught or ate or that happened to them, and consequently to think of disease as something apart from themselves" (Engel, 1962, p. 241). An example would be insufficient insulin as the cause of (rather than the mechanism involved in) diabetes. Some of the other complications of diabetes are calcification of arteries, protein urea, hypertension, and other changes in the vascular system. Some lesser types of complications of diabetes are edema of the ankles, which corrects itself in the early treatment of juvenile diabetics, and a proneness to an earlier menses in children with juvenile diabetes. There is reason to believe that fertility is unimpaired in girls with diabetes but the outcome of their pregnancy may have some complications.

Consideration for Age

The toddler or preschooler with diabetes will begin his medical regimen by having his parents take total responsibility for his care. This necessitates the parents' being fully aware of their responsibilities for the child and it requires that the medical personnel spend a great deal of time in educating the parents. As the child grows older the medical personnel must assume direction along with the parents for getting the child to assume some of the responsibility for his care. As was mentioned in the discussion earlier, the school-age child may assume some of the responsibility for testing of his urine and giving of his injections, or he may even assume total responsibility for this care. The parents' role is then decreased in that they will not be assuming the tasks to be performed—but their responsibility will be increased in relation to supervision of the child in his own management. As the child grows older the parent must be helped to relinquish control to make the child feel total responsibility for his own personal management. This is frequently very difficult when the parent has assumed all of the care for a large number of years. However, it is very important to have the child feel as normal as possible and normality requires that he begin to establish his own identity and responsibility for himself. The diabetic regimen should become part of the child's daily routine and should not necessitate a great deal of additional time to accomplish. However, it should not be treated so simply that the child is not given credit for assuming the responsibility. When the child nears adolescence it is hoped that he will be mature enough to assume the largest responsibility for his care. However, in relation to the rebellion that the adolescent is entitled to, we must make allowances and not be too critical when the child decides to rebel against his plan. The adolescent will also need additional information about his disease over and above what he was given in earlier stages. It is much easier for him to get medical information and his curiosity may stimulate him to read far in advance of what he is able to digest. The information should be discussed with the medical personnel responsible for his care so that he is able to understand the implications of what he reads. The adolescent who reads that most juvenile diabetics have early vascular changes may decide to give up as he sees his course becoming progressively worse. We must help him to understand the implications of what he reads and especially the implications to him personally.

Even though the parent has been told why the child cannot be treated with oral agents, the adolescent will need his own explanation. As he grows to adulthood it will be even more significant as he may talk to his fellow-workers and find someone who developed diabetes later in life and is being treated solely with oral agents. The importance of educating the diabetic to his disease cannot be overemphasized. If he has an understanding of *why*, then he is more apt to be willing to go along with the regimen. In making the foregoing statement it is assumed that the personality development of the adolescent is commensurate with his age and that he has had a somewhat positive experience with his disease up until this time. It is also assumed that the reactions of his family have been such that he does not feel inferior for having the disease and that his disease has not been too debilitating to him over the years. When more responsibility for care of the disease is given to the adolescent, outward or less overt signs of lack of interest in assuming this role should be monitored by the parent. Such signs as decrease in academic achievement, withdrawal from interaction with his peers, a need for self-gratification by such means as overeating, or an increase in aggressive behavior are all indicators that the adolescent is not ready to assume this increased responsibility. The adolescent may wonder about going to college. There is certainly no reason directly related to his diabetes why he should not attain a higher education. In relation to vocational planning, the diabetic may have some limitations due to the fact that he is prone to having insulin shock. Such vocational plans as being a driver for a group of people may not be realistic, or a job which necessitates climbing on buildings or joining the ranks of policemen or firemen may be out of reach. However, most of the professional areas are now open to the diabetic—including the areas of medicine and nursing. The adolescent may be deeply concerned about the possibility of getting married. Here the hereditary factor plays an important role. This should be discussed frankly and truthfully with the diabetic adolescent. Both partners in the forthcoming marriage should be aware of the consequences of such a marriage and then be allowed to make the decision for themselves.

Education Extended

PARENTS

Parent education is a most significant segment of the overall plan of care of the handicapped child. It is particularly relevant to parents of children with diabetes in view of the hereditary aspects of the illness. Parent education can be achieved by many avenues. One is the large lecture approach. In this method, an expert is usually available to give a prepared speech describing the disease process. In addition, he may cover aspects of child care, implications of the disease to the family, information regarding services offered in the community, and perhaps a brief explanation of some of the current research in the field. From this lecture, the parent utilizes the process of *selective perception*. He filters out those aspects which are easy to accept, digest, and use and apply in his own situation. This educational approach is a good stepping stone to other processes which involve a greater participation of the parent. Lecture can also be supplemented by written information on the topic. Again, this written material lends itself to selective perception. The parent can easily ignore the pamphlet completely or skim it and find areas which enhance or support his knowledge of the topic. He is still able to avoid areas which may be particularly uncomfortable to him.

The smaller group meeting lends itself to another type of parent education. In this approach, the parent is afforded the security of a group to help him express his hostility, fears, fantasies, inadequacies, and expectations regarding the handicapped child and his family. The group provides a curtain of protection not generally found in the one-to-one relationship of parent and professional worker. This protection plays an especially significant role as the parent frequently fears alienating the professional workers who they inwardly feel they need for the care of their child. The small group eventually helps the parent to look at himself and to see the relationship of his own behavior to his handicapped child. The group can also be valuable in exposing the parent to new ways of handling the child and provide him with very concrete suggestions for day-to-day living. In addition, the parent has a healthy avenue for release of his feelings. He may feel freer to express his hostility about the cost of insulin to parents who also share the burden than to outsiders or even relatives who may see insulin as a life-saving factor and therefore feel the parent should be very thankful for its existence rather than complaining about its cost. The other parents, with similar concerns, are often able to pick up on the clues and expand the topic to get to some of the deeper concerns.

The need for parent education is readily accepted but the avenue for providing this education is not firmly established. Experimentation and research with different techniques and procedures continue in many areas and will eventually lead to a more scientific basis for determining individual needs. In the interim, many different approaches are being taken to meet the needs of parents and children. The foregoing are some of the values derived from group meetings. They must be considered along with other information to decide if a group meeting is an answer for a particular family.

GROUP MEETINGS

The organization of groups of children with similar handicaps and groups of parents of children with similar handicaps has received attention. The question of whether a group will be beneficial to a particular family is not an easy one to answer. The first consideration should be given to the leadership of the group. Intelligent leadership is of top priority. One parent may benefit from a group led by another parent, while another one might be more comfortable if a professional person is leading the group.

The goals of the group should be explored before suggesting that a child or parent attend the meeting. If the goal of the parent group is to raise money to support research, some parents may not be interested. If the goal of the group is to share common problems relating to rearing the child with a handicap, the parent may be more interested.

Shostrom (1969) discusses groups in relation to the currently popular sensitivity training. Some of his remarks are extremely applicable because the focus of many groups designed for handicapped children or their parents really deal with the way the individual feels about the disease and the ways of coping with it. The group frequently makes the individual focus on very "touchy" points. In this aspect, some groups can be destructive rather than constructive. The points which seem relevant to this discussion are the size of the group, the leadership, timing of joining a group, and avoidance of a group composed of close associates.

Size of group. To be fruitful, a group of less than six persons is not suggested. It is believed that a larger group is needed to work effectively with problems. A group of more than sixteen is considered too unwieldly for a leader to handle, even with assistance. Therefore, the parent or child should also use the size as a determinant in whether or not to join a particular group.

Leadership. Shostrom (1969) makes reference to a study by Margaret Rioch that found that "natural leaders," without benefit of group work, can be as effective as highly trained workers. This point merely relates back to my comments about leadership and discourages professional workers from "downgrading" a group simply because it does not have professional leadership.

Timing of Joining a Group. In relation to timing, Shostrom (1969) suggested that one should never join a group as a "fling, binge, or surrender to the unplanned." He suggests that a crisis (such as a handicap) deserves more consideration and planning and that a decision to join a group should get the same consideration.

Avoidance of close associates in the group. Due to the nature of the group interaction, it is suggested that a person not join a group with a composition of close social or professional acquaintances. The nature of the discussions may be embarrassing under these conditions. Shostrom (1969) suggests that emphasis be placed on the confidentiality of the interactions in the group to guarantee the participants a measure of privacy.

Groups can be a most rewarding experience if utilized effectively. The parent or child should decide if the group meets his particular need.

Timing plays an important role in the adjustment of a parent or child to a group. He may not be ready for a group at the onset of the handicap but may be ready for it after a period of adjustment.

For instance, the school-age child may not benefit from hearing about another child's difficulties in getting regulated on insulin during the adolescent growth spurt if he is just learning to give himself injections. The other child's difficulties may be more anxiety-producing to him than beneficial, but this same child may benefit greatly by meeting with other adolescents with similar problems when he reaches adolescence.

In the same vein, a parent who is overwhelmed with the problems of adjusting to a new handicap may find other parents' problems more than she can handle. As time goes on, she may receive satisfaction and consolation by knowing that other parents have had difficulties similar to her own and have been able to "get over the hurdle."

The personalities of the parent and child may also influence their interest or lack of interest in joining a group. Some people do not enjoy being a part of a group whereas others flourish with this type of activity.

As professionals, we should share with the parent and child the groups that are available and their functions. The decision to join or not to join should be made by the individuals involved.

Regardless of the type of intervention utilized, whether it be group or some other process, the aim should be to help the family or child gain a conscious appreciation of the crisis situation in order to problem-solve the situation creatively. This attempt at grasping the situation will help these people to achieve mastery of the difficult precipitating situation which resulted in the "crisislike" situation.

By learning to cope with the precipitating cause, the child or parent may be able to prevent further crises from developing.

This does not mean that groups are indicated only when the situation has reached crisis proportions. I am merely suggesting that any situation that deviates from the parent's or child's "normal expectations" has the potential of resulting in a crisis situation.

In an attempt to prevent crisis from occurring, help should be directed at the precipitant factors, identified by the parent or family.

Case Presentation of In-Patient, with Study Questions

John is a 12-year-old boy admitted to the hospital with an acute upper respiratory infection. He has been unable to retain fluids for the past 24 hr. He is a diabetic of two years' duration. He is admitted for parenteral fluids, treatment of his acute infection, and evaluation of his diabetic status.

After the initial history is taken by the nurse, a plan of care is designed. (See Chapter 3 for an example of nursing history-taking and Appendix I for an example of the information gathered.) Additional information for consideration when one is establishing goals includes the following:

1. What is the meaning of the acute illness to John?
2. What is the meaning of the chronic illness (diabetes) to John?
3. What have been John's past experiences with hospitalization? On the nursing intake you have found that John has been hospitalized on four other occasions. Where was he hospitalized? Does he know this particular agency? What were the nature of the hospitalizations? Were they linked to his diabetes?
4. What cultural factors may be influencing the frequent hospitalizations?
5. Does the information regarding family constellation offer any clues which might need exploration?
6. How is John doing in school? Perhaps a call to the school nurse will be helpful.
7. How is John getting along with his peers? Have there been any recent changes in his living conditions? Perhaps a move to a new area?
8. What aspects of diabetic care need emphasis during this hospitalization? How much does John assume of his own special care?
9. What aspects of the acute illness need to be explored? Did the home atmosphere contribute to the illness? Are there other children in the family who are sick? Is the mother at home to care for the child or does she work outside the home?
10. What other members of the health team are needed to meet the objectives of comprehensive patient care?

Nursing tasks included in John's care will include the following:

1. Bathing
2. Skin care

3. Mouth care
4. Taking temperatures and administering specific therapy for elevations
5. Check of intravenous fluids; restraints as necessary for protection
6. Oral intake, if allowed
7. Providing warmth
8. Describe vomiting—amount, frequency, nature
9. Changing position while on bed-rest
10. Passive exercises to extremities
11. Record intake and output
12. Pulse and respiration: note variations
13. Note emotional responses
14. Provide appropriate play

After the acute phase, John's care will be changed to incorporate the medical regimen and plans for discharge. The dietician may be contacted to review John's dietary intake. She can make suggestions for changes, if indicated. The nurse will review John's knowledge of his disease and evaluate how he is coping with giving his own injections and testing his urine. The nurse will utilize information gathered to help the doctor decide on John's readiness for discharge. A follow-up report of John's hospitalization should be sent to the community health nurse.

To show how the history-taking forms can be adapted to other situations, I will use an in-patient nursing history-taking form to collect the information on a child in an out-patient setting. The example follows.

Case Presentation of Out-Patient

Mary A. was referred to the school nurse by a substitute teacher in the exceptional education class. Mary is a 10-year-old retarded child who was adopted as an infant. The possibility of diabetes and/or retardation were not discussed with the adoptive parents, prior to adoption.

NURSING INTAKE HISTORY

I. Appearance on first sight. Mary is a small, pale, and "dull-appearing" child.

II. Patient's understanding of illness. Mary had a limited understanding of her disease. She knew she received "shots" for "sugar."

III. Events leading up to referral. Mary is in an exceptional education class at a demonstration school. She was admitted to the school one year prior to the referral to the school nurse. The teacher in this particular class was "extremely efficient" and she did not use other professional members in meeting the needs of the children. Arrangements for the child's admission were made with the mother, teacher, and principal.

At the time of admission, the teacher told the mother there was no provision possible for testing the child's urine in school. Therefore, the mother sent a collection bottle daily for the child's noon specimen. The specimen was not refrigerated. The child took the specimen and the mother tested it when she arrived home.

IV. Place in family constellation. Mary is an only child adopted by a middle-class white family.

V. Significant information relative to

(a) *Feeding.* Mary is on a regular diet without a large concentration on carbohydrate. She has a bottle of orange juice in the classroom refrigerator. Mary's mother provides her with a half sandwich to eat on the long bus ride home. Mary feeds herself and likes most foods. She does not question why she does not have candy and desserts.

(b) *Toileting.* Mary is toilet-trained. Her training was delayed with complete continence being achieved only at age five.

(c) *Sleep.* Mary sleeps 9 hr a night. She has a 15-min rest period during school. She frequently requires a nap after her long bus ride.

(d) *Play.* Mary has limited experience with social contacts her own developmental age. In school, she was slow to socialize but this is improving with time.

(e) *Language development.* Mary also developed slowly in speech. It is easy to understand her but she communicates more like a five-year-old.

(f) *Independent and dependent activities of daily living.* Mary is completely dependent on adults for the management of her diabetes. However, she is able to dress and undress herself. She takes little interest in her personal hygiene or grooming and her mother assumes much responsibility for this.

VI. What is important to this child to make her feel secure and comfortable in this situation? Mary's diabetic condition was simply explained to the class. The children are aware that Mary sometimes needs orange juice. The children have been most willing to get this for her. Mary's previous teacher took the responsibility of getting Mary to the lavatory to obtain the noon specimen. Mary seemed to accept this procedure without question, and the other children did not seem aware of this special need. Mary seemed to be comfortable in the classroom. The advent of a new teacher was the precipitating factor for the referral to the school nurse.

VII. What are the policies of this institution which interfere with or promote the well-being of this child? In this situation, the teacher had assumed a lack of provision for testing the child's urine. After the referral, the school nurse and physician saw the child. The mother was contacted to check the child's medical plan. The "assumed policies" were adjusted to meet the child's needs better.

VIII. What is the medical plan of care which will influence the nursing plan of care? The child was receiving Ultra-Lente and regular insulin daily. The mother adjusted the dosage in accordance with the urine results. The noon results were probably not accurate as the specimen was old. The new plan was for Mary to report to the school nurse each day and the nurse would test the urine. A weekly report of the results would be sent home. Mrs. A. was very eager to have the results and requested daily telephone reports until she was convinced Mary was "controlled."

IX. What are the short-term goals for this child? Mrs. A. was interviewed and it was well-established that she thoroughly understood the disease process and its control. She was aware of "danger signals" and knew how to proceed if they occurred. Close contact with Mrs. A. by telephone was decided upon. This was at Mrs. A.'s request rather than because of an identified need. Mrs. A. was delighted that the urine would be tested at school. She was also appreciative of the additional professional interest in Mary.

X. What are the long-term goals for this child? The school nurse explored Mary's interest in testing her own urine. Mary did not seem interested but eventually urine testing will be taught. Health teaching will also be done regarding skin care, foot care, diet, and insulin. Due to the child's retardation, training for insulin administration will not be started for sometime.

Mary relates well with the school nurse and it is hoped that during her daily visits to the nurse's office she will begin to assume more of a direct role in relation to her health problem. The nurse will also work with the substitute teacher to help her with her anxiety over having Mary in her classroom.

The school nurse will also make contact with the medical source responsible for Mary's care and request a medical summary. Mrs. A. signed a consent for the release of this information. A telephone contact will also be made to the community health nurse in Mary's outlying district to familiarize her with the family. A formal referral will not be sent at this time, but Mrs. A. is interested in a resource close by in case of a future emergency.

EVALUATION

The foregoing example points out the willingness of parents to accept help when offered. Despite a situation which was tolerable, more help was welcomed by the mother. A teacher's insecurity was responsible for revealing to the school nurse a child with a major health problem, which to this time she had no previous knowledge of. As there was no major precipitating crisis, it was fairly easy for the nurse to make a positive contact with the mother. The nurse was able to offer help which the mother wanted and thereby establish a positive working relationship.

If a major crisis had precipitated the referral, it might have been more difficult for the nurse to establish a positive relationship. An example might be one in which a teacher suggested the child be excluded from class for health reasons. The nurse, who had no previous contact with the mother, might get a very negative response with this initial contact's being triggered by "unhappy news."

This situation also demonstrates that the person most qualified to be of help to the family is sometimes overlooked in delivering services. Even though the nurse is very effective in her position, there may be times when her expertise is not sought. This is more likely to happen when the teacher has been used to functioning without a full-time school nurse for a long period of time, which is the case at this school.

This case presentation also demonstrates the use of an outsider, in this instance a substitute teacher, to identify areas of concern which are considered routine by those in close proximity to the problem.

The use of the school nurse to do teaching in relation to the disease process will also help to gear the teaching to the child's readiness. The child was not ready for this teaching in the hospital. However, she may be ready before another hospital admission is necessary.

The school nurse can also keep the hospital's out-patient department up-to-date on the child's progress. The mother has not returned to the local medical doctor since Mary was hospitalized. However, Mrs. A. still wants a report to be sent to him. The school nurse will serve as a coordinator and leader of the team during the child's healthy periods and attendance at school.

References

Andersson, B. The crisis arising in pregnancy. Abbottempo, 2:4–7, May 15, 1964.

Dube, A. H. Diabetes—the three polys. Health News, Oct. 1968, p. 1–8.

Duncan, G. Diseases of Metabolism. Philadelphia, Saunders, 1964, Chapter 15.

Engel, G. L. Psychological Development in Health and Disease. Philadelphia, Saunders, 1962, p. 241.

Gallagher, J. R. Medical Care of the Adolescent, 2nd ed. New York, Appleton-Century-Crofts, 1966, pp. 216–234.

Gellis, S. S. Infants of diabetic mothers. In Nelson, W. E., ed. Textbook of Pediatrics, 7th ed. Philadelphia, Saunders, 1960, pp. 1214–1215.

Hughes, J. Psychodynamic aspects of chronic disease and childhood diabetic management. Ohio, Report of the Fifty-first Ross Conferences on Pediatric Research, 1965, pp. 97–100.

Isenburg, P. L., and others. Psychological problems in diabetes mellitus. Med. Clin. N. Amer., 49:1126, July 1965.

Jackson, R. L. Management of the young diabetic patient. Ohio, Report of the Fifty-first Ross Conferences on Pediatric Research, 1965, pp. 101–109.

Juvenile Diabetes. Michigan, The Upjohn Co., June 1967.

LuKens, K., and Panter, C. Thursday's Child Has Far to Go. Englewood Cliffs, N. J., Prentice-Hall, 1969.

Metheny, N. M., and Snively, W. D. Nurses' Handbook of Fluid Balance. Philadelphia, Lippincott, 1967, pp. 218–219.

Moore, M. L. Diabetes in children. Amer. J. Nurs., 67:104–107, 1967.

Moss, J. M. Management of juvenile diabetes. Family Physician, 15:46–50, 1968.

Nelson, W. E. Textbook of Pediatrics, 7th ed., Philadelphia, Saunders, 1960, p. 1205-1221.

Shostrom, E. L. Group therapy: let the buyer beware. Psychology Today, 2:37–40, May 1969.

Weil, W. B. Current concepts juvenile diabetes mellitus. Medical Intelligence, 278:829–831, 1968.

——— Diabetes mellitus in children. In Barnett, H. L., ed. Pediatrics, 14th ed. New York, Appleton-Century-Crofts, 1968, pp. 433–447.

White, P. Childhood diabetes. Diabetes, 9:345–355, 1960.

Pamphlets Useful for Teaching

A Handbook for Diabetics, Squibb.

Clinilog, Ames Company, Elkhart, Ind.

Diabetes and the Eye, No. 111, Commission for the Blind, New York, State Department of Social Welfare.

Diabetics Unknown, by Groff Conklin, Public Affairs Pamphlets No. 312.

Foot Care for the Diabetic Patient, U.S. Department of Health, Education, and Welfare, Public Health Service Publication No. 1153.

Keith and Ellen Win A New Look on Life! Vol. 1, No. 1, Eli Lilly and Co.

The Three R's of Diabetic Care, Arlington Laboratories.

You and Diabetes, Upjohn.

13 SHIRLEY STEELE

Nursing Care of the Child with Cardiac Conditions Requiring Long-Term Care

In developing a chapter in relation to cardiac conditions, one is immediately faced with the problem of what cardiac conditions still require long-term care. This question arises from the recent advances in cardiac surgery and pediatric anesthesia which make it possible to operate on children at a much younger age and get outstanding results. In working on such a chapter one then has to look at whether the cardiac surgery is palliative or corrective in nature. If it is only palliative, then one can say the cardiac surgery is but one phase in the therapy of the medical regimen for the child. The child, then, would require long-term medical care for his cardiac condition. The child with corrective repairs would fall into another category. With the current progress in cardiac surgery, some conditions such as patent ductus arteriosus would better fit into a text concerned with the nursing care of conditions requiring short-term care. However, many of the more complicated repairs require long-term supervision after the original surgical correction. The child frequently requires rehospitalization during some period of his childhood either for more surgery or for medical follow-up.

In this chapter I will begin with the emphasis on the nursing care related to cardiac surgery. Then I will illustrate the nursing care of a medical cardiac condition, rheumatic fever.

A diagnosis of anything's being wrong with the heart usually evokes a severe emotional response, so that the way it is presented to the family is particularly important. Most lay people have the idea that the heart is the most important organ of the body, and their emotional reactions will be based on this idea. The initial reaction of parents to

503

a diagnosis of congenital heart disease may be one of fear and anxiety. These two reactions do not necessarily diminish with time because the thought that the defect is still there is always in the parents' minds. Fear and anxiety may very well increase as the child shows signs of his illness. Such signs may be the appearance of cyanosis, becoming easily fatigued, inability for the child to drink his formula, periods of dyspnea, or overt fainting spells. These symptoms are periodic reminders to the parent that there is something wrong with their baby's or child's heart.

Some Initial Considerations

THE MOTHER

In a study by Glaser and others (1964), some interesting facts are brought out about the emotional implications of congenital heart disease in children. A key point was that the mothers seemed to live in constant fear that the child would die. This idea was strengthened by the slow and poor physical development of the child, the frequency of illness, and the somewhat undesirable personality of the child. The child was frequently negative, whiney, and irritable. Despite his undesirable behavior, the mother felt unable to punish him because of the fear of aggravating the cardiac condition. Because of these findings, it is imperative to help the parent, and particularly the mother, better understand her responsibility to her child. The mother needs an explanation of the disease in simple terminology. She also needs assurance that sudden death is not a threat. The old idea of "keeping the child as quiet as possible" must be eradicated.

The mother should be encouraged to treat the child as normally as possible. She should be encouraged to set limits for this child just as she does for her other children.

FEEDING THE INFANT

How can we as nurses help to decrease the anxiety the parent has about the child? One way is to help the parent to learn to feed the child, causing the least amount of fatigue. This can be done by making sure that the nipple holes are adequate, that the baby is held in a semi-upright position, that the formula be such that the child receives the greatest amount of carbohydrate intake in the least amount of fluid, that the child be bubbled frequently and gently, that he be allowed to rest more than the normal child, that he be given frequent small feedings, and that the mother be given adequate time to adjust to the feeding of this child while there is professional help available. By this I mean that during the hospital stay the mother should have a nurse available to answer questions or to take over if the mother seems to be getting too anxious about the feeding procedure. It is impossible to set a time table suggesting when the mother will be able to assume the total responsibility for the feeding of the baby. Early initiation in a positive manner is essential as a beginning. Frequent problems with the feeding delay the mother's ability to assume the feeding role independently. The mother needs to know that these problems would be present even if the nurse fed the baby. It is imperative that the mother be given all due consideration at the beginning so that she is able to carry out this plan of feeding for a prolonged period of time. A community health nurse referral is especially helpful to give the mother continued guidance with feeding at home. It is also helpful as the mother may not retain much of the information she has been given in the hospital.

If a referral is not made, the nurse should provide the mother with a telephone number to call for assistance. The number should be written down and clearly marked with the agency and persons to contact. Any clues as to how to "cut through the red tape" of the telephone system of the agency should be included. Every attempt should be made to make the utilization of the number free of anxiety. It is frequently difficult for the mother to seek assistance, so her attempts should be rewarded by a positive response. This will give her confidence to call again.

The preschooler with a congenital heart disease may need help from his mother to supplement his feedings because he may tire too soon and not complete an adequate nutritional intake. While we do not want to encourage the mother to take away the child's opportunity to feed himself, she must be aware of her responsibility to lend a hand, when necessary. The child with a congenital heart disease will still need to establish the same autonomy as any other child and his own self-limitations are the best guide in judging how much he is able to assume for himself. Helping the child when he is tired will give him a sense of trust in his adults. This sense of trust will be of utmost benefit when the child is subjected to periods of hospitalization and especially if the child is faced with surgical correction. If the child has had positive experiences with adults helping him when it is necessary, then he will trust them when he knows he is going to need help when hospitalized. As the child grows older, he can sense the anxiety of his parents. This anxiety may cause the child to be apprehensive. The child then is prone to excessive fears and fantasies about what is wrong with him and what his future holds. In an attempt to alleviate the child's anxiety and fears, the parents may overindulge him and overprotect him. This overprotection often leads the parent to expect less of the child and to encourage him to develop below his emotional and physical potential.

PHYSICAL DEVELOPMENT

I should like to emphasize physical development because I think it is less generally recognized that parents can be an influence on the physical development or physical retardation of their child. The emotional aspect is usually well accepted. The child with congenital heart disease is frequently a smaller child than his normal peers and this may be secondary to his pathological condition. In addition, the child who is not stimulated to be active and have the same routines and exercises of the normal child is less likely to mature physically. This lack of encouragement on the part of the parents may have an influence on the child's total development. The restrictions that the parent puts on the child may influence his self-image. Green and Levitt (1962) have studied this constriction of self-image in cardiac children. They found that children with cardiac conditions draw themselves smaller than normal children. Also, when a normal child draws himself in relation to a peer, he always draws himself larger. The child with a cardiac condition draws himself the same height as his peer.

As stated, the child with a cardiac condition is frequently smaller than the normal child in physical development. This may influence his drawing. However, the effects of social and perceptual experiences are also thought to influence his body image. The small size of his drawing may be the result of his feelings of needing continual help and being dependent on his parents. He views himself as small and insignificant as an individual.

In another study (Neuhaus, 1958), the cardiac child was felt to have a much higher incidence of neurotic behavior and dependency feelings than the normal child. This tendency seemed to decrease as the child gets older. The higher incidence of neuroticism in the young child may be explained on the basis of their shorter period of time living with a chronic disease. It may also be explained on the basis of the parents' anxiety and overprotection.

In both studies it is evident that the child with a cardiac condition needs a great deal of support and guidance to see himself as a significant person. The parents must be helped to avoid making the child so dependent on them that he cannot see himself as a significant being. The parents need guidance to give assistance only when necessary and to be able to relinguish the protective role as the child matures. The other siblings must also be included in this discussion as the effects of the child with the cardiac condition also affect them. A general rule of thumb is to let the child determine his own activity tolerance level. The child usually stops when he is tired. Very strenuous competitive sports may be excluded from his physical activity as a precautionary measure. However, the old idea of severe restriction of physical activity is now considered obsolete. These restrictions only lead to severe emotional and social deprivation which interfere with the child's future adjustments.

Cardiac Surgery

Despite the many daily anxieties created by having a child with congenital heart disease, the parents are not always willing or ready to accept cardiac surgery as therapy. It is the responsibility of the physician and also some of the other members of the health team such as the social worker or religious advisor to help the parents to understand the rationale for surgery and to help them make the decision regarding it. The parents frequently find it difficult to make the decision for the younger child as he is too small to help in the decision. The older child can be included in the discussion and his reaction can be evaluated as part of the decision-making process.

Many factors can influence the parents' decision regarding surgery. When the newborn is severely handicapped and gasping for breath the parent may be eager to have surgery as they see it as an only chance for the baby to survive. For a toddler or preschooler who has been severely incapacitated by the heart defect, the parent may look at the surgery as another stressful situation to which they would rather not subject the child. This is an especially common reaction when the child is hospitalized frequently and reacts poorly to hospitalization.

When the child's physical appearance mimics the severity of the defect, the rationale for surgery is more evident. However, when the child looks and acts "normal" it is more difficult to understand the necessity for the surgery.

Another factor which may influence the parents' attitude toward surgery is the medical information they have received regarding the defect. Due to the difficulty in making definite diagnoses in infants, the mother is frequently given conflicting or false information. If she has been told the child will "grow out of it" she may reject the surgery on this basis. She may also doubt the competence of the medical personnel who have not been able to give her an exact explanation of what is wrong with her child's heart.

Another realistic factor in the decision-making process is the financial strain the surgery might cause. A social worker can be helpful in discussing this concern.

The availability of a facility equipped to do pediatric cardiac surgery is another factor. Traveling long distances may make the decision especially difficult, especially if it means separating the mother and child from the rest of the family for a long period of time. The risk which surrounds the surgery procedure as well as the projected life expectancy can also be relevant factors in the decision. Also the reactions of relatives and friends as well as the parents' experience with other families who had similar surgery cannot be underestimated.

In the study by Glaser (1964) it was also brought out that the parents had a great deal of anxiety about the cardiac catheterization preceding the surgery. Here again, the parents were very concerned about death.

From this point on, I will proceed on the assumption that the parents and child have consented to the surgery.

PREPARATION FOR SURGICAL REPAIR

The student should avail herself of the very excellent study by Florence Blake (1964), entitled "Open Heart Surgery in Children." Miss

Blake describes her work with children undergoing open heart surgery and her findings and suggestions are most appropriate for the student, who will be caring for a child undergoing open heart surgery. As always, the age of the child is one of the primary factors in the preparation for cardiac surgery. The younger children do not seem to be as eager to participate in their preoperative teachings as the older children. It is most appropriate to identify the child's ability to understand the preoperative preparation and to adjust it accordingly. While I will make the assumption this will be done, the plan of care I will now describe will probably best fit the school-age and adolescent child.

The child should be made aware of the environment in which he will find himself immediately preoperatively, and during his convalescent period. Depending on the clinical facilities this may be two different places or it may be one and the same. The child who is admitted for cardiac surgery has usually been hospitalized previously because the child usually has a cardiac catheterization as part of his preoperative evaluation. This procedure is usually done in the same hospital as his cardiac surgery. However, the child may have been on a completely different unit than any of the ones he will be subjected to on this hospitalization. The preparation of the child is best done in small sessions and when the child is fairly well rested. Therefore, it is good to plan his sessions after the rest period that normally takes place on the hospital unit. The preparation should give the child an opportunity to ask questions, to act out his fears, and to digest new information. In keeping with normal developmental factors the teaching will best take place when accompanied by the use of toys or books appropriate to the age of the child. The child should be exposed to the same types of things that he will be exposed to postoperatively. He should be introduced to tourniquets, to syringes, to blood pressure cuffs, to oxygen equipment, to suction equipment, to blow bottles, and to the intensive care unit if it is to be utilized. The child will have previous experience with some of these things but reintroducing them will give the child an opportunity to express how he feels about them. For instance, it would be quite rare for a child with a congenital heart disease not to have had his blood pressure taken. But this does not mean that a blood pressure cuff should be omitted from his preoperative teaching. A good way of seeing how he feels about the blood pressure cuff is to have him apply it to a doll and to see how he explains to the doll what he is going to do or how it is going to feel. This will give us valuable clues regarding how to introduce blood pressure taking to the child postoperatively. In the same manner each of the other items should be introduced to the child. In addition to this equipment, puppets can serve a valuable role in preoperative preparation. It is sometimes much easier for the child to express through a puppet on his hand how he feels than it is to express to a professional person, eye to eye, how he feels. With a puppet, he finds it perfectly legitimate to explain to you that he does not like being stuck with needles, or that he does not want to have his surgery done, or that he fears separation from his parent. Giving the child an opportunity to express these things makes it easier for us to do anticipatory guidance. It also suggests to us ways that the child may be able to express his anxiety postoperatively. For instance, if he used the puppet effectively preoperatively then why not give it to him postoperatively to see if he can again express his fears?

If the child was unable to utilize the puppets for self-expression preoperatively, then postoperatively we would know they were not the answer. If the child seemed to need a mode of expression and was not able to communicate verbally then we can be especially attuned to nonverbal clues. The nurse should record on her nursing notes the reaction of the child to the equipment so that the people caring for him immediately postoperatively will have the advantage of this information.

The child needs to be taught how to deep breathe and how to turn postoperatively. The degree to which he will participate postoperatively may be influenced by how creative the nurse is in introducing these things to him. Postoperatively the nurse can then reap the benefits of this preoperative teaching. For instance, if the child was taught deep breathing by blowing plastic bubbles then this toy should be available postoperatively to achieve the same purpose. If the child was taught deep breathing by blowing up balloons, a good supply of balloons must be available postoperatively. If the blow bottles were utilized with a particular color water in them preoperatively, the same color water should be used postoperatively. If we expect the child to carry over his preoperative teaching to his postoperative period then the mechanism should be the same so the child recognizes what it is we are asking him to do.

When we are teaching turning as a preoperative exercise it is imperative to tell the child that postoperatively it may hurt to turn because of the chest tube(s). If we neglect to tell him about the chest tube(s) then postoperatively he may refuse to turn because he does not want to dislodge it (them) or he may quickly find that it hurts when he turns, concluding that it is best not to turn at all. Simple truth will aid in the postoperative period. The inclusion of the aspect of pain will help negate the child's using it as an excuse for not turning. The child is quick to point out the nurse's weaknesses and he may blame you, the nurse, for the pain, if he is not cautioned that it will be present. The child should also know he can receive medication to reduce the pain.

The child who is to be cared for in an intensive care unit deserves the right to be oriented to that unit preoperatively. The child will benefit from being introduced to his nurses and being called by name by them. This helps him to realize that they know him and that he will not get lost. This is especially important for the younger child who fears separation and fears the possibility of getting lost. The school-age child will also benefit from this because he appreciates people knowing who he is and he also appreciates people knowing his nickname—so this should be utilized freely. The child is not accustomed to being called by his last name until he gets to high school, so it is a mistake for nurses to call him Jones or Smith or so forth. The child will respond best to that which he is used to.

Plastic canopies distort the child's vision. It is helpful to have him get in a tent prior to surgery so he will be aware of these distortions. He is frequently better able to cope with this experience before he has the added stress of surgery. It is also possible to explain the pipes, machinery, and noise caused by the tent during this preoperative preparation (see Fig. 1 and 2).

SLEEP

Another valuable preoperative evaluation would be that of the child's sleep patterns. The nurse should keep a record of the child's sleep during the day as well as at night (see Table 1).

A preoperative sleep pattern would give clues as to how the child ordinarily sleeps. It would help in postoperative positionings for comfort. The comfort measures would also be altered by specific positioning in relation to the surgery.

The sleep pattern would also show how long the child ordinarily sleeps during a certain period. We could then plan our nursing care so it would not interrupt these normal sleep patterns. For example, if the

TABLE 1

JOHN AGE 8	TIME	EXAMPLE	MEDICATIONS & TIME
12/8/69	7:00 A.M.	Sleeping, left side, soundly	None
	7:15 A.M.	Beginning to awaken	
	7:20 A.M.	Fully awake & alert	
	2:00 P.M.	Took 15 min to fall asleep Brown teddy bear	Digitalis—10:00 A.M. Phenobarbital ¼ gr. 10:00 A.M. and 2:00 P.M.
	3:00 P.M.	Awake & bright	
	9:00 P.M.	To bed at 8:00 P.M.— tossed, restless—asleep on left side 2 stuffed toys Prayers at bedtime	Phenobarbital ¼ gr. 8:00 P.M.
	11:00 P.M.	Very restless—awake	None

FIG. 1. Photo taken from inside an oxygen tent. Note the distorted image the child receives. Also try, with a child's sense of fantasy, to imagine what significance each of the parts play.

child usually takes an hour afternoon nap then why wake him in 45 min to take his blood pressure? Why not let him complete his normal sleep and perhaps complete a satisfying dream?

One of the major nursing objectives should be to provide the child with adequate rest. This is achieved by planning treatments and medications to meet the child's individual needs as opposed to meeting the hospital routines. This will necessitate good organization so that the child will only be disturbed on a limited basis.

FIG. 2. Inside an oxygen tent, note the additional obstacles in this photo which interfere with the child's visual field.

ELIMINATION

Preoperatively the child is frequently up and around. After his initial urine specimen is collected, his elimination does not seem to be important unless he is on intake and output ordered by the physician. The child is free to go to the bathroom and does not get adequate practice using the bedpan. It is helpful to have him use it a couple times to familiarize him with how it feels and the adjustments needed to void or defecate in a less than adequate position.

It is also important to record the words used by the child to describe his need to eliminate. If new words are taught, they are frequently forgotten during periods of acute stress, and the child will revert to his familiar words.

Foley catheters are frequently used postoperatively and they should be explained to the child during the preoperative preparation.

Constipation is guarded against both pre- and postoperatively as it is not favorable for the child to strain to defecate. If fluids cannot be forced to aid in this process, then the physician frequently orders a stool softener to be given.

DIAGNOSTIC PROCEDURES AND PREPARATION OF THE CHILD

There are a great number of diagnostic procedures which can be done to establish the diagnosis of heart disease and the child's readiness for surgery. Two of the more common ones are the electrocardiograph and the cardiac catheterization.

EKG (ELECTROCARDIOGRAPH). The electrocardiagram records the activity of the heart. This is accomplished by having the child lie in a supine position in his bed or on the table in the treatment room. The child is prepared by explaining the reason for the recording. For example:

"John, the doctor wants a drawing of your heart action. This does not hurt and will not take long. We have a special machine to do this drawing. It looks like a brown box but when the cover is open you will see it is a very special box. It is equipped to draw lines. You might think it is scribbling or you might think it looks like the 'Etch-a-Sketch game.' [If you have an Etch-a-Sketch game this can be used to demonstrate to the child.] Special paper will come through the machine and it will be a very long line picture when we are through. To get this picture we must place special pieces of metal on your body. [Show the child an electrode.] Before we do this we put a special liquid, which comes from a tube and may feel cool, on several parts of you—like your arm. We will point out the areas as we go along. The liquid and the metal will be removed after we get the drawing. You can help by lying still while we make the drawing. Do you have any questions?"

After the procedure is completed the electrode compound is washed off and the child can resume his usual activity.

CARDIAC CATHETERIZATION. The cardiac catheterization provides a much clearer picture of the specific defect than the electrocardiogram. This clearer picture is not obtained without an increased risk. The procedure is usually considered a surgical procedure requiring parental consent. It may be done in a special cardiac catheterization laboratory or in the operating room. The parents must have a clear understanding of the procedure and be given sufficient time to ask questions. The thought of anything entering their child's heart can be an especially threatening situation. Their fear can be easily transmitted to the child.

The explanation given the child will, as always, depend on his age and level of understanding. The toddler or preschooler needs to know he will not be able to eat or drink the morning of the procedure. He will also be medicated as it is necessary for the child to be as relaxed as possible for the procedure. The school-age child and adolescent may enjoy seeing a diagram of the heart and the pathway the catheter will pass. They also need reassurance that the procedure will not cause undue pain or discomfort. The chief discomfort the child will experience is the local pain created by doing the cut-down. A common site for the cut-down is the groin in younger children or the arm in older children.

The nurse or technician accompanying the child doing the procedure should wear a lead apron to protect herself from the x-ray being used to follow the direction of the catheter. The nurse should stay at the head of the table and attempt to provide diversional activities during the catheterization. The time needed to complete the procedure varies greatly but the nurse should be prepared to entertain the child for as long as 3 hr. In the early periods, when the child is not yet bored, story telling or reading books will be effective. Later, the child gets tired of lying supine and more creative things such as magic tricks can be tried. During the procedure, the child needs assurance that things are progressing satisfactorily. If possible, he needs to know approximately how much longer it will take. Such an explanation follows.

"Henry, the catheter is now in your heart and they are beginning to get the answers they need to their questions. This part will take another twenty minutes. You are cooperating very nicely. Do you have any questions?"

If the child is of school age or adolescent he may also enjoy learning the names of the various equipment in the laboratory such as the flouroscope, the electrocardiogram (which is probably familiar to him), the pressure recorders, oscilloscopic apparatus, and blood analyzing equipment. It must also be understood that this equipment can be extremely frightening as its size is overwhelming and the space provided is usually minimal, making the room appear very "cluttered" and "official." The use of pictures, mobiles, brightly colored walls, and friendly personnel helps to lessen the negative impact of such an area.

After the catheterization is completed, the cut-down is removed and a dressing applied to the area. The child's vital signs continue to need monitoring for the next 24 hr. The dressing is observed for signs of bleeding. A drop in vital signs or bleeding at the site of the cut-down may indicate internal bleeding and necessitate prompt attention from the physician. It is not common, but it is entirely possible that, despite the most careful maneuvering, the catheter can rupture a vessel or cause phlebitis. The risks involved in left heart catheterization are higher than in right heart catheterization because of the increased difficulty in reaching the left side. It must also be remembered that the more serious and complicated heart conditions run a higher risk rate as the physicians cannot always predict the defects prior to catheterization. These defects may allow the catheter to pass in other areas than expected. Also, younger children run a higher risk due to the smaller size of the heart, which causes more difficulty in passing the catheter and in visualizing the parts. Children included in these categories will need more constant observations.

The child is usually permitted a regular diet and increased fluid intake after the catheterization. It is usually common to have the child remain quiet the day of the catheterization and then return to normal activity the day afterwards.

In addition to the visual observations made, the physician will obtain blood samples from the heart chambers for oxygen analysis and he will have pressure recordings within the chambers to help him identify the defect and its severity.

The parents and child, if he is old enough, both deserve an explanation of the findings as soon as possible after completion of the catheterization. If the catheterization is postponed for any reason, the parent and child should be told the reason so they will not worry unnecessarily. The stress related to this procedure should not be underestimated by the professional team.

THE INTENSIVE CARE UNIT

The intensive care unit has both positive and negative aspects in caring for the child undergoing cardiac surgery. Some of the positive aspects are that the nurses are usually more knowledgeable about the equipment and acute aspects of the postoperative period. The equipment is readily available for any emergency (see Fig. 3). Medical personnel usually respond quicker to a call from this area. The unit usually is in closer proximity to the operating room if an emergency does arise and

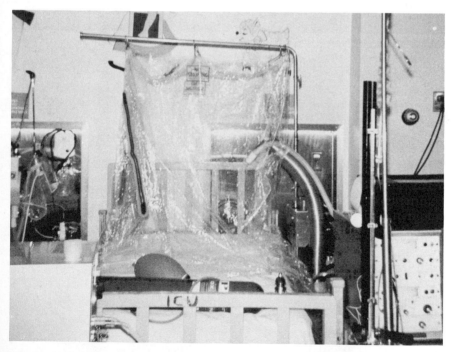

FIG. 3. An intensive care unit ready for a child returning from cardiac surgery. Emergency equipment is readily available.

the child needs to return to surgery. The negative aspects are usually concerned with the fact that the nurses frequently are so overly involved in the physical care of the child that they relegate to lesser importance the emotional aspects. Also, the visiting permitted within this unit is usually very short and the parents are usually left out in another area where they receive little in the way of progress reports on their child. Another negative aspect is the fact that the child is in an area where all of the children are acutely ill and when he is awake he is repeatedly exposed to the seriousness of the condition of the other children. He seldom has the advantage of seeing some children up running around or hearing the cheerful laughter of children at play. He is frequently in an environment which is more sterile in nature than the rooms on the convalescent floors. This "sterility" can be somewhat alleviated by making the environment more conducive to the care of the children. For the child in an oxygen tent, this can be easily achieved by hanging mobiles inside the tent, by placing toys in the tent (ones that are appropriate, such as rubber or wooden ones), by adding musical toys to the tents to cut down on the amount of motors the child is exposed to, by making the visual field that the child can see more colorful and less distorted (see Fig. 4 and 5). The child who is somewhat immobilized should have some type of toy or book within his visual

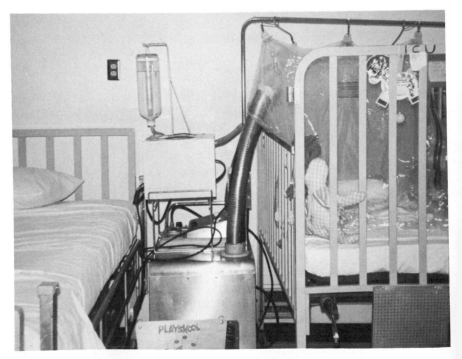

FIG. 4. Intensive care unit combining children's world and medical world.

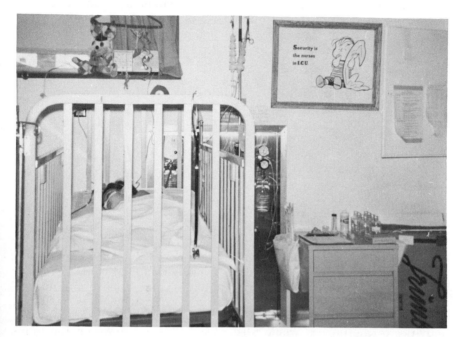

FIG. 5. Try to imagine what the child across the room thinks when he wakes up and sees this acutely ill child. Note the attempts to brighten up the environment. What additional things can be done?

field so that he does not have to turn around to find it. When he wakes up he sees color or animals or things he is ordinarily exposed to in his immediate vicinity. (Refer to Chapters 2 and 4 for a more complete discussion of toys and children's perceptions.)

The parents should also have the opportunity to be introduced to the intensive care unit, if they so desire. Some parents have stated that the visit to the intensive care unit has produced so much anxiety preoperatively that they felt less able to cope with their child's anxieties than if they had not visited it. Other parents have felt that it is a very important part of helping them to be more relaxed postoperatively. If they are not taken to the unit they should at least be told where it is and the easiest way of getting there. They should also be well aware of the restricted visiting hours, if they exist. There is no easy answer as to what amount of time the parent should spend with the child postoperatively and many of the hospital policies seem particularly restricted in this aspect. I think we need to ask ourselves, as nurses, what reasons we have for restricting visiting hours and who benefits most by the restriction—the child and his family or the personnel responsible for his care. If it is honestly the child and family who are benefiting then I think it justifies the limited visiting. If it is the medical personnel who seem to be gaining the most then I think it behooves us to reevaluate the restrictions and to make necessary adjustments. I am addressing myself now to the practice of allowing 5 min out of every hour, which is in effect in many agencies. I question whether a parent should be asked to sit for a total of 3 hr to spend a total of 15 min with his child or whether he might spend 15 min with his child and then go home and feel more relaxed having seen 15 min of care. The idea that during the 5 min the parents visit we do nothing for the child is an unrealistic one. The child who has undergone cardiac surgery frequently needs continual monitoring by professional personnel and leaving him alone even 5 min for the parent to be with him may be an unrealistic goal.

Parents are relieved to see that their child is receiving expert care. They also can ask more relevant questions if they can see actual care being given. Perhaps a viewing window would be more satisfactory than even entering the room, immediately postoperatively—especially if the child is dozing during the 5-min period that is allocated for visiting. A nurse, viewing with the parent, can then point out particular things about the child and his care. For instance, the parents may be so distracted by the equipment that is being used that they may benefit more by an explanation of this first. It takes time and courage for the parents to look past the equipment and to the child. Their 5 min may be up before this reaction takes place. If a viewing window is available, more time can be allocated without interfering with the ordinary activities of the unit. It would also conceivably cut down on the numbers of people in the area at any one time, and therefore, diminish the possibility of infection. It would also allow a discussion of equipment and the child's progress to take place away from the bedside of the children. This would be beneficial to both the child involved and the other children in the unit who may overhear conversations and think it is their progress being discussed.

Actual visiting in the unit would then have the specific purpose of communicating directly with the child. All communication with professional personnel could be done more effectively outside the intensive care unit. It is also difficult for the staff to establish any type of a meaningful relationship with the parents in a 5-min period. Meeting them outside would make it possible to spend a longer time with them (Fig. 6).

The viewing window should be accessible only with professional personnel available. If the parents were able to use this without supervision, it could heighten anxiety of both the parents and the professional staff.

PREPARATIONS

Is Preparation for the Emergency Situation Necessary? In the preoperative preparation of the child, I have not included the use of a doll with a tracheostomy. I am aware of previous writings about using a doll with a tracheostomy in preoperative preparation. My feeling in

FIG. 6. A mother and father view their acutely ill child through the intensive care unit window. The nurse is available to answer their questions and give support.

relation to this is that it may cause unnecessary anxiety in the young child and even in the school-age child to expose them to the possibility of emergency situations. The tracheostomy is not a routine postoperative condition and, therefore, I do not advocate preparing the child for this condition. If the doctor has indicated that the child will absolutely have a tracheostomy, then utilization of a doll with a tracheostomy in place can be of benefit to the child. The child will have an opportunity then to question why the tube is in place and will also be introduced to the idea of suctioning through the tracheostomy opening. In preparing the parents of the child, the procedure can be mentioned and explained and the rationale for not explaining it to the child given as honestly as possible.

The surgical procedure should be explained to the parents by the physician. The nurse is then in a position to explain the nursing intervention needed and to support the physician's explanation. She also uses this time to do significant teaching.

Preparation for Anesthesia. In many agencies the physician from the department of anesthesia will assume the role for preparing the child for anesthesia. In agencies where this is not done, the nurse can incorporate this into her preoperative plan. She needs to include an explanation regarding the mask that will be put over the child's face, the mode by which the child will get to the operating room, the clothes that the people in the operating room will be wearing, a description of what the operating room will look like, and a statement that the child will not be awake during the operation. An attempt should be made not to tell the child that he will be asleep but rather that it is a special type of a sleep that is induced by medication, so that the child will not fear going to sleep after the surgical procedure. The child should also be told that a doctor will watch him very closely during the entire time he is in this special sleep and will take responsibility for awakening him from his special sleep at the end of his surgery. The child should be told exactly when he will be separated from his parent. For instance, if the child can be accompanied to the operating room by the parent, he should know this. If the policies of the hospital do not permit a parent to accompany the child, then the child and parent should both know this. The child should know by what means he will be taken to the operating room, and who will take him there. For instance, if he is to go on an adult-type stretcher, then he needs to know this. If a small carriage will take him to the operating room, then he needs to know this (see Fig. 7). If a person dressed in a green outfit comes to get him he should know this, or if a nurse that he is very familiar with will take him then he needs to know this. The child should also choose a toy or toys which he would like to take to the operating room with him. A notation should be made on the Kardex regarding his choice so the toy or toys are included in the preoperative check list. This is all based on the idea that the more the child knows, the less fear there will be of the unknown and the less possibility there will be for misunderstanding.

The foregoing information can be applied to children undergoing any type of cardiac surgery. In addition, the nurse must be able to make additions or modifications to meet the special nursing responsibilities in relation to the child's specific diagnosis. For instance, there may be much more preparation needed for a child who is scheduled for open heart surgery with utilization of the heart lung machine than with a child who is having a closed cardiac procedure. I will not attempt to go through the many types of cardiac defects in this book. For this information, the student should refer to a book on pediatric surgery that explores the cardiac conditions.

Postoperative Care

In the postoperative period it is important to utilize the preoperative preparation of the child. For instance, as soon as he returns to the intensive care unit or area for his immediate postoperative care, he should be introduced to it in the following manner:

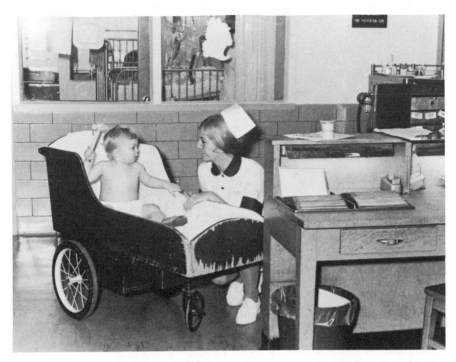

FIG. 7. Carts such as this one cut down on the fear of going to the x-ray, operating rooms, and to play activities. They allow the child to sit up and to take favorite toys along.

"Johnny, this is the intensive care unit you visited yesterday. I am your nurse, Miss Jones. Remember, I called you Johnny yesterday and said, 'See you tomorrow.' You are going into the oxygen tent that you saw yesterday. This oxygen tent may feel a little cool and may feel a little damp. That is to be expected. If you are cool, let me know so I can cover you, or wipe you off if you have moisture dripping on you. You now have the chest tubes you saw on the doll, Johnny, they are on your left side. Do not touch them. Soon I will ask you to breathe nice and deep. I will give you a balloon to blow, like you had upstairs. It will not be as easy to blow today as it was yesterday, but each day it will get easier."

In this way the child will be quickly reintroduced to his environment and to what has gone on prior to surgery. Consistent use of this technique will aid the child in his recovery and will aid the nurse in gaining the child's cooperation. The child should be repeatedly reminded that while he has pain now, each day he will have improvement and less pain. He needs more encouragement that he will get better than the adult patient does. He is usually more interested in himself and his immediate environment than he is in the future and, therefore, he needs more reassurance that this pain is transient in nature. The child will also want immediate gratification of his needs and he should know how to get this gratification. If he must call for the nurse, then he should know the means of calling for the nurse. If a nurse will be with him continuously, then he should know there is a nurse by his side and that perhaps even a hand motion is all he needs to gain her attention.

During his immediate postoperative period, the child will derive a great deal of satisfaction from getting his physical needs met adequately. However, as he begins to come along in the convalescent period, he will need more and more attention given to his emotional needs. As he begins to improve, he will begin to question, verbally and nonverbally, reasons for the nurse's activity. A simple, truthful explanation is always the rule in guiding the nurse. The child who has undergone cardiac surgery frequently is exposed to a large number of people delivering care immediately postoperatively. Due to this, he is not always aware of who is directly responsible when he wants something. The nurse can play a key role in this by always identifying when she is responsible for his care and who is responsible when she is not available. In addition to meeting the emotional needs of the child, the nurse will be responsible for many of the other procedures which are done to and for the child during the immediate postoperative period.

CHEST TUBES AND SUCTION

The student will usually have had experience with chest tubes with adult patients prior to seeing them in the pediatric patient. The same principles apply to the pediatric patient as the adult patient. First, the tubes should be checked to make sure there is no kinking; second, the bandage around the tube should be free of drainage, and if drainage does appear, it should be encircled and watched for increase in drainage; third, a Kelly clamp should be available for each tube that is in place. In case of emergency, the student would clamp off the tube as close to the chest wall as possible. Fourth, the tube should be connected to some type of drainage. Frequently the three-bottle suction is utilized for drainage. One of these bottles is the drainage bottle, the second bottle the control bottle, and the third the safety bottle (see Fig. 8).

The tubes must also be securely anchored to the bed to help prevent undue tension on them. This can be achieved by placing adhesive tape around the tubes, without constricting them, and then using a safety pin to pin the adhesive to the sheet.

The tubes also need special attention when the patient is turned. Care must be taken not to have the patient's weight resting on the tubes. The tubes must also be replaced after turning to reestablish adequate draining. (For a detailed explanation of three-bottle suction, the student should refer to Dr. Jensen's textbook entitled *Introduction to Medical Physics*.)

The nurse must also know who is responsible for emptying and measuring the chest drainage. The procedure may vary from one institution to another. Some measure drainage after each tour of duty and others measure it daily.

PATIENT   SUCTION

DRAINAGE   WATER SEAL   SUCTION CONTROL
BOTTLE   BOTTLE   BOTTLE

FIG. 8. Three-bottle system for closed chest drainage.

VITAL SIGNS

The immediate postoperative period will demand a great deal of the nurse's energy. She will be kept busy monitoring many things. Not the least of these is the child's vital signs. Vital signs are usually learned early by the beginning nurse and may seem like "just old hat" after a period of practice. However, for the child who has undergone cardiac surgery, the vital signs may be more of a challenge.

Preoperatively, the vital signs were recorded by both physicians and nurses. Each had an opportunity to cross-check their results. In addition, vital signs could be obtained under differing sets of conditions. These results should be carefully recorded so they can be effectively utilized postoperatively (see Table 2).

The variations in rates with activity can be used as gauges in planning postoperative activity. The use of varying areas for counting the pulse rate can also be useful postoperatively. If preoperatively all

TABLE 2

JOHN AGE 8	TIME	ACTIVITY	PULSE AREA	BP	R
	8:00 A.M.	Just awakened	100-Radial (lt)	100/62	16
	11:00 A.M.	Active play	110-Radial (lt) 122-Carotid (rt)	104/64	20
	12:30 P.M.	Following self-feeding	110-Radial (rt)	104/64	24

the pulse rates were taken on the left radial pulse, and postoperatively the child has a cut-down or intravenous infusion in that area, then the child's routine has to be disrupted. It is better to teach him that pulses may be obtained radially, apically, femorally, carotidly, or on the feet (dorsalis pedis). You can then explain to the child that anyone of these areas may be used to get his pulse. Letting the child count his own pulse or the nurse's pulse is also helpful in gaining his cooperation.

Pulse rates vary from cardiac condition to cardiac condition and from one age child to another age child. This creates problems in knowing what is "normal" for a certain child. The child's rate may also change due to the nature of the surgery. For instance, a child with coarctation of the aorta may lack pedal pulses. Postoperatively this rate is established by improvement in blood flow. The beginning student will need to read in relation to pediatric surgery to become familiar with each cardiac anomaly and its particular influence on the child's vital signs.

The blood pressure is another invaluable monitor, if it is taken correctly. The key to correct recordings is to select the appropriately fitting cuff. This is usually two-thirds of the child's upper arm. If possible, the child's pressure should always be taken with the same cuff. This is usually fairly easy to accomplish in a small well-equipped intensive care unit, but may be more difficult on a bigger patient unit, where only one or two cuffs are available for use with numerous children.

The limited distribution of the cuff also cuts down on the possibility of cross-contamination, which is so important both preoperatively and postoperatively with children having cardiac surgery. (The area of protection from infection is covered more thoroughly in a separate section.)

In addition to being of the right size, the cuff should be applied snugly and anchored securely before being inflated. This can be easily achieved if you have adequately prepared the child and gained his cooperation. The child should know that it will feel tight on his arm when you pump up the cuff. The child may enjoy holding the dial so you can read it. This makes him feel a responsibility for helping with his own care. The acutely ill child may not be able to participate but may benefit from having a toy to hold during the procedure. If it is necessary to recheck the reading, be sure to tell the child you are inflating the cuff again. Frequent rechecking may cause anxiety to the child, so optimal conditions should be achieved prior to beginning. These optimal conditions include proper positioning of the child and the cuff, removal of clothing between cuff and arm, as much quiet as possible, and turning off any motors which may safely be eliminated during the short period of time needed.

When in doubt of a recording, ask another nurse to check it. No one should put her pride before the child's welfare. If a recording is not easily obtainable, it may very well be an early sign of distress.

The respiratory rate is probably more variable than either the pulse rate or the blood pressure. The respiratory rate can be significantly decreased during sleep or due to postoperative medication. Respiratory rate can be significantly increased by apprehension. It can be quite irregular when the trachea needs suctioning. Sternal retractions can develop when there is respiratory distress. Some of the variations obviously hold little significance while some of them are real clues for the nurse. A simple suctioning procedure may clear the passageway and reestablish a normal respiratory rate after rest. A rapid shallow rate may indicate more serious difficulty and coupled with other unfavorable vital signs, such as a decrease in blood pressure, may need immediate medical intervention.

OTHER RECORDINGS

The central venous pressure (CVP) is also monitored closely. This is done to be sure that the child is not receiving too much intravenous fluid or losing too much blood.

The child is on intake and output and may also be on urinary specific gravity recordings.

Each hospital has its own procedure for recording these nursing observations. In addition to those specifically ordered by the physician, the nurse has several more significant observations which will be useful in determining the child's progress or lack of progress.

Nursing Observations

One observation will be in relation to the warmth of the child's body. Is it only warm to touch on the trunk, despite a slight postoperative temperature elevation? What is needed to warm the child's cold extremities? Is a pair of cotton socks or mitts adequate? Does he need three cotton blankets inside the tent to rest comfortably? Or does he toss and turn and try curling up to get warm despite the use of three blankets?

In relation to medication for pain, does the child rest quietly after absorption or does he still have the look of anxiety in his eyes? Does he seem to need medication to achieve his much needed rest? Does he seem to need medication after visits from the doctor, or his parents, or the laboratory technician? Does he cough better if he receives his medication prior to coughing or should it be withheld for better results? Does any one procedure, such as suctioning, trigger his need for medication? Does his pain interrupt his sleep? Any of these recordings can be valuable guides to the physician responsible for ordering adequate doses of medication.

As a student, you should ask yourself what other observations are significant in caring for this child. Are vital signs, warmth, and pain the only indicators necessary to achieve effective nursing care? This necessitates an evaluation process which is extremely important. The evaluation process will include such factors, such as providing a safe environment, maintaining adequate fluid and electrolyte balance, and maintaining adequate oxygenation.

OBJECTIVE: SAFE ENVIRONMENT

On the subject of meeting the objective of providing the child with a safe environment, we have already discussed the precautions in regard to chest tubes, the rechecking of vital signs by two competent persons, and the safe administration of intravenous fluids. As yet we have not included the use of side rails when the nurse is not at the bedside, the positioning of the oxygen tent for protection if the siderail cannot be pulled up, the precaution of not using woolen blankets in oxygen tents, and the correct positioning of electrical equipment to avoid contact with the oxygen tent.

The child should be placed in an area where he will be exposed to the least amount of cross-contamination. This contamination may be the result of drafts due to opening doors, open windows, or other patients, staff, or family. His care should be limited to a few well-qualified professional personnel who are in optimum health.

The safe environment should also include a check of the child's toys. Toys with sharp edges should not be left in the crib as he might roll on them and hurt himself or puncture a tube.

Providing a safe environment also includes the use of restraints as a protection for the child. Younger children sometimes have mitts applied, rather than restraints, to protect them from pulling at the tubes.

OBJECTIVE: FLUID AND ELECTROLYTE BALANCE

The objective of maintaining adequate fluid and electrolyte balance has been partially covered in the discussion of CVP recordings and intake and output. In addition, depending on the postoperative course, it will soon be the nurse's responsibility to provide the child with adequate oral intake. This intake should be divided to allow for evening and night personnel to also offer the child fluids. Spacing of the allowed oral intake will decrease the child's possibility of extreme thirst on any one tour of duty. It will also diminish the possibility of the night nurse's feeling obliged to get the child to take all the remainder of the fluid intake for the 24-hr period.

Urinary output is usually not difficult to obtain from children. Depending on their age, they are used to voiding more frequently. However, many children will have indwelling catheters immediately postoperatively. This will necessitate additional care of the perineal area. A doctor's order is not needed to give perineal care. The measuring of urinary output may be on an hourly basis during the immediate post-operative period. As the child progresses, it may be measured on each shift or daily. Again, it is the nurse's responsibility to be aware of the policy being followed as accurate reporting of intake and output is essential.

The student is referred to Fig. 9 for a comparison of the adult and infant extracellular water turnover for a day. This will help to emphasize the extreme importance of keeping accurate account of all the fluid entering or leaving the child's body.

Normal individuals of all ages require 100 to 150 ml of maintenance water per 100 calories metabolized. Since the infant and child have higher metabolic rates per kilogram than does the adult, the younger patient needs more water per unit of weight than the older patient (Statland, 1963). (See Table 3.)

In addition the student should be aware of the ordinary maintenance requirements of fluid. According to Statland (1963), the amount of water given should approximate the fluid expended for ordinary physiologic activity. Studies in both infants and adults indicate that these losses are roughly proportional to energy expenditure (see Table 4).

FIG. 9. Body water partition and comparison of daily water turnover to the extracellular fluid volume in the newborn and the adult. (Courtesy of Statland, 1963.)

TABLE 3

APPROXIMATE ENERGY EXPENDITURE DURING PARENTERAL FLUID THERAPY[1]

| | | CALORIES EXPENDED | | MAINTENANCE WATER |
AGE	WEIGHT (IN KG)	TOTAL (PER 24 HR)	PER KG PER 24 HR	PER 100 CAL (IN ML)
4 Months	5	500	100	100
2 Years	15	1250	83	100
10 Years	30	1700	57	100
Adult	60	2300	38	100

[1] After Statland (1963).

I should like to reemphasize that this is only *maintenance require-ments* for the child. The intake will also include fluid to replace losses during the operative and postoperative period.

For information about intravenous equipment, the student is re-ferred to a pediatric nursing textbook and to the company supplying the intravenous equipment in a particular hospital.

The nurse should also aid the physician in determining losses which are not easily measured—the loss by perspiration, drainage, or bed-wetting. The wet sheet may be a poor way to estimate loss as fluid quickly spreads in sheets and gives a false impression of a large loss. However, it is important to include this information in the nurse's notes. For example: "Sheet changed—moderate amount serosanguineous drainage in area of chest bandage. Drainage appeared between 8:00 and 10:00 A.M."

In addition, the nurse needs to observe the child for perspiration. It is not enough to assume that if his johnny shirt is dry, then he is not perspiring. The perspiration may show on his forehead or the palms of his hands. A flushing of the child's face is also significant, as it may be a clue to additional water losses.

TABLE 4

USUAL EXPENDITURES OF WATER PER 100 CALORIES METABOLIZED[1]

	ML H_2O PER 100 CALORIES
Insensible perspiration	45
lungs	15
skin	30
Sweat (sensible perspiration)	20
Stool	5
Urine	30 to 80
Total	100 to 150

[1] After Darrow and Pratt (Courtesy of Statland, 1963).

OBJECTIVE: ADEQUATE OXYGENATION

The child will usually receive oxygen immediately postoperatively. This can be achieved by using an isolette with an infant or an oxygen tent with an older child. Infrequently an adolescent may receive nasal oxygen. The nasal administration of oxygen dries the mucus membranes and is more irritating to the child. Oxygen administered by other methods is given with mist and this lubricates the mucus membranes. If for any reason, the child has to be transported to another area for x-ray, nasal oxygen or mask oxygen can be used during the transporting.

The administration of oxygen by isolette provides a fairly constant oxygen supply unless the top of the isolette is opened. Most nursing care can be effectively administered through the portholes. If the top is opened, the infant may become hypoxic. If so, the isolette should be closed and a high concentration of oxygen delivered to resaturate the isolette. The liter flow of oxygen should be prescribed by the doctor. The 40 percent concentration may be in effect if it is a very small infant; however, it is not nearly so important if the child's blood supply to the eyes is mature.

The oxygen tent does not guarantee as good a supply of oxygen for the older child. There is a wider area involved, the light weight plastic canopy is less effective than the harder plastic, and there is more possibility for oxygen to escape because the tent is only tucked under the mattress or bed linens. For making an oxygen bed, the student should refer back to a pediatric nursing textbook.

Just a word about ultrasonic nebulization as it is frequently used with oxygen administration and is only now beginning to get some scrutiny. According to Crocker (1970), continuous ultrasonic nebulization should never be used in infants and probably not in older children either, as it may supply as much as 6 ml per minute of fluid to the child and particularly in intubated infants, water intoxication may occur. It is possible to supply the infant or child with his total daily water requirement by ultrasonic nebulization.

The nurse should observe the child for signs of cyanosis. Cyanosis usually appears first in the child's fingernails. For this reason, any nail polish should be removed prior to surgery and left off during the child's postoperative period. Another area to observe is the child's lips or around the oral orifice. Cyanosis may be an expected symptom due to the child's cardiac condition and it may not disappear as a result of a palliative cardiac procedure. The student will familiarize herself with the cardiac defects to know whether this cyanosis is expected.

Adequate suctioning is also necessary to provide an adequate oxygen supply. The nasal passages should be kept clean and mucus suctioned from the trachea. Sterile technique should be adhered to during suctioning to cut down on the possibility of infection. Deeper suctioning may be necessary, and this is again determined by the policies of the hospital and the nurse's training. In some hospitals only physicians do the deeper suctioning, but it is becoming more common for nurses to be taught this procedure.

Crocker (1970) recommends that assisted ventilation be performed prior to suctioning episodes when a tracheostomy is in place. This ventilation is done with a suitable bag and adaptor for 3 to 5 minutes prior to suctioning in order to prevent the rapid aspiration of oxygen from the airway with resultant hypoxia.

COUGHING, TURNING, DEEP BREATHING

It is now that the nurse reaps the benefits of the preoperative teaching. She utilizes the same techniques used preoperatively to get the child's cooperation. These procedures aid in the maintenance of oxygenation and are routine postoperative procedures.

Intermittent positive-pressure therapy is frequently used in addition to the administration of oxygen. In the less serious cardiac conditions, the child may not receive continuous oxygen therapy but may receive IPPB to help loosen secretions and clear the bronchial tree.

Pain must not be forgotten as a possibility of causing respiratory problems and diminishing oxygen supply. The child may intentionally choose not to breathe deeply in order to decrease the amount of pain. It is the nurse's responsibility to evaluate the child's pain and to administer narcotics to keep him comfortable. Narcotics can decrease the respiratory rate and this should also be kept in mind.

It is quite evident that the independent nursing activities play a big role in the maintenance of adequate oxygenation.

MONITORS

Monitors of various types may be utilized to chart the patient's postoperative course. These monitors may be of varying degrees of complexity and the company information in describing their use should be investigated. A clear understanding should be made as to the nurse's responsibility in relation to the monitors.

The nurse's role in emergency measures is determined by her training and education in relation to the procedure, the policies of the hospital, and the legal implications to the nurse. Student nurses should not assume or be expected to assume the full responsibility for a child with a cardiac arrest. The most skilled person should begin the mouth-to-mouth resuscitation or use the emergency equipment available.

REORIENTATION TO TIME AND PLACE

The intensive care unit should be equipped with clocks and calendars to help reorient the child to time and place. The younger child will enjoy having a children's clock. The type wound by pulling chains can be fun. The older child will benefit by an ordinary clock. The clock should be close by the bedside, so the child can refer to it easily. For older children, the calendars can be of the conventional type, with scenes depicting areas of the child's interest. For the younger child a calendar can be made and large numbers used. The numbers can be added daily so he knows the last one up is the day's date. In addition, clouds, rain, sun, or snow pictures can be added so the child knows the weather. This is especially important if the child cannot see out of the window. Changes of the weather can be made during the day if changes occur outside. This is helpful too if the parents are unable to get to the hospital because of inclement weather, the child has already been oriented to that possibility.

CONVALESCENCE AND DISCHARGE

The convalescent period will depend on the surgery and its follow-up supervision. The degree of activity will be prescribed by the physician. The parents and child must be fully informed of the activity allowed as well as any restrictions. They should be fully aware of their follow-up appointments. They also need to know any adverse signs which necessitate immediate medical care.

The child who has received a significant improvement in his physical condition due to surgical repair may have a difficult time adjusting to his new status. Glaser et al. (1964) notes that the child and the parent may have a difficult time adjusting to the more vigorous physical activity now possible for the child. The child will need time to adjust to the extended privileges of independence with his peers. He may also have difficulty adjusting to the more strenuous educational goals now open to him.

If the surgery has been less successful, the parents and child have to learn to accept the permanency of the condition and to readjust their goals in relation to the limitations imposed by the cardiac condition.

A STUDENT'S CONTINUITY-OF-CARE EXPERIENCE

A composite picture of Larry, age 7 years, preparing for a repair of a ventriculoseptal defect. The student planned for the experience by reading and talking with the cardiac surgeon and the nursing faculty. She visited the patient's home prior to surgery and taperecorded her interview. The tape was later reviewed by the nursing faculty and the student. The student admitted Larry to the hospital, did additional preoperative preparation, and cared for him postoperatively. After discharge she again visited the home and taperecorded her interview. The nursing faculty then sent a questionnaire to the mother eliciting her feelings regarding the student's participation in their hospital experience. The results were very favorable (see Figs. 10–14).

FIG. 10. Carolyn visits Larry and "Rover" in their home prior to hospitalization. (Courtesy of Carolyn Voght.)

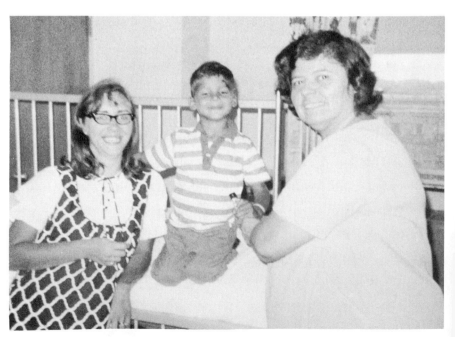

FIG. 11. Larry and his family seem delighted to see Carolyn as they begin the admission procedure. (Courtesy of Carolyn Voght.)

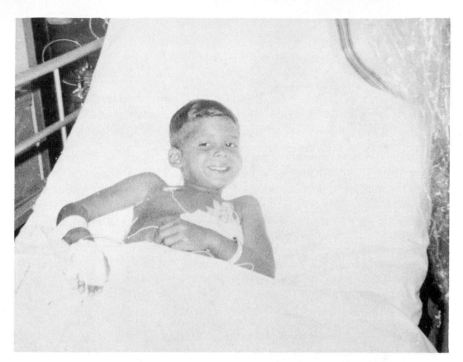

FIG. 12. Larry, one day post-operative from open-heart surgery. (Courtesy of Carolyn Voght.)

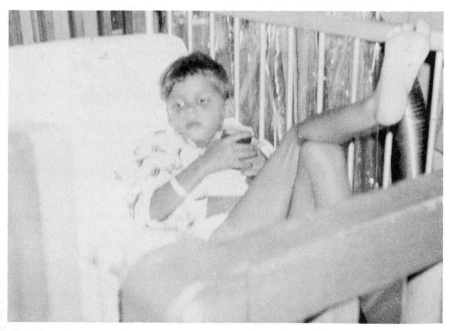

FIG. 13. Larry enjoys using the transistor unit to change his TV program on his second day post-operative. Note the positioning he chooses for comfort. (Courtesy of Carolyn Voght.)

FIG. 14. Larry returns home to some familiar surroundings and some surprises. (Courtesy of Carolyn Voght.)

Rheumatic Fever

I have chosen rheumatic fever to illustrate a medical condition requiring long-term care. It was chosen because of its high incidence of related carditis and the extended care needed even without carditis.

The length of the period needed for treating the disease as well as the fear generated by repeated susceptibility to the disease are factors contributing to the respect given the disease. Also, the knowledge that the disease is responsible for the majority of heart disease in persons under 40 years of age makes it a particularly "dreaded" disease. It is also responsible for a significant number of deaths in children.

Rheumatic fever is a long-term disease that illustrates the significance of the *host* factor in relation to disease. Two factors which play a part in the disease are economics and environment. The child from a lower socioeconomic family is more prone to the disease. This may be related to the child's physical environment. If the house is crowded or damp, which are frequently conditions of the lower socioeconomic housing, the child is more susceptible to rheumatic fever. After the child becomes infected by the streptococcus organism, he is less likely to be able to combat the attack, and rheumatic fever follows. The child from a crowded home is more likely to be exposed to more bacteria because of his close associations with other people in the household or building. Also, in conditions of overcrowding, minor infections such as pharyngitis are less likely to receive medical attention.

Age is another factor. Children between the ages of five and fifteen years are most commonly affected. The children in this age range are also more susceptible to streptococcal infections. Latitude and altitude are also considered to affect the incidence of rheumatic fever. The disease has a higher incidence in temperate zones and in seasons when respiratory infections reach their maximum peak—late winter and early spring.

The age factor seems to also play a role in reinfection. As the child gets older, he is less likely to suffer rheumatic fever as a result of reinfection with the streptococcus organism.

Heredity may also play a role in the disease as there is a higher than usual incidence of the disease in more than one family member.

Rheumatic fever seems to be decreasing in incidence as the standards of living are improved. Another important factor in the apparent decrease is the use of antimicrobial therapy. Stronger statements regarding decrease cannot be made, as the disease is not always reported; therefore, its true incidence is really not known.

Another factor which makes reporting difficult is the problem of making a definite diagnosis. The Jones criteria have been developed as a guide for physicians (see Table 5).

PRESENTING SYMPTOMS

The child who has had a Group A hemolytic streptococcus infection may recover with little attention to the illness. Approximately four weeks later, the child may have any one of a number of symptoms. He may report to the school nurse with a headache, or a sudden sore throat, or he may develop abdominal pain with nausea and vomiting. The headache or sore throat may receive little attention as the school nurse or parent may not link them to the child's previous illness. The abdominal pain may get better attention as it closely resembles the pain of appendicitis. The child frequently has a temperature elevation of 101° to 104° F.

On closer examination by a physician the child may show additional signs such as a reddened throat, a rash on the trunk, or subcutaneous nodules.

TABLE 5

JONES CRITERIA (REVISED) FOR GUIDANCE IN THE DIAGNOSIS OF
RHEUMATIC FEVER[1]

MAJOR MANIFESTATIONS	MINOR MANIFESTATIONS
Carditis	Clinical
Polyarthritis	Previous rheumatic fever or rheumatic heart
Chorea	disease
Erythema marginatum	Arthralgia
Subcutaneous nodules	Fever
	Laboratory
	Acute phase reactions
	Erythrocyte sedimentation rate,
	C-reactive protein, leukocytosis
	Prolonged P-R interval

SUPPORTING EVIDENCE OF STREPTOCOCCAL INFECTION
Increased titer of streptococcal antibodies
ASO (antistreptolysin O)
Other Antibodies
Positive throat culture for Group A streptococcus
Recent scarlet fever

[1] The presence of two major criteria, or of one major and two minor criteria, indicates a high probability of the presence of rheumatic fever. Evidence of a preceding streptococcal infection greatly strengthens the possibility of acute rheumatic fever. Its absence should make the diagnosis doubtful (except in Syndenham's chorea or long-standing carditis).
From Jones Criteria (revised) for guidance in the diagnosis of rheumatic fever, © 1967 American Heart Association.

If a physician is not available at school, the parent should be instructed to seek a medical opinion. Treating the child at home with aspirin may only mask the symptoms and delay the therapeutic regime.

THE ACUTE PHASE

The nursing responsibilities during the acute phase center around astute observations of signs and symptoms and alleviation of pain. The child admitted without a previous history of rheumatic fever will have diagnostic tests prior to instituting medical therapy. During this period, the child may be extremely uncomfortable due to pain in the large joints. The mother may say to you, "Please give him an aspirin, it helped his pain at home." It is important to explain to his mother and to the child that proper use of drugs is dependent on the tests which are scheduled. In the interim, the doctor has not prescribed aspirin. The mother and child may benefit further by talking with the doctor.

Nursing measures can help to make the child more comfortable. The affected joint or joints may feel more comfortable when supported on pillows. When the child turns he may appreciate support to the limb. The child will benefit by a properly fitted foot board, one that supports the feet and not merely the bed clothes. The foot board must be placed so the feet can easily reach it without effort on the child's part (see Fig. 15).

If the bedclothes seem to be causing pressure on the affected parts, a bed cradle may be used. If it is, the child might enjoy a small, light-weight receiving blanket next to his body (his "security blanket").

During the acute phase, the child will frequently have a temperature elevation. This makes him more prone to perspire. A comforting measure is to bathe the child more frequently with tepid water. He will also need more frequent changes of bed linen. Skin care is also important. The child may try to "overprotect" his involved arms by not moving them at all. This will increase the possibility of irritation under the axilla due to perspiration. Cleaning, drying thoroughly, and applying a light dusting of talcum powder will help to prevent skin breakdown and also odor. The older child may try to discourage the nurse from washing under the axilla. The child offers a can of spray deodorant and tries to have just this used. He needs to know that repeated application of deodorants, without washing, will only add to the irritation problem. An explanation that you will move the limb as gently as possible will usually win the child's approval or at least his cooperation.

The observation of signs and symptoms will aid the physician in his attempt to diagnose the illness adequately. One of the responsibilities of the nurse is the accurate taking of a pulse rate. This is counted for a full minute to get as accurate a count as possible. The pulse is usually taken every 4 hr. In addition a sleeping pulse is frequently ordered during the night. The nurse must be very gentle so she does not awaken the child. If the child does wake up, the pulse should be scheduled for a later hour and the actual time recorded.

Another observation the nurse can make is in relation to the rash which is sometimes present in children with rheumatic fever. It frequently appears during the child's bath and then disappears. The rash should be described and the areas involved clearly spelled out in the nurse's notes or progress record.

During the bath it is also possible to check for any nodules and

FIG. 15.   Proper placement of footboard for maximum utilization.

describe their location. Any limitation of movement of limbs can also be evaluated during the bath. The bath is usually given by the nurse during the evaluation period, on the assumption that the child has the disease. After diagnosis the bath is usually given by the nurse until all signs of acute infection have subsided and the laboratory results are returning to normal or near normal ranges.

BED-REST

The child with acute rheumatic fever is usually placed on complete bed-rest. This therapy is beginning to be questioned. Some physicians are now allowing the child out of bed after 48 hr on medication while others still maintain bed-rest for several weeks. However, the physician will prescribe the activity restrictions for the individual child. The nurse will be responsible for trying to maintain this order. During the acute stage, the child is usually in pain and bed-rest is maintained easier than during the convalescent stage. During the convalescent period, it becomes increasingly difficult to provide activities that will make him content, despite his restrictions. (This will be discussed in greater detail in relation to the convalescent period.)

Positioning of the child is extremely important because of the possible circulatory involvement and the effects of bed-rest. Rubber rings and donuts are *not* indicated. Careful attention to the bed linen to get rid of wrinkles is very important. Also, children are prone to drop crumbs, crayons, and other small objects, like paper clips in their beds. These items can cause pressure and lead to decubitus. The child will also benefit from having the head of the bed elevated. The degree of elevation needed for the child to be comfortable should be included in the observations. In the more acute circumstances, the child may be placed in an oxygen tent.

MOUTH CARE

The child who is having pain frequently breathes through his mouth. This will cause drying of the mucus membranes and perhaps cracking at the corners of the mouth. Mouth care should be given, using the child's toothbrush and paste from home. If these items are not available, a hospital mouthwash and cleaning with cotton tip applicators can be done until a toothbrush and paste are available. Some mineral oil or cold cream can be applied sparingly to the lips if they are cracking. Children are not usually receptive to the common lemon and glycerin offered adults for mouth care. A scientific rationale for selectively using lemon and glycerin is illustrated in a study by Van Drimmelen and Rollins (1969) on elderly people. Lemon and glycerin one-to-one dried the oral tissues at the first few days after instituting care. This drying can be very uncomfortable to a child who breathes through his mouth. It is also contraindicated in children immediately postoperatively when you are attempting to keep the mucus membranes moist. The lemon and glycerin tended to increase the moisture in the mouth after four or five days of use, but by this time the child is frequently well enough to resume brushing in the usual manner. The study did show, however, that cleansing with lemon and glycerin did improve the general condition of the mouth and the findings support the rationale for mouth care. (The prepared applicators for oral hygiene are saturated solutions of glycerin and lemon one-to-one.)

If the child uses an electric toothbrush at home, this may provide a nice link with home, if it can be brought in. It is necessary to make this judgment after exploring the type of electric toothbrush used.

The battery-operated types can be used if oxygen is in use but the ones that require electric cords should not be used when oxygen is in use.

TRIAL WITH ASPIRIN

After the preliminary laboratory tests are completed, the physician may begin a trial period with aspirin. Nursing responsibilities include administering the drug on a prescribed time schedule, noting relief of pain from the drug, noting the recurrence of pain if any, and noting side-effects such as ringing in the ears or nausea.

This trial period is especially important as it may provide very essential information to the diagnosing physician. Very detailed nursing notes are essential during this period.

DRUG THERAPY

After the diagnosis has been established, the child is started on drug therapy. This may include a combination of salicylates, adrenal corticosteroids, and, occasionally, barbiturates. The steroids may be withheld to see if there is cardiac involvement and how severe it is. In approximately 50 to 70 percent of initial cases, cardiac involvement may not be an issue. The steroids have been found to be more effective than aspirin in combating the acute inflammation but they do not seem to cut down the cardiac scarring. For this reason, they are frequently omitted and aspirin given alone. The use of barbiturates is dependent on how anxious or active the child is during the acute phase. They are used more when carditis is present. Digitalis and diuretics may also be ordered for treatment of the heart failure during acute rheumatic fever. A course of penicillin is given to combat the Group A streptococci. The penicillin therapy is usually administered through adulthood on a prophylactic basis.

The length of time the aspirin or cortisone therapy is continued varies from six weeks to twelve weeks, with the more involved forms lasting six months or more. The drugs are withdrawn on a gradual basis with close attention being given to the C-reactive protein and the sedimentation rate. The C-R protein gradually disappears from the blood and the sedimentation rate should decrease.

In long-term salicylate therapy, poisoning is a frequent occurrence. Toxic symptoms include nausea, vomiting, tinnitus, blurred vision, and headaches. Salicylates also interfere with prothrombin synthesis and signs of hemorrhage (such as ecchymoses) are common.

The nurse is responsible for checking with the child regarding any of these side-effects and notifying the physician before continuing therapy. Some children need enteric-coated aspirin to stop the nausea and vomiting due to irritation rather than poisoning.

(The side-effects of cortisone are discussed in Chapter 13.)

LABORATORY TESTS

SEDIMENTATION RATE AND C-REACTIVE PROTEIN. The sedimentation rate and C-reactive protein are both blood tests. They usually necessitate a venous puncture and therefore can be a threat to the child. The sedimentation rate is also referred to as the ESR (erythrocyte sedimentation rate). The sed rate is a nonspecific test, but it is frequently used when one is monitoring inflammatory processes. It is an estimate of the suspension stability of erythrocytes. In conditions such as rheumatic fever, tuberculosis, and cancer, there is an increased speed of sedimentation. The cause of this increase is not clear. However, sedimentation is known to be the result of the greater density of the erythrocytes than of plasma. The test has more value in following the prognosis of the disease than in actual diagnosis.

The normal values vary according to the many different techniques available to the laboratory. The normal values are higher for females than males, and they also vary with age. For the normal values in a particular agency, the student should contact the laboratory. In some instances the normal values are printed on the lab sheet reporting the child's results.

The C-reactive protein or CRP is an indicator of inflammation or infection. Again, the change in the results is useful for prognosis and in evaluating the therapeutic plan of care, but the test is not specific for any disease entity. In some agencies a micro method has been devised for performing this test and a finger prick, earlobe prick, or heel prick will give the necessary blood. The child still needs adequate and honest preparation before the specimen is taken. The readings vary from 0 to +4. The +4 rating is given for maximum precipitation and the 0 reading for no precipitation. In persons free of disease there is no CRP in the blood serum. When there is an active inflammatory process the protein will be found. It can be found in the joint fluids as well as in the blood serum. The amount of the protein found is an indicator of the severity of the inflammatory process. Therefore, if a child had a +2 CRP, it indicates that his disease is presently less severe than the child who has a +4 CRP. When a child is first admitted with rheumatic fever, it is not uncommon for him to have a +4 CRP. After therapy is instituted, the CRP will decrease and eventually not be present.

ANTISTREPTOLYSIN O TITERS. The antistreptolysin O titers, also known as the ASO titer or ASTO titer or ASLO titer are agglutination tests again done from the venous blood sample or by the micro method. An elevated level is present when there has been a recent streptococcus infection. Usually a titer is considered significant if it remains elevated over a period of time. An elevated titer, according to Shaeffer and Goldin (1969), is 166 Todd units or higher. If the child has suspected rheumatic fever, a series of ASO titers will be drawn. If they produce low readings, the diagnosis of rheumatic fever will be ruled out. If the readings are elevated, they will be used along with the other clinical evidence to make a definitive diagnosis.

THE CONVALESCENT PHASE

In most cases, the convalescent phase provides many more challenges to the nurse in providing care. The child is now usually free from pain and he no longer is happy to remain in bed. Ideas for helping to pass the long hours can be found in Chapter 2 and Chapter 11.

During the convalescent phase it is necessary to make arrangements for the child's discharge. These arrangements may be complicated by the reluctance of the physician to return the child to living conditions which might predispose him to another attack. A medical social worker as well as a community health nurse can be valuable team members in preparing the child for the discharge and preparing the home for the child.

Sometimes the home is not the answer and other living arrangements have to be made. Foster home placement or convalescent hospitals have been effectively utilized when the child's home cannot meet his needs.

Basically, the home needs to be well heated and the child should have a bed of his own. Ideally he should have a room of his own. If he is discharged on bed-rest or modified activity, the room is best placed on the first floor of the house. This will make it easier for the mother to grant his needs. The room should be equipped with the same type activities for occupying his time as were provided in the hospital. In addition, quiet times need to be provided for the child to do school work.

The mother will need assistance in understanding the child's impatience with his restricted activities. She will also need an explanation of the importance of follow-up for medical supervision and penicillin therapy. The mother can be supplied with a pamphlet, such as *Home Care of the Child with Rheumatic Fever*, for helpful hints about caring for the child.

It is less common for children to be placed outside of the home after hospital discharge. The usual plan is to return them to their place in their own family.

When the child is ready to return to school, the school nurse and teacher must be made fully aware of the child's limitations in activity, if any. The teacher should understand that the child should avoid exposure to infections and if he gets a minor cold he will be kept out of school as a precautionary measure.

The mother and teacher might appreciate reading the pamphlet entitled *Heart Disease in Children* to help them understand the disease process more fully.

FOLLOW-UP

In both the medical and surgical cardiac conditions, follow-up care is indicated. It is very easy for the mother to forget to continue the medication when the child appears well. The mother needs to know the reasons for the medication. She needs to develop an appreciation for a drug such as lanoxin, so she does not become lax in its administration. The financial strain of the illness needs to be periodically explored so that help can be sought if necessary. A social worker is usually well informed of the current funds available from local, state, and federal sources.

In both the medical and surgical cardiac conditions it will be necessary to help the child master the developmental tasks he has lost and to proceed to achieve new developmental tasks. If the child has relinquished trust as a result of hospitalization, he must be helped to master it again and move on to the next stage of development. The child who has been so restricted by disease that he did not have the opportunity to pass through the developmental stages at the expected time will need assistance to master them after his convalescent period.

As nurses we can begin this "restoration" of developmental achievement while the child is still hospitalized. There is reason to suspect that after a long hospitalization, with or without surgery, the child can begin to mistrust adults. This mistrust may just be caused by the child's feeling that his parents have deserted him. The nurse can begin to help the child to reestablish trust by emphasizing that the parents have him in the hospital because it is the best place for him to get well. The nurse emphasizes the fact that the parents want the very best for him and that they also want him back home as soon as possible. The child needs to know that, despite the many painful procedures he has had, the hospital is really making him better. The parents should be encouraged to use a similar approach during their visits. If they come in and say, "I want to get you out of this terrible place as soon as possible," the child cannot help but mistrust adults. They all say different things.

Parents need guidance not to cast the medical personnel in a "poor light" hoping to win the child's approval. The child then wonders even more why the parents have "put him in the hospital."

One only has to ask a child, "Why are you here?" to appreciate how confused children really are about their hospitalization. Adults should not confuse them more.

The other factor which needs special emphasis is not to try to "fool" the child. Children deserve an honest and simple explanation so they can feel comfortable. As the child gets older he deserves an explanation of his cardiac status so he can make realistic vocational, educational, and social goals.

Case Presentation and Study Questions

John is a three-year-old admitted for evaluation of a heart murmur discovered during routine physical examinations done on children of migrant farm workers. He has been in the area two weeks and is residing in a mobile home with his mother, father, and six other children. Both of John's parents work long hours and the length of their stay in the area is dependent on the crops. They estimate they will be here approximately one to two weeks before moving to another area.

John is being exposed to medical personnel and facilities for the first time. Despite his young age, he will be expected to cope with most of the experiences without the support of his family.

1. What types of things can you do for John to help overcome the effects of hospitalization?

2. Are there any past experiences which John has had which will help in his adjustment to the hospital.

3. What types of things might be done to help maintain contact with John's family?

John is scheduled for a cardiac catheterization on his third day of hospitalization. His parents have agreed to come to the hospital at 5:00 A.M. to sign the consent on the day of the catheterization. They have not visited John since admission.

1. What explanation do you have for the parents not visiting John?

2. Why would the parents arrive at the hospital at 5:00 A.M.?

3. Should a nurse be available to talk with the parents on their arrival?

4. Will the parents be able to see John at this hour? If so, what preparation will be necessary for the visit? Is preparation considered necessary?

The diagnostic workup is completed and John is found to have a ventricular septal defect. A telegram is sent to the parents requesting them to come for an appointment with the physician. Both parents come in for the interview. Despite a thorough and careful explanation, the parents deny their child has a heart defect.

1. Why do you think the parents denied the heart defect?

2. Was there anything the physician could do to change the parents' initial reaction?

3. What additional things are necessary, if any, to be done to help the parents understand?

4. What social problems do you think will be created by this diagnosis? (Include aspects in relation to the migrant family.)

The physicians have decided that John needs open heart surgery. They are aware of John's lack of previous medical attention. He has not even had beginning immunizations and his hemoglobin is low due to dietary deficiencies. The physicians feel pressured by time as they know the family, in their future work, will be located in rural areas without easy access to a large medical facility. They decide to ask the family to allow John to have his corrective surgery during this hospitalization. After a great deal of discussion, it is decided that John and his mother will remain for the surgery. The rest of the family will move southward for the next harvest.

1. What provisions will need to be made for John's mother? What other members of the health team can be utilized in making these plans?

2. John's preparation will include emphasis on nutritional aspects. What information will you want to gather? What teaching will be included?

3. How will you prepare John for surgery? What aids can you use in this preparation? When will the preparation be done?

4. During the surgical procedure you spend some time talking to John's mother. You learn, for the first time, that she is pregnant and fears the expected baby will have a heart defect.

5. What immediate responses will you make?

6. What follow-up will you arrange?

7. Why do you think his mother revealed this information at this time? Will the added stress of pregnancy need to be considered when discussing John?

John returns from the intensive care unit on his fifth day postoperatively. He has been progressing adequately with only minor complications which responded readily to therapy. His mother will remain just three more days and then she will join her family. John will stay additional time in the hospital to compensate for the limited medical supervision he will receive at his next residence.

1. What preparations will need to be made before his mother leaves?

2. What suggestions should be made regarding John's future discharge?

3. How will John be prepared for his mother's departure? What changes can be expected in John's progress when he learns he will be left alone? How will you offset these changes?

References

Barnes, C. M. Working with parents of children undergoing heart surgery. In Nursing Clinics of No. Amer. Philadelphia, Saunders, Vol. 4, No. 1, March 1969, pp. 11–18.

Blake, F. G. Open Heart Surgery in Children. U.S. Department of Health, Education, and Welfare, Children's Bureau Pamphlet number 418, 1964.

Crocker, D. The critically ill child: management of tracheostomy. Pediat., 46: 286 (Aug.), 1970.

Darrow, D. C., and Pratt, E. L. Fluid Therapy: relation to tissue and the expenditure of water and electrolyte. J.A.M.A., 365, 432, 1950.

Diagnosis, Therapy, and Prophylaxis of Streptococcal Pharyngitis in the Control of Rheumatic Fever. Wyeth Laboratories, May 1965.

Doyle, E. Congestive heart failure in infancy. Sanchez Panorama, Vol. 5 No. 3, Mar. 1968.

Fink, C., and others. Differentiating rheumatic fever from juvenile rheumatoid arthritis. Patient Care, pp. 71–81, Nov. 1968.

Glaser, H. H., Harrison, G. S., and Lynn, D. B. Emotional implications of congenital heart disease in children. Pediat., 33:367–379, Mar. 1964.

Green, M., and Levitt, E. E. Constriction of body image in children with congenital heart disease. Pediat., 29:438–441, March 1962.

——— and Haggerty, R. Ambulatory Pediatrics. Philadelphia, Saunders, 1968, pp. 666–674.

Heart disease in children. Amer. Heart Assoc. rev. 1956 (pamphlet).

Home care of the child with rheumatic fever. Amer. Heart Assoc. 44 East 23 Street, New York, N.Y. 1959 (pamphlet).

Jackson, K. Psychological preparation as a method of reducing emotional trauma of anesthesia in children. Anesthesiology, 12:293–300, May 1951.

Jensen, J. Introduction to Medical Physics. Philadelphia, Lippincott, 1960, Chapter 8, p. 90.

Maxwell, G. M., and Gane, S. The impact of congenital heart disease on the family. Amer. Heart J., 64:449–454, Oct. 1962.

Neuhaus, E. C. A personality study of asthmatic and cardiac children. Psychosom. Med., 20:181–186, May–June 1958.

Pidgeon, V. The infant with congenital heart disease. Amer. J. Nurs., 67: 290–293, Feb. 1967.

Pitorak, E. F. Open-ended care for the open heart patient. Amer. J. Nurs., 67:1452–1457, July 1967.

Prevention of rheumatic fever. Amer. Heart Assoc. 1964 (pamphlet).

Raffensperger, J. G., and Primrose, R. B., eds. Pediatric Surgery for Nurses. Boston, Little Brown, 1968, Chapter 3.

Rogoz, B. Nursing care of the cardiac surgery patient. In Nursing Clinics of No. Amer. Philadelphia, Saunders, Vol. 4, No. 4, Dec. 1969, pp. 631–644.

Ross, J. The nurse and the patient with open-heart surgery. J. Nurs. Educ., 7:25–32, Sept. 1962.

Shaffer, J., and Goldin, M. Serodiagnostic tests in diseases other than syphilis. In Todd-Sanford Clinical Diagnosis, 14th ed. Philadelphia, Saunders, 1969.

Statland, H. Fluid and Electrolytes in Practice. Philadelphia, Lippincott, 1963, Chapter 14, p. 193.

Stollerman, G. H. Connective tissue disease. In Barnett, H. L., ed., Pediatrics, 14th ed. New York, Appleton-Century-Crofts, 1968, pp. 548–562.

Swendsen, L. Nursing care of the infant with congestive heart. In Nurs. Clin. of No. Amer. Philadelphia, Saunders, Vol. 4 No. 4, Dec. 1969, pp. 621–630.

Van Drimmelen, J., and Rollins, H. F. Evaluation of commonly used oral hygiene agent. Nurs. Res., 18:327–332, July–Aug. 1969.

14 SHIRLEY STEELE

Nursing Care of the Child with Terminal Illness

In this chapter I have used the term "terminal illness" in its broadest sense. Much time can be spent in discussion of when an illness with a fatal prognostication becomes terminal. Rather than spending time on this academic endeavor, I will use the term to signify the fatal illnesses as opposed to the long-term illnesses which do not have a fairly predictable finality.

The nurse caring for the child with a terminal illness needs to be ready to cope with many situations. She may be the person settling the ward after the death of a child. She may be called upon to give support to the grieving family. She may find herself giving support to other staff or students.

To be able to meet these challenges effectively, the nurse should know the normal grieving process, she should be aware of the many ways that adults view death, she should know at what ages children understand death, and she must have constructive means to cope with this knowledge.

The adult (and also the child) undergo a predictable sequence of events when going through the grieving process. According to Engel (1964), the individual first goes through a stage of shock and disbelief, then through a stage of awareness, then through a restitution state, and finally resolves the loss. The student is referred to the article for a more thorough explanation of this process.

The child with a "terminal illness" frequently evokes an immediate feeling of sympathy from the adults in his environment. After the initial reaction the adult gradually rearranges his feelings in accordance with other significant factors he learns about the child. Feelings of sympathy may change to impatience if the child's behavior is disruptive, or sympathy may change to overprotection if the child is afraid and insecure.

It is important to consider the conditions under which the adult is functioning in order to appreciate his reactions. The parent who has recently undergone other stressful situations may feel like he is being treated "unfairly." He may become quite upset and shout obscenities at the physician giving the information. He may also be very hostile toward the nurse, who seems to support the doctor's position.

The parent who has recently gone through a similar grieving process may have that experience immediately revived, and begin crying hysterically.

Reactions to Children with Terminal Illnesses

As nurses we need to examine our different reactions and the factors which influence these reactions. Certainly age is a major factor in influencing reactions to terminal illness. When the child is a newborn, people frequently remark it is not so bad because the parents did not get a chance to know him. This is certainly far from the case because the parents have been planning for this child, either positively or negatively, since they knew of the child's conception.

The young healthy child is frequently considered the greatest loss. Statements such as, "He didn't have a chance to get started in life" are common.

The adolescent who has entered college seems to have everything to live for. His shortened life is considered a tragedy. On the other hand the adolescent who has "copped out" or was taking narcotics is frequently written off as "no loss."

The nature of the disease entity is another factor. Adults often find it more acceptable for a handicapped child to die than they do for a "normal" child to die.

There are also diseases which have a particularly tragic connotation to the lay public. One of these diseases is cancer. People still view it as a brutal disease and sometimes even contagious or a disgrace. People also think of cancer as a disease of "old age" and find it particularly difficult to accept in children.

Environmental conditions play a part. Why is it that when a child of a prominent family is fatally ill there seems to be more concern by the professional staff than when it is a child from a deprived family? There seems to be some misconception that children from "better" homes have more reason to be spared "terminal" illness. This may be partially based on the fact that these parents have supposedly given better medical supervision to their children and therefore the child should not be prone to serious illness. It may also be partially based on the fact that the nurse is more closely associated with other professional people, and she therefore wants to believe that it cannot happen to professional people.

A person from a culture that permits its people to "act out" its grief is less likely to be tolerated than people from cultures which are "stoic" and "quiet" about their grief. It is even possible to be more specific: on a busy, understaffed unit a terminally ill child may be resented because he demands so much care. Or a terminally ill child may dampen the cheerful attitude of a small pediatric unit which prides itself on keeping the children happy and minimizing effects of hospitalization. In a well-equipped intensive care unit the child with a terminal illness may be taken so as a part of the expected routine that the nurses may become too impersonal and neglect his psychological needs.

Particular seasons may influence people's reaction. People seem to be more involved if a child is very sick around a special holiday such as Christmas. If death occurs the neighbors and friends are especially sympathetic. "What a shame to spoil their Christmas. Every Christmas they will remember this."

People frequently feel that the family who has only one child has a greater loss than families with more children. Or, the loss of a boy is more difficult than that of a girl. Or the child with a superior intelligence is a greater loss than one of lesser intelligence.

Some feel that it is easier for a woman of child-bearing years to lose a child than one who is too old to have more children.

Availability of loved ones to be with the dying child is another factor. If a father is in the armed forces and cannot be with his child, everyone feels quite sympathetic. If the relative is on his way home, everyone seems to "hold their breath" hoping that he will arrive before the child's condition worsens or before death actually takes place.

This by no means exhausts the factors influencing persons' reactions which nurses might encounter personally or in their co-workers. It is merely a small sample. Realizing that we are all human, we must set realistic goals for nurses who are expected to give the best possible "comprehensive care" to these children.

REACTIONS OF STUDENT NURSES

The student nurse caring for the child will frequently have some of the same responses as the parents of the child. As the student is usually of child-bearing age, she feels a real closeness to the situation. At first learning the diagnosis, the student may experience the same type of disbelief and denial that the parents have. Students may shy away because they are not able to "cure" the child. The student is in a period when having children is foremost in his or her mind. Their own close association makes it difficult for them to handle the situation as a professional person rather than a parent. If the students have children of their own, they frequently see the patient as if he were their own child. Students will frequently wish or request not to be assigned a child with a terminal illness. They fear they will be incapable of handling the situation and unable to talk to the parents. They are especially fearful that the child will die while they are caring for him.

The student will frequently use her own faith as a means of coping with the situation. He or she will also be influenced by recent experiences with other terminally ill patients or with death. Some may never have had experience with death and they fear the unknown. Others will have seen adult patients die. This does not necessarily mean that they will be better prepared to face the death of a child.

The student frequently needs a faculty member close by when he or she is caring for the child. It seems to help just to have "moral support." Frequent conferences are also indicated to help the student express his or her anxiety and concerns. The student should also feel free to cry if he or she feels the need. Again, they should be aware that the child will sense their emotions and they should try to use "control" in the child's presence. These periods of release usually make it easier for the student to continue to function effectively. If the student feels he or she cannot continue caring for the child then the assignment should be changed.

Professional personnel must not feel that they can always be therapeutic in every situation. If terminally ill children cause them too much despair, they should not attempt to care for them.

The nursing student who is assigned to the child with a fatal illness should have time to adjust to the idea prior to her assignment in the clinical area. Hopefully theory on terminal illness should precede the assignment. Then the student should be given her patient assignment including the child's age, medical diagnosis, medical therapy, present condition, and family constellation, if known. This will help her to formulate a plan of care drawing upon her past experience in the various clinical areas. Emphasis is placed on the comfort of the child rather than the cure. The tentative nursing care plan is then altered as necessary factors present themselves during the time she cares for the child.

A frequent mistake in caring for the child with a terminal illness is to expect the child to act like he is terminally ill. Children usually do not want to be sick and they camouflage their illness very well. The adults in their lives should also try to keep this in mind. I have watched again and again children in for diagnostic work-ups who run and play in the play area, and their parents seem to be relatively relaxed prior to the time a diagnosis of a terminal disease is made. The parents then change their approach, the child is overprotected, the parents cry when they look at the child, they darken the rooms, turn off TVs or radios, and begin an oversolicitous role. Often the diagnosis is definitely determined at surgery and the child may be quite sick postoperatively so that he does not immediately object to this environment. However, the child with a medical condition, such as leukemia, is greatly concerned by the new situation. The introduction of a large number of medications, painful diagnostic procedures, or irradiation therapy is difficult enough for the child to accept without the changes in the environment and adults in his life.

The first step in developing realistic goals will be to consider the developmental tasks for the age of the child, taking into account the regression which may accompany hospitalization. Another factor which weighs heavily on the nursing student's decisions are the plans which have already been formulated by the permanent staff in the clinical area. Abrupt changes are never wise. I have heard nurses dogmatically say, "I'll just go in and change that!" This type of change is rarely accepted by the child, the parents, or co-workers. Gradual changes which show results are much more readily accepted—such as suggesting the child have periodic play periods with the shades raised, or periods of TV which include his favorite programs. The child's enthusiasm during these "trial" periods will usually guarantee more of these sessions until the environment is returned to its normal state.

The parents of the child with a terminal illness usually play a big role in the hospitalization. The other relatives and siblings may not be included until the child is discharged, but they should not be excluded from the long-range plans. In fact, the child would greatly benefit during extended hospitalizations from visits from his siblings and pets. This is a two-way process. The other children also are aware of their hospitalized family member's condition and it helps to keep them reality-oriented. Too often when a child dies the other children only remember the "well" sibling who went to the hospital to die, as they never saw the child as he progressed through his illness. The hospitalized child also feels very isolated by the hospitalization periods. He is not used to the individual attention of the parents and has learned to share them with his other siblings. A more natural state would be to continue this plan. If the hospital does not permit children to visit, then each time the child is discharged from the hospital the parents and children must make a readjustment to the usual family routine and this is often quite difficult. The other relatives should also be included as much as possible in the long-range plans. They often put pressure on the parents to change decisions which have been realistically made in the hospital. Many a well-meaning grandparent has forced the family to seek another medical decision in a far-off place which has publicized a "cure" or new method of care. This medical shopping can be expensive and disrupting to the child and the family as a whole. The shopping can have the positive effect of relieving some of the family's "guilt feelings" as they gain satisfaction from "knowing they have done all they can."

A Review of Some of the Significant Literature

A helpful study by Bozeman et al. (1955) done on parent's reactions to their terminally ill child should be a required reading. It helps the student to understand how parents progress through a series of reactions as they learn to cope with the threatened loss of their child. Such initial reactions as denial, self-injury, refusal to believe the diagnosis (or reversing it), and disbelief were common. Denial was used to try to blank out the diagnosis or to reverse the diagnosis. Most mothers were more concerned with improving the prognosis of the disease. Then feelings of guilt began to appear, with self-blame. Many felt if they had recognized signs earlier they could have prevented the disease.

Of particular significance to nursing personnel is the searching parents do for any and all information on the disease. They seem to have to know all the current facts about the disease and its prognosis. The parents frequently present all this information to the nurse who then may become threatened. If the nurse reacts negatively the parent may become angered and resent the nurse. This creates a chain reaction which impedes care, unless ways are provided for the parents and nurse to utilize each other effectively. Parents should be given avenues for using their energies effectively and while the child is hospitalized this may be accomplished by establishing a care plan which allows the parents to be with their child and help meet his emotional needs for love and comfort. It is important during the early stages to help the parents to learn to cope with the diagnosis. At this stage the child is still not incapacitated and the parent is certainly able to provide a great deal of his care. Parents must not be abruptly separated from the child. Helping them to feel they are an integral part of the care is an excellent way to help them to cope with the problem. Then, as the disease progresses, they will be better able to assist. They are introduced gradually to the progressive deterioration in the child's condition and see first hand the added responsibilities this deterioration will produce. The parents become increasingly willing to let the nurse take over as the child gets increasingly difficult to handle.

It was also brought out that none of the mothers ever gave up hope until their child was actually moribund. This is especially essential to keep in mind when giving care to the child. Because the parents have a great deal of hope until very late in the child's illness, they will not understand a nurse's early pessimism. They do not want to realize that nurses have had more experience with the disease, either through literature or experience, and may have a pessimistic outlook. The parent's attitude is based solely on their involvement with and their hope for their own child.

It is important to have the nurse understand that what we consider to be a "realistic attitude" for the parents is not necessarily that they accept the fatal diagnosis. A "realistic attitude" may only be to accept that their child is sick. It is not our place to deny the parents hope. As the disease progresses they become painfully aware of the irreversibility of the disease and their hope for recovery diminishes. It is not necessary to insist the parent's relinquish all hope for research to find a cure for the disease before their child's life is ended. None of us is in a position to take such a negative position strongly.

The parents cannot help but have some appreciation of their child's serious illness as the medical intervention is begun.

The study brought out another point that may be more pertinent to some clinical areas than others. First, rivalry between the mothers and nurses took place for the possession of the child when areas such as feeding, affection, and discipline were taken over by the nurse. It is my opinion that this factor may apply more readily where visiting hours are limited and parents take a very minor role in their child's hospitalization.

One other factor brought out seems primarily the same. The mothers were most upset when they were disturbed during visiting hours. They did not accept interruptions even when they were for the benefit of their child. In facilities where visiting hours are extended, I do not believe this is such a problem.

The study also found that the parents received their greatest support from parents of other children with the same disease. Although it is seldom necessary to introduce these parents to one another, it might be relevant in an area in which the diagnosis of terminal illness is rare. In an area which services many children with terminal illness, parents seem to find one another very readily.

Another study (Geis, 1965) which should help to plan nursing care is one in which mothers were interviewed after the death of the child to get their impressions of the care their dying child received. All the mothers seemed interested in the human element when asked what information nurses should have when caring for a dying child. They also wanted the truth and seemed to want more time to ask questions. One of the questions asked of these mothers was in relation to who they felt was the most helpful person after they learned their child would not recover. Of 21 parents interviewed, only one said the nurse was the most helpful. This information makes one wonder if the nurse can be more useful at this time. Then 33 parents were asked who was the most helpful when the child died, and five parents said it was the nurse. A mere five, despite the fact that eight mothers stated there was a nurse with their child at the time of his death.

Although this was a small sampling it is a study done by a nurse to see how we might improve services to families with terminally ill children. The answers to the interview might have been more positive for nurses if the term "most" were modified, but, nevertheless, nurses can benefit by strengthening areas of concern expressed by the mothers.

The mothers expressed their appreciation for talking to the nurse interviewer. They might also benefit by periodic talks with staff nurses prior to the child's death. One way of making ourselves more accessible to parents is to schedule short informal coffee breaks with them. Another way is to have an occasional lunch with them. Or if you cannot plan times away from the unit, at least include a few minutes of private conversation for the parents to vent their feelings. Remember that privacy is imperative as the child can easily grasp the tone of the conversation and may draw very false conclusions from it.

Another interesting finding was that little comment was made in relation to those technical skills that have been highly regarded by many nurses as their most significant contributions to patients. I feel this factor bears emphasizing. Technical skills are necessary to the nurse because she feels more comfortable if she can perform them skillfully. However, the parent needs support during the crisis and technical skills, in and of themselves, do not fill the bill. The nurse who prides herself on technical competence is frequently one who hurries in and out without giving herself time fully to evaluate the situation. She may set up a blood transfusion with great dexterity but forget to explain to the mother that John's blood count is down, but not dangerously low. Parents derive a great deal of support and satisfaction from explanations. Likewise the child feels more secure when he receives explanations. The additional time spent while doing or after completing procedures is a source of great comfort to the parents and child. It indirectly aids the nurse also, as there is less parent anxiety and resulting questioning when this procedure is routinely carried out.

In another study by Sister Mary Christopher Meurer (1962), it was found that 22 of the 47 mothers interviewed said that the nurse helped them the most in the immediate adjustment to the hospital. This is a rewarding finding but in viewing the two studies it would seem that nurses realize their responsibility to the newly admitted patient but not to the terminally ill child if only five mothers felt the nurse played the most important role.

These are both small studies and Sister Mary Christopher Meurer's population was solely mothers of children with leukemia while Miss Geis included mothers whose children died from other causes. Their major contributions are, however, in terms of looking at ways of improving nursing services through interviewing the consumers of the product.

A study by Friedman and others (1963) on a population similar to the Bozeman study brought out some other interesting facts. They found that parents seemed to accept the diagnosis intellectually rather than manifesting the great amount of denial described in the Bozeman study. The parents in this study expressed guilt for not reacting quicker to the early signs of illness. The parental guilt seemed to be alleviated by learning that the long-term prognosis for children with leukemia was about the same regardless of when the diagnosis was made. It was also pointed out that parents did not seem to recall what they were told about the diagnosis, originally. They needed explanations later after the medical plan of care was decided. The parents seemed to need assistance in carrying out immediate details and appreciated the help of the physician with this aspect. This might also carry over to nursing in helping the family with such simple things as a telephone or a private area to discuss plans.

Another point made in the study was that parents become confused and anxious if they receive varying reports about their child. This factor is a very good reason for team conferences, including all disciplines, to be held regularly on each child.

Another benefit derived from these team conferences is that the staff has an opportunity to undergo some of their grieving process during the child's course of illness. Then they are better able to help the parents cope when death actually occurs. Some of the team members are in a position to help other members begin the grieving process. This is especially important for the young students as they need a great deal of support when dealing with the dying child. It is helpful for team members to know that they can get support and even be relieved, if necessary, by team members who fully understand the child and his parents.

Both the Bozeman et al. (1955) and Friedman et al. (1963) studies brought out the need for nurses to work with the parents rather than be in conflict with them. The hospitalized child readily transfers the change in authority from parent to hospital personnel and every attempt should be made to make this situation tolerable for the parents.

Friedman et al. (1963) also pointed out that when the child nears the terminal stage parents often begin to care for other children on the ward. This is good to keep in mind as nurses might misinterpret this as lack of interest in their own child because he is no longer providing the parent with the gratification he or she needs. Friedman sees this as a part of the grieving process just prior to the imminent death of the child.

The role religion plays in the lives of the parents with children with a terminal illness is less well documented in both the Bozeman et al. (1955) and the Friedman et al. (1963) studies. While both devote a small section to evaluating the role religion plays, it is difficult to get a real feeling regarding the contributions of religion. This may be attributed to the fact that religion is frequently a private feeling. It is less common for people openly to express their true feelings about spiritual matters. Members of certain religions are more likely to express their beliefs than others. Many hospitals and agencies have eliminated from their admission data the religious preference of the family, and this makes it even more difficult for the nurse to ascertain information about a family's religious background or current religious beliefs.

The role religion plays in any family's life may vary greatly during certain periods. Even devout families may question their religious beliefs in the face of impending death of their child. Other families may turn to the church for more support.

The child facing death may well benefit from continuing fellowship with his clergyman. The young child has a limited understanding of religion, but anything which offers a continuance of his life pattern may give him added support.

The older child and adolescent are better able to make their wants known regarding spiritual counselors.

It has been my experience that at the time of death many parents "blame God" for deceiving them. In talks with parents after a period of time following the death of a child, several stated that after the death religion helped them to accept the finality and give them needed answers to "why it happened."

The student should make it known to the parents and the child her willingness to call spiritual counselors if the family wants them. She should take her clues directly from the parents and the child. In hospitals where clergy visit routinely, the role of the clergy should be explained to both the parent and the child so they will not misinterpret the professional service.

The student also should make herself accessible when a visiting clergy comes to the unit, as he may be in need of assistance in rendering professional services. He may also need a report on the child's progress to be most helpful to the child and family. A clergyman can be a most helpful member of the health team and his role should not be solely in relation to the period surrounding the death of the child.

The following statements were made with regard to implications for physicians, but they are also extremely beneficial implications for nurses.

> Each parent of a child with a fatal disease reacts to the tragedy in a unique manner, consistent with his particular personality structure, past experiences, and the individualized meaning and specific circumstances associated with the threatened loss. In general, optimal medical management depends on the physician's awareness and evaluation of certain aspects of this specific background information. However, the parents of children with leukemia do share many similar problems that are adherent in the situation, and certain modes of adjustment commonly occur in a characteristic sequence. The parental behavior, though not stereotyped, is therefore predictable to some degree (Friedman et al., 1963).

Specific In-Patient Nursing Care

According to a pamphlet prepared by the New York State Department of Health, the leading causes of death in childhood are: accidents 36%, cancer 12%, pneumonia 9%, diseases of the nervous system 6%, infectious diseases 5%, diseases of the digestive system 4%, and all other 25%. In studying this information it becomes apparent that many of the children with terminal illness will have a diagnosis of cancer of some type. As the deaths from accidents are frequently immediate, the nurse may not even see the child. The most common type of cancer of childhood is leukemia with an occurrence of 40%. The next most common sites are the brain with 24.1%, and the kidney and lymph gland with 9.6%. Bone cancers account for 3.4% of childhood cancers, endocrine system 3.0%, digestive system 1.7%, and all others 11.4% (*The ABC's of Childhood Cancer*).

In light of this information, the student will probably most readily be exposed to children with leukemia, brain tumors, or Wilms's tumors during her clinical experience. She will be formulating a plan of care focused around such medical orders as increased medications, control of temperature, relief of pain, diagnostic or therapeutic procedures, and surgery.

The child health nurse often needs special skills in administering medications. Depending on the age of the child even oral medications can be refused. Creativity—such as making a game of the task—is often wise. Bringing the known such as a favorite TV character into the picture helps to make the unknown medication more acceptable. The added threat of injections increases the demands on the nurse. The best approach is to restrain the child as needed for his protection, be truthful that it will hurt, and then give the injection quickly and skillfully. Always allow ample time following the administration to comfort the child.

The control of temperature may necessitate skills for lowering or raising the temperature. Institutions vary but such techniques as tepid sponges may be used, hyper- or hypothermia mattresses or pads may be used, blankets may be added or removed, hot water bottles may be used with caution, fans may be used, and medications ordered for PRN administration. If a child has a constant indwelling thermometer every precaution must be utilized to protect the rectal area from irritation during turning procedures. All the protection given adults' skin during these same procedures must be given—but more so. Children's skin is much more easily irritated and must be watched more frequently. The reasons for this may be attributed to the thinness of the child's skin, or the fact that the skin is less cornified and less hairy, thereby cutting down on some of the natural defenses found in the adult's skin. The child's skin also contains more water and electrolytes than the adult's. In addition, the sweat glands are underdeveloped so the child sweats less and is more prone to infection.

In relation to diagnostic procedures, the student may be expected to hold a child for a lumbar puncture or assist in a bone marrow aspiration. Both of these procedures are frequently done on children with leukemia. In my experience, the parents have been excluded from the area where the treatment is done. The rationale has been that the parent is often "hurt" more by the procedure than the child. However, it does not seem realistic to believe that a parent can never share an experience of pain with his child. They have certainly experienced many with him in the past when he has been injured at play or taken to the dentist. Certain parents could offer much consolation to the child and perhaps even diminish the need for restraining procedures by minimizing the child's fear. Separation of parent and child is an anxiety-producing experience. Each time the child has the procedure done he should be given a simple, truthful explanation of it. It should not be assumed that the child remembers from the last time or that someone else has prepared him. The nurse in the immediate situation must do the preparation. Frequently medication is administered prior to these procedures. It is important to remember that the child who is deceived may begin to associate sleep with painful procedures and eventually not be able to sleep from fear.

Another area directly related to telling the child the truth is in diagnosis. It has been my experience that the doctors in the clinical areas did not feel the child should know his diagnosis. In one hospital setting the doctors told the child he had anemia, which was usually true. They further explained that the child would need frequent transfusions and medication to control the anemia and this would even take precedence over school. For the most part, this adequately prepared the child for absence from school and repeated hospitalizations. The nurses in the clinical area were all aware of this procedure and were encouraged to talk to the child and encourage him to talk about himself. The fact that communication was not cut off completely and everyone gave the same information seemed helpful. The theme of anemia was even carried over for inclusion in the Kardex as children occasionally went into the nurses' station and flipped through the Kardex.

Another program which seems to have much more potential, especially with school-aged children and with adolescents, is one in which social workers actually work with the child to face the problems of critical illness, hospitalization, and death (Vernick and Lunseford, 1967). The parents are encouraged to tell the child his diagnosis and then professional people are available to help the child work through his feelings. The professional personnel involved in this program are involved only if they prefer to be.

In contrast to these two methods is one in which the child is not given an explanation and the nursing staff is not permitted to discuss the problems with the child. This method encourages the child to be afraid and distrust adults. When his questions about his condition are ignored or side-tracked he stops asking them and this may give the erroneous impression that all is well with the child. Only when he begins to display emotional problems is it evident that he is concerned and that these problems might readily have been avoided if he knew the truth.

While there is no simple answer to how this should be handled, the main considerations must be the age of the child, the wishes of the parents and the physician, and the past ways in which the child has been able to cope with stressful situations. In a study by Natterman and Knudson (1960) on 33 children with leukemia and related diseases, it was stated that in the age group zero to five years separation was the most severe reaction observed; in the age group five to ten years, reactions to procedures were most intense; and in the group ten years and over, the reactions to death were the strongest. This agreed with findings reported by Nagy (1948) that children from three to five years of age denied death and felt that it was not permanent, that it was only a change of some kind and could be temporary, and that the five- to nine-year-old children recognized death but without exception regard it as a person. From nine on, children achieve a realistic conception of death as a permanent biological process. The fact that they can and do understand death and its meaning supports the idea of providing these children with more than empty excuses for the death of other children on the unit. It validates the idea of support for them during their illness.

It should be remembered also that the child may very well learn his diagnosis from neighbors, medical staff, or medical records, and that if the diagnosis is withheld, much precaution has to be undertaken to keep the diagnosis a secret. The adolescent may very well come to the out-patient department alone rather than with his parents. If he is assuming a major role in his medical care, then the physician and nurse may decide to discuss his disease process and prognosis without the parents consent. Adolescents are entitled to honest discussions and will need periods to ask questions.

In relation to the overall nursing care, the parents' role has been well documented in the literature. When the mothers help to care for the child, the nurses serve as a teacher, counselor, friend, and stabilizer rather than a mother-substitute (see Fig. 1). Therefore, the reactions nurses often feel at the death of a child may be minimized by the parent participation. The reactions nurses have include sympathy, sense of a loss of a loved one, fear of death, anger at "failing" the child, inadequacy, guilt, and repression. It seems beneficial not only from the parent's and child's standpoint but also from the nurse's standpoint to involve parents actively in the care.

One very important point to remember is to gauge parents' participation as carefully as possible, changing their participation readily just as the nursing care plan is adapted readily to meet the changing needs of the child. Many factors may influence the degree of participation the parent is able to give in any one day—such things as how well the mother was able to sleep the night before, or whether she was able to eat enough to have the strength to be of help, and what reports she received from the physician. Mothers frequently can participate more when the reports are somewhat encouraging or at least do not seem too discouraging. Her participation may also be influenced by what her responsibilities are at home. If she is being expected to carry the full responsibility for the family, she may not feel up to any activity which involves physical effort. Her participation will best be utilized as emo-

FIG. 1. Pediatric rooming-in provides an excellent opportunity for the family and nurse to learn from one another.

tional support for the child. The parent should be helped to participate in the role of a parent rather than trying to play the role of nurse. Too frequently nurses will ask the mother to monitor the intravenous flow. This is not within the range of mothering tasks. It aligns her with a painful or tiresome procedure and changes the child's perception of why she is visiting. While it may seem to the nurse to be a perfectly logical request, I think we should try to see the implications to the child-parent relationship, and then we would not consider it logical (see Fig. 2).

The roles the mother ordinarily has such as bathing, feeding, disciplining, and most important *loving,* are her vital contributions. The mother is more comfortable assuming tasks she already knows. She has been perfecting these skills since the child was born and she is the expert in the area and can utilize her expertise to its fullest.

The nurses' expertise includes the intravenous infusions, the Foley catheters, and the maintenance of the suction equipment, to name a few. However, the nurse is also able to do the mothering tasks in the absence of the mother. She should try to do them as consistently as possible with the pattern the mother established.

Again, if there are positive changes to be made, they should be introduced slowly. The parent should also be aware that changes have been introduced to try to gain their cooperation in following through on them. This is especially important if there are changes made in disciplining the child. In order for the child to benefit substantially,

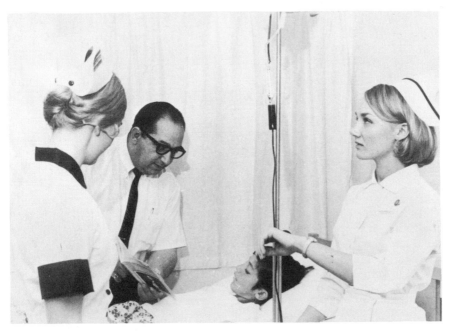

FIG. 2. This acutely ill boy benefits from the nurse's expertise in monitoring the blood transfusion. The father's expertise is used in providing diversional therapy.

all the adults need to be aware of the program and carry through consistently.

Role of the Nurse After the Death of a Child

Following the death of a child on a hospital unit, it is imperative
to restore the unit to normality as quickly as possible. The school-age
and adolescent children understand death and a simple explanation
should be given to them. The parents of the children should know what
has happened and how you explained it to the child. Frequently nurses
try to make excuses to "cover-up" death on a unit. This violates the
simple principle of telling children the truth. It also encourages the
child to mistrust adults.

In a book by Bergmann (1965), it is brought out that although
the nurses did their very best to protect the other children from the
death of a child, the nurses themselves were so upset by the death that
the children sensed it from the nurses' reactions. The other children
then began to act out in accordance with what they felt their role was
in relation to their dead peer. Although the acting out was not completely in tune with the situation, it pointed out that children can and

do have a concept of death and are entitled to a simple explanation which will satisfy their curiosity.

The child who has an attachment to the dead peer may exhibit some of the following things during his mourning process. He may cling to an object from home so he feels more secure that he will not die. He may have periods of insomnia and need more support during bedtime hours. He may refuse to eat for a period of time. The child may go through a period of acting out and be quite obnoxious. His games and songs may center around the death of the child and he may seem quite callous in his approach.

It is important to keep in mind that children have less experience with death and therefore very little past experience to draw upon in resolving their grief. Mourning involves a departure from the ordinary, and a child may become so enveloped in mourning that he has very little energy left over for any other interests. It is best to tell the children "Mary has died" soon after her death. This will usually give the children an opportunity to ask questions. The child's questions may be related to their past experiences with death, such as, "We flushed my dead goldfish down the toilet, will you flush Mary down the toilet?"

The child with a long-term illness may have more reason than other children to fear that death will also claim him. He will probably need more time, on an individual basis, to express his anxiety. He may have the same doctor as the deceased child and he begins to question the competency of his doctor. He may question why the nurses let Mary die.

The child with a long-term illness may possibly have more experience with death because of his more frequent hospitalization and greater exposure to medical situations. But these experiences may not have helped him in learning to cope with death—they may only have served to make him feel less secure.

An example follows. Jim was ten years old when his hydronephrosis became extremely incapacitating. An ileoconduit was scheduled and the proposed surgery was explained to Jim. He had been hospitalized several times and was presently hospitalized three months because of problems with continuing his foster home placement. Jim's preoperative preparation was started and the thought of death became utmost in Jim's mind. One day he was overheard talking to another school-age child. Jim was relating all the deaths of children which had taken place, on this busy hospital unit, since his admission. At the end of the list he added his own name.

Fortunately this conversation took place in plenty of time to get professional help for Jim prior to surgery.

A factor which helps to restore the unit to normal is children's capacity to "forget" the death. They are quick to return to the ordinary daily activities and are thought to complete the grief process in much less time than adults.

The children will, of course, be reminded of the death of the adults in their environment continue to show signs of unrest. This is another reason for professional personnel to be able to function under the stress created by death on the pediatric unit.

The child's misconceptions about death frequently revolve around the idea that death is a punishment for wrong doings. Therefore, the child who has been "bad" may fear death as his "punishment."

The child with a long-term illness may have secretly or openly wished the other child would die so he did not get so much of the staff's attention. This death wish is frequent in children, but the wished-for death rarely happens so the child does not have to feel the guilt associated with receiving his wish. If the child does die, the child making the wish feels very guilty for his thoughts. The child will need help to understand that he did not really cause the child's death. He will also need assurance that children do sometimes wish people would die.

The death of another child, while it may be frightening, is usually less traumatic to the child than losing one of his parents or perhaps even a pet.

The student is referred to the pamphlet entitled, "Helping Your Child to Understand Death" by Anna W. M. Wolf for answers to questions regarding death.

Out-Patient Services

The intermittent nature of some of the terminal illnesses such as leukemia necessitates attention to the care offered in the out-patient clinics, especially when the children are treated in a clinic which bears the name of the disease entity. Even children who previously received private medical supervision are frequently referred to the specialty clinic for their follow-up care. This often changes the whole pattern of care for this child and his parents. In one study (Bozeman et al., 1955), it was shown that parents were often quite hostile toward the clinic. The common complaints about clinic care include long waits, impersonal approaches, exposure to very sick children, lack of specific appointments, and lack of privacy, to mention but a few.

A concern by the professional staff in one clinic servicing children with leukemia was that the children get to know other children with the same disease and soon lose this attachment by the death of the other child. The appointment days were staggered so the child did not expect his friend to come on the same day, thus eliminating the possibility of strong peer relationships being formed. It was believed that the parent, rather than a peer, could better serve as the stable figure during clinic appointments.

It is important to remember that children with long-term illnesses learn to integrate their specialty clinic into their normal life style. For the school-age child his social groups then include his family, his community, his peers, his school, and his clinic. The way he perceives the clinic is largely dependent on interpersonal relationships. This places a great responsibility on the nurse in the clinic to become acquainted with the patients and to assume a large role in making the clinic experience as positive as possible. In addition to personal identity, the nurse should be sure that privacy is guaranteed each child, that he is accompanied for painful procedures, that he is prepared for all clinic procedures, and that his next clinic appointment is scheduled to least interfere with his personal plans. With pediatric care rapidly moving to the out-patient departments which are physically not ready to accept the large influx of patients, good interpersonal relationships can be a great compensation.

Other nursing contributions to personalizing the out-patient care of terminally ill children might include the following techniques.

The regularly scheduled visits to the clinic should be known in advance. All professional personnel should review the old records prior to visiting the child for his clinic examination. Children should be approached in the waiting area and addressed by name. Facts which are easily compiled, such as birthdate or upcoming special events, can further add to the individualizing of patient care. A comment such as, "Birthday wishes are in store for you this week!" can be helpful. A

FIG. 3. Long waiting hours in the out-patient department can be fun when recreational therapy is provided. Student nurses can gain knowledge of normal growth and development from making observations about play activities.

handy supply of children's birthday cards can be kept on hand to be signed by the child's physician and nurse. Other similar occasions can be acknowledged in the same manner. Children enjoy surprises, and small inexpensive gifts can be wrapped and put into a grab bag for boys and one for girls. This will further suggest to the child the professional personnel's interest in children. To any particular child it will signify a direct interest in him.

The waiting area should be well equipped with toys and activities to make the waiting period seem shorter. A donated supply of magazines can be useful for the parents (see Fig. 3 and 4).

Films, filmstrips, posters, and pamphlets can also be utilized in the waiting area. Some of this material can be geared to the children, while others may appeal to the parents and the children can utilize the time playing in another area (see Fig. 5).

The waiting area should have comfortable seats for both the children and the parents. It should have a crib or play pen available for infants who could not be left at home.

The waiting area should also be equipped with machines offering nutritious food items, such as fruit juice, milk, and crackers. Coffee is also considered a "friendly" offering and, if possible, it should be offered free of charge to the parents.

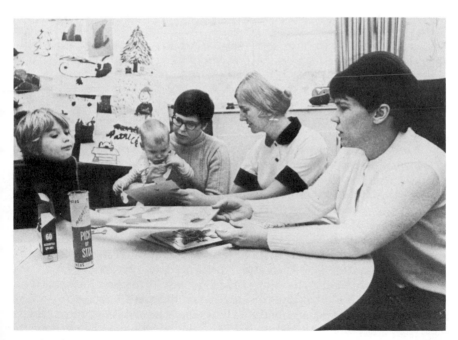

FIG. 4. The use of teen-age volunteers in the out-patient department waiting room helps to increase interest in child care. It also frees the parents to talk privately to the professional personnel.

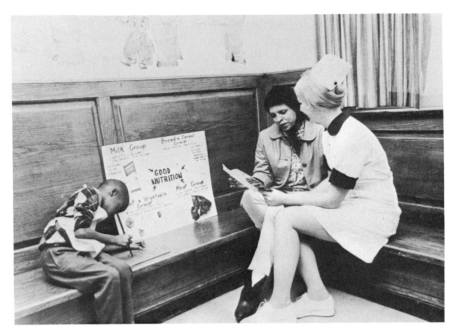

FIG. 5. Visual aides utilized in teaching during waiting time in out-patient department.

It also helps to have the waiting area clean and aesthetically appealing. This will diminish the complaints of attending an out-patient service.

Out-Patient Nursing Intake Interviews

The nurse in the out-patient department should do intake interviews with the parent and child on each visit. It is important to know how the child is adjusting or coping between visits. The nurse is able to elicit this information by offering the patient and parent an acceptable situation in which to verbalize. This situation should provide for privacy and be carried out in a relaxed manner. If the interview seems hurried, appropriate information may be withheld. It is important to know how much of a strain this long-term or terminal illness is having on the family. If it is reasonable, the whole family should come for visits rather than just the patient and parent. This can serve several purposes. One, the other children learn to appreciate some of the stress placed on their affected sibling. They also can see that the child is receiving excellent care and that everything possible is being done to prolong his life. Another important point is that the other children frequently suffer when there is a child in the family who needs a great deal of attention. Counselling may be indicated for the other children to help them understand what is taking place with their brother or sister. They may also need explanations for their parents' behavior. If possible, the interview should precede the physical examination so that the information gathered can be shared with the physician and other team members.

The following are examples of forms which can be utilized for out-patient nursing intake interviews. The first one is suggested when one is interviewing parent and child together. The second is for interviewing school-age and adolescent children without their parents. The third form is suggested for planning effective nursing care during the visit and also for determining needs for referral to other agencies.

As the majority of these children return frequently to the clinic, a Kardex is especially useful in compiling the information.

In addition, an example of collecting interim information on admission to the in-patient service is illustrated in Appendix II. Appendix III gives an example of an in-patient Kardex. It can be adopted for out-patient use, also.

The simple guideline in utilizing these tools is to give as "comprehensive" a picture of this child and his family as possible.

FORM 1.

UNIVERSITY HOSPITAL
U.S.A.

NURSING INTAKE INTERVIEW (OUT-PATIENT)

NAME _____ AGE _____ DATE _____

   I. Reason for appointment

  II. Previous appointment or hospital admissions
       (date, reason, action taken)

 III. Family constellation

 IV. Habits:
       Eating (describe amount, how often, types of food, likes, and dislikes)
       Elimination
       Sleeping
       Language development
       Play—peer groups

  V. Allergies

 VI. Activities of daily living
       Independent
       Dependent
       School
       Social interests

 VII. Special needs, fears, problems

See example of information gathered, Appendix I.

FORM 2.

UNIVERSITY HOSPITAL
U.S.A.

NURSING INTERVIEW OF CHILD (OUT-PATIENT)

NAME _____ AGE _____ DATE _____

   I.   Reason for appointment

  II.   Preparation for visit

 III.   Habits:
         Eating
         Elimination
         Sleeping
         Play—peer groups

 IV.   Activities of daily living
         Independent
         Dependent
         School
         Social interests
         Relationships with siblings

FORM 3.

UNIVERSITY HOSPITAL
U.S.A.
OUT-PATIENT NURSING INTERVENTION

NAME _____ AGE _____ DATE _____

   I.   In relation to child (incorporating principles of normal and
       development)

  II.   In relation to family

 III.   Community resources available to meet nursing objectives

 IV.   Follow-up plan of care

OUT-PATIENT EXAMINATION

When the child's turn comes to go to the examining room, the nurse should greet the child and his parents (see Fig. 6). The child will then be encouraged to help in his preparation. He will be encouraged to guess how much he weighs, to take his own oral temperature, and to undress and get into the proper garb (see Fig. 7). He will be offered all the privacy he desires during this procedure.

Questions which the child can adequately answer will be asked of

FIG. 6. The out-patient waiting room provides the nurse with an opportunity to meet the entire family.

him directly. An attempt should be made to have the child feel he is an integral part of the visit, not just an appendage.

The child and parents should be introduced to the physician, if they have not previously met him. They are also introduced to students of any profession who may be present during the examination.

Many of the procedures which formerly necessitated hospitalization now are done in the out-patient department. These include bone-marrow aspirations, blood counts, blood transfusions, and paracentesis. In a busy clinic the nurse must be able to teach the parent what signs to observe while the child is receiving a transfusion; she must also be able to organize her work load to permit her to drop in on the child who is spending a period of time in the OPD and offer support and a listening ear. If any of the procedures are done in a different area, the nurse should be very sure to give the parents and child adequate directions to the area. This will cut down on the amount of anxious activity spent in finding the area.

Referrals to community health nursing can contribute effectively to help the family deal with grief, to help with treatments or medications, and to encourage follow-up visits. The referral should try to indicate where in the grieving process the parent is at this time. If the parent is still in the period of denial, it is imperative for the community health nurse to know this. If the referral is sent after the death of the

FIG. 7. John is a mentally retarded boy who enjoys having his height and weight monitored. (Courtesy of Cantalician Center, Buffalo, N.Y.)

child, it is important for the nurse to know when the death occurred and also what the parents were told about the post-mortem, if one was done. Home visits after death can be most helpful in identifying things that the parent felt were positive or negative about the care given their child. The community health nurse can also be an effective listener long after many of the family's friends and relatives have stopped letting the parents vent their feelings. The community health nurse is also in a position to evaluate how the family unit is beginning to function without the deceased member. She may also be able to help with the fears of the other children in relation to death.

Group meetings of parents of children with long-term or terminal illness may be very beneficial. Parents can discuss their feelings as well as problems they are having caring for the child. Professional personnel should be a part of these groups so they can help the parents work through some of the difficult situations and also to help correct any false impressions the parents may have about the disease process. For a more thorough discussion of groups the student is referred to the appropriate section in Chapter 12.

Home Care

As home care programs are developed, the admission of the terminally ill child has not created any great problems. Depending on the particular home care program, the child has received in the home the services of laboratory technicians, oxygen therapists, and medical, nursing, physical, and occupational therapists. The parents who have participated in the program seem to receive satisfaction from keeping their sick child at home as long as possible. The added security of knowing they can telephone a professional person any time during the day or night lessens their anxieties. The child benefits greatly by not being separated from his home and family for long periods. As more home care services are established, the out-patient departments may feel some relief from all the additional services they are now offering.

With this added comprehensive home care it becomes evident that the community health nurses in any area may be seeing a great deal more patients with acute illness than they have in the past. Children may one day go to the hospital only for surgery and immediately return home for their postoperative care. This will necessitate better and faster communication between the hospital and home and perhaps monitoring apparatus will eventually be part of our home care program. The nurse may one day push a button to get a doctor's order for handling pain, push another to connect the doctor to the local pharmacy, answer the door bell to receive the delivered drug, administer the drug while teaching the mother the technique for the next time, and provide the psychological support to the child.

Is it any wonder that the nurse working with the terminally ill child must be one who is technically competent in the art and science of nursing?

Clinical Material—In-Patient Service

Nursing care may be influenced by the setting in which the child received his medical care. Children who are segregated according to their disease process are more prone to be in constant contact with other children who are terminally ill. This creates an atmosphere of solemnity which is not found in a generalized setting. Continually during the day the child is exposed to very sick children or children who show dramatic side-effects from medical therapy such as loss of hair, distortion of their bodies, or marks on their bodies to indicate the place for radiation to be administered. In a general hospital, the child is able to seek out children whom he may see as being "free from illness." He also meets parents who are relieved by the improvement in their children. Another big problem which arises in the specialty hospital is that the adult patients he meets when he goes off the pediatric unit may be extremely disfigured by surgery and it is impossible to protect the child from these repeated exposures. One child, returning from radiation therapy with new purple marks on his face, told the nursing student that he was upset because "they painted more marks on my face." An adult patient riding in the same elevator reacted immediately by saying, "Don't be upset—look at all the marks I have," exposing a chest covered with markings. The child became quite restless at this point, and it was necessary to spend a great deal of time assuring him that this patient was receiving very different medical treatment than he was receiving.

Another problem created when accompanying the child patient to various hospital areas is the frequency with which people ask, "He is not a patient, is he?" The very young child, who does not realize the nature of the hospital or unit becomes confused by such a question and may soon begin to wonder what is wrong with being a patient here. He is not able to interpret the question as, "I hope this child does not have cancer," as the adult intended it. The older child, who is very suspicious of being in this unit or hospital, may interpret this question as meaning, "Does this child have cancer?"

It becomes increasingly evident that you cannot protect the child from inquiring adults, so the next best possible solution is to be sure that the child is accompanied by a professional person who can readily help the child contend with the many problems he will encounter when he leaves the unit. Despite these problems, children seem to need to leave the unit and take trips to other areas in the hospital where they know no one will hurt them, such as a gift shop or snack bar.

Satisfactory use of the play area is essential to the child in a specialty unit. It should never be used to perform treatments on the child. He should be able to feel very safe in this area. This is especially necessary as so many other areas in the hospital are a constant threat to him. He needs his bed and his play area to stabilize his environment. It is a great challenge to the nurse or play therapist to provide games, toys, and activities which the child can use to act out his aggressions, express his fears, or just have fun. Tricycles are an excellent means for using excess energy created by the confined area and also for pretending to be able to get away. Games which allow the child to "hit out" also help to release pent-up anxiety. The use of stuffed toys such as a wolf or other seemingly "bad" characters to punch or toss around have been useful in letting the child feel that now he is able to "hurt" something like he is frequently being hurt with needles and painful procedures.

It is important not to have the extremely ill children dampen the other children's play time. The empathy which children have for one another must be considered. If the child who is nearing death is sleeping in the play area and not receiving any benefit from being with the other children, he should be returned to his room. This eliminates one barrier to the effective use of the play area by temporarily eliminating children who are too sick to participate.

The play area should be supervised by adults who are atuned to the children's conversations and needs. It is of little use to provide children outlets for expressions if there is no one to help them work through their feelings effectively. The child may only need to know that it is all right not to like the hospital or it is all right to be angry with his mother, or he is not going to lose his hair like Mary did.

One observation I have made during play time is that the children seldom bring their own beautiful new toys out of their rooms. They play in the play area with the hospital toys. One interpretation might be that the child wants his connections with home free from "contamination" by the hospital, another might be that he is not willing to share these prized possessions with other children, another that the hospital provides such nice toys that he does not need the others, or still another that too many gifts quickly bestowed on the child have little meaning to him. The major use of this observation is not to be too quick to try to make the child bring these toys out for use as he may have some real reason for leaving them untouched and if he has not verbalized this reason it is best not to probe.

In a specialized area such as a cancer unit, the play area may easily become a place where parents hold a "mock wake" for their dying child. The parents may bring the child to the area and then sit and cry as they view their own child and other children in a similar condition. It is necessary to intervene when this situation exists. Other children readily pick up the feelings of tearful parents and become concerned. It is also necessary to help the parent realize that the laughter of other children cannot be eliminated because their own child is seriously ill. In the general hospital, the parents who are grieving actively rarely select the play area, so this is not as big a problem. It is necessary to keep in mind that children do not expect adults to cry. They may never have seen their parents cry before. This is a source of great anxiety to the child and he needs an explanation to help him understand the reason for the behavior. It is best if the parent is able to give this simple explanation. If they are not enough in control to do so, the nurse can help by saying, "Mommy is very unhappy because you're sick. She hopes you will be better soon."

Another factor in the specialty hospital is that parents may suddenly become upset because they are exposed to children who are all terminally ill. It may not be their own child who makes them "break down" at the moment. For instance, one parent started crying when she saw a recently diagnosed child which brought back memories of when she received the diagnosis, another cried when she recalled that her child was once as attractive as a child who was not yet showing the effects of medications, another cried when she saw a child much sicker than her own. Thus a place such as the play area where parents and children meet should be well staffed to supply support and to make changes which are necessary.

Areas of Great Concern to Children and Parents

X-RAY OR RADIATION THERAPY. The use of the x-ray equipment, which is usually given little consideration "because it does not hurt the child," was a threat to some children. The size of the equipment was overpowering, the fact that the child had to be left alone was frightening, and the varying times that children had to wait to see if the films had to be repeated were all sources of concern. The child needed good preparation and activities to make the time pass by more quickly.

BLOOD WORK. The "pricking" of fingers for complete blood counts was not considered "painful" by the children probably because they were "conditioned" by frequent sticks. However, they were concerned when they saw the blood being removed and when it was diluted they thought this larger amount was all their blood. The children were able to correlate loss of blood with replacement of blood as it was given so frequently, and some wondered if they didn't take so much if they would not be spared the transfusion! Again, the need for careful, simple, periodic explanations for the child is borne out.

DIAGNOSTIC PROCEDURES. Some of the children spent a significant amount of time worrying about their medical regimen. For instance, one would say, "I think it is time I had a bone marrow." This statement could evoke many responses from the adults to whom it was said. One might be to the effect that the child was so smart to know this, another to respond to her with a positive or negative reply immediately, another to ask her why she thought this, and so forth. If the child was encouraged to talk more about it her responses often showed that she wanted to know if she was well enough to go home, or if she needed blood, or that she was concerned because one of her friends was sicker. If the child was not encouraged to talk more about it she became restless, interrupted other children's games, or would withdraw and go to her room or sit in a corner.

TRIPS TO THE TREATMENT ROOM. The treatment room, as would be expected, was a serious threat to the children. They were very concerned when other children went there, as well as themselves. They quickly picked up any crying and they needed to be reminded that it was all right to cry. In their anxiety they frequently laughed at the other children who acted out. They took great delight in telling the story to others, indicating that they would like to have been able to do this themselves but did not dare to let down their defenses that much. They frequently labeled another child "bad" for crying or resisting therapy. In addition to wanting to know what was going to be done in the treatment room, the children also seemed to need someone to accompany them and remain with them while they were there. This need seemed to far exceed the damage done to a relationship between a child and a nurse because the nurse assisted in a painful procedure. The nurse should, however, always be aware that the child might change his attitudes towards her after she has assisted and be prepared to have to reestablish this relationship if it deteriorates.

SIDE-EFFECTS OF MEDICATION. Children with terminal illness can be receiving a variety of medications. Some of the medication may be experimental, in the sense that it is given as a last resort. Other medications may be given despite the fact that they produce side-effects, and this may cause as much concern to the child, parent, visitors, and professionals as the disease process itself.

An example would be the side-effects of the folic acid antagonist, methotrexate, which is given to achieve remissions in children with acute leukemia. In addition to the remission the child may lose his hair. This is a very dramatic side-effect. The child probably has seen other children without their hair and he hopes this will not happen to him. It is difficult to assure the child that he will not lose his hair because you know he may eventually be treated with the same drug. The use of wigs helps to cut down the unattractiveness of the girls. However, some children have to wait a significant amount of time before the wig is available, others refuse to wear them, and still others do not have access to them, especially the boys. The children have to be encouraged to put them on early in the morning and to wear them during their wakeful hours. The more natural the situation is made, the better the children adjusted to the wig. The availability of wigs and toupees to meet today's fashion fad has helped in the adjustment for the child. However, the wig still may be uncomfortable for the child and it also has a tendency to cause the scalp to itch, which makes the child resist wearing it.

Another example is the weight gain and Cushoid effect of steroids. The child was frequently referred to as "fatty" by other children and adults. This distortion of body image was very painful for the child. He did not have time to internalize the changes in his body and frequent attention was being given to them by others. The child was teased about clothes which no longer fit him due to his increase in weight. Parents frequently showed "before" and "after" snapshots of the child to other people and this embarrassed the child. The child needs to know that it is not his fault that he has gained all this weight and that his parents still love him.

While earlier we considered the empathy children can have for one another, we must now consider that children can also be very cruel to one another and that the school-age child is especially prone to this. Therefore, it is not uncommon for them to point out changes in one another and to make a joke of it. One day a severely sick child had become jaundiced and the children laughed at him, told him how yellow he looked, and repeatedly took the opportunity to stare at him. The child was too sick to fight back and chose to close his eyes and try to ignore them.

COMMUNICATION.   During the time material was being collected for this book, it became increasingly evident that verbal and nonverbal communication were key factors in giving effective nursing care.

The nursing students frequently would communicate to the child in front of the parent. Such a seemingly innocent statement as to what the child wanted to be when he grew up, would elicit almost a shock response in the parent. One child showed a student her notebook in which she was recording money, which she received as gifts. The student reacted by saying, "Oh, you're going to be rich when you grow up!" The child's mother was very upset by this and her whole facial expression was one of shock. The students soon became aware that their everyday conversations with the child had to be altered when the parents were present. Such expressions as, "I thought I'd die," commonly used in the vernacular, had to be eliminated from vocabularies as the parents tended to overly react to the word "die." Children playing with guns and telling other children to die after being playfully shot also affected some highly sensitive parents. While it is unrealistic to expect that we can completely alter all conversation so parents do not react negatively, it is realistic to aim for improved communication by being more sensitive to parent reactions. We can also improve communication by getting feedback from other staff and parents regarding situations which disturbed parents. I believe parents are in the best position to help us identify things which were stressful to them and they can usually supply kinds of situations which displeased them.

INTRODUCTION OF NEW EQUIPMENT.   One can not overestimate the fears and fantasies that families and children have regarding "serious-looking" equipment. The sounds of equipment coming down the corridors can make the family and child extremely anxious. They secretly hope and occasionally express their hope that the equipment is not coming into their area. The child may even chose to hide, hoping not to be found until after the imagined crisis is passed.

Anxiety can be lessened if families and children are given a simple explanation of equipment which echoes its arrival and if it is destined for their child they need additional preparation.

An example would be the need for an oxygen tent. The machinery often jangles and the plastic hood may rustle. These are familiar sounds to hospital personnel but different and frightening sounds to persons less familiar with the hospital environment. The family and child should be told that the child is either being placed in the oxygen tent or it is being kept close by in case it is necessary. The other children and families in the room also need to know who the tent is in readiness for so they do not falsely assume it is for them or their child.

A more dramatic piece of equipment and one less well known to children and families is the portable x-ray machine. Children need a great deal of preparation before being subjected to this evaluation. The size of the machine may be greatly exaggerated by a small child who is lying frightened and feeling alone. If not prepared he can misinterpret the machine and even imagine he is going to be "sucked up" like an object in a vacuum cleaner. The requests to remain very still for the x-ray can be misinterpreted, too. The child gets very tense and finds it difficult to relax until the machine and its technician leave the area.

SCHOOL.   Several of the children missed attendance at school, and when it was not provided during their hospitalization they were concerned. They seemed to need more than play to occupy their time. The self-discipline needed to do school work seemed a healthy thing. School work is readily associated with "normal" children and provides a means for the seriously ill child to maintain contact with normality. When planned school programs were not provided it was more difficult to get the child interested in school work. The children who were sick for long periods seemed to miss the continuity of school the most, and they frequently talked of returning to school. The school-age child who was deprived of school work frequently received some satisfaction by having jobs to do on the unit, such as putting away the linen or putting together new charts.

General Ideas Collected from Clinical Contacts, and Possible Implications

1. In relation to staffing a unit specifically designed for the care of terminally ill children, the nursing service administration has a great challenge. It would seem important to revitalize the staff periodically so that the nurses do not become too insensitive to the children's needs. Revitalization might be achieved by rotating the staff periodically. This is a procedure which has been discontinued in many places to decrease staff dissatisfaction. I feel it should be reevaluated because continual exposure to terminally ill children is too much of a strain when continued over long periods of time.

2. Parents frequently voiced their appreciation of student nurses who seemed to have more time to spend with the children and aides who were quite free in their responses.

3. One of the biggest challenges I found as an instructor was in helping the students realize the seriousness of the child's illness and then being able to help them continue to function effectively after they thoroughly realized it. The students had a tendency to deny the prognosis in the same way that parents responded when they first heard it. It was brought out in the Natterson and Knudson (1960) study that parents deny the diagnosis at first but then take the death rather well, whereas the staff accepts the diagnosis rather blandly but take the death poorly, because they have only recently learned to know the child as a person. I think the same factors play a part with the student. She has

just learned to know the child and she can not bear to have anything happen to him, so she denies the seriousness of his condition.

4. When a hospitalized child has a weekend pass, parents would frequently say that they had an argument after the child's pass was up about whether to return the child to the hospital. This points out the necessity of discussing with the parent the ambivalence the child may develop to hospitalization if he knows the parents are ambivalent. If the child has heard the argument, he will usually take the side of the parent who favors not returning him to the hospital and this can create many child-parent conflicts.

5. While children seem to benefit a great deal from weekend passes, they are often quite lonesome on Monday after their return to the hospital. Therefore, more people should be available on Monday to help them in the readjustment period and perhaps painful treatments should be kept at a minimum on Monday.

6. Whenever possible, holidays should be spent at home. But if the child is hospitalized both parents and children seem to respond to extra preparations made to celebrate, and staffing should again provide for extra time to prepare for the celebration.

7. Children who live long distances from the hospital need support during visiting hours by volunteers, staff, or other parents who frequently "adopt" them. The effects of long separations have been discussed in the current literature, so I will not include them here.

8. In a small unit one child assumes the leadership role and it is useful to work through him in getting the cooperation of the other children.

9. Volunteers and people not consistently in the area are readily accepted by the children and are more effective if they are given a report to help them better fulfill their particular function. The child whose body may have been drastically altered since the volunteer's last visit, may be very upset because the volunteer does not call him by name. If she was told that this was Jimmy, it would save the child the disappointment and also help the volunteer adjust more easily.

10. Consistent discipline is needed by the terminally ill child as much as any other child. It is very difficult to maintain consistent discipline when so many people are responsible for the care of the children. Therefore, good Kardex notations are imperative and team conferences are necessary to be sure everyone understands the developmental needs of the child as well as the medical needs. The parents should be included in these conferences so they are actively participating in the overall care—which includes discipline.

11. Better selection should be made of television programs as the children too readily associate with the many medical programs and often misinterpret what they see and hear.

12. Many of the children seem much older than their stated age, perhaps as a result of all they have been through. Nurses must be care-

ful not to expect too much of these children because they seem more mature.

13. Several of the parents developed headaches and other symptoms as a result of their child's illness. The parents must be permitted time to vent their feelings in relation to themselves as well as their children.

14. The mothers of children who are sick a long time begin to wonder what they are going to do with all their free time once the death has come. If parents have been helped to understand the nature of the illness, if they have been taught new techniques for caring for sick children, and if they have been helped with general child-rearing practices, they may well be able to look back on the experience and have positive as well as negative memories of the long illness. Hopefully, family ties may be strengthened by this threatening condition, rather than weakened.

15. Students and staff may become very frustrated because they can not do more to help the children during their hospitalization. Staff conferences may be helpful, as staff members can be supporting influences to one another. If a staff psychiatrist is available, it is helpful to have him sit in on these sessions.

16. The children seem to be always seeking answers to their unasked questions. Consequently, any clinical discussions should be out of the child's seeing or hearing range. Also, the nurses' station should be out-of-bounds for the child. The child should be given enough of an explanation about reports, conferences, and clinical sessions that they are not suspicious that we are talking about them. They need to understand that these are medical discussions that they would not understand, and that medical personnel need to have these sessions so that each child can receive the best possible care.

17. Intravenous infusions and transfusions become a source of concern to the children and they compare the rate of flow with one another. Concern is shown if the rates are not synchronized. Again, a simple explanation is indicated to allay their fears.

CONCLUDING STATEMENT

I have made an attempt to collect ideas from the clinical area and the literature to be used by nurses to improve nursing care to the terminally ill child and his family. While I have not attempted to exhaust the topic, it is hoped that these general ideas can be applied to the care of the terminally ill child in a variety of settings.

Case Presentation and Study Questions

Susan is admitted to a four-bed unit on a busy medical floor. She is six years old and an only child. Her mother and father are both college educated. Her mother is a nurse and her father an engineer. Susan has received all her conscientious medical supervision from the same pediatrician. She has had one other hospitalization, for a fractured arm, approximately one year ago.

This admittance was precipitated by a series of minor symptoms which the pediatrician recognized as being consistent with lymphocytic leukemia. Susan has been bruising easily, has had numerous epistaxis without provocation, and is more irritable than ordinary. The pediatrician did a hemoglobin determination in his office and found it to be 8 g. The admitting diagnosis is anemia, unknown etiology.

1. What additional tests will be done to determine a more exact diagnosis?

2. Considering the host factors, is Susan a candidate for lymphocytic leukemia?

3. Are Susan's presenting symptoms congruous with other types of cancer? Are they related to conditions other than cancer?

4. Is Susan's room placement appropriate? Are there any changes you might suggest?

5. What factors will determine who prepares Susan for her diagnostic evaluation?

The bone marrow aspiration confirms the diagnosis of lymphocytic leukemia. The private pediatrician verifies the findings by additional consultation with the hematology department. He learns that the hospital laboratory is functioning at maximum capacity and that Susan's needs would better be met at a specialized hospital for the care of children with cancer. Susan's pediatrician is not affiliated with the other institution, so her care will have to be transferred if she is to go there.

1. What changes might be expected in the parents' attitude when they hear the diagnosis?

2. If Susan is transferred to the other hospital, what preparation needs to be done? How can you assist in the preparation?

3. How would you explain the transfer to Susan?

Susan is transferred to the other hospital and admitted to a four-bed unit not significantly different than her previous room. Susan's mother comes out to the desk and vehemently rejects the room placement. She wants Susan transferred to a private room immediately.

1. What do you think precipitated the mother's response?

2. What can be done to help the parents and child adjust to the new situation? Is a private room a good solution? Who can help to make this situation more tolerable? Will the "settling-in" situation be delayed under these conditions?

3. How will the mother's anxiety influence Susan? How can you give Susan additional support during this time?

During the nursing intake history Mrs. M. tells you Susan is here for treatment of her anemia. She further states that Susan will only be here two or three days so she will assume the responsibility for Susan's total care.

1. What information will you pass on to the physician from your interview?

2. Is it "normal" for a professionally educated parent to completely deny a diagnosis of leukemia? How soon do you think Mrs. M. will begin to be affected by the impact of her daughter's illness, or is she already affected?

3. What do you think Mrs. M. means when she states she will assume Susan's total care? What aspects of care should be delegated to the parent? How are these aspects altered because the mother is a nurse?

Susan is started on medication and begins to respond to therapy. For a period of time, Susan feels sicker than she did on admission. Mrs. M. and Susan complain about many things during this time. Included in their complaints are alternating periods of being too hot or too cold, too much noise in the corridors, too little variation in the food, and too many visitors to the other children in the room.

1. What should you do about the complaints?

2. Why do you think they are being so hard to please? Are there ways of getting to the problems which are at the root of the complaints?

3. Are these complaints very different from expected behaviors under similar conditions? Will some of the complaints resolve with the passage of time? If so, when can this be expected?

4. What anticipatory guidance should be given during this time? What is the rationale for providing anticipatory guidance?

Susan is now in remission and is ready for discharge. Mrs. M. and Susan present candy and thank-you's to the staff for their excellent care. You feel especially pleased as you recall the change in their attitudes since admission.

1. Do you feel Mrs. M. and Susan are sincere? If so, what factors influenced their "change in attitude"?

2. When Susan is admitted again, can you expect them to be as gracious as they are on this discharge?

3. What notations will you want to keep regarding this hospitalization experience? Why?

Two-and-a-half years elapse and Susan is hospitalized with severe hemorrhaging. She has been hospitalized for short periods on three other occasions and each time she has responded to therapy. This time it is evident that Susan will not respond. Mrs. M. has been very capably caring for Susan but now seems more interested in the other children and their parents than she is in Susan. Mrs. M. leaves the hospital for long periods and also spends extended time in the coffee shop. When she is on the unit she is usually found giving assistance and support to other parents.

1. How do you evaluate Mrs. M.'s behavior?

2. Is this behavior significantly different than other parents' reactions to their dying children?

3. What support can you offer Mrs. M? What other members of the medical team can give support?

4. How is Mrs. M.'s activity influencing the other parents?

5. Is Mrs. M.'s activity a part of her grieving process? How do you think this will contribute to Mrs. M.'s behavior when Susan dies?

References

ABC's of Childhood Cancer. New York State Department of Health, 1959 rev. 1966.

Ariel, I. M., and Park, G. T., eds. Cancer and Allied Diseases of Infancy and Childhood. Boston, Little, Brown, 1960.

Bergmann, T. Children in the Hospital. New York, International Universities Press, 1965.

Bonine, G. N. Student's reactions to children's deaths. Amer. J. Nurs., 67:1439–1440, July 1967.

Bowlby, J. Grief and mourning in infancy and early childhood. Psychoanal. Stud. Child, 15:9–52, 1960.

Bozeman, M. F., Orbach, C. E., and Sutherland, A. M. Psychological impact of cancer and its treatment. The adaptation of mothers to the threatened loss of their children through leukemia: Part 1. Cancer, 8:1–19, Jan.–Feb. 1955.

Brauer, P. H., Cockerill, E., and Kutner, B. A Constructive approach to terminal illness. New York, National Foundation, Inc.

Bright, F., and Sister M. Luciana France. The nurse and the terminally ill child. Nurs. Outlook, 15:39–42, Sept. 1967.

Carpenter, K. M. Parents take heart in the city of hope. Amer. J. Nurs. 63:82–85, Oct. 1962.

Dargeon, H. Tumors of Childhood. New York, Hoeber, 1960.

deBenneville, A. K. Nursing services in home care. In Schultz, E. D., and Rudick, E., eds. Nursing in Ambulatory Units. Dubuque, Iowa, Wm. C. Brown Co., pp. 33–38.

Engel, G. L. Grief and grieving. Amer. J. Nurs., 64:93–98, Sept. 1964.

Fagin, C. Why not involve parents when children are hospitalized? Amer. J. Nurs., 62:78–79, June 1962.

———— The effects of maternal attendance on the post hospital behavior of young children. Philadelphia, Davis, 1966.

Family program in childrens cancer unit. Hospitals, 39:66–69, March 1965.

Ford, L. C., and Silver, H. K. The expanded role of the nurse in child care, Nurs. Outlook, 15:43–45, Sept. 1967.

Freidman, S. B., Chodoff, P., Mason, J., and Hamburg, D. Behavioral observations in parents anticipating the death of a child. Pediat. 32:610–625, 1963.

———— Karon, M., and Goldsmith, G. Childhood leukemia: a pamphlet for parents. U. S. Dept. of Health, Education, and Welfare. U. S. Government Printing Office, 1963.

Geis, D. F. Mother's perceptions of care given their dying children. Amer. J. Nurs., 65:105–107, Feb. 1965.

Green, W. A. Jr., and Miller, G. Psychological factors and reticuloendothelial disease: observations on a group of children and adolescents with leukemia; an interpretation of disease development in terms of the mother-child unit. Psychosom. Med., 20:124–143, 1958.

Hamovich, M. B. Parent and the Fatally Ill Child. Duarte, Calif., City of Hope Medical Center, 1964.

Hays, J. S. The night Neil died. Nurs. Outlook, 10:801–803, Dec. 1962.

Knudsen, A. G., and Natterson, J. M. Participation of parents in the hospital care of terminally ill children. Pediat., 26:482–489, 1960.

Meurer, Sister Mary Christopher. Working with the mother to improve nursing care of the child with leukemia: nursing in relation to the impact of illness upon the family. New York, American Nurses Association Series No. 2, 1962, p. 14–21.

Micheal, P. Tumors of Infancy and Childhood. Philadelphia, Lippincott, 1964.

Morrissey, J. R. Death anxiety in children with fatal illness. In Parod, H. ed. New York, Crisis Intervention, Family Service Assoc. of Amer., 1965, pp. 324–338.

Nagy, M. The child's theories concerning death. (Cited by Natterson and Knudsen.) J. Genet. Psych., 73:3, 1948.

Natterson, J. M., and Knudson, A. G. Observations concerning fear of death in terminally ill children and their mothers. Psychosom. Med., 22:456–465, 1960.

Ohman, E. W., and Walans, D. An approach to the nursing diagnosis of behavior in a pediatric specialty clinic. Nurs. Science, April 1964.

Quint, J. C. The threat of death: some consequences for patients and nurses. Nurs. Forum, 8:287–299, 1969.

Rudick, E. Nursing and the new pediatrics. Nursing Clinics of North America. Philadelphia, Saunders, March 1966, Vol. 1, No. 1. p. 75–81.

Scahill, M. Preparing children for procedures and operations. Nurs. Outlook, 17:36–38, June 1969.

Sharp, E. S. Experiment in family-centered nursing in a pediatric out-patient service. The Alumnae Magazine, 63:66–80, Sept. 1964.

Smith, Margo. Ego support for the child patient. In Rudick, E., ed. Pediatric Nursing. Dubuque, Iowa, Wm. C. Brown Co., 1966, pp. 60–70.

Solnit, A. J., and Green, M. Psychological considerations in the management of deaths on pediatric services. Pediat., 24:106–112, 1959.

Truth sustains leukemic children. Med. World News, Sept. 1964, p. 62.

Vernick, J., and Lunceford, J. L. Milieu design for adolescents with leukemia. Amer. J. Nurs., 67:559–561, March 1967.

Wolf, A. W. Helping your child to understand death. New York, Child Study Association of America, 1958.

Wu, R. Explaining treatments to young children. Amer. J. Nurs., 65:71–73, July 1965.

APPENDIX I

Example of Nursing information gathered in Nursing Intake Interview, Out-patient. Data collected by Miss Virginia Siuidara, Class of 1969.

Name: Jane Jones
Age: 3 years
Date: 10/30/68

I. *Reason for appointment.* Upper respiratory infection coughing, runny nose, has had problem since March 1968 when was brought up North from South by parents. Had had difficulty breathing at night. Breathes through mouth. Mother doesn't know why child keeps getting colds. Denies child goes outside without coat on or plays in dress.

II. *Previous appointment or hospital admissions.* Patient was admitted to this clinic previously for pneumonia during winter months, January 1968. Was given drugs here to alleviate symptoms. No hospitalization. Has been coming to clinic regularly when child develops runny nose, coughing, sneezing which might possibly lead to pneumonia. When patient gets sick she gets irritable, cries a lot, and does not eat. Has been to clinic also for immunizations.

III. *Family constellation.* Jane lives in a small two-room apartment with maternal grandmother and her two-year and five-year-old cousins. Mother brings child to grandmother's house on Mondays and takes her home Friday night. Mother is separated from husband who previously worked in a shoe store. Mother, 20 years old, works in a clothing factory. Child seems to communicate and talk more freely with maternal grandmother, who seems very protective of child. Grandmother would not let child play with one particular toy as she thought it might hurt her. Child sees father on occasion but not very often.

IV. *Habits.*   *Eating:* Child prefers to eat with fingers and likes warm foods. She is left-handed and likes vegetables, especially green. Likes all meats except fish. Has to have food cut up for her. Drinks from a cup. Child likes candy and frequently eats between meals—especially

585

cookies, candy, potato chips. Doesn't always eat with family. Eats when hungry. Meal time often in front of TV. Child has most of baby teeth. Has never been to the dentist.

Elimination: Child is partially toilet-trained. Will have accidents when unable to get clothes unbuttoned or when too busy playing. Mother seems to have lenient attitude toward toilet training, states, "accidents can happen." Diaper at night time. No trouble with constipation, occasionally diarrhea, usually takes drug ordered by the doctor for it, but this is rare.

Sleeping: Sleeps with dolly in her large bed. Goes to bed at 8:30 P.M. and gets up at 7:30 or 8:00 A.M. Sleeps in room with grandmother; usually sleeps soundly throughout the night unless she has to get up to go to the bathroom. Does not fall out of bed. Has no trouble in going to sleep. Quiet when put to bed. No prayers or rituals such as story telling, etc., at that time.

Play—peer groups. Child plays well with two-year-old boy cousin and five-year-old girl. Occasionally fights over possession of toys. Likes to imitate grandmother in play activities such as sweeping the house. Plays with dolls, Raggedy Ann. Likes to be their mama. Very active, likes to run, jump, climb. Shares tricycle with two cousins.

Language development: Child talks in one- or two-word sentences; responds to commands—how old are you, or open your mouth, or stay here. Stutters occasionally when excited, shy with strangers but jabbers constantly at home. Laughs freely, talks with Southern accent and slowly. Started saying "mama," first word, at 8 months. Can count to five.

V. *Allergies:* Allergic to tomatoes. Breaks out in a rash when the food is eaten. No allergies to feathers, dust, flowers, drugs, etc., noted by the mother or the grandmother.

VI. *Activities of daily living:* Independent. Is able to go to the bathroom by herself. Opens doors, climbs stairs, eats fairly well by herself except that foods must be cut up for her. Is able to dress herself, wash her hands and face—tries to brush her own teeth.

Dependent: Has to have help buttoning coat, zippering zippers, tying shoes, bathing, and combing hair.

School: child wants to go to nursery school. Mother wants to send her to school next year. Five-year-old cousin goes to kindergarten and tells child about it. Mother is saving money to enroll child in nursery school.

Social interests: Enjoys TV—especially cartoons. Has been looking forward to Halloween for past two weeks. Likes to play the game of hide-and-seek with five-year-old cousin. Likes story books, especially to look at the pictures.

VII. *Special needs, fears, problems:* Child likes all kinds of foods. Mother says child eats all the time, especially between meals. Has been trying to stop the child from doing this by punishing her, but this has been done inconsistently as grandmother spoils the child. Needs consistency in diet instruction. Fears dogs and cats. Was scratched by a dog once. Grandmother and mother have no pets. Doesn't have fear of the dark. Mother tries not to use the term "boogy man." Doesn't usually have nightmares. Fears strangers until she gets to know them. Child is left-handed, has trouble handling eating utensils. Is very clumsy.

APPENDIX II

Example: Partial Information Gathered on Interim Admission

John M. is a four-year-old white male with a diagnosis of lympho-cytic leukemia. He is admitted to the pediatric unit of a large local hospital. His condition was diagnosed twelve months ago, in the same hospital.

Important factors to consider in planning nursing care:

1. age of child
2. sex of child
3. previous hospitalization
4. disease process
5. length of illness

Developmental factors:

1. *Age:* preschooler's preoccupation with fantasy
         need for parents
         limited concept of time
         need for appropriate toys
         need for connection with home
         self-feeding skills
         dressing skills—appropriate clothing
         language development
         bedtime ritual
         nursery school experience, if any
         sleeping arrangements at home
         number and sex of siblings

Information gathered:

1. *General.* Mother housewife. Father employed 3:00 to 11.00 P.M. at a local steel mill.

   John has an imaginary friend named Henry. His favorite toy is a fire engine. Likes to sleep with a teddy bear. He shares a room with two brothers. He has his own bed but frequently gets in bed with James, age six years. Five children in family—William,

589

age nine; James, age six; John, age four; George, age two; Mary, age six weeks. John has not attended school. Prior to his illness he played with two boys next door. Since his illness he stays close to home, withdrawing from outside contacts, children or adults. John's vocabulary is advanced for his age but he has regressed during his illness. He prefers to point and whine to make his needs known. His communication with his mother has not been affected. At bedtime John recites his prayers to his mother. His favorite prayer is "Now I Lay Me Down to Sleep." After the prayer John drinks a glass of warm milk. Since his illness, he likes to have a light on while he sleeps. John frequently asks how long he has to stay at the hospital.

2. *Sex.* John is most familiar with living with boys. His placement in the ward should be in a multiple bedroom with other boys.

3. *Previous hospitalizations.* John has been hospitalized on four occasions. He had an adenoidectomy at the age of two years. He was hospitalized for three weeks at the time he was diagnosed as having leukemia. Since then he has had two admissions, one of four days' duration for infected fingers and a temperature elevation, the other for an evaluation of hematuria which subsided and he was discharged two days later.

Mrs. M. roomed-in for the overnight admission for the adenoidectomy. She roomed-in for one week during his three-week hospitalization. On all other admissions she visited daily from 1:00 to 8:00 P.M. Mr. M. visits at least four times a week for approximately 1½ hr, in the early afternoon before work.

4. *Disease process.* John's second hospitalization was triggered by an elevated temperature of three days' duration. He had many bruises which could not be related to trauma. He also developed enlarged lymph nodes. He was admitted with a diagnosis of fever of unknown origin. The diagnosis was made following a complete work-up including bone marrow evaluation. John was treated and went into remission. He has been followed in the out-patient department in between hospitalizations. He has been comparatively comfortable until two days ago when he developed soreness in his knees. The morning of admission he developed a severe headache and admission was advised.

5. *Length of illness.* The length of illness is best described as twelve months in duration. However, John has not felt ill for a good portion of the time. In interviewing him he states he was only sick two days. He does not admit knowing anything about the previous hospitalizations. (Although this seems extremely hard to believe, it is important to start at the point the child feels free to admit to.)

Plan of action:

1. Orient child and mother to unit

   (a.) choose appropriate bed, near nurses' station

2. Introduce child and mother to staff and other children in his room
3. Provide written information regarding the hospital routines to supplement verbal information
4. Complete routine admission including physical aspects
5. Record appropriate information in patient's chart
6. Begin Kardex utilizing appropriate information
7. Check doctor's orders pertaining to child
8. Complete nursing tasks related to doctor's orders
9. Familiarize mother with plan of action and expected role
10. Review past hospital record in relation to nursing observations and information—especially nursing history taking form

(Example of Kardex, utilizing information gathered to this point from interview and past record, follows.)

APPENDIX III:
SAMPLE KARDEX

NAME	John M.			Dr. Jones	

G & D—DEVELOPMENTAL STAGE (check)

Infant		Toddler		Preschooler |x| School-age		Adolescent	

Identify developmental stage of this child including social milieu: preschooler—third of five boys. Mother, housewife, father, steelworker employed 3–11 P.M. Has imaginary friend, Henry.

Deviations from "expected" developmental level: will be evaluated after working with child

Goals for maintaining or expanding developmental tasks during hospitalization or between out-patient visits: will be identified after working with child

MEDICAL PLAN			NURSING INTERVENTION
Diet: Regular 3X daily with supplements			Identify likes and dislikes
			Eat with other boys at small table
			Chocolate milk shake at 3:00 P.M. and bedtime
Medications	5 mg. po.	qid	
Prednisone		10-2-6-10	Mother crushes and gives him fruit
Methotrexate	IV by MD	Daily	Administered in treatment room at 1:30 P.M.
Treatments:	(frequency)	(time)	(how done)

Independent nursing activities: observe mucus membranes for lesions daily. Note and chart bruises daily. Record any bleeding. Mother bathes child, needs supplies.

Bottle		Pray. |x| Light |x| Siderail		Toys |x| Snack |x| Toilet |x

NAME	AGE:	WORKING
Johnnie (nickname)	4 years	DIAGNOSIS: Lymphocytic leukemia

After the first day of care the developmental level of John is evaluated.

Deviations from the expected developmental level were as follows:

1. Refused to feed self—need to encourage mother to have John feed himself

2. John needs help in toileting—unable to snap pajama bottoms

Goals for maintaining or expanding developmental tasks were established.

1. Work with mother to let John start feeding himself. When he tires, administer help.
2. Encourage John to play with both boys and girls in the playroom.
3. Teach toothbrushing. This has been neglected as mother feared bleeding gums. Adapt cotton applicator if toothbrush too harsh.
4. Encourage verbalization.

Goals will be expanded and adjusted as daily nursing plan is established.

APPENDIX IV: HOME CARE EVALUATION SHEET

Cystic Fibrosis

Name: .... Age: .... Hospital No.: ......

Date: .... Weight: ...... Height: ....

Date of last visit: .... Weight: ...... Height: ....

Date of next clinic visit: .... Weight: ...... Height: ....

General Condition:

Better: ....

Same: ....

Worse: ....

Appetite:

Good: ....

Moderate: ....

Poor: ....

Activity and Emotional Status:

1. Exercise tolerance:
   Plays hard all day: ....
   Plays but tires easily: ....
   Listless, lies around: ....

2. School attendance for past 6 weeks:
   Number days absent: ....

3. Attitude:
   Happy and alert: ....
   Happy and quiet: ....
   Fussy and irritable: ....

595

Gastrointestinal Status:

1. No. of B.M. daily: ...... 4. Change of color of lips or nails with activity of coughing:

2. Type: Yes .... No ....
   A. Normal: ....
   B. Soft yet formed: .....
   C. Mushy: ....
   D. Mushy and greasy: ...

3. Prolapse: Yes ... No ...

Respiratory Status:

1. Respiratory rate per min. ....

2. Acute flare-up of respiratory infection: Number ....
   A. Severe: .... Number .... Dates: ....
   B. Mild: .... Number .... Dates: ....

3. Cough:
   A. Frequency: Night only: .... Early A.M. .... Day and night ....
   B. Type:
      1. Loose, productive ....
      2. Dry, hacking ....
      3. Blood-tinged mucus: Yes .... No ....
      4. Color of mucus:
         a. Yellow ...... b. White ...... c. Greenish yellow ......

4. Postural drainage:
   Effective: Yes .... No ....
   Youngster cooperative: Yes .... No ....

Medication:

1. Antibiotics:
   A. What antibiotic is patient on at present? ....
   B. If patient has had an acute respiratory illness (as noted above) that required a change of antibiotics, what was used? ....
   C. Give dosage: ....
   D. Give length of time on this: ....

2. Inhalation Therapy:
   A. Mist tent:
      1. Used: Yes .... No ....
      2. Number of hours per day: ....
      3. Type of solution used in nebulizer: ....
   B. Intermittent aerosol therapy:
      1. Used: Yes .... No .... No. of times daily: ....
      2. Are antibiotics used? Yes .... No ....
      3. What antibiotics used? ....

3. Pancreatic Supplement:
   A. Name of supplement used: ....
      1. Number of capsules with each meal: ....
      2. Multi-vitamin: Type: .... Dosage ....

   B. List all the medications used either by name or description: ....
   ....

REMARKS:

PLEASE NOTE: When this form has been completed, please mail to
....

Courtesy of the National Cystic Fibrosis Research Foundation, New
York, N.Y.
....

Index